Fertility Counseling

Clinical Guide and Case Studies

Fertility Counseling

Clinical Guide and Case Studies

Edited by

Sharon N. Covington

Psychological Support Services, Shady Grove Fertility Reproductive Science Center, Rockville, MD;
Intramural Research Program on Reproductive and Adult Endocrinology, National Institutes of Child Health and Human Development (NICHD), National Institutes of Health (NIH), Bethesda, MD;
and Department of Obstetrics and Gynecology, Georgetown University School of Medicine, Washington, DC, USA.

CAMBRIDGE
UNIVERSITY PRESS

CAMBRIDGE
UNIVERSITY PRESS

University Printing House, Cambridge CB2 8BS, United Kingdom

Cambridge University Press is part of the University of Cambridge.

It furthers the University's mission by disseminating knowledge in the pursuit of education, learning and research at the highest international levels of excellence.

www.cambridge.org
Information on this title: www.cambridge.org/9781107643116

First published 2015

A catalog record for this publication is available from the British Library

Library of Congress Cataloging in Publication data
Fertility counseling : clinical guide and case studies / edited by Sharon N. Covington.
p. ; cm.
Includes bibliographical references and index.
ISBN 978-1-107-64311-6 (paperback)
I. Covington, Sharon N., editor.
[DNLM: 1. Infertility – psychology. 2. Counseling.
3. Reproductive Techniques, Assisted – psychology. WP 570]
RC889
616.6′92 – dc23 2014046700

ISBN 978-1-107-64311-6 Paperback

Additional resources for this publication at www.cambridge.org/9781107643116. Password provided in relevant chapters.

Family, like a lotus, may struggle to grow, pushing through murkiness before reaching the light and, then, blossom into unique beauty and strength.

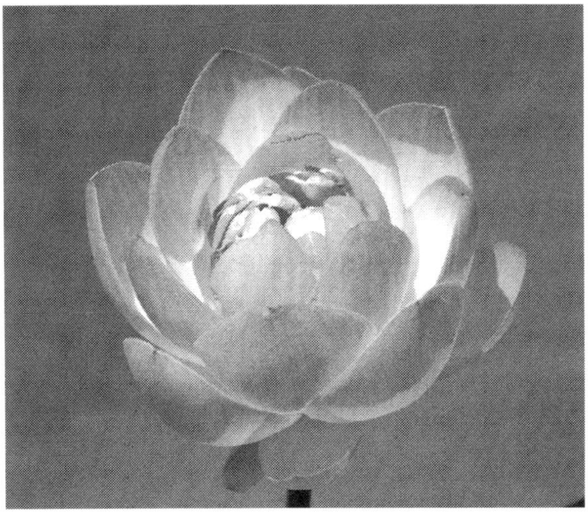

Dedicated to:

My patients who have allowed me the honor to share in their struggle through the murkiness of infertility and witness their growth.

My husband, Barry, and our growing family: Laura, Brendan, Darlene and Luke Covington; and Michelle, Scott, Sean, Michaela and Liam Harmon.

Lotus photo by Michelle Covington Harmon, used with permission

Contents

Section 6: Practice issues

Online resources and tools for fertility counseling practice available at www.cambridge.org/9781107643116.

Contributors

G. David Adamson, MD
Medical Director, Palo Alto Medical Foundation Fertility Physicians of No. California, Palo Alto, CA; Clinical Professor, ACF, Stanford University, Stanford, CA; and Associate Clinical Professor, University of California San Francisco, CA, USA

Linda D. Applegarth, EdD
Clinical Associate Professor of Psychology and Director of Psychological Services, The Ronald O. Perelman & Claudia Cohen Center for Reproductive Medicine, Weil Medical College of Cornell University, New York, NY, USA

Jean M. Benward, MS
Psychotherapist, Counseling Offices of Jean Benward, San Ramon, CA, USA

Jacky Boivin, PhD
Professor, Cardiff Fertility Studies Group, School of Psychology, Cardiff University, UK

Eric Blyth, MA, PhD
Professor of Social Work at the Centre for Applied Childhood Studies, University of Huddersfield, Queensgate, Huddersfield, UK

Laura S. Covington, MSW
Clinical Social Worker, Shady Grove Fertility Reproductive Science Center, Rockville, MD, USA

Sharon N. Covington, MSW
Director of Psychological Support Services, Shady Grove Fertility Reproductive Science Center, Rockville, MD; Associate Investigator, Intramural Research Program on Reproductive and Adult Endocrinology, National Institutes of Child Health and Human Development (NICHD), National Institutes of Health (NIH), Bethesda, MD; and Assistant Clinical Professor, Department of Obstetrics and Gynecology, Georgetown University School of Medicine, Washington, DC, USA

Eileen A. Dombo, MSW, PhD
Assistant Professor and Assistant Dean & BSW Program Chairperson, The National Catholic School of Social Service, The Catholic University of America, Washington, DC, USA

Sofia Gameiro, PhD
Lecturer, Cardiff Fertility Studies Group, School of Psychology, Cardiff University, UK

Megan Flood, MA, MSW
Licensed Independent Clinical Social Worker; Faculty, Washington School of Psychiatry, Washington, DC, USA

Joann Paley Galst, PhD
Psychologist at Independent Practice, New York, NY, USA

Hilary Hanafin, PhD
Licensed Psychologist at the Center for Surrogate Parenting, Encino, CA, USA

Sarah R. Holley, PhD
Assistant Professor of Clinical Psychology, San Francisco State University, San Francisco, CA, USA

Judith E. Horowitz, PhD
Licensed Psychologists, Independent Practice, Coral Springs, FL, USA

Janet Jaffe, PhD
Co-founder and Co-director of the Center for Reproductive Psychology, San Diego, CA

Laura Josephs, PhD
Clinical Assistant Professor of Psychology at the Center for Reproductive Medicine, New York-Presbyterian Weill Cornell Medical Center, New York, NY, USA

Susan C. Klock, PhD
Professor, Departments of Obstetrics and Gynecology and Psychiatry, Northwestern University Feinberg School of Medicine, Chicago, IL, USA

Irving G. Leon, PhD
Adjunct Associate Professor of Obstetrics and Gynecology, University of Michigan Health System, Ann Arbor, MI, USA

Anne F. Malavé, PhD
Clinical Psychologist and Psychoanalyst, Private Practice, New York City, and Faculty, Supervisor, and Graduate, William Alanson White Institute of Psychiatry, Psychoanalysis and Psychology, New York, NY, USA

Erica J. Mindes, PhD
Licensed Clinical Psychologist, Covington and Hafkin & Associates, Richmond, and Shady Grove Fertility Reproductive Science Center, Annandale, VA, USA

Lauri A. Pasch, PhD
Assistant Professor at the Department of Psychiatry, University of California, San Francisco, CA, USA

Brennan D. Peterson, PhD
Associate Professor of Psychology at the Faculty of Psychology, Crean College of Health and Behavioral Sciences, Chapman University, Orange, CA, USA

William Petok, PhD
Licensed Psychologist at Independent Practice, Baltimore, MD, USA

Allison B. Rosen, PhD
Clinical Psychologist, New York; NY, Adjunct Assistant Professor at the Department of Obstetrics and Gynecology, New York Medical College, Valhalla, New York; Program Psychologist at the Institute for Fertility Preservation, Rye, NY, USA

Patricia L. Sachs, MSW
Clinical Social Worker, Shady Grove Fertility Reproductive Science Center, Rockville, MD, USA

Tara H. Simpson, PsyD
Licensed Psychologist, Shady Grove Fertility Reproductive Science Center, Rockville, MD USA; Adjunct Professor at the Department of Psychology, University of Maryland Baltimore County, Catonsville, MD, USA

Margaret Swain, RN, JD
Attorney in Private Practice, Riderwood, MD, USA

Petra Thorn, PhD
Social Worker, Social Therapist, Family Therapist in Private Practice, Moerfelden, Germany

Carol B. Toll, MSW
Clinical Social Worker, Shady Grove Fertility Reproductive Science Center, Rockville, MD, USA

Uschi Van den Broeck, PhD
Clinical Psychologist and Researcher and Family Therapist, University Hospitals Leuven, Gasthuisberg, Leuven University Fertility Center (LUFC), Leuven, Belgium

Katherine Williams, MD
Department of Psychiatry & Behavioral Sciences, Stanford University SoM, Stanford, CA, USA

Julianne E. Zweifel, PhD
Clinical Psychologist, Adjunct Professor at the Department of Obstetrics & Gynecology, University of Wisconsin School of Medicine and Public Health, Madison, WI, USA

Foreword

The ever-changing world of reproductive medicine has introduced a new cohort of individuals and couples to the possibility of parenthood. A burgeoning of innovative technologies and the introduction of third party reproduction have given hope to a diverse group of would-be parents including patients beyond reproductive age, cancer patients seeking fertility preservation, same-sex couples and a growing number of other family configurations wanting children. The spectacular growth of this discipline has ushered in a host of social, psychological and ethical complexities that has increased the need for fertility counseling and collaboration between clinicians working in this field.

This book is a boon to mental health professionals and other practitioners struggling to keep pace with this rapidly evolving field. Sharon Covington and her contributors have provided an excellent reference source for the management of patients entering this new world. Each chapter, written by a distinguished international scholar or clinician, begins with a case study – a uniquely effective model. Medical schools, law schools and business schools have recognized that case studies are the best way to learn because they offer the complexity and feel of an authentic clinical encounter. Each case addresses an issue particularly salient today to patients, fertility counselors and the medical treatment team and underscores the psychological, ethical and medical aspects of assisted reproduction. The cases vary widely, exploring issues and problems once considered rare and unusual but now rapidly becoming mainstream. By focusing on actual cases (altered only to protect privacy) the challenges and nuances of these issues can be explored in detail.

The foundation of the book is based on the concept of collaborative reproductive healthcare, so superbly introduced by Sharon Covington and David Adamson in the opening chapter. This is the model that we followed when we started our work together in 1982 in the Yale fertility program, shortly after the first IVF baby in our program was born. Decherney, already a well-established reproductive endocrinologist with years of treating the infertile, upon hearing the hue and cry from a public trumpeting ethical concerns about "test tube babies" and recognizing the impact of emotional uncertainty and anguish that accompanies infertility, decided that it made sense to have a mental health professional on the team to provide counsel and support. Greenfeld, a newly graduated social worker who knew nothing about infertility and its treatment and certainly nothing about infertility counseling (a term that had not yet been coined), readily joined the team and learned, as most novice clinicians do, from colleagues and from the patients themselves.

As we reflect back on those early days of IVF, we consider the factors common to the cases we shared at that time. Typically, patients with a long history of infertility often traveled great distances at considerable expense for that one last chance at pregnancy at a time when success rates were low. We were providing new medical technology and grappling with the short-term stresses of the treatment as well as its longer-term psychological and social implications among this hopeful, yet vulnerable, early group of patients. As major advances have transformed the field since those early days, the psychological, ethical and legal challenges faced by our patients have steadily increased, requiring ever more knowledge and clinical skill. This text provides an accessible review of these changes and the clinical techniques for addressing them.

As editor, Sharon Covington draws on her years of clinical experience and astute observation, broad theoretical background and precise communication skills to bring together a pivotal volume capturing the state of the field today. Her expertise is evidenced by her selection of topics and formatting of the chapters, which provide the experienced clinician or the novice trainee new insights into this exciting field. She has created a volume that will continue to be a training and reference tool for years to come.

Alan DeCherney and Dorothy Greenfeld

Acknowledgments

Writing, for me, has always been like giving birth. I contemplate endlessly, experience great anxiety and anguish as I start; slowly and painfully labor away until I finally can push the finished work out – and then wait, wonder and hope others will love what I have produced. Creating this book has been more like assisted reproduction. The process began with hopes and dreams that couldn't be completed, which led to a treatment decision and new approach. With the help, support and advice of many I was able to formulate a plan for a text that would be strong clinically and yet personal and relevant. I had been hearing in the fertility counseling classes I teach to mental health professionals that they wanted tools to help them in their practice (so they would not have to "reinvent" the wheel) as well as learn how clinicians do their work through illustrative case material. *Fertility Counseling* is the culmination of this vision, conceived and gestated with the assistance of many helping hands.

The process would not have begun without the steadfast support, assistance, patience and good nature of my editor, Nick Dunton, and Cambridge University Press. In addition, each of my esteemed contributors was enthusiastic and committed to tackling this new project, which made moving forward possible with renewed energy. Reading their chapters, I was not only enlightened but challenged to think more critically about my own clinical work with infertility patients. I also realized just how far this field has come since I began working in reproductive medicine over 30 years ago. Wanting to use the collaborative reproductive healthcare model as a foundation of the book, I am greatly appreciative of my friend Dr. David Adamson agreeing to write it with me. David is one of the most highly regarded (and busiest) reproductive endocrinologists in the world and has long been a proponent of the integration and coordination of psychosocial care within the American Society of Reproductive Medicine (ASRM) and the European Society of Human Reproduction and Embryology (ESHRE). I also was honored that Dr. Alan DeCherney and Dorothy Greenfeld MSW agreed to write the Foreword, as I believe they established one of the very first practices of this model at Yale Fertility Center many years ago. Alan had a vision early on that his patients needed specialized assistance with the psychological demands of infertility and treatment, and therefore sought Dorothy out as a social worker in one of the hospital's clinics. Alan, who is the head of my department at the National Institutes of Health (NIH) and former Editor in Chief of *Fertility and Sterility*, was an early supporter of "The Mentals," a term I recall he good-naturedly used for fertility counselors. Dorothy has been my good friend since we met at my first ASRM meeting in 1986. She has been a pioneer and leader in infertility counseling as a clinician, researcher, writer, educator and social networker as she is always so welcoming to new clinicians to the field. To each and every colleague who contributed to this text, I am deeply grateful and appreciative.

Many other hands helped to make it possible for me to do this project. My practice with Shady Grove Fertility Reproductive Science Center has formulated my work and has expanded beyond my wildest imagination since we began almost 25 years ago. With an outstanding staff of 33 doctors, nurses and administrative assistants (now totaling over 550 staff, in 18 offices extending to 4 states), there is not space to acknowledge all who hold my gratitude, yet a special thanks to: Drs. Robert Stillman, Michael Levy and Eric Widra; and nurses Michele Purcell, Margaret Ann Conners and Marsha Deweese. I am blessed to have an amazing staff of social workers and psychologists, several of whom have shared their wisdom and extensive experience in chapters here on third party reproduction: Patricia Sachs, Carol Toll, Ellen Eule, Erica Hanson, Michelle Hester, Erica Mindes, Tara Simpson, Mia Joelsson and my daughter, Laura Covington. These extraordinary women have sustained and bolstered me throughout the years, and I am eternally grateful to have them in my life and work. I also want to acknowledge my research team on Primary Ovarian Insufficiency (POI) at the NIH, headed by Dr. Larry Nelson, whose commitment, compassion and leadership I greatly admire. For 50 years, my friend first, then co-therapist and partner, Nancy Hafkin PhD has been there to listen, support, encourage and, when necessary, hold me accountable – all of which have made me a better clinician, for which I am most thankful. It has also been a joy and sustenance to share the journey in this field with my friends and colleagues, Linda Applegarth EdD and Susan Klock PhD. Linda and I became friends before sharing our personal experiences with reproductive loss and were drawn to specialize in this work at the same time. It is a precious gift to have a friend who truly knows and understands all the personal and professional struggles, and is always there for you. Sue is a soul mate; like-minded in the way we approach our work and our fun, she has guided me in gaining confidence in our shared interests of research based in clinical practice. As I have said before, I feel so lucky to have the opportunity to do the work I love, with people I love to work with.

Finally, and foremost, is my love and gratitude to the hands that help and hold me at home. My family has been by my side throughout my career and with every book I have done, assisting in so many ways. There has never been a greater supporter in my life and in my work than my husband, Barry. He is a man of kindness, courage and intellect, who loves with his whole heart and gives selflessly to others, setting an example for our children. All my children have jumped in whenever I needed it: my oldest daughter, Michelle, with technology challenges, editing advice, design decisions and always a good ear; my son, Brendan, with all my computer struggles, graphic designs and internet problems and my daughter-in-law, Darlene, who willingly shared her expertise in writing and marketing; and my youngest daughter, Laura, who has developed the same passion for this profession and has brought me great joy to share it with her – I appreciate her team spirit at work, while being knee-deep in her doctoral program. My son-in-law, Scott, and our four beautiful grandchildren, Sean, Michaela, Liam and Luke were there to offer a welcome distraction and a perspective on what is important in life. It has also brought me happiness and pleasure to share my profession, and now this field, with my sister-in-law, Bonnie Cochran LCSW. Bonnie is a cheerleader in life, encouraging, caring and taking the initiative to do what needs to be done. And to my "chosen" sisters, Virginia Frederick LCSW, Sandra Takai MD and Sheila Cave, who listened to my struggles, understood my needs and always encouraged me to bring out my best throughout this process, a special thank you!

To all my respected contributors, colleagues, friends and family, I give my heartfelt thanks, deep appreciation and gratitude for your support and assistance in this journey.

Sharon Covington

Chapter 1

Collaborative reproductive healthcare model

A patient-centred approach to medical and psychosocial care

Sharon N. Covington and G. David Adamson

Katie and Paulo are a highly successful, driven couple, who have worked hard in their careers to get established. Katie, 34, and Paulo, 36, met five years ago while in an MBA program, dated for three years as they concentrated on their jobs, and then carefully planned a wedding to be followed a year later by starting a family. They are used to working hard, setting goals, achieving them and moving on to the next. They are young, healthy and in control of their lives. However, the one thing they have never anticipated and could not foresee was difficulty getting and staying pregnant. After all, they have spent most of their adult life judicially using birth control and trying not to become pregnant.

Katie has been off the pill for over a year. They have been using an ovulation predictor kit, carefully timing intercourse, yet no pregnancy. Each month there is hopeful anticipation mid cycle followed by sadness when Katie's menstrual cycle begins. As the months tick on, Katie becomes more obsessed with trying to conceive, reading books and searching online, and upset when it doesn't happen. Paulo doesn't understand why she is responding this way, as he believes it will occur in time. However, the more he tells her "don't worry, it will happen," the more distressed she becomes. Sex, which always had been a great source of pleasure and comfort for them, now has become like work, with demands and deadlines. Both their families have started to ask about when they will be having children and they find their social circle getting smaller as they see their friends having kids seemingly without any difficulty. Feeling stressed, distressed and helpless, Katie and Paulo set up an appointment with a reproductive medical practice to find out what is going on.

Introduction

While this case vignette illustrates many common issues of patients seeking reproductive medical assistance, there is nothing "typical" about the average patient who seeks out fertility treatment today. Rapid advancement in technology and changes in societal views of reproductive rights have created choices and options for family building few could have imagined one generation ago. Heterosexual couples, while still the norm, are being joined by a diverse group of adults who also long for children. Older couples, single men and women, same-sex couples, people facing life-threatening medical circumstances or serious genetic conditions and transgender individuals have access to reproductive techniques that will allow them to have a child or children. In addition, a new group of patients are presenting, not for infertility treatment, but to preserve fertility options for the future through cryopreservation of their gametes.

This chapter will lay the foundation for subsequent chapters in this book regarding the medical and psychosocial assessment and treatment of individuals and couples needing reproductive medical assistance. As a physician and a mental health professional (MHP), we believe that optimal patient care involves the collaboration of numerous healthcare professionals (doctors, nurses, laboratory scientists, paraprofessionals, administrative staff, as well as counselors) working together to provide reproductive medical services. Over the last 30 years, we have observed a dramatic change in the recognition of the psychological consequences of infertility and the role fertility counselors play as an integrated part of the

Fertility Counseling: Clinical Guide and Case Studies, ed. Sharon N. Covington. Published by Cambridge University Press.

treatment team. Today, there is international consensus that the complex psychosocial issues of infertility patients' experience cannot be separated from the extraordinary reproductive technologies physicians use to treat these problems (i.e.,"you can't separate *what is being done* to your body, from how you *feel* about what is being done to your body"), and thus necessitates a collaborative approach to care. The American Society for Reproductive Medicine (ASRM) and the European Society for Human Reproduction and Embryology (ESHRE), as well as numerous other professional organizations and governmental policies, recognize this multidisciplinary method [1,2]. In addition, there is increasing recognition that, for patients seeking medically assisted reproduction (MAR), "optimal care" requires attention to their psychological vulnerability as well as the impact of negative interactions at the clinic between staff and patients [3]. These two issues can create a psychological burden for patients, affecting compliance and their ability to make decisions about continuing with treatment. Thus, "best practice" in reproductive healthcare will include ways to minimize patients' emotional and psychological distress, while providing effective clinical care in a positive environment.

As clinicians and colleagues, we have spent our careers advocating for the medical and psychosocial integrative care proposed by Covington with the "collaborative reproductive healthcare model" [4] and by other authors as "patient-centered care" [5] or "integrated approach" [6]. This model has a biopsychosocial approach in which the diagnosis and treatment of impaired reproduction are considered in terms of a variety of aspects impacting an individual/couple's experience with infertility: physiological, psychosocial, interpersonal, familial, spiritual, cultural and societal. A patient's overall health, functional status, emotional well-being and quality of life are influential factors in how s/he is able to navigate the condition. This approach emphasizes the importance of healthcare providers and patients as collaborators in diagnosis, treatment and health maintenance in order to achieve optimum results. The collaborative model integrates the best medical and psychosocial patient care, and is responsive to patient values and needs. Our approach in this chapter will be to present this model through a medical and psychosocial overview of the evaluation and treatment of infertility, following Katie and Paulo as they pursue their wish for a child.

Overview of infertility

In our modern world, most people think that getting pregnant is easy. They think this because a combination of sociologically driven delayed parenting, effective contraception and societal silence regarding infertility creates the perfect storm for disbelief when pregnancy does not occur almost immediately when they "try to get pregnant." Everyone is different, so some couples are highly *fertile*, others less so but still normal, some have sufficiently impaired fertility that they can be considered *subfertile* (although there is no agreed definition for this term) and some do not get pregnant within one year of having regular unprotected intercourse and, by the World Health Organization (WHO) definition, are considered *infertile* [7–9]. Since almost half of couples with no identifiable fertility problem will get pregnant in the second year of trying without any medical intervention, these couples often need and/or receive very little diagnosis and treatment [10]. Couples who fail to get pregnant after five years can be considered *sterile*, although very rarely pregnancies will occur without medical intervention even in these couples [11].

The WHO has defined infertility as a "disease." *Primary infertility* means that the patient has never been pregnant. A woman experiencing infertility after having ever been pregnant, regardless of the outcome of that pregnancy, has *secondary infertility*. *Recurrent miscarriage*, historically defined as three spontaneous pregnancy losses, but now defined as the spontaneous loss of two or more clinical pregnancies and usually investigated at that time, is not considered to be infertility, but is a different disease classification [8].

It is very difficult to determine the prevalence of infertility. However, studies that have been done suggest that about 7–9% of couples are infertile at any given time [12,13]. Traditionally, the causes of infertility in younger patients (<35) are ovulation problems about 15% of the time, tubal/pelvic pathology about 35%, male factor 35%, unexplained 10% and other 5% (Figure 1.1). However, over the past two decades, as women and men have delayed attempts at pregnancy, ovulation and hormonal problems, along with decreased egg quality, affect about 40% of the couples, pelvic problems occur in about 30%, cervical/combined factor (e.g., vaginal/cervical abnormalities and failure to have sex) in about 5% and primarily male factor in about 25%. In addition, reduced sperm quality would affect an additional 25%

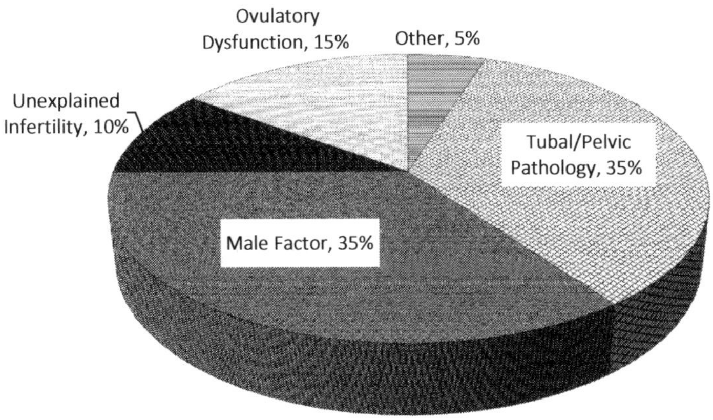

Figure 1.1 Causes of infertility in couples.

of couples in which a female factor is the primary cause. Some, but not all, studies suggest that decreased ovarian reserve associated with the older age of women attempting pregnancy is much more common in developed countries and pelvic factors, such as fallopian tube adhesions and occlusion, are more common in low-resource countries.

In developed countries a very common cause of difficulty getting pregnant is advanced age. The increased educational and economic opportunities for women have, understandably, resulted in many women delaying childbearing in order to pursue other life goals and interests. However, the female reproductive system has not changed. A baby girl is born with about 700 000 to one million eggs, the number of which continues to decrease over time. At puberty there are approximately 350 000–500 000 eggs (Figure 1.2) [14]. Women's fertility is at its peak from about age 23–31, and then begins to decrease because of a declining number of eggs and reduced percentage of eggs with a normal number of chromosomes (fewer euploid, i.e., normal number of chromosomes in the eggs and more aneuploid, i.e., abnormal number of chromosomes in the eggs). This results in a decreased pregnancy rate of approximately 3% per year from age 31–34, and 8% per year to age 39, so that at age 39 the average woman has about half the chance of getting pregnant than she did at age 31. From age 39–42 the chance of pregnancy is reduced about half again (Figure 1.3) [15]. Therefore, the chance that a woman in her mid 20s will get pregnant is about 30% on the first cycle without contraception, dropping gradually to about 10% on her 6th cycle and 3–5% by the 12th cycle. Each of these numbers is approximately half as high for a 39-year-old woman and one-quarter as high for a 42-year-old woman [16]. While there is a wide range of ovarian reserves in women at any given age, age remains the most important predictor of the ability to get pregnant and deliver a healthy baby [17].

Male fertility is less well understood. Fertility decreases with age in men, but much less than in women, with a man in his 50s having about 70% the capability of creating a pregnancy that he had in his 20s. Additionally, rates of autism, schizophrenia and bipolar disorders may be higher in children born to older fathers [18]. Most of the time when sperm quality is poor a cause cannot be found. Situations that can cause male infertility include prior testicular surgery for cancer, chemotherapy or radiation treatment for cancer, serious testicular injury, undescended testicle(s), mumps after childhood, social and prescription drugs that interfere with spermatogenesis, sexually transmitted infections, obstruction of the vas deferens duct that transports sperm from the testicle to the penis, complications of hernia operations, exposure to environmental toxicants, possibly large varicocoele and testicular exposure to high temperatures for prolonged periods of time.

General lifestyle and other factors can affect fertility. The commonest of these in developed and even many developing countries is obesity, which reduces fecundity through hormonal and ovulatory dysfunction [19,20]. Excessive exercise and/or decreased weight for women can reduce fertility also. Other factors can include excessive use of alcohol, smoking, social drugs, certain prescription medications, exposure to environmental toxicants, radiation exposure,

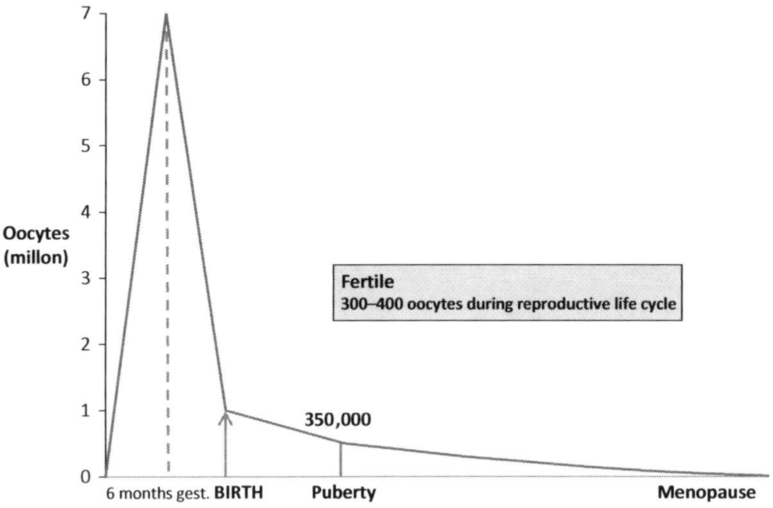

Figure 1.2 Oocyte numbers over a lifetime [adapted from Ref. 14].

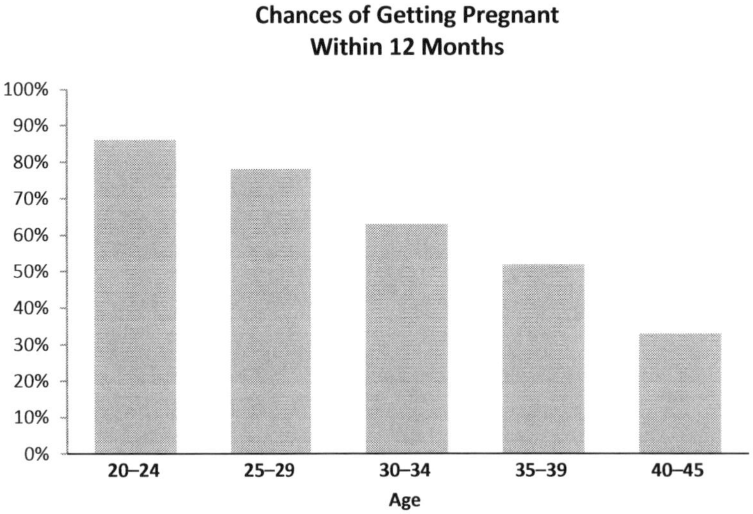

Figure 1.3 A woman's chance of getting pregnant by age [adapted from Ref. 15].

or excessive heat for men. It is important to emphasize good health habits with respect to diet, exercise and sleep. All reproductive age women would benefit from taking a supplemental multi-vitamin, iron, folate, vitamin D and calcium [21,22].

Generally, women who are younger than 35 and don't get pregnant after one year of unprotected intercourse should seek professional assistance from their gynecologist or a reproductive endocrinologist. Because of the reduction in fertility that occurs with age, women aged 35–40 should see a physician after about 6 months of no contraception, and women 40 or older after 3 months. Of course, if a couple has a history of an issue that might contribute to fertility problems, they should see a fertility specialist when they start attempting or, even better, when they decide that they will want to have a family. Examples of such problems are prior chemotherapy or radiation, irregular menstrual cycles, known hormonal problems, history of pelvic surgery, endometriosis, ruptured appendix or surgery on the cervix and, for the male, history of penile, testicular or hernia operations, or exposure to heat, environmental toxicants, chemotherapy, radiation or other drugs that can affect sperm production.

The goal of fertility treatment is to optimize the number of healthy eggs that can potentially be fertilized in any given cycle and result in implantation of embryos and birth of a healthy singleton baby.

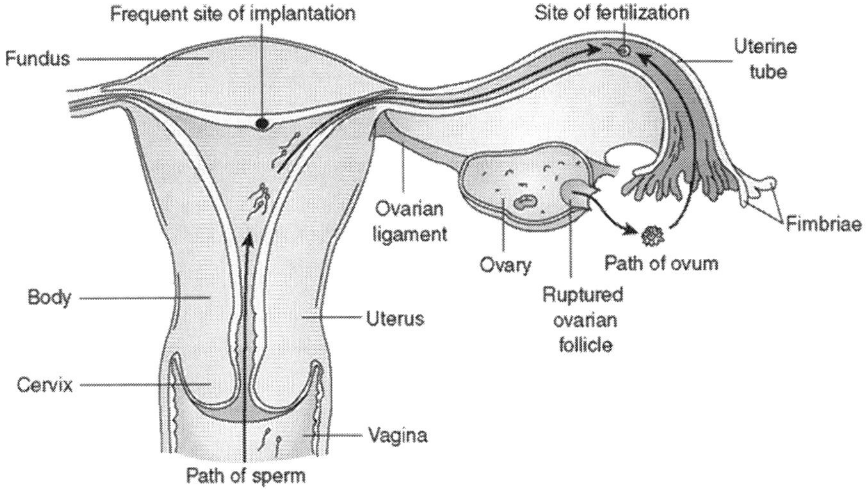

Figure 1.4 Female reproductive anatomy and physiology. Source: http://what-when-how.com/nursing/normal-pregnancy-maternal-and-newborn-nursing-part-1/.

Treatment of patients with low ovarian reserve can be done by using oral or injectable medications that increase the number of eggs ovulated. However, the quality of the eggs is not changed by these medications. Additionally, the risk of miscarriage and of having a baby with a birth defect increases with age. Fertility treatment can be used to overcome some, but not all, of this decrease. Modern testing can help to identify babies with problems during pregnancy, and sometimes with in vitro fertilization (IVF) even before pregnancy, by testing embryos using preimplantation genetic diagnosis (PGD) technology.

When patients present to the physician with infertility, it is important to recognize the reason the patient is there. It is not to diagnose, not to treat, but rather to intervene to obtain the desired outcome – a healthy singleton baby. The barriers to achieving this patient goal are several: medical conditions in the female and/or male, the patient's age, financial barriers and psychological stress. Approximately 50–60% of patients seen in a tertiary care center will have a baby. About 10% will decide not to pursue treatment because the prognosis is very poor, while about 30% will not achieve their goal because of financial and/or psychological barriers: 10% financial reasons alone, 10% psychological reasons alone and 10% a combination of the two. Additionally, even the patients who do get pregnant will often experience significant financial and/or emotional challenges during their treatment. If the physician is to optimize intervention, these issues must be actively addressed.

Reproduction: physiology and pathophysiology

In order for pregnancy to occur a healthy egg must be released from the ovary (ovulation) and be fertilized by a healthy sperm. Sperm are deposited at the cervix and make their way up through the endocervical canal and uterus to meet the egg, which has been picked up by a normally functioning fallopian tube from the ovarian surface or pelvis. The uterus must be functional and the endometrial lining must be able to respond to the estrogen and progesterone hormones secreted by the ovary so that the endometrium is prepared for implantation of the blastocyst. The blastocyst results from the fertilization of the egg and its development into a zygote and then an embryo and then the blastocyst by day 5 after fertilization (Figure 1.4).

The process of ovulation begins with the pulsatile release of gonadotropin releasing hormone (GnRH) from the hypothalamus at the base of the brain. This pulsatile release can be affected by weight, stress and other factors. The frequency of pulses changes during the menstrual cycle to cause the production of Follicle Stimulating Hormone (FSH) by the pituitary gland, causing the follicles in the ovary to develop. The ovary must have follicles (the number of which become reduced with age) containing cells that make estrogen in the follicular phase (the first half of the menstrual cycle leading up to ovulation). During the follicular phase, approximately 10–20 follicles begin to grow, but eventually one exerts dominance over the others through a process of natural selection (the best one grows and the others stop growing). The rapidly increasing estrogen level from the cells in this enlarging follicle stimulates the release of luteinizing hormone (LH) by the pituitary gland which causes the egg in the follicle to mature and to be released from the follicle (ovulation).

The egg is released into the pelvis and is picked up by the fallopian tube. The egg only lives about 12–24 hours so it is important for sperm to be present when the egg is ovulated. The sperm, which have swum up from the cervix, fertilize the egg in the fallopian tube. Sperm will live 2–4 days in the female reproductive tract. The fertilized egg is called a zygote. The cells divide and at 3 days, the 8 cells are called an embryo. The embryo continues to grow in the fallopian tube and enters the uterus at 5–6 days, comprises about 150–250 cells, and is called a blastocyst. The blastocyst floats in the uterus for about a day before implanting in the endometrium. The endometrium has been stimulated to grow by the estrogen from the follicle.

After ovulation, the follicle collapses on itself and becomes more vascularized and is called a corpus luteum ("body yellow"). This structure then makes progesterone under the influence of LH and some FSH that is produced by the pituitary gland. The progesterone is essential for the endometrium to develop properly so that implantation of the blastocyst can occur. If implantation and pregnancy occur, the trophoblast (early placenta) secretes human chorionic gonadotropin (hCG) which is the hormone tested for to detect pregnancy. The hCG stimulates the corpus luteum to continue producing progesterone until the placenta takes over with progesterone production at approximately 8–10 weeks of pregnancy. Progesterone is necessary to maintain the developing pregnancy.

Understanding the physiology of reproduction, it is no wonder there may be many things that impede, diminish or get in the way of fertilization and implantation. While there are many specific causes of infertility, the general categories are fairly simple:

1. *Female factors*:
   a. Egg and hormonal factors: decreased ovarian reserve based on age or other factors; ovulation abnormalities from hypothalamic/pituitary gland dysfunction, polycystic ovarian syndrome (PCOS – diagnosed by the presence of two of three of irregular ovulation, clinical or biochemical hyperandrogenism, or antral follicle count greater than 12 in each ovary) or abnormal weight; hormonal problems such as thyroid disease, hyperprolactinemia or renal gland disease; and endometrium problems affecting implantation.
   b. Pelvic/anatomic factors: uterine problems such as fibroids, adenomyosis, polyps, adhesions or congenital abnormalities; tubal problems such as adhesions, internal fibrosis or obstruction; pelvic peritoneal problems such as endometriosis or adhesions; cervical or vaginal abnormalities preventing deposition of sperm at the cervix and/or access of sperm into the uterus and fallopian tubes [23,24].
2. *Male factor*: azoospermia, oligospermia, decreased motility or morphology; genetic disorders (e.g., Klinefelter's) erectile dysfunction (ED), ejaculatory dysfunction or other problems affecting the delivery of sperm to the cervix at the appropriate time.
3. *Combined factor*: having intercourse at the wrong time with respect to timing of fertilization; using lubricants that harm sperm.
4. *Unexplained:* In about 10–20% of cases a definitive cause of infertility is not identifiable and the diagnosis is "unexplained infertility." However, this diagnosis is commonly thought to represent an undiagnosable egg or sperm problem.

Evaluation of infertility: colloborative care

Medical management

Initial assessment of infertility includes a history and physical examination of both male and female partners [25]. The *female* history involves asking about menstrual history, prior pregnancies and attempts at prior pregnancy, fatigue, constipation and other symptoms of thyroid disease, breast secretions, acne and hirsuitism. Use of exogenous hormones such as estrogen found in soy-based products and alternative medicine such as herbs or other supplements are potentially important because these bioactive compounds can interfere with the patient's own hormones. History of issues affecting pelvic factor, such as prior abdominal/pelvic operations, sexually transmitted infections (STI) and pelvic pain with

Table 1.1 Ovarian reserve testing [27].

Blood levels:
Anti-mullerian Hormone (AMH: normal ~> 1 ng/ml)
Follicle Stimulating Hormone (FSH: normal ~ <10 miU/ml)
i. Estradiol (E2: normal ~ < 80 pg/ml)
Thyroid Stimulating Hormone (TSH: normal < 2.5 miU/L)
Prolactin levels (PRL: normal ~ 25 ng/ml).
Ultrasound:
Antral Follicle Count (AFC: normal ~> 7)

menses, intercourse or bowel/bladder function, is also significant. *Male* factor should be assessed by history of prior pregnancies created and/or exposure to pregnancy, sexually transmitted infections, urethritis, prostatitis, reproductive injuries, accidents, operations or diseases, undescended testicle(s), environmental toxicants, excessive heat, erectile dysfunction, obesity, genetic causes, hormonal abnormalities and other reproductive problems [26]. *Combined* factor history includes cervical operations, frequency and timing of intercourse and use of lubricants. General questions regarding weight, diet, exercise, sleep, smoking, alcohol or drug use, exogenous hormones, alternative medicines, other medications, general health and prior fertility testing and treatment are important for both female and male patients.

Female testing

Physical examination includes general health, height and weight, blood pressure and respiratory rate. Visual examination of the external genitalia, vagina and cervix should be performed followed by bimanual examination of the uterus, ovaries and rectovaginal area. The thyroid should be examined, along with the breasts for galactorrhea (nipple secretions) and the skin for acne or hirsuitism (abnormal facial hair, peri-areolar hair).

Initial testing for causes of infertility is fairly simple. Table 1.1 lists common blood work used to test for ovarian reserve and the normal levels [27]. In addition, hyperandrogenemia (increased male hormone levels) can be tested with testosterone and possibly other androgenic hormone levels in selected situations. The clomiphene citrate challenge test (CCCT) is a more sensitive test of ovarian reserve than cycle day 3 FSH alone and is occasionally helpful. Karyotype (chromosome testing) is occasionally indicated to rule out genetic problems. Endometrial biopsy to date the endometrial development is a traditional test that has been shown not to be helpful and is no longer performed.

Pelvic factor is usually assessed initially with ultrasound to obtain information about the uterus (e.g., uterine myomas, which are benign muscle tumors of the uterine wall), congenital abnormalities (septate uterus may be associated with infertility, single and double uterine abnormalities with pregnancy complications) and endometrial thickness and characteristics; the ovaries (size, antral follicle count, ovarian cysts); the fallopian tubes (hydrosalpinx or complete distal obstruction of the fallopian tube), paratubal cysts and possibly endometriosis (only endometriomas which are ovarian cysts of endometriosis and deeply infiltrative endometriosis can be seen on ultrasound). A saline infusion sonogram (SIS, also known as a sonohysterogram or SHG) provides additional sensitivity (ability to detect a real abnormality) to identify intrauterine polyps, myomas or adhesions. After an ultrasound, the most common test of the pelvic organs is a hysterosalpingogram (HSG). The HSG is a radiological procedure that is better at documenting whether or not the uterine cavity is normal shape and whether or not the fallopian tubes are open and/or have intratubal damage or peritubal adhesions. Very occasionally magnetic resonance imaging (MRI) or computerized tomography (CT) may be used to help define abnormalities of the uterus or ovaries or other pelvic masses. Surgical procedures that can be used to further diagnose and then to treat problems that have been identified by imaging technology include hysteroscopy (passing a small telescope through the cervix to look into the uterine cavity) and laparoscopy (passing a small telescope through a sub-umbilical incision into the abdomino-pelvic cavity to look at the internal organs) with hydrotubation (injection of colored fluid through the fallopian tubes to check for patency), which are minor surgical procedures that usually require anesthesia.

Male testing

Male testing is almost always initiated with a semen analysis to measure volume of semen, pH, liquefaction, count, motility and morphology. Normal parameters by the World Health Organization Standard (5th Edition) count is $\geq$ 15 million/ml, progressive motility $\geq$ 32% and strict morphology $\geq$ 4% [28]. Morphology is especially difficult to assess and many men have slightly decreased morphology. Antisperm antibody and other male tests rarely add additional useful information except perhaps for men with prior vasectomy considering reversal [29].

Tests for combined factor generally involve sexually transmitted infection testing for HIV 1 and 2, HTLV (Human T lymphotropic virus) I and II for men, hepatitis B and C, syphilis, chlamydia and gonorrhea. The traditional test for combined factor, the postcoital test, has been shown not to be helpful and is no longer performed [30–32].

General/systemic tests for hematology (blood, spleen), biochemistry (liver, kidneys, parathyroid), blood sugar (pancreas) are generally indicated if not done within the past 1 to 2 years. Obese patients or those with family history of diabetes mellitus should be tested with fasting blood sugar (normal <100 mg/dl) and HgA1c (a measure of glucose metabolism, normally less than 5.7%).

The purpose of testing is not to do tests or, in fact, to simply make a diagnosis. The purpose of testing is to determine the prognosis for the patient given the test results, and how that prognosis can be improved by: intervention with lifestyle or other general/systemic changes; hormonal treatment of specific ovulation or other hormone problems; controlled ovarian stimulation to increase the number of eggs ovulated in a given month; surgical intervention to improve the pelvic organs; male factor treatment with drugs or surgery; or combined factor treatment to get more, better sperm closer to the egg(s) at the right time. All diagnostic tests and medical or surgical interventions should be focused on improving the patient's quality of life by better disease management and, specifically, meeting the desired wish of delivering a healthy singleton baby.

> Katie and Paulo meet with the Reproductive Endocrinologist (RE) who takes a thorough medical history and then orders a series of diagnostic tests. Katie is diagnosed with Polycystic Ovarian Syndrome (PCOS) and Paulo's semen analysis indicates a low sperm count. A course of intrauterine insemination (IUI) with Clomid is planned.

At this planning visit, their physician explains to them that infertility represents the 5th highest burden of disease globally in reproductive-age individuals, and that learning one is infertile often carries an emotional impact equivalent to that of a diagnosis of HIV or cancer. Additionally, this is a condition that often has to be dealt with by the couple alone because it is generally not discussed socially, even while there can be significant pressures from other family members to have children. Infertility is often the first major challenge a young couple face together, so it is important to communicate clearly to each other how they feel and what they want to do. The husband can be educated about the fact the woman almost always experiences much more pressure and emotional stress than the man, and so the man must support his wife personally and socially; while she needs to express appreciation for his efforts, even though they cannot completely resolve her emotional burdens. The importance of obtaining the best available evidence, asking questions and making logical decisions can be emphasized. The value of emotional support through good nutrition, sleep and exercise as well as meditation, prayer, yoga, acupuncture, mindfulness, or other mind–body exercises and support groups is emphasized. The important role of individual, couple and/or group counseling during treatment is explained. They are provided with written materials on the medical and emotional aspects of infertility, support resources and information, and the psychological services available at the clinic.

Psychosocial management

Despite the media attention often given to infertility, few people ever anticipate they will have problems getting pregnant or carrying a baby. There is mounting evidence that men and women frequently underestimate their reproductive time clock [33] as well as lifestyle issues that can affect childbearing (e.g., smoking, body weight, alcohol, drug and caffeine consumption), and it is suggested that people should be encouraged to think about parenthood goals in a similar way as one does other important life goals, like education and careers [3]. In addition, advances in technology in cryopreservation of ooyctes have opened a new area of counseling for women needing to preserve their fertility due to a medical problem, usually cancer treatment, or by choice to use in the future (see Chapter 15). Hence, MHPs in all types of practice settings can play an important role in helping their clients understand and consider preconception issues, fertility awareness and reproductive options.

The intention and planning of family creation is something that takes place psychologically long before it ever occurs physically. Individuals and couples begin thinking about having a child and being a parent often while still children themselves, as the imaginary journey towards parenthood begins. The longer one walks down this path, the stronger the attachment to the "wished-for" baby. If difficulties occur along the road, assistance may be needed in order to achieve the dream of a child. These difficulties may be caused by medical or genetic issues, which result in infertility, or by other life circumstance, such as not finding a partner or sexual orientation, whereby people are technically not "infertile" but nonetheless need medical assistance to have a child. No matter what the path is that has brought an individual or couple to seek MAR, every person brings a history that will impact how he or she experiences impaired reproduction (see Chapter 2).

Psychosocial Context

Reproduction is a basic human need, influenced by strong psychological, cultural and social drives. Griel and colleagues [34] describe infertility as a "socially constructed reality" rather than purely a medical condition with psychological consequences. Individuals and couples must embrace the role of parenthood as a desired social role or they would not seek medical assistance. For couples, it is a condition that affects them both, no matter who is identified as impaired, and is most evident as a state of "absence" (i.e., no child) rather than disease or symptoms. In addition, there are strong sociocultural influences in both developed and developing countries that shape how an individual or couple experience infertility. In pronatalist cultures, childlessness is surrounded by shame and stigma, while in developed societies not having a child may be viewed as a voluntary, viable choice. Griel et al. state, "The experience of infertility is shaped by the social context... [and] best understood as... a process whereby individuals come to define their ability to have children as a problem, to define the nature of that problem, and to construct an appropriate course of action" [34, p. 141].

In a controversial revision of Maslow's hierarchy of needs theory, Kenrick and colleagues [35] renovated the pyramid by replacing "self-actualization" and putting "parenting" at the top, reflecting new findings from the fields of neuroscience, developmental and evolutionary psychology. They contend that reproduction is not just about producing children, but also raising and parenting them so they, in turn, will reproduce. Therefore, all the effort that goes into parenting (e.g., caring, feeding, nurturing, educating children) is based in deep-rooted psychological urges that are a hallmark of being human and are passed down from generation to generation.

Thus, parenthood is not only a desired social role, but also a biologically driven need, creating the "perfect storm" for psychological distress when thwarted. It is well established in the literature (and throughout this text) that infertility is an inherently stressful experience that creates great emotional turbulence in the individual and/or couple the longer it goes on. So whether by impairment or circumstance, patients presenting for MAR will need psychological support and assistance throughout the treatment process. While most couples presenting to clinics are emotionally well-adjusted and not fundamentally different from others, they are more likely to experience distress over time, affecting self-esteem and life satisfaction, as a result of infertility [34].

Men and women will experience infertility differently in both the way they feel and the way they cope. Most studies indicate that women experience greater infertility related stress, reporting more symptoms of depression and anxiety than men. Men also experience infertility stress, but with less emotional affect and more indirectly, through the effect it has on their partner and concern about her [34]. The emotional context changes when infertility is gender-specific (i.e., female-factor or male-factor), with the diagnosed individual within a couple having a more negative response typically reflecting negative feelings surrounding diminished self-esteem, self-image and body-image [36]. Consequently, shame may become a defining force as an individual feels there is something inherently wrong or defective about themself. Feelings of grief and loss, well documented throughout the literature, are the emotional response and continue when treatment is unsuccessful and, finaly, when moving on to third party reproduction.

Regarding coping strategies, women display higher levels of seeking social support (e.g., talking to friends and family), avoidant behavior of painful situations (e.g., baby showers, pregnant friends) and information-seeking. Men tend to use distancing from the pain of infertility and problem-solving [37]. These different gender-related coping strategies may give rise to additional stress within a couple's relationship, as women seek more ways to obtain emotional support, while men attempt to problem-solve and, when not effective, distance themselves out of frustration. This dynamic can be played out further in their sexual relationship, which is explained in the adage: "Women need to feel loved (i.e., emotionally supported, feeling truly understood) in order to have sex, and men need to have sex (i.e., take action, physical response) in order to feel loved." Thus, infertility can have a powerful effect on a couple's sexual relationship not only due to the repeated, time-sensitive, performance demands of procreation, but also because of the differences in the ways men and women cope with distress (see Chapter 4).

Assessment

Infertility is not experienced in a vacuum and needs to be understood within the context of the history a patient brings to it. Just as physicians would not begin to treat a patient without comprehensive history taking and doing a thorough medical examination, fertility counselors also must take a similar approach. There are a number of tools available to help the counselor gather information, as well as self-administered interventions used to identify patients in need of additional emotional support.

The *Comprehensive Psychosocial History of Infertility* (CPHI) provides a framework for the clinician to gain knowledge about a patient's history, stressors and current and past functioning relevant to infertility [38]. It covers the spectrum of issues relevant to an infertility patient's emotional status as well as a couple's functioning and covers reproductive history, psychiatric history, marital, family and social relationship history. Past history of loss, trauma, instability and psychological dysfunction may be rekindled and exacerbated by parallel feelings brought out during infertility evaluation and treatment. It is also important for the fertility counselor to gather information and gain an understanding of the interaction between reproductive stages/events and psychological symptoms, such as during puberty, menstrual cycles, pregnancy, or while on oral contraceptives; the psychological side effects of medications used during treatment; and considerations for patients with a psychiatric history and on psychotropic medication (see Chapter 6).

Besides standard instruments used in the screening of depression and anxiety, a number of infertility specific screening tools have been developed that help clinicians identify how patients are doing and their level of distress. These tools are validated, self-administered instruments, quick to take, and can be easily interpreted by clinicians. *FertiQoL* can be completed online by patients (http://www.fertistat.com/fertiqol), is currently available in 31 languages with others in progress, and takes about 10–15 minutes to complete [39]. It assesses the impact of fertility problems and its treatment on a patient's quality of life along domains of personal, social and relational life. *SCREENIVF* has been found to be highly predictive of those at risk for treatment distress, which helps in directing patients towards additional psychological support [40]. The *Fertility Problem Inventory* (FPI) is another validated tool that measures an individual's infertility related stress as well as the impact on a couple's relationship [41]. Any of these screening tools will help the fertility counselor in the assessment of a patient's current functioning and need for support as treatment progresses.

Anticipation, prevention and support

For patients entering treatment, it may feel like embarking on a journey and entering a strange land where you don't speak the language or know the terrain you must travel. In this sense, fertility counselors, along with other members of the treatment team, will serve as guides. Metaphors like this abound that relate to the struggles and issues faced by patients, from the "emotional rollercoaster" of monthly or treatment cycles, "road maps" of where one has been and is going, and "bridges" that need to be crossed to reach a goal or connect to divergent paths or views. Since both words and visualizations are used, metaphors can be a powerful tool to open ways of thinking, evoke emotions, help understanding and change perspective with infertility patients.

Preparatory counseling is seen as both helpful and a valuable service for new patients entering treatment [42]. Patients need to anticipate what is ahead, and should be provided with information and reading materials regarding medical conditions, treatment options, the emotional experience of infertility, support services and resources. It is ideal if these materials are available in printed versions for view in the office or to share during a counseling session, or to have as an electronic file that can be emailed to patients prior to meeting. These educational materials and resources become the fertility counselors "tools of the trade" and having them readily available and organized is important. Being able to anticipate what is ahead emotionally, where and how difficulties may arise and what strategies might help can prevent more serious problems. Helping patients understand that "an ounce of prevention is worth a pound of cure" may help them be more adaptive and resilient to the distress of infertility.

Support becomes a pivotal piece of care for all members of the treatment team. Patient-centered care is supportive and focuses on positive communication with staff – empathy, respect, sensitivity, trustworthiness and responsiveness. As all MHPs know, these interactions are the basis of forming a therapeutic relationship in counseling. While individual and couple counseling should be easily accessible for patients, the reality is that only a small minority will follow on their own and those given a referral for counseling during a "crisis" often deem it as another example of their inadequacy [43].

Research has shown that the most effective psychosocial intervention is group counseling [43], normalizing the emotional response to infertility, teaching effective coping strategies and educating patients on various aspects related to treatment and family building. These groups can consist of periodic (weekly/monthly), open-ended gatherings more emotion-focused on dealing with treatments (e.g., general infertility, recipients of donor gametes, intended parents or gestational carriers, secondary infertility, etc.), skill-building (e.g., mind–body techniques, cognitive-behavioral strategies, etc.), or specific topics providing more psycho-education (e.g., adoption discussion, disclosure assistance, etc.), yet all will be offering patient support. Patient organizations, such as Resolve, continue to provide support, advocacy and information, while the Internet has dramatically changed the way patients access information, seek support (chat rooms, blogs, social media, etc.) and obtain education [44]. (For an in-depth discussion of group work in fertility counseling, please see Reference [45].)

Spirituality is another form of support, often overlooked by clinicians, which should be explored by fertility counselors yet (see Chapter 5). Religion and spirituality usually occur within a cultural context of the patient going through treatment and may provide important information about how infertility is perceived. Patients with a strong spiritual foundation utilize this belief system to cope with the sense of loss of control, to help in decision-making and to find meaning and purpose from the experience. While many clinicians, both medical and psychological, are uncomfortable with addressing religion and spirituality, research continues to show this is a neglected area that fertility patients wish was discussed [46].

Treatment of infertility: colloborative care

Medical intervention

There are multiple potential medical interventions for infertility, but they can, generally, be grouped into three categories: observation, standard/conventional treatment and in vitro fertilization (IVF). While recurrent miscarriage is not strictly a category of infertility, the management during treatment will also be addressed. A fourth category of medical intervention, third party reproduction (donor sperm, donor egg, gestational carrier), is not technically a treatment for infertility and will be discussed in the next section.

Lifestyle choices to optimize pregnancy

Patients can optimize their chance for pregnancy by healthy lifestyle choices [21]. People attempting pregnancy should get 8 hours of sleep, eat a healthy, balanced diet, get a moderate amount of exercise and maintain normal weight. Studies show that women with a body mass index (BMI) of greater than approximately 30 begin to have decreased pregnancy rates. Women with a BMI less than about 19 can also experience ovulation disorders and less chance of pregnancy. Women should not do more than about two hours of aerobic exercise per week, but there are no limits on non-aerobic exercise such as weights, yoga, walking and swimming. Men should avoid exercise that might cause significant increase in testicular heat, for example, long bicycle rides or excessive use of hot tubs or saunas, as well as excessive heat from laptop computers, the proverbial really tight underwear, or other sources of heat. For women, alcohol should be avoided or at least limited to small amounts in the follicular phase before ovulation, although there are no good studies on how much, if any, alcohol is entirely safe. Men may have small amounts of alcohol, definitely less than two standard drinks of beer or wine or other alcohol per day although, again, there are no studies that prove any specific amount is entirely safe. Two to five cups of coffee or similar amount of caffeine per day from other sources is acceptable for women or men. Similarly, drug and medication use should be limited to that which is absolutely necessary. Any questions should be directed to the patient's personal physician. Social drugs, toxicants such as pesticides, paint sprays, hair/cosmetic sprays, industrial chemicals and radiation should be avoided. Pre-natal vitamins with calcium, iron and folate for the woman and a male multi-vitamin with anti-oxidant are recommended. Appropriate vaccinations for rubella, chicken pox, whooping cough and other diseases should be obtained according to Centers for Disease Control (CDC) recommendations.

Observation/no treatment

Observation alone is sometimes appropriate in young women with a short duration of infertility and no obvious causes of infertility after at least an initial history, physical examination and simple testing that show normal menstrual function, normal sperm and appropriate timed intercourse. Usually not more than 3–6 months of observation alone is indicated. Intercourse should occur every 2 days plus or minus half a day (i.e., every 1.5 to 2.5 days, or every 1 to 3 days at the outside). Intercourse should begin not later than 16 days before the expected menses based on the woman's shortest cycle in the past 6 months. (i.e., if shortest cycle in the past 6 months is 26 days, intercourse should start on day 26–16 = CD 10 where CD 1 = the first day of the last menstrual period) [47,48]. Basal body temperature charting can occasionally be used retrospectively to confirm ovulation, urinary LH sticks (Ovulation Predictor Kits) can be used to help time intercourse, but intercourse should begin several days before an expected rise. Assessing cervical mucus for viscosity can be informative but generally not sufficiently so to be the primary method of timing intercourse [49]. Pre-Seed, canola oil or mineral oil can be used as a lubricant but other lubricants should be avoided because they may reduce sperm function. Position of intercourse does not matter and the woman can remain supine after intercourse for 10 or so minutes if she chooses, although the potential benefit of this is unproven.

While mind–body/integrative care programs, yoga, acupuncture and other holistic approaches likely can improve the patient's sense of well-being and enhance their ability to comply with and manage their fertility care, thus boosting their chances to take home a baby, there is no credible evidence that these alternative medicine approaches will intrinsically increase biologic pregnancy rates. Herbal medicines and other alternative ingestions can reduce pregnancy rates if they contain bioactive ingredients that interfere with normal ovulation or controlled ovarian stimulation (COS).

Standard fertility treatment

After undergoing the tests noted above to assess sperm, eggs, uterus and combined factors, specific problems should be treated. Thyroid disease should be managed with thyroid supplement or appropriate treatment of hyperthyroidism. Hyperprolactinemia can be treated with bromocryptine or cabergoline after pituitary assessment for markedly elevated prolactin levels rule out a pituitary adenoma. Hyperandrogenism can be treated with dexamethasone or other appropriate medications. Insulin resistance can be treated with weight loss/metformin/insulin or other appropriate medications.

After testing and management of general lifestyle factors and general health conditions, treatment of specific fertility problems usually involves the use of hormones and/or minor or major surgery for the female, treatment of the male with hormones or minor surgery, or treatment of both with intrauterine insemination (IUI), IVF or use of donor sperm, eggs or gestational carrier. The goal of treatment is to increase the chance of pregnancy in each menstrual cycle by bringing more egg(s) together with more sperm in the best possible pelvic environment at the right time.

Female factor

(See Figure 1.5.) Oligo-ovulation can be treated with clomiphene citrate (Clomid or Serophene) usually starting with a dose of 50 mg per day cycle day 5 through 9 and increased as necessary [50]. Empiric controlled ovarian stimulation (COS) is usually performed with clomiphene 100 mg for 5 days starting on cycle day 3, 4 or 5, with similar pregnancy rates regardless of start day. Letrozole 2.5 to 5 mg per day can be used if clomiphene is not successful or in place of clomiphene if patients experience side effects from clomiphene. Letrozole is likely superior to clomiphene in PCOS patients and should be the first line of treatment [51]. Metformin can be considered as first-line treatment in selected patients [52]. COS should be monitored with ultrasound on approximately cycle day 11 to assess response to treatment with at least 1 or 2 maturing follicles ($\sim >15$ mm) but not an excessive number that could lead to increased risk of multiple pregnancy (< 4 mature follicles) [53]. The risk of twin pregnancy with clomiphene is approximately 8% and

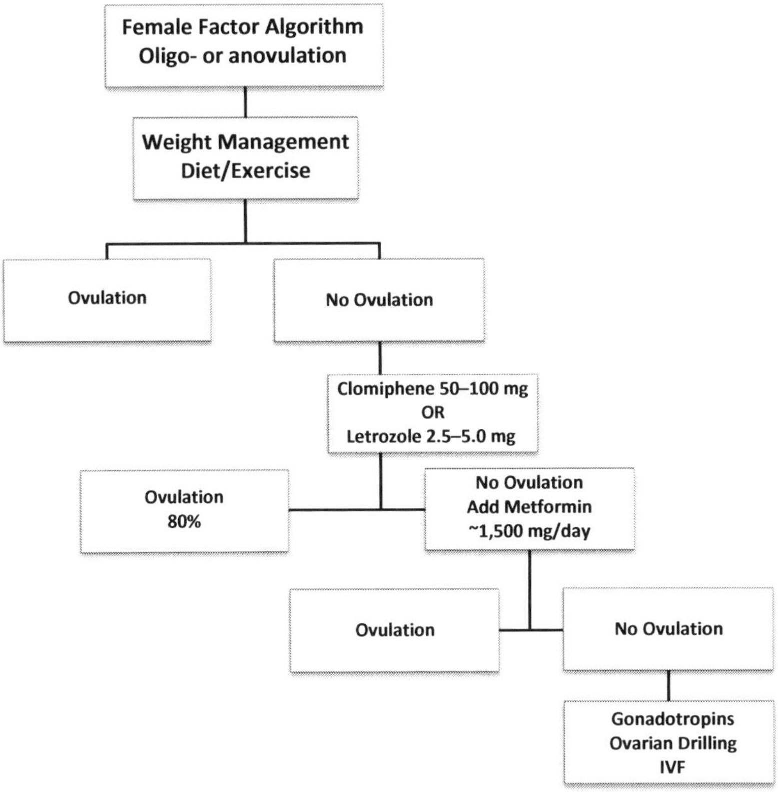

Figure 1.5 Female factor algorithm.

triplets 0.5%. Other side effects of clomiphene include thinning of the endometrium, headaches, hot flashes, vaginal dryness, mood changes, breast tenderness and occasionally photophobia or other eye symptoms. The cause of the latter are unknown, but thought possibly to be vascular in nature, and are sufficient to merit discontinuation of clomiphene use. Ovarian hyperstimulation syndrome (OHSS) with ovarian cysts is very rare with clomiphene.

Cancer, such as breast, ovarian and endometrial, is more common in women with infertility. The evidence does not support a relationship between fertility drugs and an increase in these cancers, though more studies are needed. However, there may be a small increase in the slower-growing, less-invasive borderline tumors in women treated with clomiphene.

Type 1 amenorrhea, which is very uncommon, can be treated with very low dose gonadotropins. Patients undergoing any type of gonadotropin treatment must be carefully monitored with ultrasound to follow the follicle number and size, and usually also with blood estradiol levels [54–57]. Ovarian hyperstimulation syndrome (OHSS) affects 1–3% of women treated with gonadotropins, and occurs following administration of hCG. (See the section below on IVF for more details.) More importantly, while gonadotropins can be very effective, they also carry the risk of twins and even triplets and higher order multiples [53]. Such pregnancies have much higher risks of a baby with a serious medical problem and also of maternal pregnancy complications. Prematurity, which occurs much more frequently in multiple pregnancy, is the major, but not only, cause of these problems. Today, there are very few patients who benefit from gonadotropins that are used outside of Type 1 amenorrhea or in IVF cycles. The increased pregnancy rates, decreased risks, shorter time to pregnancy and increased cost-effectiveness of IVF almost always make it a better treatment choice than gonadotropins and IUI [58,59].

Some patients have lesions in their uterus that reduce or prevent the chance of pregnancy. Intrauterine polyps, which result from excessive growth of the endometrium from estrogen stimulation, can be identified by ultrasound and treated by hysteroscopy. Hysteroscopy involves passing a small telescope through the cervix, usually as an office procedure or a short, outpatient procedure with intravenous sedation and monitored anesthesia care, and then using scissors or forceps to remove the polyp. A dilatation and curettage (D&C) is often done at the same time. Myomas, also called fibroids, result from excessive growth of a single cell in the muscle wall of the uterus. Myomas can occur in any number, location and size in the uterus: pedunculated (on a stalk outside the uterus), subserous (just under the outer layer of the uterus), intramural (in the wall of the uterus), submucous (protruding into the uterine cavity) and intracavitary (almost completely into the uterine cavity). Myomas that distort the uterine cavity reduce pregnancy rates and should be removed before fertility treatment. Large and/or multiple intramural myomas may reduce IVF pregnancy rates and removal should be considered before IVF. Myomas that cause pain or abnormal bleeding should also be removed. Intrauterine myomectomy can be accomplished with a hot electrosurgical loop resection or sometimes scissors and forceps. Intrauterine scarring or adhesions can also be diagnosed and cut or removed at hysteroscopy. Such adhesions are not common and usually result from complications of a pregnancy associated with trauma to the endometrium and infection. Severe adhesions are called Asherman's syndrome.

Some patients have an abnormally developed uterus. Most congenital abnormalities do not reduce pregnancy rates but may be associated with increased complications of pregnancy because the uterine cavity is either too small or abnormally shaped, leading to problems with the functioning of the placenta during pregnancy and/or premature labor. However, a relatively common abnormality called a septate uterus – in which there is a fibrous septum in the middle of the uterus – is possibly associated with increased miscarriage rates and should be removed before attempting pregnancy. This is easily done by resection with scissors during a hysteroscopy. After some, usually more extensive, hysteroscopic procedures the patient has a balloon catheter left in the cavity for a few days, antibiotics and/or estrogen hormones to help the endometrium regrow and reduce the risk of adhesions forming inside the uterus.

Other uterus, fallopian tube or pelvic problems can reduce pregnancy rates and can be treated by laparoscopy or laparotomy. Both of these operations require general anesthesia. Laparoscopy involves passing a small telescope into the abdomino-pelvic cavity through the umbilicus. Laparotomy usually involves a small "bikini" incision. If a very small abdominal incision is made, this is called a mini-laparotomy. Myomas that distort the uterine cavity, but cannot be removed by hysteroscopy, can be removed at laparoscopy or laparotomy [60]. Adhesions around the uterus, ovaries or fallopian tubes can usually be removed at operative laparoscopy. Different energy sources such as electrosurgery, laser or scissors can be used depending on surgeon preference, with no difference in effectiveness. Blocked fallopian tubes can be repaired, although if damage is severe and the tube is blocked at its distal end near the ovary (hydrosalpinx), then pregnancy rates are still very low afterwards (10–20%) and ectopic pregnancy risk is high, so IVF is more appropriate. Very badly damaged tubes with hydrosalpinges should be removed because their presence reduces IVF pregnancy rates [61]. Endometriosis is a common disease of the pelvis that can result in different types of inflammatory lesions on the pelvic peritoneum, adhesions around the uterus, tubes and ovaries, cysts in the ovaries (endometriomas), invasion into the uterine wall (adenomyosis) and deeply infiltrative endometriosis (DIE), especially in the pelvic cul de sacs and between the rectum and the vagina. Surgical treatment of endometriosis increases pregnancy rates and reduces commonly associated pain symptoms [62–64]. Some women who have had bilateral tubal sterilization may benefit more from tubal reversal (microreanastomosis) than from IVF.

Male factor

(See Figure 1.6.) Male factor problems also need attention. Healthy lifestyle behaviors are usually the most important. Some men may benefit from clomiphene citrate 25 mg per day continuously, or treatment of chronic prostatitis or other infections. Surgical treatment of varicocoele, which is a varicose vein of the testicular vein, may be indicated if the man has pain symptoms associated with the varicocoele and/or it is very large. The role of varicocoele in infertility and its treatment has been controversial for decades. Current recommendations are to offer varicocoelectomy to the male partner when all of the following are present: a varicocoele is palpable, the couple has documented infertility, the female has normal fertility or potentially correctable infertility and the male has one of more abnormal semen analyses or sperm function test results [65]. Other serious anatomic abnormalities are rare but should be treated. Men with obstructive

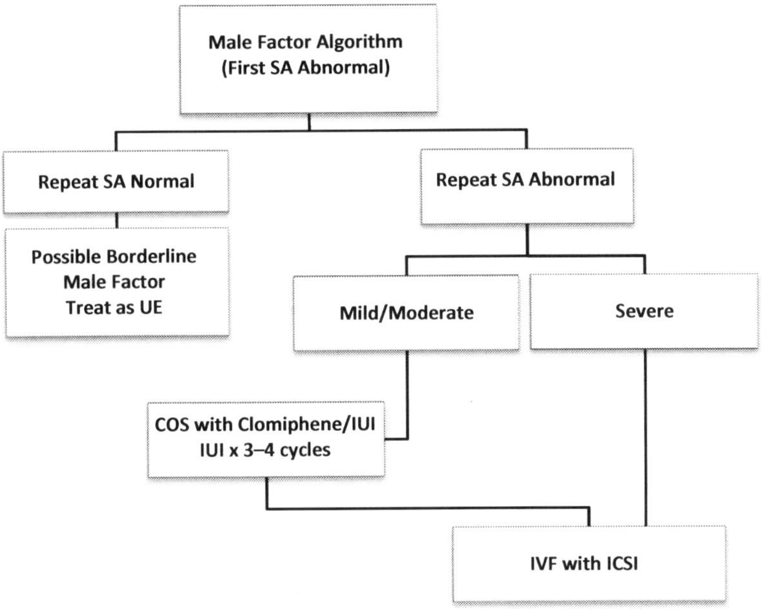

Figure 1.6 Male factor algorithm.

azoospermia may benefit from testicular or epididymal biopsy and cryopreservation of sperm or, for men with a vasectomy, a surgical reconnection of the vas deferens (vasovasostomy) [66]. Male fertility decreases slightly with age and the risk of having a baby with a problem, especially autism-related disorders, increases very slightly, but there are no known specific diagnostic tests or treatment for these changes.

Combined factors can be treated with sperm washing and intrauterine insemination [67]. This procedure enables more motile sperm with normal shape to be placed closer to the egg(s) at the right time in the cycle when ovulation is occurring. Depending on the clinical situation, this can increase the pregnancy rate only a small amount to up to 2–3 times. It can also be used when intercourse is difficult for psychological reasons in the male or female. Of course, such situations should also be addressed with counseling to identify and treat underlying psychological issues.

Unexplained infertility

(See Figure 1.7.) Up to 10–30% of couples have unexplained infertility, the diagnosis typically being made after the basic evaluation fails to reveal an obvious abnormality [68]. Unexplained infertility can be treated with IUI alone which increases the pregnancy rate per cycle from approximately 2% in control cycles to 5% in treated cycles. The use of clomiphene by itself produces a very small but significant increase in pregnancy. It would seem, therefore, that the use of clomiphene and IUI together would be at least as beneficial as either treatment alone. While probably the most common treatment, there are no well-designed trials that actually confirm its benefit [69–71]. Gonadotropins and IUI together result in pregnancy rates approximately twice as high as for either gonadotropins or IUI alone, which in turn are twice that of intracervical insemination alone. However, it is not clear if treatment does any more than speed up the time to pregnancy as opposed to increasing cumulative live birth rates. ART pregnancy rates for unexplained infertility are similar to other diagnoses, dramatically higher than with no treatment and not increased by adding ICSI. The adverse risks of treatment are primarily multiple gestation and OHSS. When considering treatment options for couples with unexplained infertility, it is prudent to consider simple treatment before complex treatment and to balance what is known about effectiveness against the cost and adverse effects of different treatments [68]. Nevertheless, clomiphene and/or IUI are generally never used for more than 3 to 6 cycles and gonadotropins and IUI more than 3 to 4 cycles before proceeding to ART, simply because they are almost never successful after that number of cycles. In recent years, excellent studies confirm that IVF is more cost-effective than gonadotropins and IUI, and so it is usually the most appropriate treatment after failed clomiphene and/or IUI [58,59].

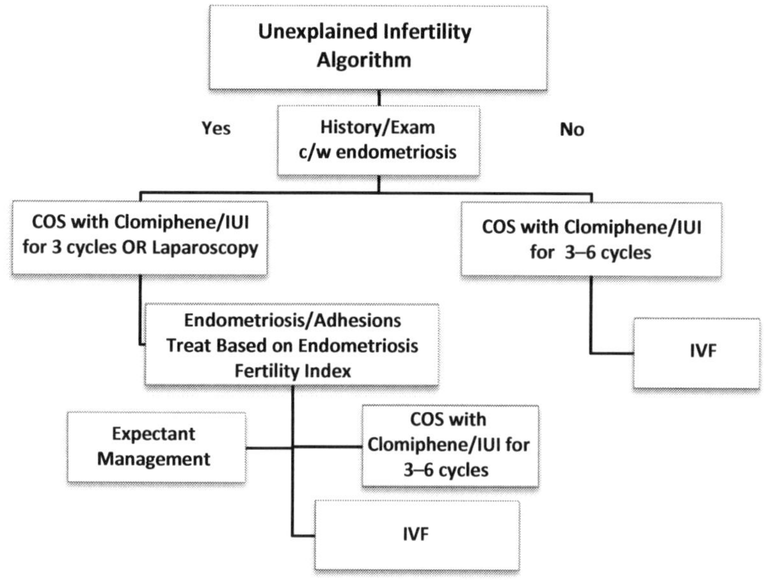

Figure 1.7 Unexplained infertility algorithm.

Recurrent miscarriage

Recurrent miscarriage or recurrent pregnancy loss (RPL) is often the most difficult clinical situation for both patients and physicians to manage. This is so because of the emotional trauma associated with miscarriage and our inability to identify the reason for pregnancy loss in 50–75% of the patients [72]. It is important to counsel patients that, even with three or more prior pregnancy losses, the chances for a successful live birth are 50–60%, depending on maternal age and parity, even with no treatment. The majority of pregnancy losses are sporadic and caused by random genetic factors that increase with age. It is appropriate to investigate RPL after two consecutive clinical pregnancy losses. Assessment of RPL focuses on screening for genetic factors and anti-phospholipid syndrome, assessment of uterine anatomy, hormonal and metabolic status and lifestyle factors. Investigation may include karyotype screening of potential parents, screening for anticardiolipin antibodies, lupus anticoagulant, and anti-beta 2, glycoprotein I, sonohysterogram, hysterosalpingogram and/or hysteroscopy, thyroid and prolactin screening and karyotyping of products of conception with the second or additional miscarriages. Identified problems should be treated when possible. Women with persistent, moderate to high levels of circulating antiphospholipid antibodies can be treated with a combination of prophylactic doses of unfractionated heparin and low-dose aspirin. Psychological counseling and support is especially important for couples with RPL.

In vitro fertilization (IVF)

Generally, after diagnostic tests are done, systemic problems addressed and specific causes of infertility identified and treated, standard treatment is performed for 3 to 6 months if there are no identifiable issues that suggest only IVF can solve the medical problem. Issues that usually should result in immediate referral to IVF include advanced maternal age, diminished ovarian reserve, significant tubal damage, two or more ectopic pregnancies, moderate to severe male factor, failed prior treatments and/or prolonged infertility. If 3 to 6 months of standard treatments do not result in an ongoing pregnancy, most patients are candidates for IVF. Occasionally, in younger patients or those with miscarriages, standard treatment can effectively be used for a longer period of time. IVF is a very successful treatment for most, but not all, patients. IVF does not improve uterine factor and cannot change egg quality. All patients considering IVF need to be thoroughly counseled regarding IVF. Issues about which the patients need to be made aware and decisions they need to make are discussed below.

An IVF cycle generally consists of suppressing the ovaries with oral contraceptives for three weeks so that all of the eggs start maturing at about the same time when ovarian stimulation begins. Different types of ovarian suppression and stimulation cycles include long luteal suppression with the gonadotropin releasing hormone (GnRH) agonist leuprolide acetate (Lupron), leuprolide acetate flare cycles and GnRH antagonist cycles with cetrorelix (Cetrotide) or ganirelix (Antagon). No studies show any protocols are superior to long luteal suppression protocols with GnRH agonist and there are no studies that demonstrate any specific protocol will increase pregnancy rates in poor responders.

Injectable fertility medications can be human menopausal gonadotropins (HMG) that contain both FSH and LH and are sold as Repronex or Menopur. Follitropins are recombinant FSH, sold as Follistim and Gonal F. The scheduling and protocols for monitoring these subcutaneous injections are complex and need to be explained in detail and specific written instructions given to patients. Ovarian cancer risk is of historical concern but reasonably good data conclude there is likely very little risk of ovarian carcinoma and/or very few patients are ever affected. However, absolute confirmation of gonadotropin safety with respect to cancer may yet be several decades away. Additional medications such as dexamethasone, bromocryptine and/or growth hormone may occasionally be used in selected patients.

The goal of fertility treatment is to optimize the number of healthy eggs that can potentially be fertilized in any given cycle and result in implantation of embryos and birth of a healthy singleton baby. It is not possible to know with certainty how any woman will respond to ovarian stimulation medications until they are actually used. There is a risk of either not responding much at all with very little or no benefit from the ovarian stimulation, or the risk of responding too much with the risk of large ovarian cysts, pelvic pain and/or OHSS. The potentially significant medical risks of OHSS include pelvic discomfort from large ovaries, nausea, vomiting, accumulation of fluid in the peritoneal, pleural and/or pericardial sac resulting in a distended abdomen, difficulty breathing and/or cardiac problems. Significant fluid imbalance in the body can result in a very high concentration of red blood cells in the vascular system, cause blood clots, kidney and/or liver failure or affect other vital organs. Hospitalization is needed in about 1 in 300 patients and in the rarest of cases, death can occur. If pregnant, a second wave of OHSS can occur, and complications can be more severe with multiple pregnancy [73]. Minor side effects include inflammation and bruising at the injection site.

Use of these fertility medications does increase pregnancy rates but does not reduce miscarriage rates, the risk of pregnancy complications, or birth defects/abnormal babies. Women experiencing infertility generally have approximately 1.5 to 2 times the risk of pregnancy and baby complications regardless of whether they use fertility drugs or the method of getting pregnant. Approximately 10–15% of cycles are cancelled before egg retrieval because of low response to gonadotropins or hyperstimulation/OHSS.

After ovarian stimulation, which lasts about 8 to 12 days on average, human chorionic gonadotropin (hCG) is used to trigger final maturation of the eggs. Trade names for these drugs are Novarel, Ovidrel and Pregnyl. Leuprolide acetate (Lupron) trigger can be used in antagonist cycles to avoid OHSS. It is essential to time carefully this injection with respect to time of egg retrieval procedure, the interval being about 35–36 hours.

The egg retrieval procedure involves monitored anesthesia care with conscious sedation performed in a procedure room or surgery center. A small needle is passed through the posterior vaginal wall into the ovary using transvaginal ultrasound guidance. Each follicle is entered and the follicular fluid is aspirated into a small test tube, which is passed to an embryologist who looks at the fluid under a microscope to identify and separate any eggs into a separate small dish. The procedure takes approximately half an hour. The patient goes home about an hour after the procedure. The risks of the procedure include anesthetic complications, drug reactions, breathing or heart problems, neurologic problems, bleeding, infection, or blood clots. However, the procedure is, overall, very safe. Rarely, no eggs are retrieved or the eggs that are found are not viable. This happens about 3% of the time, usually in older patients. Additionally, on average only approximately two or three of the eggs retrieved will be of appropriate maturity to be fertilized. Furthermore, even eggs that have normal maturity do not all have normal chromosomes. At age 35 less than half of the eggs have normal chromosomes and at age 40 the percentage of normal eggs is approximately 10–20%.

While eggs are being retrieved from the patient, her partner will provide a sperm specimen by masturbation. The sperm specimen will then be prepared in the embryology laboratory for insemination of the partner's eggs. In situations in which the male has erectile dysfunction or any other type of problem that might make it difficult or uncertain that he can collect sperm on the day of egg retrieval, it can be arranged for the male to come in the day before to the laboratory and collect a specimen that will be kept overnight and used for insemination the next day. Alternatively, the male can collect a specimen days or weeks in advance and have it frozen in the laboratory and stored until the day of egg retrieval. In very selected cases of men with very poor sperm quality or other obstructive ejaculatory duct problems, sperm can be obtained surgically from the testicle or epididymis by a urologist using procedures called testicular sperm extraction (TESA) or microsurgical epididymal sperm aspiration (MESA) at the same time as the female partner is having eggs retrieved. However, if the male partner is sterile or the female patient has a same-sex partner or is single, donor sperm will be used for fertilization of the eggs.

Eggs can be fertilized by standard fertilization in which case about 50 000 to 100 000 sperm are placed around the eggs. In cases in which there is concern about the sperm quality, or occasionally for other reasons, intracytoplasmic sperm injection (ICSI) or injection of one sperm into one egg can be performed. This procedure is done in approximately 70% of cycles in the United States. ICSI increases the chances that at least some eggs will be fertilized, but ICSI does not increase the fertilization rate if the sperm function normally. Unfortunately, some men have normal semen analysis but their sperm do not function normally, and thus ICSI can be helpful for them. Approximately 70–90% of normal appearing eggs will fertilize. In cases in which it is not clear if ICSI is needed, the eggs can be split into both types of fertilization if sufficient mature eggs are retrieved. Eggs are checked one day after fertilization to see if normal fertilization has occurred, called the 2 pronuclear (2 PN) stage.

Embryos can be cultured to day 3 at which time they are at a cleavage stage or approximately 8-cell stage. On day 3, embryos are graded by the number of cells and the appearance of those cells. Embryos can also be grown from day 3 to day 5 in culture, at which time they are a 150–250-cell blastocyst. The probability a blastocyst will implant and result in a baby is about 1.3 to 1.4 times higher than a cleavage stage or day 3 embryo. However, only about 50% of the embryos grow in culture from day 3 to day 5. Most, but not necessarily all, of the embryos that fail to grow are abnormal. Therefore, patients who choose to continue with culture to blastocyst stage will have fewer blastocysts to choose from than day 3 cleavage stage embryos, and some patients, especially older patients, might have no blastocysts to transfer. Additionally, there are some concerns that embryos remaining in culture might experience "imprinting" problems where the expression of genes is influenced, and some studies suggest that babies born after culturing to blastocyst may have more abnormalities. However, the vast majority of babies born from blastocysts are healthy and the pregnancy rate for each blastocyst transferred is significantly higher than for an embryo. There are clinical reasons to transfer on either day 3 or day 5 and these must be discussed and decided upon with each patient individually. There is no convincing evidence that cumulative live birth rates are increased by growing day 3 embryos to blastocysts and transferring them on day 5. There is now a system on the market approved by the FDA called Eeva™ (Early Embryo Viability Assessment) that increases our ability to predict which embryos will grow from day 3 to day 5, and therefore should improve pregnancy rates with day 3 transfers to be approximately equivalent to blastocyst transfer without having to grow to blastocyst. The optimal role for day 3 versus day 5 transfer is yet to be determined and requires more well-designed clinical research studies.

Preimplantation Genetic Diagnosis (PGD) can be done to identify selected known genetic problems in the patient and/or her partner. It has proved to be 95% to over 99% accurate. Preimplantation Genetic Screening (PGS) is technically the same procedure as PGD in terms of putting a small needle into the blastocyst and removing 5 to 15 cells; however, the cells are then sent to a very specialized laboratory to do Comprehensive Chromosome Screening (CCS) using one of the modern genetics platforms that analyzes thousands of genes in the chromosomes from the blastocyst. While CCS can identify abnormal blastocysts, it is not yet clear that performing CCS increases the live birth rate. Because of its cost of approximately $5000 it has limited application at this time. When PGS is performed, usually all the blastocysts are cryopreserved on day 5 to give time to do the PGS test and get the results before doing a frozen/thaw cycle a month or two later. The optimal role of PGS for CCS is yet to be determined in well-designed clinical trials, but there is a lot of interest in this clinical approach.

Multiple pregnancy is the major complication of IVF and results from many factors. Approximately 70% of infertile patients say they would like twins.

Nevertheless, twins have approximately 1.2 to 2 times the risk of serious, permanent physical and/or mental abnormalities or death. The risk of serious pregnancy complications for the mother is also increased about twice as much. Therefore, it is important to have as a goal the birth of a healthy singleton baby and patients need to be carefully counseled about the risks. The best way to ensure this is to perform elective single embryo transfer (eSET). eSET can be performed with either a day 3 cleavage stage embryo or day 5 blastocyst. For patients in their late 30s it can be appropriate to transfer two day 3 embryos, but the risk of twins is too high to transfer more than one blastocyst in most patients unless the patient is in her 40s. Each patient will have the number to transfer finalized after the number and quality of the embryos are determined during the cycle [74,75].

Assisted hatching is a technique that involves making a small hole in the embryo cell wall with a laser beam on day 3 if the patient meets certain criteria, namely age 38 or more, prior failed IVF cycle(s), cryopreserved/thawed embryos, or thickened outer cell wall (zona pellucida). Reasonably good studies suggest, but have not entirely proven, an increase in pregnancy rates as a result of assisted hatching. The procedure may be associated with a small increase in identical twin pregnancies, which are associated with a lower chance of a healthy baby.

The embryo transfer procedure is done under abdominal ultrasound guidance and is painless. Sometimes the procedure just takes a few minutes and sometimes it can take longer because of difficulty passing the catheter into the uterus. Patients are usually asked to limit their activities significantly for the day following embryo or blastocyst transfer, primarily for emotional reasons because it has been claimed, but not proven, that this will increase pregnancy rates. No anesthesia is required for the embryo transfer.

It is necessary to provide progesterone or other hormonal support to the endometrium in the luteal phase, because the ovary has been suppressed by the GnRH agonist or antagonist. Progesterone can be given intramuscularly in the buttock, which has been proven effective for over 50 years, yet can be painful. Vaginal suppositories or capsules can be used instead and are not associated with pain but are found to be messy by some patients and have been shown to be equivalent, but not superior to, intramuscular progesterone. Progesterone taken for a short period of time generally does not have serious side effects, but some patients do experience nausea, constipation, breast enlargement and tenderness, headache, fluid retention and depression.

Approximately 12 to 14 days after the embryo transfer a serum pregnancy test is done to determine if the embryo(s) has implanted and is developing. It is best not to be overly active during these two weeks because the ovaries are usually enlarged from the gonadotropin drugs and a high degree of activity will potentially increase pelvic discomfort and risk ovarian cyst leakage and pain or ovarian torsion.

Approximately two-thirds of patients who have a positive pregnancy test following IVF will deliver a baby. The proportion who will miscarry in the first trimester, or lose a baby in the second or third trimester, ranges from about 15% for patients around age 25 to 75% for a woman age 45. About half the pregnancy losses will occur in the first two weeks after the first positive pregnancy test and most of the remaining losses will occur before 12 weeks of pregnancy. After 12 weeks of pregnancy only about 5% of pregnancies will be lost. Ectopic or tubal pregnancy occurs in about 2–4% of patients and must be carefully diagnosed and managed with either methotrexate injections or surgery. The vast majority of IVF babies are healthy, but the risk of an abnormal baby is about 1.2 to 1.6 times higher than the general population. The risk increases for all women who have a multiple pregnancy and for all women who are older. Tests, most but not all of which are non-invasive, can be performed to help assess the baby during the first and second trimester. Cell-free DNA blood tests, quadruple testing, chorionic villus sampling (CVS), amniocentesis, and ultrasound testing are the types of tests that are generally discussed with and performed by the patient's obstetrician.

Induced fetal reduction, also known as pregnancy reduction, is a difficult topic to discuss because of the emotional and ethical/societal aspects associated with it. Nevertheless, it is a relatively easy, safe and effective procedure that can significantly reduce the risk of multiple pregnancy, especially high order (triplet or more) pregnancy, and increase the probability of a healthy mother and baby. The risk of losing the entire pregnancy as a result of the procedure is approximately 5% but the improvement in pregnancy and fetal outcome is greater than that, especially for triplet or higher order pregnancies.

It is possible to cryopreserve by vitrification (an ultra-high-speed freezing process) any viable embryos or blastocysts that were not transferred in the fresh cycle. Pregnancy rates in frozen/thaw embryo transfer cycles (FET) following vitrification are similar to fresh transfer and appear to be as safe with respect to good outcomes with healthy babies. Embryos or blastocysts have been kept frozen and successfully thawed for 10–20 years. It is important to discuss the eventual need to use the embryos or blastocysts to attempt a pregnancy or to dispose of them in the future if they are not needed. Disposition options include transfer into the patient's uterus, donation to research, donation to another patient or discarding.

Either natural FET cycles or medicated FET cycles can be used to transfer thawed embryos. The natural cycle requires no medications but more monitoring than the medicated cycle and has a higher chance of being cancelled because the time of ovulation cannot be adequately determined or the endometrial lining does not seem adequate. The medicated cycle does require medications but is more predictable. Both types of cycles have similar financial cost and pregnancy rates.

Live birth rates per cycle start for both fresh transfer cycles and FET should be discussed with the patients. Future treatments depending on whether the cycle goes well or poorly and whether the patient is pregnant or not should be discussed before the cycle starts. The health of babies born from IVF should be discussed. A large number of studies have concluded that babies born after IVF and ICSI have a slightly higher (approximately 1.2 to 1.6 times) risk of being abnormal. It is not entirely clear, but most experts think this is primarily due to the patient population being treated, that is infertile patients, who will have slightly higher reproductive risks and slightly less good outcomes than patients with no reproductive problems who get pregnant without difficulty. It is not thought that the IVF procedure itself creates much risk, although there may be some small risk that could come from handling eggs and sperm and from culturing embryos outside the body. The risk of abnormal babies with ICSI appears to be slightly higher than that with conventional or standard IVF fertilization, and is likely related to the population of patients needing ICSI to get pregnant. A condition called hypospadius in which the urethral opening on the penis is on the underside of the penis may occur slightly more often. The major risk from IVF is having multiple pregnancy, which increases the risk of having a baby with a problem about 1.2 to 2.0 times from 2.5% to 4% for major problems or death. However, it is important to note that most IVF and ICSI babies are healthy.

The average number of IVF cycles done by patients in the United States is approximately two. Many patients will do three or four fresh cycles, but few do more than that. Patients should know that fewer than half of all patients get pregnant on their first cycle. However, even on the sixth or seventh cycle the pregnancy rate is about half as high as it is on the first cycle in populations of patients who have continued to undergo IVF cycles for that long. Most patients find that frozen/thaw cycles are much less demanding and cost much less so that they can do more of them, although there are still emotional costs associated with doing multiple cycles and patients do drop out of treatment for both financial and/or emotional reasons. Besides further IVF cycles, the patient needs to be informed about other options including donor egg and/or sperm, adoption or child-free living.

Patients need to know that, while concerns have been expressed about long-term risks of IVF treatment associated with ovarian stimulation or egg retrieval and anesthesia, there are no confirmed known longer-term risks. Additionally, there are benefits from pregnancy, including reduced risk of breast, ovarian and other cancers. Patients should be informed about additional sources of information including the American Society for Reproductive Medicine (ASRM) website (www.asrm.org), the European Society of Human Reproduction and Embryology (ESHRE) website (www.eshre.org), the ASRM patient website (www.reproductivefacts.org), the Society for Assisted Reproductive Technology (SART) website (www.sart.org), the Centers for Disease Control site for ART results (www.cdc.gov), RESOLVE (www.resolve.org) and other legitimate fertility websites.

Katie and Paulo's first cycle of IUI is quite simply medical, involving taking oral tablets at home and a simple office procedure, but it is unsuccessful. The stress associated with raised expectations, sperm collection in the clinic and the intensity of the "artificial insemination" in the office, followed by the two weeks of waiting and negative pregnancy test, leave Katie and Paulo very depressed. Nevertheless, the plan was for three cycles, so they try again and are thrilled to learn Katie is pregnant after completing the second cycle. Katie is followed up with blood tests, then ultrasound, and released to her Ob/Gyn. However, at her first appointment at 10 weeks she learns there is no heartbeat and she must have a D&C. Katie and Paulo are devastated, having been so excited with the "success" of pregnancy that they had already told all their family and friends, and find themselves grieving alone. Katie becomes very anxious, begins to research all the reasons why a miscarriage could happen and asks for genetic testing. Even though her physician tells her the miscarriage is almost certainly just a random event that occurs in approximately one-third of pregnancies in infertile couples, she insists on testing despite the fact her insurance will not cover the cost. The testing revels Katie is a carrier of MTFHR, a disorder of a gene-related protein but one that is not clinically significant in Katie's situation and, based on the best evidence available, did not contribute to her pregnancy loss [73].

They decide to continue IUI treatment and have another pregnancy loss at 6 weeks. Katie becomes even more anxious, and insists on more testing. A karyotype (chromosome analysis) of the products of conception (POC) identifies common, random, chromosomal abnormalities that are associated with miscarriage. They meet with the RE and discuss the fact that there is no way to change the chromosomes but that IVF with ICSI and PGD could potentially reduce the risk of another miscarriage, although it has not been shown yet to increase live birth rates. The stress of the failed treatment, and especially the two miscarriages, make Katie and Paulo decide to take money from their "house fund" to pay for IVF with PGD. The RE notes how sad and anxious Katie has become, and how helpless and withdrawn Paulo appears, and recommends they set up a consultation with the clinic fertility counselor.

Psychosocial intervention

Therapeutic approaches

The longer patients like Katie and Paulo pursue treatment, the more difficult it becomes. Each cycle or new approach to treatment comes on the heels of failure, which takes an emotional toll. The fertility counselor can offer a safe haven to process feelings of anxiety, sadness and loss as well as assist with coping strategies to deal with the next cycle of treatment. Just as physicians must take an evidence-based approach to their work, fertility counselors also need to know how to evaluate and assess the most effective way to address their patient's needs to help them comply with treatment and heal emotionally (see Chapter 19). For patients that are crossing borders to seek reproductive service, fertility counselors also must be aware of cultural, legal, religious and social influences that others bring with them from their countries (see Chapter 22).

Katie and Paulo are struggling with a number of emotional issues as a consequence of treatment – repeated miscarriages, diagnosis of infertility factors related to each partner and the shift to assisted reproductive technology. While both are struggling, Katie's pain and needs are more evident, which precipitates the referral to the fertility counselor. However, in the course of meeting with Katie, the fertility counselor and Katie will need to decide if it is best to work on these issues in individual therapy (see Chapter 3), couples counseling (see Chapter 4), or a combination of both. Whatever modality is chosen, the fertility counselor will need to help them work through the grief from the pregnancy losses (see Chapter 16) in order to be at a stronger emotional place to move forward with the next phase of treatment and the high-stakes nature of IVF. Unknown to Katie is the fact that the fertility counselor also experienced recurrent miscarriages when she was trying to have a family. While it has been many years since the miscarriages and she has since had two children, hearing Katie's anguish over these losses quickly brings her back in time (see Chapter 17).

Promoting resiliency

Resiliency refers to the concept of an individual's ability to adapt to adversity and cope flexibly with life's challenges, thus reflecting how one copes with stress and one's emotional hardiness. It is seen as a process and not a character trait, and thus is not a personality characteristic one is born with but rather can be a learned behavioral adaptation to a distressful event or significant trauma. Resilience has been studied extensively in the literature with regard to loss and potential trauma [76] and, more recently, with regard to health and illness. Individuals with chronic health conditions (e.g., cancer, heart disease, pain) who were more resilient have less depression and anxiety, as well as decreased disease susceptibility, improved prognosis and adaptation to their condition. Limited research has been conducted to examine resiliency regarding distress from infertility, another chronic health condition, and found resilience in women undergoing infertility treatment was lower than the general

Table 1.2 Promoting resiliency during infertility.

- Emphasize behavioral skills which enhance resiliency:
  - Learning relaxation techniques
  - Teaching cognitive re-appraisal
  - Identifying active coping strategies
  - Practicing health-enhancing behaviors
  - Promoting optimism and acceptance
- Encourage social connections and sharing of feelings
- Increase self-esteem, self-acceptance, and self-adequacy
- Identify spiritual resources and "the bigger picture" beyond oneself
- Find a positive meaning and purpose to the experience of infertility

population [77], men tended towards less distress indicating more resilience, and higher resilience correlated with higher quality of life in infertile couples [78].

Drawing from this research, fertility counselors should consider ways to enhance resiliency as indicated by Table 1.2. Having programs that teach cognitive–behavioral techniques (e.g., cognitive restructuring, positive thinking, etc.) ideally in a group setting, which allows for social connections, is essential. Clinics should also have tools available to help with times known to be especially stressful for patients, specifically the two-week waiting period after treatment and before getting pregnancy results. The Positive Reappraisal Coping Inventory (PRCI)[79] is a low-cost, easy to administer, self-help intervention that increases positive affect during the two-week waiting period and helps in coping with uncertainty in other stressful situations. (Readers need to contact the authors if they wish to reproduce this card for use in their practice.)

Integrative/complementary care programs, specifically for fertility patients, are becoming increasingly popular, offering classes in yoga, breathing, graduated relaxation, mediation, mindfulness, guided imagery and nutrition counseling, as well as offering acupuncture services. Helping patients develop active coping skills, such as self-care or breaking problems down into manageable pieces, and drawing upon spirituality has been shown to be effective in building resiliency. Rebuilding self-esteem and being able to find meaning in the infertility experience, with both thought and action, is also an important part of the counseling process. In sum, incorporating cognitive-behavioral skills, active coping, spirituality and finding ways to put meaning and purpose to the adversity enhances resiliency.

Third party reproduction: colloborative care

More than another aspect of infertility care, third party reproduction requires the coordinated, collaborative approach of numerous professionals (i.e., medical, psychological, legal, and donor/gestational carrier agencies) together with multiple participants (intended parents, gamete donors/carriers and their partners) to help in family building.

Medical issues

Sperm donation has been performed since biblical times. Until the past century, this involved sperm deposition with intercourse, and until the last few decades fresh sperm placed around the cervix (cap insemination) or into the uterus after sperm washing (IUI). However, improvements in sperm freezing technology and concerns over sexually transmitted infections, particularly HIV, have resulted in almost all inseminations now being done with cryopreserved sperm from screened individuals. This procedure was for many years called artificial insemination or AI, but now is called partner insemination (HI) or donor insemination (DI). Donor insemination has most commonly been used for heterosexual couples with severe male factor infertility. However, since IVF became more available in the mid 1980s, and especially ICSI in the early 1990s, severe male factor can be treated by IVF/ICSI. That technology development, along with other societal changes, has resulted in a more common use of donor sperm being with single women and lesbian couples who wish to have children. The use of donor sperm and donor eggs is regulated by the Food and Drug Administration (FDA) and requires sexually transmitted infection and other screening of both anonymous and other donors. The intended recipients receive donor sperm specimens from regulated sperm banks and choose the donor based on physical characteristics and qualities they value and desire. Further, at the request of intended parents, offspring and in some cases national legislation, sperm banks have initiated an "identity released" donor program where sperm donors agree to allow the release of personal information and even contact with donor-conceived children when they reach the age of 18. The sperm can then be shipped in containers that keep the sperm frozen until it is used or placed in a more permanent cryostorage tank. Known sperm donors can still be used, but this is less commonly done and more often carried out in a non-medical environment.

Egg donation is a recent development since IVF became more available in the mid 1980s. From a medical perspective, the process of egg donation is more involved than sperm donation. Different characteristics of egg donors, the basis on which they can be chosen, characteristics of different agencies, ASRM and ESHRE guidelines, the process of assessing donors by patients and the important characteristics for the patient and her husband need to be discussed with patients [80].

Egg donor screening involves a detailed history, family history, physical examination and specific gynecologic examination, in particular for antral follicle count, antimullerian hormone (AMH) and follicle stimulating hormone (FSH) and estradiol (E2) levels, general hematology and biochemistry tests, genetic testing and screening, sexually transmitted infection screening and testing, drug and nicotine screening and testing, psychological screening and counseling, and an explanation of management of the egg donor during the cycle.

Legal issues, including consent forms, control and management of the eggs and embryos, split donor cycles, requirements for establishing parenthood, potential changes in law over time and situations and issues to be considered and avoided need to be discussed with the intended parents. Psychological issues such as anonymous versus known donors, legal issues surrounding anonymity, the potential for telling the child and other family members about egg donation and reproductive choices the couple would face over the child's lifetime should be addressed by both the physician and the fertility counselor. Also, discussion of financial issues including the cost of egg donation, insurance and payment options need to be addressed.

Recipients need to understand medical management during the cycle, including the fact the egg donor is also a patient, the screening and timeline for the donor, medical management of the donor and other aspects of the relationship with the donor. Medical management of the female recipient, who will undergo what amounts to a medicated cycle getting her uterus ready to receive an embryo, is important to understand. Options such as freezing all the embryos for later transfer and the obtaining of cryopreserved eggs from an egg bank are also possible options for consideration. The male role involves screening and the provision of the sperm.

Egg donation, in many countries, is generally anonymous now and so issues of anonymity and disclosure must be discussed and resolved before starting a cycle. When known egg donors are involved, the nature of the ongoing relationship needs to be determined and finalized to the extent possible. The medical process for egg donors is the same as for IVF patients, with careful coordination of the cycle with the female recipient and sperm from her male partner.

Other options that are performed much less commonly but that are appropriate for some patients are embryo donation and gestational carrier. *Embryo donation* is an excellent option but the problem is that not many people decide to donate embryos. This occurs because embryos are generally donated by patients who have had successful IVF treatment, in which case they have children from the cohort of embryos that are frozen and so often consider the embryos to be siblings of their living children, making embryo donation more psychologically difficult.

Gestational carrier (GC) is an option for patients who don't have a uterus because of developmental or disease problems, or who have a non-functional uterus, history of pregnancy losses or underlying medical condition that makes pregnancy dangerous. GCs may be recruited or altruistic and are known to the intended parents (IPs). All of the considerations of egg donation apply, plus the added issues of pregnancy in another person and longer-term relationship issues, all of which need to be discussed, agreed upon and finalized in writing before undertaking a gestational carrier cycle. Psychological assessment and counseling for all parties involved in third party reproduction – intended parents, donors and GC participants – should be mandatory.

Psychosocial issues

When patients move on to third party reproduction, they do so either out of an experience of loss and often repeated treatment failure, or because life circumstance necessitates the need for reproductive assistance. Whatever the reason, there is a common thread to the experience because using a donor or GC correlates with "loss," be it genetic connection or biological connection by carrying a pregnancy and giving birth, which must be grieved. For couples who have exhausted all treatment options for a genetically or biologically shared baby, third party assistance is their last hope. For gay or lesbian couples, or single individuals, these treatments offer hope for the family of their dreams, yet also the realization that it will not happen without the assistance of another person or people, whether known or anonymous. Because of the multifaceted issues (medical, psychological, legal, ethical, social, etc.) involved in third party reproduction, the ASRM, ESHRE and numerous other regional and legislative organizations recommend that all participants receive counseling and psychological education before undergoing treatment. Today, as many as five individuals may come together in these arrangements – intended mother and father (or same-sex couple), a sperm donor, ovum donor and a woman who will carry the pregnancy – which generates a complex psychosocial minefield to maneuver during the counseling process.

All that goes into counseling for third party assistance is covered extensively in Sections III and IV of this book. The reader is referred to the chapters covering recipients of anonymous donor egg and/or donor sperm (Chapter 7), the counseling and assessment of men and women wanting to donate their gametes (Chapter 8) as well as intended parents and gestational carriers (Chapter 9). Participants who have an existing relationship, usually a family member or friend, and come together to help create a child need additional assistance in understanding how to make these relationships work and the implications for the future (Chapter 10). When "older" (the definition of which is hotly debated among clinicians) individuals or couples seek ART treatment, how to optimize counseling raises unique issues of what might be in the best interest of a child versus the right to parent (Chapter 11). In addition, single women and men are choosing to use reproductive technology to have children today in increasing numbers (Chapter 12), as are gay, lesbian, bisexual and transgender people (Chapter 13), accessing care that requires a sensitivity and understanding of their needs during treatment. And for all patients using third party assistance, a critical aspect of counseling will be helping them understand the importance of discussing with offspring the origins of their creation, an ongoing conversation that most parents find daunting and need help with from the counselor with direction and words to use (Chapter 18).

Decision-making in infertility: colloborative care

Reviewing family building options

Throughout the treatment process and during times of decision-making, it can be helpful to reconsider all family building options. To review, couples wishing to get pregnant have, in general, six potential options from which to choose, although not all options apply to all patients. These options begin with no specific fertility treatment but an approach in which patients optimize their chance for pregnancy by healthy lifestyle choices with respect to sleep, diet, exercise, alcohol, drug and medication use, along with prenatal vitamins with calcium, iron and folate for the woman and a male multi-vitamin with anti-oxidant. Timing of intercourse every 1 to 3 days and the potential use of urinary LH test kits to confirm ovulation may be helpful. Basal body temperature recording and mucus testing are not generally helpful but might be used in selected couples.

A second option is standard fertility diagnosis and treatment. Patients undergo diagnostic tests for hormonal/ovarian reserve, pelvic, male, combined and systemic factors that affect fertility. After testing, treatment can involve management of identifiable problems of the female by use of hormones, minor or major surgery; treatment of the male; the use of intrauterine insemination and/or management of general health conditions. The goal of treatment is to increase the chance of pregnancy in each menstrual cycle by bringing more egg(s) together with more sperm in the best possible pelvic environment at the right time.

A third option is IVF, the treatment with the highest chances for pregnancy for almost all infertility patients regardless of the cause of their infertility. However, it is more involved for the patient and more expensive, so it is not always the best choice for a given patient. With IVF, ICSI is the single most effective treatment for male factor infertility of almost any severity. However, IVF does not improve egg quality and does not treat problems with the uterus.

A fourth option is egg donation, sperm donation or gestational carrier that can be used in situations in which the egg and/or sperm number and/or quality is very low or unavailable from a partner, or the uterus is absent or severely abnormal. Another person can provide eggs, sperm or a uterus (gestational carrier), as third party collaborators. The major barriers to third party reproduction are personal values, psychological considerations for the patient and financial cost. The cost of an egg donation cycle is approximately $30 000 to $35 000 although the chances for a baby are 65–75%. Sperm donation is cheaper at generally less than $1000 per cycle but pregnancy rates are approximately 10% per cycle. GC costs are approximately $75 000–125 000.

A fifth option is adoption or foster care. Adoption can be a very successful way for patients to have a family, while foster care can give provide an opportunity to care and parent both in the short and long term. Public adoption can take a long time and is often more available to younger patients. Private or international adoption is often chosen by patients but is quite involved and can be expensive, costs being approximately $25 000 to $75 000. Adoption specialists, including agencies and attorneys, are available to educate and guide about the process and various options (see Chapter 14).

A sixth option is child-free living. Child-free living, which means a conscious decision not to have children or, in some cases, to continue with the number of children already born but not attempt to have more, is a very reasonable choice for many people. While children are wonderful and may be critical to many people's happiness, not everyone has to be a parent, and certainly not if they choose not to be. Child-free living has some economic, time and lifestyle advantages that balance off some of the benefits of having children. Thus, this is a choice all patients should at least consider before pursuing fertility diagnosis and treatment.

Cost–benefit analysis

With so many options, all very different, making decisions can be difficult for patients. A framework for this that can be helpful is performing cost–benefit analysis of the different treatment options.

The **benefit** of any treatment choice is equal to the value of that choice to the patient/couple, multiplied by the probability of a successful outcome, which is a healthy baby. The outcomes are potentially different with the different options: her or his own biologic child, a child resulting from involvement of a donor, an adopted child or no child at all. The value of each outcome to patients is unique to the couple and can only be determined by them, not the physician. The physician's role is to provide patients with information and guidance to help them make the best reproductive decision for themselves. The probability of a healthy baby is a prognosis that can be approximately estimated by the physician by applying the best available evidence in the literature to the patient's unique clinical situation. Interpreting the literature can be a difficult exercise given the plethora of studies, many of them not well designed and/or with other biasing factors. Utilizing national and/or professional guidelines is generally the best approach [81]. Patients also need to be directed to legitimate sources of information so that they do not waste time, money and emotional energy pursing inappropriate tests and treatments (e.g., www.reproductivefacts.org). Together, the patient and physician can determine the level of benefit for the different options and start to prioritize approaches to treatment. For any treatment option to be appropriate it must, therefore, have both reasonable value to the patient and reasonable chance of occurring if treatment is undertaken.

The benefits of any treatment must be balanced by the **costs**. There are four types of costs. The first cost is *financial* (**$**). Financial cost is important because approximately two-thirds of patients who don't have a baby don't because they have to drop out owing to financial barriers. This occurs because some infertility treatments are expensive, but more so because many insurance plans do not provide much infertility coverage. To manage this problem, many fertility clinics have financial counselors who will ascertain as best they can the insurance coverage the patient has, and explain to them other financial packages, plans and financing to help deal with the financial challenges many patients face with fertility treatments. The second cost is *time* (**T**). Patient's fertility becomes reduced over time, and is often much reduced even when the patient is first seen because of her age and duration attempting pregnancy. Therefore, the time treatment takes is an important consideration in making choices. The third cost is the potential *health risks* of diagnosis and treatment (**Rx**). Fertility treatment is generally safe. The biggest risk, by far, is the risk of success, that is, a pregnancy confers more risk on the woman than any of the tests or treatments that are generally undertaken in fertility management. However, risks can be increased significantly if the patient has an underlying medical condition such as obesity, has a multiple pregnancy, or has complications from fertility drug use, such as OHSS, or from a surgical procedure. Long-term risks are thought not to occur, or to be very minor, or to occur in a very small proportion of patients treated. The fourth and often biggest cost is emotional or *psychological* (Ψ). Patients with infertility can suffer emotional stress equivalent to those of other diagnoses such as HIV and cancer. Infertility can profoundly affect a woman's sense of personhood, marital relationship, sexual and reproductive self, family place and responsibility and social worth. Women are almost always more severely affected than men. Strategies to deal with this situation include having frank communication and agreement with the partner, having strong partner understanding and support, obtaining accurate information about infertility and fertility treatment, asking questions of the physician and undertaking resiliency activities such as yoga, prayer, meditation, self-help groups, professional counseling or other integrative care programs. For a choice to be a good choice, a depiction of a cost–benefit analysis might look like this:

$$\textbf{Benefit} > \textbf{Cost}$$
$$\textbf{OR}$$
$$\textbf{Value} \times \textbf{Probability Success} > \$ + \textbf{T} + \textbf{Rx} + \Psi$$

After obtaining the appropriate diagnostic tests, couples who are aware of the value to them and prognosis of the different choices, and know the costs, can prioritize the choices and initiate treatment. The process of assessment of costs and benefits should be continuously carried out, and a formal reassessment with the physician performed at least every three months because the infertility situation changes over time. In this way optimal management of the patient's infertility can occur, and the maximum chance for pregnancy and a healthy baby can be achieved.

Katie met with the fertility counselor over several months while they prepared for treatment. She had the opportunity to grieve her miscarriages and learn some cognitive behavioral strategies to deal with the stresses of treatment. Understanding that stress builds during the IVF cycle, culminating in the most difficulty during the two-week wait before getting the results, she was able to use the PRCI card the fertility counseling provided to help in coping by focusing on positive aspects and challenging negative thoughts. As a couple, they decided to attend the Clinic's monthly support group, meeting other patients, and gaining strength from what they learned in the group.

Katie and Paulo went through IVF with ICSI and PGS. They had four embryos without an identified abnormality and, after discussing with their RE and counselor, chose to transfer one embryo during a FET cycle. They become pregnant and later delivered a healthy son. They are undecided about if they will return for treatment or what they will do with their remaining embryos.

Stopping treatment

When treatment has been successful, patients transition away from the reproductive medical practice, ideally, towards normalcy in pregnancy, birth and parenthood. While the pregnancy after infertility is at greater risk prenatal and postpartum, most patients navigate the process without significant difficulties [82]. For those where treatment is not successful, they will need to decide if they will remain childless (or with secondary infertility, without more children) or will seek parenthood through adoption (see Chapter 14). Ending treatment and moving on in either direction will require a process of grief and mourning made more difficult due to the invisible nature of this profound loss – the death of the dream child.

The necessity to say a formal "goodbye"

Ingrid, 41, sought individual counseling as she was struggling over whether to end treatment or pursue adoption. She and her husband, Bill, had been together for 15 years, never feeling they needed a legal bond, but had married just three years earlier after a crisis in their extended family changed their minds. Ingrid and Bill never thought they wanted children, but something changed after they got married and they decide to try to become pregnant. As months slipped on and aware of Ingrid's age, they sought medical assistance, yet still no pregnancy. After a series of IUI cycles, they agreed that they did not want to pursue ART; however, Ingrid continued integrative care approaches (yoga, acupuncture and homeopathy) while trying on their own to get pregnant. After two years of monthly disappointments, Ingrid entered therapy feeling depressed, depleted and in a quagmire over wondering what to do. The fertility counselor talked with Ingrid about "emotional inertia" being an indication of difficulty mourning an intangible, yet deep, sense of loss and recommended grief work, which would include Bill during the process.

Grieving is the hardest work one ever does in life and is made more difficult when the loss is elusive and amorphous, as with the death of the "dream" baby. After processing over many sessions all the emotions associated with infertility and with Ingrid was still feeling "stuck," the fertility counselor suggested a powerful technique to help make the intangible, tangible – writing a letter of "goodbye" to Ingrid's dream child. As the MHP described the process (naming and visualizing the child; discussing why s/he was wanted; what her hopes and dreams and wishes were for him/her; and why Ingrid must say "goodbye"), Ingrid started to weep. She was told that this "assignment" could not be dictated (i.e., "do this before our next session") but needed to be contemplated and begun when Ingrid had the time, space and emotional energy to do it. The fertility counselor also suggested that Ingrid talk to Bill about doing the same task, as Ingrid felt very alone in her grief. Over the coming weeks, Bill joined the sessions and they discussed what tackling the letter brought up, and whether they wanted to remain a family of two or pursue adoption. The next week, they both came in with their letters and read them aloud to the counselor in a very emotionally cathartic meeting, deciding they would ritualize the farewell by burning the letters and releasing the ashes in a stream near their house. As time went on they decided against adoption, focusing instead on other ways to channel their nurturing instincts (friends' and family's children), follow things they loved to do together (travel) and work together to grow a new business (an art gallery) that reflected their joint creative interests. Ingrid left therapy feeling resolved in her grief, a renewed sense of self and confidence in the future.

Exit counseling

Patients who are not successful with treatment will make the decision to end trying to have a child either consciously or unconsciously. At times a "default" decision is made when patients stop treatment, deciding they need a break (often due to the psychological stress of treatment or financial burdens) yet never to return, or to defer decision-making on alternative family building. The avoidant behavior extends over time and becomes an unconscious choice to remain childless, adding to a sense of being "unresolved." For others, like Ingrid and Bill, the emotional journey of disengagement from treatment was a conscious, emotionally charged process in decision-making. Based on a longitudinal study of infertile couples, Daniluk [83] identified four stages in the transition to childless after infertility, along a continuum of themes including: "hitting the wall," "reworking the past," "turning toward the future" and "renewal and regeneration." Each of these stages involves approximately a ten-month period, thus taking about 3.5 years to fruition, a reference point that is often very useful for patients to understand. For fertility counselors, helping patients make a conscious decision to end treatment without success may also involve assisting the physician to give their patients permission to stop [84].

Another aspect of exit counseling for all patients, whether pregnant or not, is to address the consequences that protracted infertility can have on a couple's relationship. Most notably is a couple's sexual relationship, which is discussed in detail in Chapter 4. Other issues to explore include self-esteem, marital communication and satisfaction, relationships with family and friends and overall quality of life. The good news is that infertility has the potential to teach couples life-long skills and resiliency to deal with future adversity. Long-term studies have indicated overall good psychological adjustment in both couples who achieved parenthood with medical assistance as well as those who remained childless [85].

It is also important to address the needs of single women as they leave treatment. For some, they may have progressed through years of treatment and high-stakes interventions, possibly culminating in creating embryos with donor egg and sperm (something they never imagined they would do when starting DI), and "succeed" by becoming pregnant with twins (or more). These women may find themselves with depleted finances and social supports as they embark towards their long-awaited dream of motherhood. Support groups for single mothers by choice, whether offered by the fertility clinic or self-help organization, can provide a welcome and powerful safety net through treatment and into parenting.

Conclusion

As a final note, practicing as a fertility counselor presents numerous challenges and cannot be done in isolation. Membership and participation in the Mental Health Professional Group (MHPG) of the ASRM, the Psychology and Counselling Special Interest Group of ESHRE, the British Infertility Counselling Association (BICA), Australia/New Zealand Infertility Counselling Association (ANZICA), BKiD (Germany) or another of the growing number of national organizations representing the field of fertility counseling is essential. When a fertility counselor establishes a practice, there are many things to consider from devising consents, releases, reports and so on, and not the least of which is "what constitutes competency" to practice. Chapter 21 on legal issues provides a hands-on approach to clinical management. As one's practice grows, fertility counselors are continually presented with ethical dilemmas and struggles in their work, and Chapter 20 offers a valuable context and framework to address these problems. This field of practice is dynamic and continually expanding, in tandem with the technology, and fertility counselors must stay abreast.

Reflections from the clinicians

SNC: Over 30 years ago, I moved my psychotherapy practice into an office with an Ob/Gyn who had a special interest in infertility, to share space and be able to cross-refer. This was a dream opportunity as I thought it would be great to team up and learn from each other, knowing his patients all had a psychological history and my psychotherapy patients all had a reproductive history – well, I had a lot to learn! It was a very different experience doing individual and couple therapy in a medical office versus my previous private practice space, and took some getting used to by both my patients and me. My other office space had been quiet, with a revolving door of one or two patients at a time, and often felt quite isolating. In the medical practice, there was lots of activity in the office throughout the day and interaction with medical and administrative staff on both professional and personal levels – questions about how to handle problems with patients, advice about family struggles or help with personality clashes within the office. Within a few years, the practice grew to specialize entirely with infertility and all aspects of reproductive medical treatment.

Many of the staff had a hard time understanding what I did as a social worker (some saying they thought social workers "just hand out welfare checks") other than just "chat" with the patients, as whatever I was doing seemed elusive and amorphous compared to medicine. However, over time as we worked side by side when problems or issues came up with patients, I was able to offer tangible help and understanding on how to handle patients' emotional needs, which assisted in providing effective care. I, on the other hand, was in awe of the doctors and nurses as I watched them treat scores of women in a day, each with their own personality and reproductive problems, needs and demands, yet all unique and special. It was only by working together in this close, collaborative way that we learned from each other and grew in bringing better care to our patients. It was the best, most rewarding, educational and professional experience I have ever had, and continues to be to this day.

GDA: After fourteen years of formal training to become a reproductive endocrinologist and two years in practice, I remember thinking that I had become a pretty competent reproductive medicine specialist helping infertile patients. While having a conversation with another physician I respected very much and who had been in practice many years longer, he said it took him at least five years in practice before he felt he really began understanding and meeting the needs of his patients. This comment made me reassess my perspective on the care I was giving my patients. I realized how important it was to always strive for the best, to constantly assess my performance, to critique my clinical and surgical judgment, and to constantly acquire new information, learn new technologies, teach and perform research. Even more importantly, I learned how essential it was to listen to my patients about their real needs and the psychosocial environment in which they were experiencing and dealing with their infertility. Only by doing so could I begin to provide the quality of care I wanted to give to my patients. To learn more, I became involved with the Board of Resolve of Northern California for 10 years, and then the National Resolve Board for 10 years. Recognizing how important mental health professionals are in our specialty, I also helped initiate the Mental Health Professional Group at the ASRM, and also supported the American Fertility Association. My awareness of the importance of emotional challenges and the contributions of MHPs grew dramatically. These experiences increased significantly my ability to provide quality infertility care to my patients. On the first consultation I validate and discuss the emotional aspects of infertility, give information and refer patients to national, regional and practice resources. We have three wonderful fertility counselors who have worked with our practice for 30 years and who provide incredibly useful support to our patients. We have also developed several ongoing formal "mindfulness" programs that have been very successful. I am grateful for the opportunity to share my experiences in this textbook, in the hope it will help other professionals and patients better manage their experience with infertility.

References

1. Covington SN. The role of the mental health professional in reproductive medicine. *Fertil Steril.* 1995; 64: 895–7.
2. Norre J, Wischmann T. The position of the fertility counselor in a fertility team: a critical appraisal. *Hum Fertil.* (Camb). 2011 Sep; 14(3): 154–9. Epub 2011 July 7.
3. Gameiro S, Boivin J, Domar A. Optimal in vitro fertilization in 2020 should reduce treatment burden and enhance care delivery for patients and staff. *Fertil Stertil.* 2013; 100(2): 302–9.
4. Covington SN. Infertility counseling in practice: a collaborative reproductive healthcare model. In: Covington SN, Burns LH, Eds. *Infertility Counseling: A Comprehensive Handbook for Clinicians*, 2nd Edn. London: Cambridge University Press, 2006; 493–507.
5. Van Empel IWH, Aarts JWM, Cohlen BJ, Huppelschoten DA, Laven JSE, Nelen WLDM, Kremer JAM. Measuring patient-centredness, the neglected outcome in fertility care: a random multicentre validation study. *Hum Reprod.* 2010; 10: 2516–26.
6. Boivin J, Domar AD, Shapiro DB, Wischmann TH, Fauser BC, Verhaak C. Tackling burden in ART: an integrated approach for medical staff. *Hum Reprod.* 2012; 27(4): 941–50.
7. Evers JL. Female subfertility. *Lancet* 2002; 360: 151–9.
8. ICMART and WHO. Zegers-Hochschild F, Adamson GD, de Mouzon J, Ishihara O, Mansour R, Nygren K, Sullivan E, Vanderpoel S. International Committee for Monitoring Assisted Reproductive Technology (ICMART) and the World Health Organization (WHO) revised glossary of ART terminology, 2009. *Fertil Steril.* 2009 Nov; 92(5): 1520–4.
9. te Velde ER, Eijkemans R, Habbema HD. Variation in couple fecundity and time to pregnancy, an essential concept in human reproduction. *Lancet* 2000; 355: 1928–9.
10. Snick HKA, Snick TS, Evers JLH, Collins JA. The spontaneous pregnancy prognosis in untreated subfertile couples. The Walcheren primary care study. *Hum Reprod.* 1997; 12: 1582–8.
11. Leridon H. A new estimate of permanent sterility by age: sterility defined as the inability to conceive. *Popul Stud.* (Camb) 2008; 62: 15–24.
12. Boivin J, Bunting L, Collins JA, Nygren, KG. International estimates of infertility prevalence and treatment-seeking: potential need and demand for infertility medical care. *Hum Reprod.* 2007; 22(6): 1506–12.
13. Gurunath S, Pandian Z, Anderson RA et al. Defining infertility – a systematic review of prevalence studies. *Hum Reprod Update* 2011; 17(5): 575–88.
14. Wallace WH, Kelsey TW. Ovarian reserve and reproductive age may be determined from measurement of ovarian volume by transvaginal sonography. *Hum Reprod.* 2004; 19: 1612–17.
15. Hendershot GE, Mosher WD, Pratt WF. Infertility and age: an unresolve issue. *Fam Plan and Perspect.* 1982 Sep–Oct; 14(5): 287–9.
16. Zinaman MJ, Clegg ED, Brown CC, O'Connor J, Selevan SG. Estimates of human fertility and pregnancy loss. *Fertil Steril.* 1996; 65: 503–9.
17. te Velde ER, Pearson PL. The variability of reproductive aging. *Hum Reprod Update* 2002; 8: 141–54.
18. Kidd SA, Eskenazi B, Wyrobek AJ. Effects of male age on semen quality and fertility: a review of the literature. *Fert Steril.* 2001; 75: 237.
19. Practice Committee of the American Society for Reproductive Medicine. American Society for Reproductive Medicine, Birmingham, Alabama. Obesity and reproduction: an education bulletin. *Fertil Steril.* 2008; 90: S121–4.
20. van der Steeg JW, Steures P, Eijkemans MJ, Habbema JD, Hompes PG, Burggraaff JM, et al. Obesity affects spontaneous pregnancy chances in subfertile, ovulatory women. *Hum Reprod.* 2008; 23: 324–8.
21. Practice Committee of the American Society for Reproductive Medicine in collaboration with the Society for Reproductive Endocrinology and Infertility. Optimizing natural fertility: a committee opinion. *Fertil Steril.* 2013; 100: 631–7.
22. The Practice Committee of the American Society for Reproductive Medicine. American Society for Reproductive Medicine, Birmingham, Alabama. Smoking and infertility. *Fertil Steril.* 2008; 90: S254–9.
23. The Practice Committee of the American Society for Reproductive Medicine. Endometriosis and infertility: a committee opinion. *Fertil Steril.* 2012; 98: 591–8.
24. Practice Committee of the American Society for Reproductive Medicine in collaboration with the Society of Reproductive Surgeons. Pathogenesis, consequences and control of peritoneal adhesions in gynecologic surgery: a committee opinion. *Fertil Steril.* 2013; 99: 1550–5.
25. The Practice Committee of the American Society for Reproductive Medicine. Diagnostic evaluation of the infertile female: a committee opinion. *Fertil Steril.* 2012; 98: 302–7.

26. The Practice Committee of the American Society for Reproductive Medicine. Diagnostic evaluation of the infertile male: a committee opinion. *Fertil Steril.* 2012; 98: 294–301.
27. The Practice Committee of the American Society for Reproductive Medicine. Testing and interpreting measures of ovarian reserve: a committee opinion. *Fertil Steril.* 2012; 98: 1407–15.
28. World Health Organization. *WHO Laboratory Manual for the Examination and Processing of Human Semen*, 5th Edn. Geneva: WHO; 2010.
29. The Practice Committee of the American Society for Reproductive Medicine. The clinical utility of sperm DNA integrity testing: a guideline. *Fertil Steril.* 2013; 99: 673–7.
30. Griffith CS, Grimes DA. The validity of the post coital test. *Am J Obstet Gynecol.* 1990; 162: 615–20.
31. Hull MGR, Savage PE, Bromham DR. Prognostic value of the post coital test. *Br J Obstet Gynaecol.* 1982; 89: 299–305.
32. Oei SG, Helmerhorst FM, Bloemenkamp KWM, Hollants FAM, Meerpoel DM, Keirse MJNC. Effectiveness of the postcoital test. *BMJ* 1998; 317: 502–5.
33. Peterson BD, Pirritano M, Tucker L, Lampic C. Fertility awareness and parenting attitudes among American male and female undergraduate university students. *Hum Reprod.* 2012 May; 27(5): 1375–82.
34. Griel AL, Slausen-Belvins K, McQuillan J. The experience of infertility: a review of recent literature. *Social Health Illn.* 2010 Jan; 32(1): 140–62.
35. Kenrick DT, Griskevicius V, Neuberg SL, Schaller M. Renovating the Pyramid of Needs: contemporary extensions built upon ancient foundations. *Perspect Psychol Sci.* 2010; 5(3): 292–314.
36. Petok, WD. The psychology of gender-specific infertility diagnosis. In: Covington SN, Burns LH. *Infertility Counseling: A Comprehensive Handbook for Clinicians*, 2nd Edn. London: Cambridge University Press; 2006, pp. 37–60.
37. Jordan C, Revenson TA. Gender differences in coping with infertility: A meta-analysis. *J Behav Med.* 1999; 22: 341–58.
38. Comprehensive Psychosocial History of Infertility (Appendix 3). In: Covington SN, Burns LH, eds. *Infertility Counseling: A Comprehensive Handbook for Clinicians*, 2nd Edn. London: Cambridge University Press; 2006, 563–4.
39. Boivin, J, Takefman, J, Braverman, A. Development and preliminary validation of the fertility quality of life (FertiQoL) tool. *Fertil Steril.* 2011; 96: 409–15.
40. Verhaak CM, Lintsen AME, Evers AWM, Braat DDM. Who is at risk of emotional problems and how to know? Screening of women going for IVF treatment. *Hum Reprod.* 2010; 25: 1234.
41. Newton CR. The Fertility Problem Inventory: measuring perceived infertility-related stress. *Fertil Steril.* 1999; 72: 54–62.
42. Hakim LZ, Newton CR, MacLean-Brine D, Feyles V. Evaluation of preparatory psychosocial counselling for medically assisted reproduction. *Hum Repro.* 2012; 27(7): 2058–66.
43. Boivin J. A review of psychosocial interventions in infertility. *Soc Sci Med.* 2003; 57: 2325–41.
44. Aarts JWM, van den Haark P, Nelen WLDM, Tuil WS, Faber JJ, Kremer JAM. Patient-focused Internet interventions in reproductive medicine: a scoping review. *Hum Repro Update* 2012; 18(2): 211–27.
45. Covington SN. Group approaches to infertility counseling. In: Covington SN, Burns LH, ED. *Infertility Counseling: A Comprehensive Handbook for Clinicians*, 2nd Edn. London: Cambridge University Press, 2006, pp. 156–68.
46. Roudsari RL, Allan HT, Smith PA. Looking at infertility through the lens of religion and spirituality: a review of the literature. *Hum Fertil.* 2007 Sep; 10(30): 141–9.
47. Stanford JB, Dunson DB. Effects of sexual intercourse patterns in time to pregnancy studies. *Am J Epidemiol.* 2007; 165: 1688–95.
48. Stanford JB, White GL and Hatasaka H. Timing intercourse to achieve pregnancy: current evidence. *Obstet Gynecol.* 2002; 100: 1333–41.
49. Scarpa B, Dunson DB, Colombo B. Cervical mucus secretions on the day of intercourse: an accurate marker of highly fertile days. *Eur J Obstet Gynaecol Reprod Biol.* 2006; 125: 72–8.
50. The Practice Committee of the American Society for Reproductive Medicine. Use of clomiphene citrate in infertile women: a committee opinion. *Fertil Steril.* 2013: 100: 341–8.
51. Legro RS, Brzyski RJ, Diamond MP, Coutifaris C, Schlaff WD, Casson P, et al. for the NICHD Reproductive Medicine Network. Letrozole versus Clomiphene for infertility in the Polycystic Ovary Syndrome. *N Engl J Med.* 2014; 371: 119–29.
52. Johnson N. Metformin is a reasonable first-line treatment option for non-obese women with infertility related to anovulatory polycystic ovary syndrome – a meta-analysis of randomised trials. *Aust N Z J Obstet Gynaecol.* 2011; 51: 125–9.
53. The Practice Committee of the American Society for Reproductive Medicine. American Society for

Reproductive Medicine, Birmingham, Alabama. Multiple gestation associated with infertility therapy: an American Society for Reproductive Medicine Practice Committee opinion. *Fertil Steril.* 2012; 97: 825–34.

54. The Practice Committee of the American Society for Reproductive Medicine. Birmingham, Alabama. Current evaluation of amenorrhea. *Fertil Steril.* 2008; 90: S219–25.
55. The Practice Committee of the American Society for Reproductive Medicine. Use of exogenous gonadotropins in anovulatory women: a technical bulletin. *Fertil Steril.* 2008; 90: S7–12.
56. Fluker MR, Urman B, Mackinnon M, Barrow SR, Pride SM, Ho Yuen B. Exogenous gonadotrophin therapy in World Health Organization Groups I and II ovulatory disorders. *Obstet Gynecol.* 1994; 83: 189–96.
57. Mulders AG, Laven JS, Eijkemans MJ, Hughes EG, Fauser BC Patient predictors for outcome of gonadotrophin ovulation induction in women with normogonadotrophic anovulatory infertility: a meta-analysis. *Hum Reprod Update* 2003; 9: 429–49.
58. Reindollar RH, Regan MM, Neumann PJ, Levine BS, Thornton KL, Alper MM, Goldman MB. A randomized clinical trial to evaluate optimal treatment for unexplained infertility: the fast track and standard treatment (FASTT) trial. *Fertil Steril.* 2010; 94: 888–99.
59. Goldman MB, Reindollar et al, A randomized clinical trial to determine optimal infertility treatment in older couples: the Forty and Over Treatment Trial (FORT-T), *Fertil Steril.* 2014; 101: 1574–81.e2.
60. The Practice Committee of the American Society for Reproductive Medicine in collaboration with the Society of Reproductive Surgeons. American Society for Reproductive Medicine, Birmingham, Alabama. Myomas and reproductive function. *Fertil Steril.* 2008; 90: S125–30.
61. Practice Committee of American Society for Reproductive Medicine in collaboration with Society of Reproductive Surgeons. American Society for Reproductive Medicine, Birmingham, Alabama. Salpingectomy for hydrosalpinx prior to in vitro fertilization. *Fertil Steril.* 2008 Nov; 90(5 Suppl): S66–8.
62. The Practice Committee of the American Society for Reproductive Medicine. Endometriosis and infertility: a committee opinion. *Fertil Steril.* 2012; 98: 591–8.
63. Adamson GD, Pasta DJ. Endometriosis fertility index: the new, validated endometriosis staging system. *Fertil Steril.* 2010; 94(5): 1609–15.
64. The Practice Committee of the American Society for Reproductive Medicine. American Society for Reproductive Medicine, Birmingham, Alabama. The role of tubal surgery in the era of assisted reproductive technology. *Fertil Steril.* 2012; 97: 539–45.
65. The Practice Committee of the American Society for Reproductive Medicine. Report on varicocoele and infertility. *Fertil Steril.* 2008; 90: S247–9.
66. Practice Committee of the American Society for Reproductive Medicine in collaboration with the Society for Male Reproduction and Urology. Evaluation of the azoospermic male. *Fertil Steril.* 2008; 90: S74–7.
67. Steures P, van der Steeg JW, Hompes PG, Bossuyt PM, Habbema JD, Eijkemans MJ, et al. Effectiveness of intrauterine insemination in subfertile couples with an isolated cervical factor: a randomized clinical trial. *Fertil Steril.* 2007; 88: 1692–6.
68. The Practice Committee of the American Society for Reproductive Medicine. Effectiveness and treatment for unexplained infertility. *Fertil Steril.* 2006; 86(4): S111–4.
69. Bhattacharya S, Harrild K, Mollison J, Wordsworth S, Tay CCK, Harrold A, et al. Clomifene citrate or unstimulated intrauterine insemination compared with expectant management for unexplained infertility: pragmatic randomised controlled trial. *BMJ* 2008; 337: 716–23.
70. Fisch P, Casper RF, Brown SE, Wrixon W, Collins JA, Reid RL, Simpson C. Unexplained infertility: evaluation of treatment with clomiphene citrate and human chorionic gonadotropin. *Fertil Steril.* 1989; 51: 828–33.
71. Deaton JL, Gibson M, Blackmer KM, Nakajima ST, Badger GJ, Brumsted JR. A randomized, controlled trial of clomiphene citrate and intrauterine insemination in couples with unexplained infertility or surgically corrected endometriosis. *Fertil Steril.* 1990; 54: 1083–8.
72. The Practice Committee of the American Society for Reproductive Medicine. Evaluation and treatment of recurrent pregnancy loss: a committee opinion. *Fertil Steril.* 2012; 98: 1103–11.
73. The Practice Committee of the American Society for Reproductive Medicine. Ovarian hyperstimulation syndrome. *Fertil Steril.* 2008; 90(3): S188–93.
74. The Practice Committee of the American Society for Reproductive Medicine and the Society for Assisted Reproductive Technology. Criteria for number of embryos to transfer: a committee opinion. *Fertil Steril.* 2013; 99: 44–6.
75. The Practice Committee of the Society for Assisted Reproductive Technology and The Practice Committee of the American Society for Reproductive Medicine. Committee opinion: elective single embryo transfer. *Fertil Steril.* 2012; 97: 835–42.

76. Bonanno GA, Westphal M, Mancini AD. Resilience to loss and potential trauma. *Annu Rev Clin Psychol.* 2001; 7: 511–35.

77. Sexton MB, Byrd MR, von Klug S. Measuring resilience in women experiencing infertility using the CD-RISC: examining infertility-related stress, general distress, and coping styles. *J Psych Research* 2010; 44: 236–41.

78. Herrmann D, Scherg H, Verres R, von Hagens C, Strowitzke T, Wischmann T. Resilience in infertile couples as a protective factor against infertility-specific distress and impaired quality of life. *J Assist Reprod Genet.* 2011; 28: 1111–17.

79. Lancaster D, Boivin J. A feasibility study of a brief coping intervention (PRCI) for the waiting period before a pregnancy test during fertility treatment. *Hum Reprod.* 2008; 23(10): 2299–307.

80. The Practice Committee of the American Society for Reproductive Medicine and the Practice Committee of the Society for Assisted Reproductive Technology. Recommendations for gamete and embryo donation: a committee opinion. *Fertil Steril.* 2013; 99: 47–62.

81. The Practice Committee of the American Society for Reproductive Medicine. American Society for Reproductive Medicine, Birmingham, Alabama. Interpretation of clinical trial results. *Fertil Steril.* 2008; 90: S114–20.

82. Covington SN, Burns LH. Pregnancy after infertility. In: Covington SN, Burns LH. *Infertility Counseling: A Comprehensive Handbook for Clinicians*, 2nd Edn. London: Cambridge University Press; 2006, pp. 440–58.

83. Daniluk JC. Reconstructing their lives: a longitudinal, qualitative analysis of the transition to biological childlessness for infertile couples. *J Counsel Develop.* 2001; 79: 439–49.

84. Takefman JE. Ending treatment. In: Covington SN, Burns LH. *Infertility Counseling: A Comprehensive Handbook for Clinicians*, 2nd Edn. London: Cambridge University Press; 2006, pp. 429–39.

85. Wischmann T, Korge K, Scherg H, Strowitzki T, Verres R. A 10-year follow-up study of psychosocial factors affecting couples after infertility treatment. *Hum Repro.* 2012; 27(11): 3226–32.

Chapter 2

Reproductive psychology and fertility counseling

Susan C. Klock

The English language lacks the words to mourn an absence. For the loss of a parent, grandparent… or friend, we have all manner of words and phrases, some helpful some not. Still we are conditioned to say something, even if it is only "I'm sorry for your loss." But for an absence for someone who was never there at all, we are wordless to capture that particular emptiness. For those who deeply want children and are denied them, those missing babies hover like silent ephemeral shadows over their lives. Who can describe the feel of a tiny hand that is never held?

Laura Bush, *Spoken from the Heart*, 2010

This was not how it was supposed to be. This was not what you dreamed it would be. And you don't know how it will end. It's okay if you don't know how to wrap your mind around your emotions. Be gentle with yourself for not totally having control of how you feel from moment to moment.

Steve Wiens, *Huffington Post*, August 5, 2013

The dream of having a baby is deeply embedded in most cultures, religious traditions and throughout time. As much as Western culture has evolved to include numerous roles for women, having a child continues to be an important life goal for the majority of women of childbearing age. The majority of women and couples who desire to become pregnant will conceive naturally, have a successful pregnancy and experience the transition to parenthood. But for a minority of women, the desire to become pregnant will be met with frustration, failure and unexpected challenges. Additionally, for single women and men, gay, lesbian, bisexual and transgendered individuals, the quest for a family is increasingly available via the reproductive technologies but having a child is a labyrinth of individuals (donors and gestational carriers), medical staff, money and emotions navigated over time. The experience of infertility prompts unique psychological reactions and adjustment. Mental health professionals (MHPs) are frequently called upon to provide psychological assessment and counseling to individuals and couples who are experiencing infertility and its psychosocial sequelae.

The purpose of this chapter is to provide an overview of the psychology of infertility as an aspect of reproductive psychology and the field that has emerged of fertility counseling. Reproductive psychology refers to the psychological, behavioral and societal aspects of reproductive potential, fertility control and infertility, pregnancy and birth, and parenting. Each of these areas is a focus of clinical and scientific inquiry. An area of reproductive psychology that has significantly developed in the past 30 years is the psychology of infertility. The psychology of infertility focuses on the intrapersonal and interpersonal emotional, cognitive and behavioral factors related to the experience of infertility. After some brief background information, a review of two leading theoretical frameworks for understanding the psychology of infertility will be presented, then an introduction to the history and practice of fertility counseling will be provided. The purpose of this chapter is to provide a broad review of the psychology of infertility, and to provide context for the specific counseling topics presented in this volume.

Background

Reproduction is a biological imperative for humans to perpetuate their continued existence, but in the twenty-first century, in developed cultures, the wish for a child carries other meanings. In earlier times (and still existing today in developing countries), children were needed for economic survival, providing accessible and free labor for a largely agrarian culture.

Fertility Counseling: Clinical Guide and Case Studies, ed. Sharon N. Covington. Published by Cambridge University Press.

As such, children were valued for their economic contributions to the family and in the wider social context for their contributions to the labor force. After the Industrial Revolution and the implementation of child labor laws, children were displaced from the work force. The economic value of children diminished but the social and emotional value of children grew as the child's role shifted to one of providing affection, connection, stimulation and companionship for the parents. As Griel [1] noted, children became valuable as emotional investments, providing emotional warmth and affection, particularly to their mothers.

In modern cultures, having a child represents the desire to pursue happiness and the belief that having a child is a key component to personal happiness [2]. Hoffman and Hoffman [3] discussed the motivation for parenting and described nine categories of motivation for parenting. These value categories describe the needs that a child fulfills in a parent, including adult status and social identity, expansion of the self, moral values, group ties and affection, stimulation and fun, achievement and creativity, power and influence, social comparison and economic utility. Parenthood represents an important developmental milestone in most adults' lives, indicating that they have reached a point of stability and maturity and an arrival into adulthood. Van Balen and Trimbos-Kemper [4], in a study of the motivations for parenting among a sample of infertile individuals, found that the primary motivation for wanting children was the belief that having a child would bring them happiness and well-being. In a subsequent study, van Balen [5] found that the most frequently mentioned motivation for parenthood among fertile and subfertile women was happiness in the mother–child relationship. Other motivations, such as the desire to have a child as a means of achieving adulthood and strengthen identity and enhanced partner attachment were also noted. Also, in van Balen's study among the subgroup of women with previous infertility, the average score on the desire for motherhood scale was much higher than for fertile women, as indicated by a response category corresponding to the statement, "I am willing to give up almost everything to have a child." As the infertile woman or couple begins trying to get pregnant, the desire to have a child may strengthen as the need to devote more time, emotional and financial resources to fertility treatment increases.

Given the motivation to have a child, there are several factors that interact to affect the likelihood that an individual or couple will have a child. It is estimated that 15% of women are unable to become pregnant after a year of attempts [6]. Using a nationally representative sample, the National Survey of Family Growth (NSFG) found a current prevalence of infertility of 7.4% among married women in the USA [7]. But as Thoma et al. have noted, the way in which fertility is measured affects the estimated prevalence [8]. Using survey data, a constructed approach (women who are in a relationship, not using birth control, and are sexually active over the past 12 months) yielded an infertility rate of 7%. Alternatively, the current direct approach (asking women if they were trying to get pregnant and if so for how long) estimated a 15% infertility rate. These estimates are consistent with estimates of 12% frequently cited from Mosher and Pratt [9].

There are numerous factors that affect the overall infertility rate, including the trend in US and Western cultures for delayed childbearing due to increased work, educational or financial goals [5,6]. It is estimated that approximately 50% of infertility problems are attributed to the female partner, 35% to the male and 20% unexplained or unknown [6]. The development and widespread availability of assisted reproductive technologies, including ovulation induction, ovarian stimulation, in vitro fertilization (IVF), gamete donation and gestational surrogacy, have all contributed to the effective treatment of infertility with nearly half of infertile couples seeking medical treatment for their infertility [10]. As the medical technology has developed and become more widespread, the psychological aspects of infertility have become an important field of study. The psychological adjustment to infertility and its treatment are the focus of the next sections of this chapter.

Reproductive psychology and infertility

For decades clinicians believed that infertility, particularly "unexplained" infertility, was caused by psychological distress [11–13]. This psychosomatic conceptualization was largely based in psychoanalytic thinking and focused on psychogenic conflict as a cause of infertility. Possible conflicts, such as conflict about the maternal role or feminine identity were frequently cited as causes of female infertility. In the 1980s, MHPs began to question the assumption that psychological distress caused infertility, but instead posited that infertility caused psychological distress. This change of causal direction provided a new paradigm for conceptualizing the psychological aspects of infertility. Two theoretical perspectives have guided much of the clinical and research activity since this time: grief and loss theory and the stress and coping model.

Grief and loss

Bowlby [14] described the four stages of grief after an "affectional bond" had been broken and proposed that grief was a normal adaptive response after a loss. The four stages of grief are described as: (1) shock and numbness; (2) yearning and searching; (3) despair and disorganization and (4) reorganization and recovery. Shock and numbness is the phase during which the loss is not perceived as real and feels impossible to accept. There is physical distress during this phase, which can result in somatic symptoms. Yearning and searching is the stage during which one becomes aware that the loss has been experienced and the future that had been imagined or counted on is realized as no longer a possibility. Attempts at trying to fill the void that the loss has left are common and preoccupation with the loss can persist. The third stage of grief is despair and disorganization. During this stage the individual realizes that the loss has occurred and that life will not go back to the way it was or the way it was imagined. It is during this stage that despair and hopelessness may set in. Finally, reorganization and recovery occur as one develops new routines, plans and goals. The loss recedes and adjustment to the changed life develops. Bowlby's classic model is useful in understanding the grieving that infertile individuals and couples undergo as they face the diagnosis of infertility.

A further exploration of grief and loss theory in the context of infertility was provided by Menning [15]. Menning applied Kübler-Ross's five stages of death and dying (shock, denial, anger, bargaining and acceptance) to describe the typical thoughts and feelings associated with the infertility experience. Although the grief and loss models are focused around the death of a loved one, in the infertility context the loss is of the imagined or dreamed-of child.

Expanding on the grief and loss model, an important paper on the psychological aspects of infertility was by Patricia Mahlstedt [16]. In this manuscript, based on extensive clinical observation, Mahlstedt described a series of losses experienced by infertile individuals and couples, among them: the loss of self-esteem, relationships, health and financial security. The adaptation to these losses can be conceptualized through the stages of grief theory provided above. Mahlstedt's paper provides important descriptive information for any clinician working with infertile individuals.

According to Mahlstedt, the infertile person experiences a loss of self-esteem by failing to achieve a desired goal of having a baby despite a concerted effort. The loss of the dreamed-for child can directly diminish the person's sense of self-efficacy, generativity and prompt existential anxiety. The inability to meet the goal of having a child challenges and erodes the person's self-esteem. The problem may worsen significantly if the individual has been highly successful in other areas of life and has not developed the coping skills to deal with failure and loss.

The second loss is the real or feared loss of important relationships. This includes not only the intimate partner relationship but also relationships with family, friends, co-workers and others. Significantly, the infertile partner may worry that their partner might leave them. They may also experience difficulties in discussing their thoughts and feelings about infertility and its treatment, blame one another for the infertility and have difficulty adjusting to the changes in sexual activity due to the infertility and its treatment. The changes in an infertile couple's sexual interactions have been written about extensively (see Wischmann for a review) [17,18] but constitute a significant loss for the couple. In addition to the perceived losses in the intimate relationship, the individual(s) may also experience changes or losses in their relationships with family. Women may withdraw from relationships with siblings or friends who are pregnant or who have recently given birth. Infertile individuals may avoid social gatherings during which pregnancy and childrearing are discussed, and family gathering during the holidays is notoriously difficult for the infertile couple in that the focus on family and children is very pronounced, thus highlighting the infertile person's loss. Withdrawal from others and loss of relationships diminishes social support and can compound feelings of isolation and depression.

The third loss discussed by Mahlstedt is the loss of health. The infertile couple initially undergoes numerous tests and procedures to assess their reproductive system. These tests are time consuming and often require numerous, specifically timed visits to the medical clinic. During the course of the infertility diagnostic evaluation and treatment, women and men can take on the patient role and begin perceiving themselves as ill, or at times serious medical problems, such as cancer, may be identified and they become ill. Moreover, for women taking fertility medications, the side effects of the medications can produce significant symptoms that undermine a women's feeling of health. IVF can feel like the complete medicalization of reproduction.

A fourth loss can be the loss of financial security. At this writing, 15 states in the United States mandate coverage for some type of infertility treatment, although the extent of the coverage is variable [19]. Additionally, it is unknown what the impact of the Affordable Care Act in the United States will be on the provision of coverage for infertility services. In the European Union and United Kingdom, national coverage is provided but wait times are often lengthy. IVF can cost between $10 000 and $15 000 and often several cycles are needed. Couples may assume significant debt in order to finance their infertility treatment. An extension of the concern for financial stability is the concern about loss of employment. Infertility treatment often requires frequent visits to the clinic for monitoring, tests or procedures. Frequent absences from work can leave individuals feeling vulnerable to job loss or loss of status at work. Disclosure to employers about the nature of the time away from work can in turn prompt women to worry about loss of possible promotion or advancement at work or being put on the "mommy track." Nondisclosure of the reason for the work absences can be equally stressful.

Related to the loss of self-esteem and the loss of relationships is the perceived stigma of infertility [20]. Stigma, the idea of a negative sense of social difference that is so outside the social norm that it devalues the individual, is experienced by the individual and in the context of the family, social group or larger society. The infertile individual may feel different, inferior, defective or worthless. Despite the advancement of women's rights in many areas, the predominance of childbearing as a primary value of women in culture is still the norm. Additionally, the experience of infertility for men is equally stigmatizing in masculine-dominated cultures. The stigma of infertility is evident in Western cultures but is even more pronounced in developing countries and nonsecular cultures. The experience of infertility in this context can prompt stigmatization of the individual by their family and society in addition to that by the individual him or herself [21]. This can lead to social isolation, which can compound feelings of loss, isolation and grief.

Using the grief and loss model, these losses can be identified, worked through and resolved in order to maintain psychological well-being. Working through of the emotional impact of these losses in the context of infertility may be aided by psychotherapy with a mental health professional. Clinicians should be aware of these losses, their presentation and their resolution during therapy.

Stress and coping

Another model that has provided a framework for conceptualizing the psychological aspects of infertility has been the stress and coping model. In the 1980s, as it became clear that psychological stress did not cause infertility but, instead, infertility caused psychological distress, the stress and coping model became useful for understanding the emotional response and for providing a theoretical framework to study the psychological aspects of infertility. The stress and coping model refers to the theories put forward by Lazarus and Folkman [22] and others (see Stanton for a review, [23]) to describe an individual's reaction to a stressful life event such as infertility.

A stressful event or experience is defined as one in which the person appraises the event or experience as challenging or exceeding one's abilities, or endangering one's well-being. Using this model, the infertility experience is the stressful event and the individual's characteristics (appraisal, personality style, coping) influence their response or adjustment. The appraisal of infertility can mediate the severity of a person's response. Appraisal consists of primary and secondary appraisal. Primary appraisal refers to how important the person perceives the event. Secondary appraisal consists of the person's evaluation of their ability to affect or change the event. In the infertility context, a primary appraisal has a large magnitude of importance for a woman who has tailored her life choices around parenting. In this case, the perceived threat to the woman's sense of self caused by the infertility would be high because parenthood is of high importance to her. The secondary appraisal relates to the individual's perception of their ability to change the event. For the infertile woman, she may ask herself, "Can I see my doctor?"; "Can I undergo IVF?"; "Can I modify my health behavior to alter the infertility experience?" Further, responses to stress can be both adaptive and maladaptive. In general, those events that are appraised as more threatening or important to an individual and those that are perceived as unchangeable are more likely to impair adjustment [23].

Personality characteristics can also affect a person's adjustment or response to infertility. Traits such as locus of control, trait anxiety, optimism and resilience have all been studied in reference to infertility adjustment [24–26]. For example, Sexton et al. examined the personality construct of resilience, the capacity of individuals exposed to a negative event to maintain relatively stable, healthy levels of psychological and physical functioning, as it pertains to adjustment to infertility. In their sample they found that women undergoing infertility treatment had lower than normal levels of resilience. Additionally, women with low resilience had higher reported levels of infertility distress and active coping behaviors were positively correlated with resilience.

In addition to appraisal and personality factors, adjustment to infertility is also mediated by coping strategies and behaviors [27,28]. Types of coping have been described by Folkman and Moskowitz [29] as falling into four categories which are: (1) problem-focused; (2) emotion-focused; (3) social coping and (4) meaning-focused coping. Problem-focused coping can be activity related and includes activity engagement, restraint from activity and active planning. Emotion-focused coping includes psychological denial, avoidance, distancing, disengagement via alcohol or drugs or mental disengagement. Social coping includes seeking instrumental support and seeking emotional support. Meaning-focused coping can include cognitive restructuring such as positive reinterpretation, humor and acceptance. Although these are commonly used categories to describe or measure coping, they are not definitive nor are there always clear-cut distinctions between types of coping. Individuals generally engage in problem-focused coping when they perceive that something can be done to change their situation. Emotion-focused coping is used when people feel that something must be endured.

The research on coping in the field of infertility generally indicates that various coping strategies are helpful in certain situations. As Folkman and Moskowitz point out, there are no inherently good or bad coping strategies; instead, the effectiveness of the coping is context dependent, therefore extensive study of coping in a specific context is needed before generalizations can be made [29]. Additionally, they point out that attempts to study coping in a specific context have been attempted in order to create an intervention to optimize adjustment, but determining coping effectiveness is context driven and a dynamic process.

Using the stress and coping model, the infertile person becomes aware of their infertility and appraises how challenging or threatening it is to them. For a woman for whom motherhood is a very important life goal, her appraisal of infertility is very challenging or threatening. She may ask herself, "Who will I be if I am not a parent?" or "What will I do with my life if I can't have a child?" If her answers to those questions are unsatisfactory then she may begin to formulate ways to cope. Problem-focused or active coping may include seeking information from her doctor, talking to friends, modifying her health behaviors (quit smoking, lose or gain weight), all in an attempt to alter her infertility situation. Seeking medical intervention in the form of infertility treatment can be viewed as a type of active coping. Emotion-focused coping could include avoidance, such as the person who avoids going to the shopping mall, grocery store, religious services or other places where pregnant women are likely to be seen. Alternatively, an example of social coping is an individual going to an infertility support group or an adoption education meeting, thereby creating connections with others to help them cope with their infertility. Meaning-based coping represents deeper cognitive reframing: attaching meaning to the infertility experience. A common example of this is a comment such as, "Going through infertility has made my marriage a lot stronger" or "Through infertility I have realized how much I value relationships with my extended family and friends."

Using the stress and coping model, researchers have ascertained information regarding personal, behavioral and social variables that affect adjustment to infertility. This information in turn can be used to inform clinical interventions and, as such, is relevant for the fertility counselor's fund of knowledge. Since the 1990s there have been hundreds of studies that have used this conceptual framework to improve our understanding of the psychology of infertility. These studies have investigated coping style [30–32] and personality variables as they relate to psychological distress in the forms of anxiety, both state and trait, and depression, and treatment outcome as related to ART (see Boivin and Matthiesen for reviews [33,34]). In general, studies have concluded that in the infertility situation, active coping is more adaptive than emotion-focused coping. Optimism and internal locus of control are more adaptive than pessimism and internal locus of control.

Fertility counseling

Case illustration

Ann, 34, and her husband Steve, 36, reluctantly began trying to get pregnant when Ann stopped using birth control about a year ago. She was concerned about their financial security and her wish to move to an apartment in a nicer part of town. Steve wanted to start a family and assured her that there would be no "perfect" time, so they should just let it "happen naturally." After a year Ann talked to her gynecologist who ran some preliminary tests that indicated she was "fine" so the couple kept trying for another six months before deciding to see a reproductive endocrinologist (RE). Although they lived in an insurance-mandated state, their insurance provider only gave a lifetime limit of $10 000 for fertility treatment, prompting Ann to worry more about their finances. After their consultation with the RE it was found that Ann had decreased ovarian reserve and Steve was azoospermic. During the consultation, Ann was visibly upset and stressed. Steve expressed disbelief about his infertility diagnosis. The RE referred the couple to a mental health professional (MHP) on his treatment team to: (1) discuss family building options, including adoption, donor sperm use or child-free living; (2) assess each partner's emotional well-being and (3) assess the couple's communication and coping in reference to the new infertility diagnoses.

The MHP saw the couple for an initial consultation where she described the purpose of the consultation and the boundaries of information sharing with the referring physician. During the initial history taking she gathered information about their history as a couple, their education and work histories, relevant family information, mental health history and for each partner, their thoughts about parenting and appraisal of the infertility diagnosis. Additionally, symptoms of depression and anxiety were assessed in addition to current health habits (smoking, alcohol and drug use, caffeine intake, diet and exercise). She observed the couple's interactions with one another and their communication style. At the end of the first appointment she formulated a plan which included: (1) gathering information about donor sperm use; (2) meeting again with the couple to discuss their treatment plan and provide continued guidance, as needed, to discuss the short- and long-term implications of donor sperm use for family building and (3) an individual referral for Ann to treat her generalized anxiety disorder.

This case provides a typical clinical scenario for a MHP working in the field of infertility psychology and providing fertility counseling. Understanding the psychology of infertility as well as understanding the roles of psychological assessment and intervention is critical for the MHP to provide useful service to an infertile individual or couple.

History

With the advent of IVF in 1979 and the broad application of assisted reproductive technologies in developed countries in the 1980s and 1990s, the field of fertility counseling developed. For the past 30 years, psychologists, social workers, psychiatrists, marriage and family therapists and other mental health professionals have been providing fertility counseling. Fertility counseling offers individuals an opportunity to explore their thoughts, feelings, beliefs and relationships in order to reach a better understanding of the meaning and implications of any choice of action they may make; counseling may also offer support to them as they undergo treatment and may help them to accommodate feelings about the outcome of any treatment [35]. The need for specialized fertility counseling has been identified since the widespread use of assisted reproductive technologies (ART) began in the late 1980s. Some countries mandate the provision of fertility counseling in relationship to specific types of ART (New Zealand, South Australia, Victoria) and some countries require fertility counseling to be available (UK, New South Wales and Western Australia), whereas in the majority of other countries there are professional society recommendations for fertility counseling but no legislative or other mandates for its provision (see Blyth for a review [36]).

Fertility counselors can come from many different backgrounds. Psychologists, social workers, marital and family therapists and psychiatrists are common professions for fertility counselors. Currently there are no mandated training requirements or specialized credentialing for fertility counselors. Professional societies in the United States, the European Union and Canada describe their recommendations for training and experience. The guidelines from the Mental Health

Box 2.1 Types of fertility counseling (adapted from Blyth, [36]).

1. **Implications counseling**: the exploration of personal and family implications of infertility and infertility treatments and gamete donation, requiring the skills of a trained psychosocial counselor. Undertaken prior to beginning treatment to allow sufficient time for reflection before making any irrevocable decision. Implications counseling may also be necessary after treatment.
2. **Support counseling**: the provision of emotional and psychological support throughout the process of diagnosis, investigation, and treatment and gamete donation, to assist patients to deal appropriately with the experience and/or consequences of their treatment.
3. **Therapeutic counseling**: focused on mediating the more pervasive upsetting and stressful consequences of both impaired fertility and fertility treatment. Much like traditional psychotherapy focusing on a specific problem or issue to be worked through.
4. **Decision-making counseling**: counseling available to patients at significant points in their decision-making around management of fertility treatment.
5. **Crisis counseling**: for patients experiencing a crisis or adverse outcome while undertaking fertility treatment.

Professional Group (MHPG) of the American Society for Reproductive Medicine (ASRM) are provided in Box 2.1 [37]. These guidelines provide a summary of the types of services a fertility counselor should be able to provide and recommended qualifications and training. The five components of qualification and training include a graduate degree in a mental health discipline, a license to practice, training in the medical and psychological aspects of infertility, supervised clinical experience in fertility counseling and participation in continuing education.

The Human Fertilisation and Embryology Authority, Code of Practice [38], enumerated four aspects of infertility counseling: (1) information gathering and analysis; (2) implications and decision-making counseling; (3) supportive counseling and (4) therapeutic counseling. In addition, the Australian and New Zealand Infertility Counselors Association have described five types of infertility counseling [39]. These five types have been described by Blyth (see Box 2.2 [36]) and include implications counseling, support counseling, therapeutic counseling, decision-making counseling and crisis counseling. In addition to considering these types of counseling with the infertile individual or couple, this counseling is also appropriate and relevant to third party reproduction participants, such as egg or sperm donors, gestational carriers and their partners. The provision of counseling to infertility patients can also be conceptualized and offered based on the type of treatment the individual or couple is receiving; for example, in a clinic it may be determined that all patients undergoing IVF, gamete donation or gestational surrogacy have counseling [40]. Providing counseling based on the type of treatment being offered minimizes concerns of discrimination to particular sub-groups of patients.

The Psychology and Counseling Special Interest Group of the European Society of Human Reproduction and Endocrinology (ESHRE) convened a meeting of delegates from seven countries to discuss counseling issues in infertility. This led to the document "Guidelines for Counseling in Infertility" [41,42]. The guidelines recommend the availability of psychosocial services throughout the treatment process and enumerate the patient-centered aspects of care that should be implemented by the treatment team and how professional counseling can be used when needed. Patient-centered care can include the routine provision of written or video information about the psychological aspects of infertility. Other services could be self-help groups or professional-led support groups to empower patients and normalize their experience. Additionally, the guidelines address the need for more specific counseling in certain clinical situations, such as with patients experiencing high distress, multiple pregnancy, facing the end of treatment and sexual dysfunction, third party reproduction and individuals or couples experiencing social infertility. The most recent version of the ESHRE Psychology and Counseling SIG counseling guidelines are currently under review [43]. The purpose of these guidelines is to offer best practice advice on how psychosocial care can be incorporated and implemented in infertility and medically assisted reproduction. The stated aim is to provide a framework to provide psychosocial care over the stages of infertility treatment and tailored levels of psychological care based on patient need.

The Canadian Fertility and Andrology Society Counseling Special Interest Group has also developed

Box 2.2 Qualification guidelines for infertility counselors (adapted from the MHPG of the ASRM [37]).

A qualified infertility counselor should be able to provide the following services:

- psychological assessment and screening
- diagnosis and treatment of mental disorders
- psychometric testing (psychologist)
- decision-making counseling
- couple and family therapy
- grief counseling
- supportive counseling
- education/information counseling
- support group counseling
- referral/resource counseling
- staff consultation
- crisis intervention
- sexual counseling
- psychotherapy

The following guidelines suggest the minimum qualifications and training of mental health professionals providing infertility counseling and psychological services. The mental health professional should have:

1. Graduate degree in a mental health profession.
2. License to practice.
3. Training in the medical and aspects of infertility including basic reproductive physiology, etiology of male and female infertility, testing, diagnosis and treatment of reproductive problems and the assisted reproductive technologies.
4. Training in the psychology of infertility indicating knowledge of marital and family issues associated with infertility, and the impact on sexual functioning, approaches to the psychology of infertility including psychological assessment, bereavement/loss, crisis intervention, post traumatic stress, and typical/atypical responses, family building alternatives including adoption, third party reproduction, child-free lifestyle, psychological and couple treatments and the legal and ethical issues of infertility treatments.
5. Clinical experience. The mental health professional should have a minimum of one-year clinical experience providing infertility counseling, preferably under the supervision of or in consultation with a qualified and experienced infertility counselor.
6. Continuing education. Continuing education helps ensure continued growth in knowledge and skills. Regular attendance at courses offered by the American Society for Reproductive Medicine or other professional organizations and educational institutions is recommended to provide continuing education in both the medical and psychological issues in reproductive healthcare.

counseling guidelines [44]. The guidelines were written to meet the mandate of developing standards of practice for Canadian fertility counselors. The purpose is to define the provision of care to support individuals and couples experiencing infertility and to help them examine the emotional, psychosocial, relational and ethical aspects of treatment options and to assisted in informed decision-making. Additionally, the goals of counseling include helping individuals set realistic goals and prepare for and cope with treatment and its outcome. The Canadian guidelines also describe the multiple roles of the fertility counselor, which include psychosocial support and education, crisis counseling, psychotherapy, serving as a liaison between the patient and her treatment team, providing referrals, addressing ethical issues, development of counseling protocols and interventions, documentation of services, training of others in the field and research and writing.

All of the guidelines describe the two basic types of services provided by fertility counselors: assessment and counseling. Assessment includes a clinical interview and often the administration of measures of depression, anxiety, coping, quality of life, personality and other relevant measures to provide initial assessment of individuals or couples presenting for fertility treatment. The information gathered from the clinical interview and any ancillary measures can provide useful information regarding the psychological functioning of the individual and guide further interventions, if needed. Assessment also may uncover the diagnosis of a psychological disorder requiring treatment; this may be a contraindication for or a reason to delay fertility treatment. Although the overall prevalence of a mental illness is low, women who have experienced infertility have been shown in population-based studies to be at an increased risk for dysthymia and anxiety disorders [45,46]. Assessment also includes the psychological assessment of third party reproduction participants such as gamete donors, gestational carriers and intended parents.

In addition to assessment, the fertility counselor can provide various forms of counseling. The format, timing and type of counseling are highly individualized and dependent on the needs of the client, the availability of the counselor and the situation. Peterson et al. provide a useful schemata for conceptualizing the stepwise process to determine the provision of psychological counseling [47]. They describe a stepwise progression, with the initial phase including information gathering and analysis and decision-making. If further

Table 2.1 Risk factors for high distress among infertile individuals (adapted from Peterson et al. [47]).

Personal factors	Situational	Treatment related
Pre-existing psychopathology	Poor marital relationship	Medication side effects
Primary infertility	Poor social network	Miscarriage
Female	Frequent reminders of infertility	Prior treatment failure
Avoidance coping		

intervention is needed, then additional implications counseling and decision-making counseling may be indicated as well as support counseling and short-term crisis counseling as the individual or couple moves through their medical treatment. Last, psychotherapy with crisis counseling and/or therapeutic counseling may be needed on a longer-term basis for some individuals. Peterson et al. also usefully point out the risk factors for high distress among infertile individuals that may require psychotherapy (Table 2.1).

The pros and cons of whether the fertility counselor is part of the treatment team or an outside consultant have been considered [48]. The advantages to having the mental health professional as part of the infertility treatment team are ease of access, decrease of stigmatization and facilitated communication with the medical staff. Disadvantages include perceived bias toward medical interventions and concern regarding communication boundaries with medical staff.

The impact of psychological counseling on the well-being and adjustment of infertile individuals has also been studied. Chan et al. found that a four-session group intervention was successful in decreasing anxiety among a group of women undergoing their first cycle of IVF [49]. Ockhuijsen et al. found in a randomized controlled trial that positive reappraisal intervention reduced anxiety in women waiting to find out the outcome of their fertility treatment [50]. A review of the studies of the effectiveness of psychosocial interventions in infertility was published by Boivin [51]. In this review, Boivin reported that of the 380 studies reviewed, only 25 assessed the impact of the intervention on a psychological outcome measure. Of these 25 studies, it was found that psychosocial interventions were effective in reducing negative affect but did not change interpersonal functioning. In addition, psychological interventions have not consistently been shown to change pregnancy rates in controlled studies. The need for large, theory based, controlled trials for fertility counseling interventions is shown and presents a goal for the next stage in the development of the field of infertility counseling.

There are personal, situational and treatment-linked risk factors that may leave an individual vulnerable to significant psychological distress. As risk factors for psychological distress and/or a psychological disorder are considered in the context of infertility counseling, it is important to remember the overall greater likelihood of high distress/psychological difficulty among women compared to men. A significant majority of studies assessing infertility related stress find that women cope differently and experience more stress than men [52,53].

Fertility counseling is a dynamic and ever-changing field. Significant advancement has occurred since its inception 30 years ago but change is inevitable as medical technology advances and individuals seek out advanced fertility care. Gameiro et al. described their view of optimal provision of care for IVF patients, which included recommendations specifically for the MHP [54]. These authors recommend routine pre-treatment psychological screening to identify at risk or vulnerable individuals and offer them referral to psychological care early in the treatment process. Additionally, they recommend providing clear, easy to obtain information on how to access psychosocial help and urge the provision of general psychosocial support in daily care in the IVF treatment process. Others have suggested the use of counseling to promote healthy lifestyle choices among fertility patients to improve their health and decrease negative health behaviors that may affect fertility [55]. There are many possible innovations and changes ahead for fertility counselors as we continue to improve and expand our efforts in assisting infertile individuals and couples achieve their goal of building a family. Whether in the context of assessment or the provision of therapy, providing empathy, knowledge and acceptance will continue to be the foundation of the care MHPs provide.

Reflections

Much has changed in the world of fertility counseling. During my first week as a psychology intern, in 1988, I was told to "go down to the infertility clinic and see what they want you to do." I was handed a chart; I read through the varying hieroglyphics of medical testing and notation and went into the room. I felt uninformed, anxious and ill-prepared, much like the woman I was about to meet. I met a woman in her mid 30s preparing for her first cycle of IVF. After we spoke for nearly an hour it became clear to me that she felt the profound grief of invisible loss. She talked about her husband, their imagined child, her fear of IVF, and the existential fear of never being able to have a child. At that time, IVF was a novel and relatively rare intervention. I did not know what to say or do to help her. On that day I decided to educate myself on the medical aspects of infertility, the psychology of grief and loss and psychotherapeutic interventions for individuals facing invasive medical treatments.

Now fertility counseling includes a much broader range of clinical scenarios – talking to an 18-year-old cancer patient about preserving her fertility by banking oocytes before her first round of chemotherapy; coordinating the gestational carrier and oocyte donor for a gay male couple attempting their first cycle of IVF; or coordinating across countries third party reproduction collaborations. Even as the situations become more logistically and clinically complex, I am struck by the fact that the feelings remain the same – fear, sadness and a tug of war between despair and hope. I view my job as a fertility counselor to be about being informed and prepared about the treatments, their implications and the logistical details but, more importantly, about being able to help sift through the feelings, putting words to the inexplicable and making the invisible loss visible.

References

1. Griel, AL. *Not Yet Pregnant: Infertile Couples in Contemporary America.* New Brunswick, NJ, Rutgers University Press, 1991.
2. May, ET. *Barren in the Promised Land: Childless Americans and the Pursuit of Happiness.* New York, Basic Books, 1995.
3. Hoffman LW, Hoffman M. The value of children to parents: In: JT Fawcett, ed. *Psychological Perspectives on Population.* New York, Basic Books, 1973: 19–73.
4. Van Balen F, Trimbos-Kemper T. Involuntary childless couples: their desire to have children and their motives. *J Psychosom Obstet Gynaecol,* 1995; 16: 137–44.
5. Van Balen F. Late parenthood among subfertile and fertile couples: motivations and educational goals. *Patient Educ Couns,* 2005; 59: 276–82.
6. Speroff L, Fritz M. *Clinical Gynecology, Endocrinology and Infertility* (7th edn.) Philadelphia, Lippincott, Williams & Wilkins, 2005: 1013–28.
7. Chandra A, Martinez G, Mosher W, Abma J, Jones J. Fertility, family planning and reproductive health of U.S. women: data from the 2002 National Survey of Family Growth. *Vital Health Stat,* 23, 2005: 25: 1–160.
8. Thoma M, McLain A, Louis J, King R, Trumble A, Sundaram R, Louis G. Prevalence of infertility in the United States as estimated by the current duration approach and a traditional constructed approach. *Fertil Steril,* 2013: 99: 1324–31.
9. Mosher WD, Pratt WF. Fecundity and infertility in the United States: incidence and trends. *Fertil Steril,* 1991; 56: 192–93.
10. Boivin J. International estimates of infertility prevalence and treatment seeking potential need and demand for infertility medical care. *Hum Reprod,* 2007; 22: 1506–12.
11. Benedek T. Infertility as a psychosomatic defense. *Fertil Steril,* 1952; 3: 527.
12. Mai F, Munday R, Rump E. Psychosomatic and behavioural mechanisms in psychogenic infertility. *Br J Psychiatr,* 1972; 120: 199.
13. Shatford LA, Hearn MT, Yuzpe AA, Brown SE, Casper RF. Psychological correlates of differential infertility diagnosis in an in vitro fertilization program. *Am J Obstet Gynecol,* 1988 May; 158(5): 1099–107.
14. Bowlby J. The making and breaking of affectional bonds. *BJP,* 1977; 130: 201–10.
15. Menning B. The emotional needs of infertile couples. *Fertil Steril,* 1980; 34: 313–19.
16. Mahlstedt P. The psychological component of infertility. *Fertil Steril,* 1985; 43: 335–42.
17. Wischmann T. Sexual disorders in infertile couples. *J Sex Medicine,* 2010; 7: 1868–76.
18. Wischmann T. Sexual disorders in infertile couples: an update. *Current Opin Obstet Gynecol,* 2013; 25: 220–22.
19. RESOLVE. Insurance coverage in your state. www.RESOLVE.org, retrieved January 10, 2014.
20. Miall CE. Perceptions of informal sanctioning and the stigma of involuntary childlessness. *Deviant Behav,* 1985; 6: 383–403.
21. Nachtigall R, Pitcher L, Tschann J, Becker G, Quiroga S. Stigma, disclosure, and family functioning among parents of children conceived through donor insemination. *Fertil Steril,* 1997; 68: 83–89.
22. Lazarus R, Folkman S. *Stress, Appraisal, and Coping.* New York, Springer, 1984.
23. Stanton A. Cognitive appraisal, coping processes and adjustment to infertility. In *Infertility: Perspectives from*

Stress and Coping Research. A Stanton and C Dunkel-Schetter, (eds.) New York, Plenum Press, 1992; 87–108.

24. Hjelmstedt A, Widstrom A, Wransby H, Mattheissen A, Collins A. Personality factors and emotional responses to pregnancy among IVF couples in early pregnancy: a comparative study. *Acta Obstet Gynecol Scand*, 2003; 82: 152–61.
25. Verhaak C, Smeenk J, Evers A, Kremer J, Kraaimaat F, Braat D. Women's emotional adjustment to IVF: a systematic review of 25 years of research. *Hum Reprod Udate*, 2007; 13: 27–36.
26. Sexton M, Byrd M, von Kluge S. Measuring resilience in women experiencing infertility using the CD-RISC: Examining infertility related stress, general distress and coping styles. *J Psychiatr Res*, 2010; 44: 236–41.
27. Folkman S, Lazarus R. Coping as a mediator of emotion. *J Pers Soc Psychol*, 1988; 54: 466–75.
28. Carver C, Scheier M, Weintraub J. Assessing coping strategies: a theoretically based approach. *J Pers Soc Psychol*, 1989; 56: 267–83.
29. Folkman S, Moskowitz J. Coping: Pitfalls and promises. *Annu Rev Psychol*, 2004; 55: 745–74.
30. Demyttenaere K, Bonte L, Gheldo M, Vervaeke M, Meuleman C, Vanderschurerem D, D'Hooghe T. Coping style and depression level influence outcome in in vitro fertilization. *Fertil Steril*, 1998; 69: 1026–33.
31. Schmidt L, Holstein B, Christensen U, Boivin J. Communication and coping as predictors of fertility problem stress: cohort study of 816 participants who did not achieve a delivery after 12 months of fertility treatment. *Hum Reprod*, 2005; 20: 3248–56.
32. Panagopoulou E, Vedhara K, Gaintarzti C, Tarlatzis B. Emotionally expressive coping reduces pregnancy rates in patients undergoing in vitro fertilization. *Fertil Steril*, 2006; 86: 672–7.
33. Boivin J, Griffiths E, Venetis CA. Emotional distress in infertile women and failure of assisted reproductive technologies meta-analysis of prospective psychosocial studies. *BMJ*, 2011; Feb 23: 342: d223.
34. Maththiesen S, Fredricksen Y, Ingerslev H, and Zachariae R. Stress, distress and outcome of assisted reproductive technology (ART). A meta-analysis. *Hum Reprod*, 2011; 26: 2763–76.
35. British Infertility Counseling Association. *Guidelines for Good Practice in Infertility Counseling, (2nd edn.)* London, British Infertility Counseling Association, 2007.
36. Blyth E. Guidelines for infertility counseling in different countries: Is there an emerging trend? *Hum Reprod*, 2012, 27: 2046–57.
37. Mental Health Professional Group, American Society for Reproductive Medicine. Qualification guidelines for infertility counselors, 1995. www.ASRM.org.
38. Human Fertilization and Embryo Authority. *Code of Practice*. London, HFEA, 1991.
39. Australian and New Zealand Infertility Counselor's Association Guidelines for Professional Standards of Practice in Infertility Counseling. 2003.
40. Klock S, Maier D. Guidelines for the provision of psychological evaluations for infertile patients at University of Connecticut Health Center. *Fertil Steril*, 1991; 56: 680–85.
41. Boivin J, Appleton T, Baetens P, Baron J, Bitzer J, Corrigan E et al. Guidelines for counseling in infertility: outline version. *Hum Reprod*, 2001; 16: 1301–04.
42. Psychological Special Interest Group of the European Society of Human Reproduction and Embryology. Guidelines for counseling in infertility. http://www.eshre.eu/~/media/emagic%20files/SIGs/Psychology/Guidelines.pdf. 1999. Accessed October 2014.
43. Psychology and Counseling Special Interest Group. Guidelines on psychosocial care by healthcare professionals in infertility and medically assisted reproduction. www.ehsre.eu/Guidelines-and-Legal/Guidelines/Guidelines-in-development.aspx. 2014.
44. Counseling Special Interest Group, Canadian Fertility and Andrology Society. Assisted Human Reproduction Counseling Practice Guidelines. December 2009 www.cfas.ca/images/stories/pdf/csig_counseling_practiceguidelines_december_2009_.pdf.
45. Klemetti R, Raitanen J, Shivo S, Saarni S, Koponen P. Infertility, mental disorders and well-being – a nationwide survey. *Acta Obstet Gynecol Scand*, 2010; 89: 677–82.
46. Baldur-Felskov B, Kjaer S, Albieri V, Steeding-Jessen M, Kjaer T, Johansen C, Dalton S, Jensen A. Psychiatric disorders in women with fertility problems: results from a large Danish register-based cohort study. *Hum Reprod*, 2013; 28: 683–90.
47. Peterson B, Boivin J, Norre J, Smith C, Thorn P, Wischmann T. An introduction to infertility counseling: a guide for mental health and medical professionals. *J Assist Reprod Genet*, 2012; 29: 243–48.
48. Van den Broeck U, Emery M, Wischmann T, Thorn P. Counselling in infertility: Individual, couple and group interventions. *Patient Educ Couns*, 2010; 81: 422–28.
49. Chan C, Ng E, Chan C, Ho P, Chan T, Effectiveness of psychosocial group intervention for reducing anxiety in women undergoing in vitro fertilization: a

randomized controlled study. *Fertil Stertil*, 2006; 85: 339–45.

50. Ockhuijsen H, van den Hoogen A, Macklon N, Boivin J. The PRCI study: design of a randomized clinical trial to evaluate a coping intervention for medical waiting periods used by women undergoing a fertility treatment. *BMC Women's Health*, 2013; 13: 35.
51. Boivin J. A review of psychosocial interventions in infertility. *Soc Science Med*, 2003; 57: 2325–41.
52. Greil A, Slauson-Blevins K, McQuillan J. The experience of infertility: a review of recent literature. *Sociol Health Illn*, 2010; 32: 140–62.
53. Peterson B, Newton C, Rosen K, Skaggs G. Gender differences in how men and women who are referred for IVF cope with infertility stress. *Hum Reprod*, 2006: 21: 2443–49.
54. Gameiro S, Boivin J, Domar A. Optimal in vitro fertilization in 2020 should reduce treatment burden and enhance care delivery for patients and staff. *Fertil Steril*, 2013; 100: 302–09.
55. Homan G Litt J, Norman R. The FAST study: Fertility assessment and advice targeting lifestyle choices and behaviours: a pilot study. *Hum Reprod*, 2012; 27: 2396–404.

Chapter 3

Fertility counseling for individuals

Linda D. Applegarth

Stephanie, age 42, presented as a single, divorced, PhD college biology professor. Her initial goal for individual counseling was to gain additional emotional support as she began fertility treatment, and to see herself more comfortably as a single mother, something that she had never envisioned previously. She had been divorced for five years with no children, and she had spent the last several years focused on building a successful career. Stephanie described herself as having a history of chronic, endogenous depression. She reported that she had been in psychotherapy previously, and had been taking 20 mg of fluoxetine daily for several years. She indicated that she had no intention of stopping this medication that she obtained through her internist.

Stephanie stated that she was generally aware of the limitations of her fertility, given her age. However, she had already met with a reproductive endocrinologist (RE) and was soon to begin an in vitro fertilization (IVF) treatment protocol using anonymous donor sperm. An extensive psychosocial history revealed that Stephanie was the middle of three children, and the second girl. Her parents had been divorced for 17 years, and neither had remarried. Stephanie's father had developed some significant mental health problems that were ill-defined, but consisted primarily of unpredictability, mood swings, and hostility. Her mother and older-sister were both described as "withholding" and "controlling." She apparently did not have a close relationship with her younger brother.

Stephanie and I began to meet on a once-weekly basis. Her first IVF treatment was unsuccessful, and she quickly scheduled another cycle that was also unsuccessful. At the same time, Stephanie indicated that she had been dating actively through an internet dating service, and had recently begun seeing a man (Jim) on a regular basis. Although they had discussed their feelings and ideas about children, Stephanie had not revealed to Jim that she was actively undergoing treatment. As she completed her third IVF cycle with an anonymous sperm donation, she became highly anxious about telling Jim about the cycle, and struggled with the decision whether to transfer or cryopreserve the resulting embryos. Her crisis state resulted in additional sessions with me, and her decision to "confess" to Jim. Ultimately, she decided to cryopreserve those embryos, and after about four months of dating, Stephanie and Jim decided to do an IVF cycle together. Before proceeding, Stephanie met with me to discuss this decision and her need to have a partner actively present in her life. At the same time, she was able to articulate her ambivalence about another marriage. The couple did two more IVF cycles that were unsuccessful. Shortly after their last cycle, Stephanie came into the fertility clinic for a monitored intrauterine insemination (IUI) with Jim's sperm. The IUI was successful, and Stephanie and Jim decided to marry shortly before she gave birth to a healthy girl at age 45.

Stephanie has continued to work in individual counseling. The treatment, after a 10-year period, has clearly evolved from a focus on fertility issues to a focus on her relationship with her child; her ambivalence about her marriage, about conflicts and stressors in her work setting; the death of her mother and resulting conflicts with siblings; and her tendency to place her personal friendships and her own emotional and physical needs as a low priority.

Introduction

The practice of individual counseling or psychotherapy is both a science and an art. True understanding of this art and science can only come with real-time

Fertility Counseling: Clinical Guide and Case Studies, ed. Sharon N. Covington. Published by Cambridge University Press.

exposure to therapist–patient interactions, regardless of the amount of empirical knowledge someone may have about a specific psychotherapeutic theory or technique. Psychotherapy and counseling techniques are rational and systematic procedures designed to improve the patient's mental health [1]. Ideally, counseling techniques are applied within a theoretical framework or approach. In this chapter, the terms "counseling" and "psychotherapy" will be utilized interchangeably.

In general, individual counseling or psychotherapy includes interactive processes between a person and a qualified mental health professional (psychiatrist, psychologist, clinical social worker, marriage and family theapist, licensed counselor or other trained practitioner). Its purpose is the exploration of thoughts, feelings and behavior with the goal of problem solving or achieving higher levels of functioning. Psychotherapy aims to increase the individual's sense of personal wellbeing. Psychotherapists employ a range of techniques based on experiential relationship building, dialogue, communication and behavioral change, all of which are intended to improve the mental and emotional health of a client or patient, or to improve relationships. Although society typically has been somewhat skeptical of what is considered a "soft science," it is encouraging to note that in a recent study in Germany [2] about attitudes toward psychotherapy, it was found that a significant majority of the population (ranging in age from 14 to 92 years) indicated a positive belief and approach regarding counseling.

Broadly speaking, psychotherapy may also be performed by practitioners with different qualifications. It may be legally regulated, voluntarily regulated, or unregulated, depending on the country, state, or district jurisdiction. Requirements of these professions vary, and often require graduate school and supervised clinical experience. In Italy, for example, the practice of psychotherapy is restricted to graduates in psychology or medicine who have completed a four-year postgraduate course in psychotherapy at a training school recognized by the state [3]. Germany restricts the practice of psychotherapy for adults to psychology professions who have completed a five-year course [4]. Both France and Sweden have restrictions on the title "psychotherapist" which may only be used by professionals who have specialized postgraduate training. Psychotherapists in France must be professionals on the National Register of Psychotherapists [5] and those in Sweden must be issued a license by the National Board of Health and Welfare [6]. Interestingly, in the UK, psychotherapy is voluntarily regulated. National registers for psychotherapists and counselors are maintained by three organizations: The United Kingdom Council for Psychotherapy, the British Associations for Counselling and Psychotherapy and The British Psychoanalytic Council. Following a review in 2007, the UK Health Professions Council concluded that mandatory professional regulation by the above-noted organizations was the most effective way of regulating the practices of psychotherapists and counselors, rather than statutory regulation [7]. Similarly, in Australia and Belguim, the title of "psychotherapist" is not yet legally protected. In Australia, the terms "psychotherapist," "social worker" and "counselor" are currently self-regulated with several organizations campaigning for government regulation [8,9].

In Asia, regulations regarding the practice of counseling or psychotherapy are evolving. In Japan, registration and certification as a psychotherapist is available through the Japan Federation for Psychotherapy. The government does not license or regulate practice for psychologists, but does license social workers. As a result, some psychologists work under the umbrella of social welfare licensing laws [10].

In the United States, "psychotherapist" is a general term used to describe an individual who has been professionally trained in an advanced degree (i.e., psychiatry, psychology, social work, nursing or counseling) and licensed by a state professional board to treat mental, emotional and behavioral disorders by psychological means [1]. Criteria for such licensure vary from state to state.

In sum, however, the general practice of "psychotherapy" or "psychological counseling" may sometimes be vague and ill-defined. For those who have met their state or country's requirements as a "psychiatrist," "psychologist," "social worker," "psychiatric nurse," "professional counselor" or "marriage and family therapist," there is usually a requirement of additional education and clinical training on psychotherapeutic theory and technique.

Within the framework of a broad number of therapeutic approaches to individual counseling, fertility counseling also takes an important place – one that requires experience and an additional knowledge of the many medical components of fertility treatment. Individual counseling is, in fact, the cornerstone of fertility counseling, and a solid knowledge and skill-base of psychotherapeutic approaches and clinical techniques are critical to treating the infertile population effectively.

Individual fertility counseling is defined as psychotherapeutic interaction or treatment contracted between a trained mental health professional and a client or patient who is struggling emotionally to achieve parenthood. This struggle usually includes issues that are psychological in nature and can vary in terms of their causes, influences, triggers and potential resolutions. Accurate assessment of these and other variables depends on the practitioner's experience, capability and understanding of the psychological and medical components of infertility and its treatment. Psychotherapy strategies and techniques can also change or evolve as the practitioner acquires greater knowledge and more insight into the patient's issues and conflicts. As Van den Broeck and colleagues point out, "infertility counseling has become a specialist form of counseling requiring professional expertise and qualification" [11, p. 422].

This chapter will present three key approaches to individual fertility counseling and will be explained by following the case above, as well as another example that provides anecdotal illustrations of each approach. These theoretical approaches include: (1) psychodynamic psychotherapy; (2) cognitive-behavior therapy and (3) supportive counseling. They will be described as they pertain specifically to fertility counseling and are intended to help to elucidate the theories and techniques within the context of assisting fertility patients to understand and manage the emotional and psychological consequences of their condition.

Psychodynamic psychotherapy

The theoretical foundations of psychodynamic psychotherapy can most appropriately be understood within an historical context. First and foremost, psychodynamic therapy has grown out of early psychoanalytic theory. But, as McWilliams has pointed out, psychoanalysis has never been a static theory, and is also ever-evolving [12]. Nonetheless, there are a number of key influential concepts in psychoanalysis that have significantly impacted psychodynamic psychotherapy: (1) early Freudian theory and practice; (2) ego psychology; (3) object relations theory and interpersonal psychoanalysis and (4) the self-psychology movement.

Briefly, the early work of Freud was an effort to understand and to reduce psychopathology for those diagnosed with severe "neuroses." The patients who initially "captured Freud's attention suffered from what we would now term posttraumatic, borderline, and somatoform disorders" [12, p. 72]. Although he originally used hypnosis to relieve psychiatric symptoms, Freud later began to value free association as a treatment methodology. It was within this context that the "talking cure" was born. From his patients' free associations, Freud inferred that many of their "neuroses" were the result of the expression of two contradictory internal attitudes, one or both of which were unconscious. For example, wishes for sexual gratification in tandem with moral rejection of such wishes. He thus adopted the concept of "dynamism" from physicists, and began referring to the dynamic unconscious, thus the source of the term psychodynamic [12].

Interestingly, Freud's form of psychoanalysis did not point to qualitative differences between healthy and sick, or normal and abnormal. Rather, psychoanalysis views psychological problems on a continuum, as a matter of degree, and as different aspects and expressions of universal human struggles. Although contemporary analytic therapies have diverged considerably from their Freudian base, the core ingredients in Freud's early work remain present in one form or another in almost all current psychodynamic therapies: an appreciation of dynamic unconscious processes, the assumption of a direction or tilt to all mental life, a developmental viewpoint, a sense of the ubiquity of conflict and defense and an attention to the transference process [13].

Ego psychology is a psychoanalytic approach that developed in North America in the 1930s. It was based on Freud's notion that the mind is a competing arena of demands from the *id* (primitive impulse), *ego* (sense of "I") and *super ego* (conscience and personal values/ideals). The ego was seen as mediating between id, superego and reality – using both conscious coping skills and unconscious defenses such as repression, denial, displacement and projection. Psychological and emotional health is thus equated with ego strength, the ability to cope realistically, flexibly and adaptively with life's challenges [14]. In treatment, ego psychological analysts work to make clients aware of their defenses so that they can consciously choose more adequate ways to cope. In so doing, the therapist also tries to foster a strong working alliance so that the client experiences the analyst as a warm and caring collaborator [15]. This therapeutic relationship would then lead the psychotherapist to comment upon or interpret resistances on the part of the client with the idea that the patient would consider other means of managing anxiety and other painful emotions [16]. In traditional ego psychology, interpretation was considered to be the therapist's primary therapeutic activity, and insight was assumed to be the main agent of change. McWilliams notes, "a significant, enduring contribution of ego psychology has been its emphasis on assessing underlying psychic structure before choosing a treatment approach" [12, p. 76]. Nonetheless, many analysts today have rejected sterile and strict ideas of ego psychological models and techniques. Gabbard [17], for example, suggests that post-Freudian analysts have continually modified their theories and practices in response to research developments in science, psychology and philosophy. There is now a greater attempt to address the needs of different populations, cultural contexts and other pressures on practice.

In the United Kingdom in the 1950s, a number of analysts such as Fairbairn, Winnicott and Klein began to focus on internalized relationships and their affective themes. This body of work was called object relations theory, and in the United States a similar movement led by Harry Stack Sullivan and colleagues called itself interpersonal psychoanalysis. As a result of this movement, the Freudian focus on drive, conflict and defense was considered less relevant to a client's problems than were primary relationship issues [18]. Most notably, the focus was often on one's sense of self more than, for example, on Freudian issues of gratification and frustration. Similarly, issues of basic security, closeness and an internal sense of effectiveness and control are more critical than issues of drive satisfaction. Psychotherapists who adhere to object relations theory recognize what earlier relationships the client has internalized or "introjected." McWilliams [12] notes that from an object relations viewpoint, one group of patients whom psychotherapists found easier to understand included those who are often diagnosed as borderline personality disorder. Specifically, clients with a borderline diagnosis often feel controlled and engulfed in relationships; hence, those who adhere to the object relations theory understand the significance of primary relationships and attachments in the client's life and are able to maintain empathy with them, as well as boundaries, and to be a stabilizing presence.

The self-psychology movement of the 1970s appears to have evolved from broad cultural changes, particularly in the West: rapid technological change, splintered extended families and communities and increased mobility. As a result, psychoanalysts began seeing more clients who suffered from feelings of emptiness, low self-esteem and confusion about their identity and direction in life. These clients seemed to have a broken or stunted sense of self, and tended to crave validation from outside. They tended to treat others with either idealization or devaluation, thus compensating for or offsetting their own problems of self-esteem. Through these personality dynamics, there arose a "rich clinical and empirical literature on narcissism, the psychoanalytic term for these deficient states and compensatory attitudes" [12, p. 79]. Ironically, Freud had considered these patients as untreatable [12]. Unlike Freudian theory that focused on the experience of guilt in the patient's conscious and unconscious life, in self-psychology, the dynamic of shame was seen to play a significant role in the patient's inner experience. Hans Kohut was instrumental in the self-psychology movement because his attention to empathy, nonjudgmental acceptance and authenticity, along with a focus on the client's early childhood shame experiences, played out in the therapeutic relationship [19]. Of interest, the notion of shame as described in self-psychology may be a particularly useful one in relation to the psychotherapeutic work with infertility patients. Shame is often a central emotional construct in infertility, and the therapist can assist the patient in addressing what is experienced as a broken or diminished sense of self-worth.

Over time, psychoanalysts have become increasingly aware of self-esteem issues and have seen the applicability to all clients of the self-psychology orientation. Kohut and colleagues, then and now, see empathy as an important treatment technique, and have urged clinicians to choose interventions on the basis of whether or not they will be experienced as "empathically attuned" [12].

In sum, many approaches to psychodynamic psychotherapy have evolved in response to different clinical and societal challenges. Most contemporary psychoanalytic therapists now draw from all or most of the approaches described above in an effort to respond to the distinct psychological needs of each patient. Psychodynamic therapy can be effective as both a long-term or a short time-limited, modality. It should be noted, however, that perhaps the greatest difference between this psychotherapeutic approach and others has to do with the attention to transference and countertransference. Psychodynamic psychotherapy focuses on feelings, perceptions and behaviors that are in the "here and now" – both in the session and in the patient's life. The patient may project painful feelings and negative attributions (as well as loving ones) from past key relationships onto the counselor, which may or may not be immediately interpreted and explored by the therapist. At the same time, the therapist must also be alert to his or her own feelings about the patient. The countertransference may relate either to the therapist's personal issues (such as unresolved infertility), or to the patient's issues and actions that engender strong feelings in the therapist. In either case, the countertransference is significant to the treatment process, especially if the counselor has had personal experience with infertility. (A more thorough discussion of transference and countertransference is provided in Chapter 17.)

Stephanie, part 1

Overall, the ongoing work with Stephanie has been conducive to a psychodynamic therapy approach. She is curious and psychologically minded, and does not suffer from conditions such as addiction, anti-social tendencies, obsessive–compulsive disorders, major depression, or an acute borderline state that would suggest that psychodynamic therapy would be insufficient or inappropriate. Stephanie has been verbal and adept at self-reflection. She has had previous experience with psychotherapy, and quickly connected and committed to the process. My willingness to listen respectfully and open-mindedly, and Stephanie's likeability and openness, enabled us to establish a therapeutic alliance. The intent was also to develop a working collaboration as we explored her thoughts and feelings about her infertility, as well as having a child and being a single parent. An extensive psychosocial history revealed a personality style that was deeply ambivalent, a factor that probably has contributed to her chronic, low-grade depression. Her expressed need for approval, and wish to be a "good girl" became material for interpretation and exploration within the context of being a single parent and, later, in terms of being a spouse. Stephanie grew up with a mother who had high expectations and strict moral views, thus influencing the need to win approval from those around her. Becoming an unwed, single mother was therefore a paradigm that left Stephanie feeling significant emotional conflict, and also contributed to her focused and unrelenting efforts to find a partner while also undergoing treatment.

Stephanie was generally unrealistic about her chances of conceiving a child, despite age-related outcome information from her RE, and she resisted exploring this in psychotherapy. Like many infertility patients, she saw herself as an exception to the statistics and, because she had been successful in many other areas of life (e.g., social, educational and career success), she was unable to consider the possibility of unsuccessful fertility treatment. She tended to approach her IVF treatments in a straightforward, matter-of-fact manner, tending to minimize her anxiety about the treatment process and potential outcome. Although she spoke often in earlier treatment sessions about adoption or oocyte donation, she would quickly brush these options aside as "not for me" and "too many problems." Even gentle, neutral questions about an unsuccessful treatment outcome were met with a defensive stance. When Stephanie became involved with Jim, she soon began having conversations with him about her desire to have children. She actively continued IVF treatment with anonymous donor sperm while they were dating, and as they became closer and more serious about their relationship, Stephanie began experiencing significant anxiety. Still, she opted not to confide in Jim about her fertility treatment, fearing that he would choose to end the relationship. Again, this became important material for psychodynamic exploration as it connected to her longstanding need for approval and fear of rejection – resulting from ambivalent or conflicted relationships with both parents. Talking with Jim about her strong desire for a child and aggressive fertility treatment involved significant emotional risk for Stephanie, but she was able to make a connection between this key personality characteristic and her resistance to being open with Jim. Over time, Stephanie was also able to understand how her needs for love and approval affected many aspects of her life, including her relationships at work, with friends and with me.

In working with Stephanie, a focus on the transference and countertransference was important in our work together. For example, at several points, Stephanie would be significantly late for our appointments. She would breathlessly appear in my office with "excuses" such as being held up by phone calls, student requests, difficulty finding a taxi and so on. After several of these incidences, I commented that her tardiness seemed to reflect how difficult it was for her to put herself ahead of others' needs and demands. Further exploration of this behavior led to Stephanie's acknowledgment that her need to fulfill other's needs ahead of her own stemmed from longstanding guilt and anxiety about not meeting parental expectations. Stephanie's tardiness for our sessions also created angry feelings as part of my countertransference – an indication that I was feeling that our work together was being demeaned by her need to please others outside the treatment hour. Over time, it became clearer to Stephanie that all of her efforts to win the approval of others were often fruitless, creating anger and frustration because she spread herself so thin, and ultimately leaving her feeling lonely and enervated.

Cognitive-behavioral therapy

Cognitive-behavioral therapy (CBT) is an active, here-and-now focused psychotherapeutic approach. The goal is to help clients understand the ways in which their thinking and behavior contribute to their distress, to help them develop strategies to overcome problematic cognitive and behavioral patterns, to solve their current life difficulties and ultimately to apply learned strategies to manage life's challenges after therapy has ended [20]. For purposes of this chapter, the terms "cognitive therapy" and "cognitive-behavioral therapy" will be used interchangeably.

Aaron Beck, considered by many to be the father of cognitive therapy, initially developed this therapeutic approach to treat depression [21]. Subsequently, it has become a treatment for a wide range of psychiatric disorders, including personality disorders, anxiety, substance abuse, eating disorders and suicidal behavior [22–25]. In addition, there are "many more psychiatric disorders, psychological problems, and medical conditions with psychological components" [20, p. 130] for which cognitive therapy has been demonstrated to be efficacious by empirical research. The emotional and psychological components of infertility would certainly be included in this list. A recent study by Faramarzi and colleagues found that CBT improved the social concerns, sexual concerns, marital concerns, rejection of a child-free lifestyle and need for parenthood more than the use of psychotropic medication. They indicate that CBT is a reliable alternative to antidepressant medication, and suggest that it is actually superior to psychotropic medication (i.e., fluoxetine) in resolving and reducing infertility stress [26].

Cognitive-behavioral theory and principles

Craske notes that the theories and principles of cognitive–behavioral therapy are derived from several different sources that have become interwoven with one another over time [27]. Thus, the CBT practitioner will draw from both *learning theories* and *cognitive appraisal theory* in order to conceptualize a problem and develop a treatment plan. Underlying the basic goal of CBT is the idea that problem cognitions, behaviors and emotions have been acquired in some part through learning and experience, and are likely therefore to be modified by new experiences and learning – notwithstanding other contributing factors such as genetics and temperament. Cognitive-behavioral therapy aims to teach new ways of responding and to build new learning experiences that together promote more adaptive ways of cognitive, affective and behavioral responding. Specifically, cognitive therapy, within the broader context of CBT, has the greatest depth and breadth of empirical research that supports its efficacy and effectiveness [28,29]. It is also stressed that CBT is a coherent theory in which clients' clinical presentations are understood within the context of the cognitive and behavioral components that create, maintain and exacerbate distress. According to Judith Beck and others, this method of understanding is called cognitive case conceptualization [30,31]. For example, some mental health professionals tend to view cognitive–behavior therapy as a set of techniques that treat a patient's symptoms but are not part of a coherent theory that helps to resolve the patient's underlying issues. Cognitive case conceptualization serves as a foundation for the individual patient. This template is therefore a means of organizing a client's presenting problems, and it guides the implementation of clinical interventions. In addition, the structure of the session itself allows the counselor to monitor systematically the client's progress in treatment, and build an organized approach to problem-solving. Lastly, another unique feature of cognitive therapy is its set of therapeutic techniques that psychotherapists can utilize in order to achieve "meaningful cognitive and behavioral change" [27, p. 131].

Most important, however, is the development of a solid understanding of the client's clinical presentation that takes precedence over the use of any specific techniques. Unlike other approaches to counseling, the client is actively engaged in the process of experimentation and ongoing evaluation of the effectiveness of any interventions. Evaluation of the intervention strategies not only permits revision where applicable, but also assessment of the overall progress of treatment. A key to CBT treatment is the active involvement of the client, as well as client–therapist collaboration in formulating and implementing a treatment plan.

Cognitive-behavioral therapy strategies and process

The process by which psychotherapists work collaboratively with clients is generally known as cognitive restructuring. Clients and therapists thus work to identify, to evaluate and, if necessary, to modify cognitions that are experienced in situations in which the client also experienced emotional distress [24]. The aim of this process is to assist clients to (1) recognize the ways in which their cognitions affect their mood and (2) modify inaccurate or unhelpful cognitions that are exacerbating emotional distress. Cognitive restructuring with patients is done during psychotherapy sessions in order to coach clients in acquiring and practicing these skills. The therapist also encourages clients to apply these skills systematically in their daily lives outside of the sessions. Cognitive restructuring begins with educating clients about the basic model. Described below are four techniques involving cognitive restructuring that can be utilized to assist patients in skills building. Each of these techniques can be especially useful when working with anxious and/or depressed infertility patients.

In CBT, self-monitoring is a tool for evaluating the working relationships between thoughts, behaviors and emotions, including antecedents and consequences in real time. Self-monitoring is especially valuable for recording subjective experience (e.g., "all of my friends wonder when I am going to announce that I am pregnant") along with levels of subjective distress [27]. This strategy begins with the notion that emphasizes the importance of a "personal scientist model of learning" [27, p. 88] to observe one's own reactions by using objective terms rather than emotionally loaded terminology. Work sheets and diaries are common forms of recording, and feedback from the counselor about the self-monitoring positively influences compliance as well as emphasizing progress or identifying relationships between behavior, thoughts and emotions that can be further targeted in treatment. There is infrequently any contraindication to self-monitoring, but the technique may need to be modified to suit an individual patient's needs or personality [32].

Another primary technique in CBT is *relaxation*. This can include a broad array of strategies such as autogenic training, progressive muscle relaxation, breathing retraining, as well as meditation and yoga. The data indicate that muscle relaxation is generally anxiety reducing [33], and has been used for a number of disorders such as headaches, sleep disturbance, asthma, hyperactivity and so on, as well as various forms of anxiety, including specific concerns that center on various aspects of the fertility treatment process.

A third CBT technique involves behavioral rehearsal of social skills and assertiveness. This treatment technique initially involves an evaluation of the client's skills in a number of social and assertive situations. The rationale for this useful technique emphasizes how learning more effective social and assertive skills will help patients to achieve greater personal control and respect for self and others. For example, many patients present to the fertility counselor acknowledging fears of asking specific questions to the medical team about treatment protocols or decisions; or are often at a loss as to how to manage questions from family or friends about fertility status. Their anxiety, self-consciousness and emotional sensitivity leave them feeling helpless, overwhelmed, or angry – or all of the above. In such cases, the fertility counselor may assist the patient in developing a number of behaviors for the purposes of role-playing and behavioral rehearsal.

Craske notes that patients who desire to make "assertive requests for behavior change in others include a statement of the negative impact of the current behavior, provision of a specific and reasonable alternative behavior, and a statement of the likely positive impact of the new behavior on both parties" [27, p. 91]. In turn, it is the therapist who directly models the specific skill or uses secondary models to help clients develop mastery or improved coping. Clients then rehearse the behaviors both in and out of session so that the practice involves real-life situations. The mechanisms behind behavioral rehearsal are based on principles of reinforcement and shaping, and new behaviors are reinforced by the counselor. The new or changed behaviors are intended to result in more positive reinforcers in the social environment and fewer negative ones, thus improving overall mood and functioning. Ultimately, these newly acquired skills may raise self-esteem and efficacy, and decrease negative beliefs and feelings about one's self and the world.

It should be noted, however, that there are circumstances in which behavioral rehearsal of social skills and assertiveness must be limited. Assertiveness training, for example, should be undertaken in a culturally responsive manner. Many CBT strategies are based on North American/European norms of autonomy and independence. Notably, in other cultures such as Asia, the Middle East, South America and Africa, assertiveness may conflict with values of the importance of family and collectivism [34]. Culturally sensitive assertiveness, instead, can include prefacing assertive communication with more traditional forms of deference and respect [35], or by using other CBT strategies such as problem-solving.

A very important CBT skill that has been utilized for a wide array of difficulties, including anxiety, depression, couples conflict and stress management, is problem-solving [27]. As with other strategies described above, cognitive behavioral therapists use a guided discovery approach to problem-solving, and create an environment for clients to acquire skills that will help them to solve specific problems in their lives. The focus is for clients to draw their own conclusions on the basis of problem-solving, and gain confidence so that they can address other problems in their lives that arise when they are no longer in treatment [20].

In essence, problem solving is a skill-building intervention. The work of D'Zurilla and Nezu [36] has become the framework for many CBT therapists' problem-solving approaches. The process includes approximately four distinct steps to problem-solving: (1) the CBT therapist works with the client to identify the problem using objective language, to separate facts from assumptions and to set realistic goals; (2) alternatives are developed by generating as many solutions as possible, and a list of action plans are set forth for the enactment of each solution; (3) a cost–benefit analysis is conducted of each solution to determine which are most likely to be implemented and (4) the action plan that is associated with the most effective solution is implemented, and the success of the implementation is evaluated so that modifications can be made if necessary.

Table 3.1 provides an overview of the above-described CBT strategies or techniques that can be applied to the specific needs of infertility patients. These patients can ultimately apply these skills not only to concerns, conflicts and difficulties that arise during their infertility experience, but also to other difficult or stressful challenges in their lives.

Table 3.1 Cognitive-behavioral strategies for individual fertility counseling.

Self-Monitoring	Patient records events or images (such as failed IVF treatment or sight of pregnant woman) that create emotional distress. Records resulting negative thoughts and feelings, along with cognitive distortion utilized, and alternative, more balanced ways of thinking and responding.
Relaxation and Stress Management	Patient learns an array of physiologic strategies for managing anxiety and stress. Often utilized before or during medical treatments or receiving bad or difficult news. Includes muscle relaxation, breathing exercises, meditation or yoga. Provides patient with greater sense of self-mastery.
Behavioral Rehearsal and Assertiveness	This technique emphasizes learning more effective social and assertive skills for achieving greater sense of personal efficacy and respect for self. Enables infertility patients to ask questions and discuss treatment options more effectively with medical staff, and/or manage inappropriate or probing questions or comments from family, friends, work colleagues and so on.
Problem-Solving	A skill-building intervention that allows the patient to identify the problem so as to separate fact from assumption, develop useful, alternative descriptions or solutions to the problem, and implement a more effective plan of action to deal with the problem. This treatment strategy can be very helpful for infertility patients who must consider alternative medical treatments or who must confront alternative family building options other than biologic or genetic parenthood.

Wenzel notes that a final important aspect of cognitive-behavioral therapy is the "extensive empirical basis for its efficacy and effectiveness" [20, p. 173]. Clients not only acquire strategies for managing the cognitive and behavioral aspects of their current distress, but also develop a solid understanding of the components of their life problems. This psychotherapy approach emphasizes that CBT is flexible by providing a rich framework for understanding the development of underlying unhelpful beliefs and behavioral patterns, and then shifting these patterns for clients who need to do so. Many infertile patients seeking individual psychotherapy request cognitive-behavioral therapy. Most fertility patients who enter counseling, in fact, do not wish to explore deep-seated issues or resolve past conflicts, nor stay in therapy long term.

Rather, they are asking for tools with which to manage the anxiety, fear and depression that stem from infertility diagnoses and treatment outcomes within a short-term parameter.

Lori

A typical example of individual fertility counseling using CBT strategies and techniques involves the case of Lori, a 34-year-old married woman. She and her husband of three years had been attempting to achieve a pregnancy for over a year. Seven months prior to meeting with me for the first time, Lori had become pregnant spontaneously, but had suffered a miscarriage at eight weeks gestation. Although the pregnancy loss had been "disappointing" for her and her husband, Lori said that they had been optimistic about quickly becoming pregnant again. When that did not happen, Lori became increasingly anxious and frustrated, leading her to seek out medical help from a RE. Sperm analysis and Lori's extensive fertility tests revealed no known etiology, and thus were labeled "unexplained" infertility. The RE's discussions with the couple regarding a step-by-step treatment plan that might ultimately include IVF had created greater distress for Lori. The RE had suggested that she reach out to a fertility counselor to help her manage her anxiety about infertility treatment more effectively.

Lori presented to our initial session with significant anxiety and she voiced fears that all of her efforts to become pregnant with medical assistance were likely to be a waste of time and money. The possibility of doing IVF was viewed as "the last straw" because it was the "end of the line" in terms of treatment options. Her perspective indicated that after all she and her husband might do in order to have a child together, they would still be left childless. She commented that such a thought "terrified" her. Nonetheless, underlying her anxiety were, also, clear elements of hope – something that Lori herself could articulate. Yet, her ongoing anxiety, depression and low tolerance for frustration had negatively affected her self-esteem and her marriage, as well as her relationships with her parents, siblings, in-laws and friends. She tended to make sweeping declarations such as "No one understands what this is like," and "All of my friends are pregnant – or working on having a second child. It's all been so easy for them, and they're clueless."

In general, it was apparent that Lori was functional in many areas of her life: she was intelligent, had close relationships with her family, a supportive, caring husband and a responsible job as an attorney in a small firm. Thus, adopting a problem-solving focus on the current fertility issues seemed to be sufficient to reduce her emotional distress. Using a CBT approach, Lori and I together set an agenda for how we would use our time together. At the same time, Lori was also told that she was free to raise other issues, if needed. This strategy helped to build collaboration in the therapeutic relationship. I suggested that she might want to talk more about her experience of the pregnancy loss, but the choice was hers. This was a topic that brought her to tears, but Lori tended to brush it off as irrelevant. As a CBT therapist, I respected her wish, but noted this avoidance as important information for cognitive case conceptualization, and remained aware of signs that this issue was exerting unwanted effects on Lori's cognition, emotion and behavior. My hope was that as the therapeutic relationship developed further, she might be comfortable expressing her thoughts about this event in relation to the emotional distress it engendered.

A first step in working with Lori was to clarify the meaning of her infertility. A typical question I asked is, "If you were to undertake more aggressive medical treatment for the infertility, what's the worst thing you'd be afraid of happening?" After careful thought, Lori replied that her great fear was that the treatment would be unsuccessful and that she would never be a mother, that her husband would leave her, and that she would be a great disappointment to her family. An inability to conceive would mean not only personal failure of a lifelong dream, but also rejection and abandonment by those closest to her. Ongoing discussions with Lori directly addressed these fears, and she was able to ponder how she might reconsider and handle the possibility of further treatment failures as well as the disappointment and anger she experienced when talking with family and friends. This involved cognitive restructuring that, in this case, focused on education about evidence and de-catastrophizing questions. The CBT strategy with Lori, therefore, was to assist her in acknowledging and building upon the innate coping skills and resources that she had to manage the emotional distress associated with infertilitye treatment.

Over a period of eight sessions, Lori was able to utilize CBT strategies to managing her anxiety and negativity. She kept a self-monitoring diary that enabled her to identify and evaluate automatic thoughts about her infertility treatment and outcomes, as well as about interactions she experienced with her husband, family and friends.

She was gradually able to identify her own negative thought patterns that greatly impacted her level of emotional distress. In addition, Lori gained the ability to counteract her own negative automatic thoughts with more balanced interpretations of her social interactions and treatment experiences.

As each session began, I used a typical CBT session structure that included a brief mood check and a bridge from the previous session. This approach thus modeled a systematic view to problem-solving, and helped continue the theme that ran across sessions so that the time could be used productively. As each session ended, I also asked for feedback on which aspects of the session had been helpful, and how applicable the strategies might be for her outside of our sessions.

In the first several sessions together, we also did breathing exercises and other relaxation techniques that Lori could also use outside our sessions as a means of balancing her mood, reducing stress and ensuring improved sleep patterns. These relaxation techniques were also very helpful to Lori just prior to undergoing IUI. Over time, Lori reported a significant reduction in emotional distress. She was able to communicate more effectively with her husband, who, in turn, was better able to provide support. She also demonstrated the ability to apply the strategies she had learned in therapy to her daily interactions at work, as well as with her family members and friends, most of whom, as Lori came to understand, were well-intentioned but poorly informed. She gradually became more comfortable having honest, non-defensive conversations with those closest to her.

In our last three sessions, Lori was more comfortable and able to address her more profound feelings and thoughts about her miscarriage. Further exploration of this event suggested that Lori appeared to hold a core belief that she saw herself as unworthy. The miscarriage, for her, was a powerful symbol of her unworthiness to become a mother. When she spoke about the pregnancy loss as "meant to be," she was also ultimately able to see that she really believed that she was "not meant to be a mother." Her inability to conceive immediately after this loss was further evidence, in her thinking, that this was true. In this case, it was important for Lori to be able to voice this core belief in her own words so that cognitive restructuring could be applied to her automatic thoughts about this core issue. By the time fertility counseling ended, Lori had begun to develop a healthier core belief about herself and was able use new strategies to manage this and other difficult life problems. Several months later, Lori contacted me to inform me that she was nine weeks pregnant following a third IUI cycle with clomiphene citrate. She and her husband had seen a heartbeat, and Lori was now under the care of her obstetrician.

Supportive counseling

Individual supportive psychotherapy is defined as a treatment modality designed to ameliorate or reduce symptoms, to maintain or improve the client's self-esteem, and to maximize one's adaptive capacities. It is used primarily to reinforce a patient's ability to cope with stressors through a number of key activities, such as the counselor attentively listening and encouraging expression of feelings and thoughts, in an effort to help the individual gain a greater understanding of their situation and alternatives. Some consider supportive psychotherapy to be the most widely used psychotherapy and treatment modality provided to the majority of patients seen in mental health centers and psychiatric clinics [37]. Of particular interest is that supportive psychotherapy bases much of its approach on psychoanalytic, cognitive-behavioral and learning theories [38]. Those who primarily practice supportive psychotherapy must, according to Winston and Goldstein, be able to integrate successfully various other therapeutic approaches in order to best meet the needs of the patient. Many fertility counselors will do supportive psychotherapy, in part because it tends to focus less on unconscious drives and conflicts, and in part because it is often consistent with the desires and needs of those seeking treatment. It is a common form of therapy that may be provided over the short or long term, depending on the individual and the specific set of circumstances.

In general, however, Winston [37] points out that decreasing levels of ego function and increasing levels of psychopathology are also indications for a more supportive stance. Although this is generally not the case with infertility patients, who seldom present with significant psychopathology, this type of intervention and the techniques utilized still rely on patient assessment. If supportive psychotherapeutic interventions are indicated, the techniques include "alliance building, skills building, reducing and preventing anxiety, and awareness expanding" [37, p. 7]. As in psychodynamic psychotherapy, the importance of the therapeutic relationship is also stressed in supportive psychotherapy. However, supportive psychotherapy tends to focus more on the real relationship between patient and therapist, and less on the transference as is traditionally done in psychodynamic approaches. The real relationship exists in the here and now of the therapeutic alliance, and includes a genuine liking for each other without the distortions that are a critical part of the transference. Thus, the real relationship will include the patient's hopes and aspirations for help, care, understanding and love, as well as daily interactions that occur between individuals on a social level. In any case, the therapeutic alliance is necessary to support the work of psychotherapy, in general, and in supportive therapy, Hellerstein, et al. [39] stress that an early therapeutic alliance in the therapy is predictive of outcome. These researchers also note that breaks in the therapeutic alliance occur less often than in psychodynamic therapies, possibly because the alliance in supportive psychotherapy is not threatened by difficult confrontations or interpretations that can create more patient anxiety [39].

The specific interventions or techniques utilized in supportive psychotherapy will again depend on the assessment of the client. For example, alliance-building on the part of the therapist may include expressions of interest, empathy and conversational style. Esteem-building can involve reassurance, normalizing and encouragement. Skills-building includes teaching, advice and guidance through anticipation. Importantly, normalizing, reframing and rationalizing techniques can reduce anxiety. Interventions such as clarification, confrontation and interpretation can also be helpful in expanding the patient's awareness of his or her problem or situation. Winston [37] stresses, however, that interpretation is used sparingly in supportive psychotherapy; and, when it is used, it is in a more general or indirect way. A treatment strategy in supportive therapy is to strengthen defenses, as opposed to that of psychodynamic psychotherapy, which as noted previously attempts to challenge defenses so that more in-depth conflicts, feelings and wishes become more available for exploration.

Winston and Goldstein [38] also point out that cognitive-behavioral techniques are a critical component of supportive psychotherapy, and can be utilized for specific problems such as panic, depression, obsessive-compulsive symptoms and dysfunctional thinking. The authors state that the therapeutic process in supportive psychotherapy involves identifying and challenging automatic thoughts, and testing them empirically. Patients are taught to monitor their automatic thoughts, validate these thoughts and develop alternative ways of thinking. Reframing is an additional technique often utilized to correct cognitive distortions.

Similarly, a number of therapeutic interventions used in supportive psychotherapy can be seen as a form of teaching – a way of imparting knowledge. Thus, learning theory also plays a significant part in the work of supportive psychotherapy. Etkin and colleagues [40] note that, in general, psychotherapy can be considered a "controlled form of learning" through the acquisition of a combination of skills and knowledge. In a "learning theory-informed approach to supportive psychotherapy, patients are viewed as participating in an educational process" [40, p. 150]. Preparation and homework may be necessary to enhance the learning process. Within the context of a supportive psychotherapeutic approach, patients may be encouraged to seek out additional resources, and develop strategies for using those resources to achieve objectives.

Resources may be libraries, the Internet, articles, books, videos and so forth [38]. In the process, the patient can also be involved in evaluating their own learning, and ultimately promoting the skill of critical reflection, that is, the process in which the patient questions and then replaces or reframes an assumption. Alternative perspectives are developed from previously taken-for-granted ideas or forms of reasoning. Like CBT, the goal of this technique is to enable the patient to devise alternative ways of thinking, relating to others and problem-solving.

It appears that supportive psychotherapy has many practical and effective applications in fertility counseling. Most infertility patients presenting for assistance from a fertility counselor are anxious and depressed – fearful that they cannot tolerate treatment or that they will never become parents. Often, the fertility counselor is asked to take on multiple roles within the psychotherapeutic interaction – roles that include not only traditional forms of psychotherapy, but also that of providing education and information about common responses to treatment options, perspectives on parenting alternatives, as well as information on how best to access additional support resources.

In sum, through supportive psychotherapy, counselors assist patients in learning how to move forward and make decisions or changes that may be necessary to adapt, either to an acute change, such as a pregnancy loss or a failed infertility treatment cycle, or to a chronic situation, such as depression resulting from lengthy and ongoing infertility and treatment. In this form of therapy, a trusting relationship between the patient and therapist is integral to the patient's healing process, particularly if the patient needs to come to terms with his or her life circumstances and related losses.

Stephanie, part 2

During my long-term treatment with Stephanie, there were several periods that were most conducive to supportive counseling. For example, after she became pregnant with IUI, she developed a number of medical complications during her last trimester, including gestational diabetes and hypertension, which required bed-rest and an extended leave of absence from her work. Adding to her changes and transitions, she and Jim had been married a month earlier. Stephanie asked for telephone sessions over the six-week period prior to the birth of her daughter. During that time, my focus was on providing reassurance during this period of anxiety, as well as assisting her with more "nuts and bolts" concerns such as obtaining information on future childcare options. We often discussed the impact of parenthood on her career and considered strategies for managing both in ways that would optimize her time with her child and also allow her to maintain a productive level of work. Stephanie also verbalized her increased anxiety about the work issue in part because she would be the primary breadwinner in the family and her four-month maternity leave was seen as potentially jeopardizing her work position. Rather than focus on her ambivalence about career and motherhood, or address transference issues, we focused instead on more practical approaches to finding ways that would minimize Stephanie's anxiety and maximize her work environment. This included ongoing discussions with the chairman of her biology department, which might include more grant-writing and research with fewer teaching hours. These strategies proved to be helpful to Stephanie in that her ongoing contact with her employer began to lessen her anxiety both prior to and after her baby's birth.

Stephanie and I also met, less frequently, for several months after her daughter was born. As a result, it was also an appropriate time to continue supportive psychotherapy. Within the context of an established therapeutic alliance, we focused on issues pertaining to developing an optimal childcare situation. She expressed delight and comfort with motherhood, and did not experience postpartum depression. Her husband, Jim, was also very supportive and engaged in childcare. At the same time, we again focused on ways in which Stephanie could establish a role for herself in her work setting that also allowed her to maintain as much involvement with her daughter as possible.

Table 3.2 Individual fertility counseling: three approaches to psychotherapy.

Psychodynamic Psychotherapy	Patient is appropriate for and wishes to explore longstanding emotional conflicts and concerns, significant relationships, and issues of self-esteem within the context of understanding and dealing with infertility. Treatment can be long or short term.
Cognitive-Behavioral Therapy	Patient requests skills building assistance and techniques for managing anxiety, depression, anger and other negative feelings associated with the infertility experience. Treatment is generally focused and time-limited.
Supportive Psychotherapy	Patient requests emotional support through understanding and empathy. Patient may request to be seen on an "as-needed" basis. The individual may be emotionally vulnerable or resistant to self-exploration. Psychoeducational information and resources may be provided along with CBT strategies for managing infertility experience. Treatment is generally short term.

Summary and reflections

In this chapter, I have attempted to review some central foundations, values and techniques of three fertility counseling approaches: psychodynamic psychotherapy, cognitive-behavioral therapy and supportive psychotherapy. I have not gone into specific detail about many of the techniques given the limitations of this chapter. However, my goal has been to provide basic information as to how each of these individual treatment approaches can apply most effectively to patients experiencing infertility and its treatment (see Table 3.2). The cases that I have presented involve my treatment with women in Western culture; however, all of these psychotherapy approaches can apply to men, as well as to both men and women of other cultures – as long as societal and cultural factors are understood and built into the treatment techniques.

Each of these approaches also has bodies of research that support them, and provide data on "evidenced-based" effectiveness. At the same time, although it is important for the mental health community to appreciate the value of qualitative research, process research and accumulated clinical experience, it may often be easier empirically to study more discrete elements of practice than the more subtle aspects of therapeutic process and relationship. It has been my own longstanding conclusion that the personal qualities and experience of the individual counselor are key to a successful psychotherapy outcome. In fact, Bruce Wampold [41] in his book *The Great Psychotherapy Debate* has effectively delineated factors that make psychotherapy effective. He reports that:

1. Psychotherapy is indeed effective.
2. The type of treatment is *not* a factor.
3. The theoretical bases of the techniques used, and the strictness of adherence to those techniques, are both *not* factors.
4. The counselor's strength of belief in the efficacy of the technique *is* a factor.
5. The personality of the therapist is a *significant* factor.
6. The alliance between the patient and the counselor (meaning affectionate and trusting feelings toward the counselor, motivation and collaboration of the patient, and empathic response of the counselor) is a *key* factor.

Wampold has concluded that it is difficult to pinpoint exactly why psychotherapy actually works, but there are certainly factors that make it effective, as described above. Despite the availability of valuable resources to a person experiencing the emotional distress of infertility – friends, family, religious and spiritual guides, personal reading, healthy eating and exercise, to name a few – psychotherapeutic intervention can still be most effective at healing this profound psychological and emotional injury. Critical to the psychotherapeutic treatment is the therapist's knowledge and understanding of the available reproductive technological resources, medical treatments and options that patients must confront on a regular basis.

There are many therapeutic treatment approaches that the practitioner may utilize during individual fertility counseling. This unique population, although generally psychologically healthy, often lacks sufficient coping strategies for managing the many complex, unpredictable and potentially devastating aspects of fertility treatment and outcomes. Depression and anxiety are the two most frequent emotional sequelae of the infertility experience; however, I have found through my own years of clinical work that these psychological states may stem from very different sources, depending on the personality factors and coping styles of any particular individual client. The type of psychological intervention will therefore vary not only because of various personality types, but also because of the severity of the distress. Specific requests from the patient as to what approach and treatment length is most suitable for them will also determine the counseling approach, and may mean that he or she will need to be referred to a suitable psychotherapist with not only expertise in fertility counseling but also specialized training in the required treatment modality.

Many infertility patients, however, have had little or no prior experience with psychotherapy or counseling, and are unsure of how the fertility counselor will be able to assist them. As Peterson and his colleagues have suggested, psychological care for infertility patients can include implications and decision-making counseling, support counseling and short-term crisis counseling [42]. I have found clinically that most are responsive to a supportive counseling approach in that this approach tends to be time-limited, provides strategies for managing anxiety and depression (including crisis intervention), depends on a strong therapeutic alliance and can include an important psycho-educational component as well. I have also seen in my 30-year clinical work with fertility patients that a supportive counseling approach can sometimes move into a more psychodynamic treatment approach, or likewise into a more cognitive-behavioral approach, depending on the personality characteristics and stated needs of the patient.

My own clinical experience with fertility patients has been the absolute highlight of my work and career as a mental health professional. Over the years, the work that we have done together has been not only a tremendous learning experience for me but also a gift. This chapter is intended to provide a solid overview of three individual fertility counseling approaches, and it hopefully also provides a useful glimpse into what I believe to be the breadth, depth and richness of fertility counseling as it is practiced today.

References

1. Greenberg LS, McWilliams N, Wenzel A. *Exploring Three Approaches to Psychotherapy*. Washington, DC: American Psychological Association, 2014.

2. Petrowski K, Hessel A, Korner A, Weidner K, Brahler E, Hinz A. Attitudes toward psychotherapy in the general population. *Psychother Psychosom Med Psychol* 2014; 64(2): 82–85.
3. Ossicini Act. No. 56/1989. Ordinamento della professione di psicologo: esercizio dell'attivita psicoterapeutica. www.psico.unifi.it/upload/sub/Tirocinio/L56-1989.pdf, 1989. (Accessed February 19, 2014.)
4. "Psychotherapist" may not be used by persons other than physicians, psychological psychotherapists or child and adolescent psychotherapists. http://bundesrecht.juris.de/psychthg/index.html 1998. (Accessed March 5, 2014.)
5. "Arrete du 9 juin 2010 relatif aux demandes d'inscription au register national des psychotherapeutes." http://www.legifrance.govu.fr/affichTexte.do?cidTexte=JORFTEXT000022336754&dateTexte=&categorieLien=id2010. (Accessed March 5, 2014.)
6. "Application for license to practice as a psychotherapist." National Board of Health and Welfare(Sweden). http://www.socialstyrelsen.se/applicationforswedishlicencetopractiseeea/psychotherapist. (Accessed March 5, 2014.)
7. UK Department of Health. Trust, assurance and safety: the regulation of health professionals.http://webarchive.nationalarchives.gov.uk/2013010715354/http://www.gov.uk/prod_consum_dh/groups/dh_digitalassets/@dh/en/documents/digitalasset/dh_065947.pdf White Paper, 2007. (Accessed March 12, 2014.)
8. Psychology Board of Australia – Endorsement. http://www.psychologyboard.gov.au/Endorsement.aspx 2010. (Accessed March 12, 2014.)
9. Australian Counseling Association http://www.theaca.net.au and Psychotherapy & Counseling Federation of Australia http://www.pacfa.org.au (Accessed March 12, 2014.)
10. Japanese Federation for Psychotherapy. www.counselingjapan.com/eng/eng/cs_tokyo_japan_ml20031.php 2003 (Accessed March 17, 2014.)
11. Van den Broeck U, Emery M, Wischmann T, Thorn P. Counselling in infertility: individual, couple and group interventions. *Patient Ed and Counseling* 2010; 81: 422–28.
12. McWilliams N, Psychodynamic therapy. In Greenberg LS, McWilliams N, Wenzel A. (eds.) *Exploring Three Approaches to Psychotherapy*. Washington, DC: The American Psychological Association, 2014, 71–127.
13. Pincus D. Who is Freud and what does the new century behold? *Psychoanalytic Psych* 2006; 23: 367–72.
14. Hartmann H. *Ego Psychology and the Problem of Adaptation*. (D. Rapaport, Trans.) New York, New York: International Universities Press, 1958.
15. Greenson R. *The Technique and Practice of Psychoanalysis (Vol 1)*. New York, NY: International Universities Press, 1967.
16. Brenner C. *Psychoanalytic Technique and Psychic Conflict*. New York, NY: International Universities Press, 1976.
17. Gabbard GO. *Long-term Psychodynamic Therapy: A Basic Text* (2nd edn). Washington, DC: American Psychiatric Association, 2010.
18. Guntrip H. *Psychoanalytic Theory, Therapy, and the Self: A basic guide to the human personality in Freud, Erickson, Klein, Sullivan, Fairbairn, Hartmann, Jacobson, and Winnicott*. New York, NY: Basic Books, 1971.
19. Kohut H. *The Restoration of the Self*. New York, NY: International Universities Press, 1978.
20. Wenzel A. Cognitive therapy. In Greenberg LS, McWilliams N, Wenzel A. (eds.) *Exploring Three Approaches to Psychotherapy*. Washington, DC: The American Psychological Association, 2014, 129–82.
21. Beck AT, Rush J, Shaw BF, Emery G. *Cognitive Therapy of Depression*. New York, NY: The Guilford Press, 1979.
22. Beck AT, Emery G. *Anxiety Disorders and Phobias: A Cognitive Perspective*. New York, NY: Basic Books, 1985.
23. Beck AT, Wright FD, Newman CF, Liese BS. *Cognitive Therapy of Substance Abuse*. New York, NY: The Guilford Press, 1993.
24. Fairburn GC. *Cognitive Behavior Therapy and Eating Disorders*. New York, NY: The Guilford Press, 2008.
25. Wenzel A, Brown GK, Beck AT. *Cognitive Therapy for Suicidal Patients: Scientific and Clinical Applications*. Washington, DC: The American Psychological Association, 2009.
26. Faramazi M, Pasha H, Esmailzadeh S, Kheirkhah F, Heidary S, Afshar Z. The effect of the cognitive behavioral therapy and pharmacotherapy on infertility stress: a randomized controlled trial. *Int J Fertil Steril* 2013; 7(3): 199–206.
27. Craske MG. Cognitive-behavioral therapy. In Vandenbos GR, Meidenbauer E, Frank-McNeil J. (eds.) *Psychotherapy Theories and Techniques: A Reader*. Washington DC: The American Psychological Association, 2014.
28. Dobson KS. *Cognitive Therapy*. Washington DC: The American Psychological Association, 2012.
29. Epp AM, Dobson KS. The evidence base for cognitive-behavioral therapy. In Dobson KS. (Ed.) *Handbook of Cognitive-Behavioral Therapies (3rd*

edition). New York, NY: The Guilford Press, 2010, 39–73.

30. Beck JS. *Cognitive Behavior Therapy: Basics and Beyond (2nd edition)*. New York, NY: The Guilford Press, 2011.
31. Kuyken W, Padesky CA, Dudley R. *Collaborative Case Conceptualization: Working Effectively with Clients in Cognitive-Behavioral Therapy*. New York, NY: The Guilford Press, 2009.
32. Heide JM, Marx BP. Self-monitoring as a treatment vehicle. In O'Donohue W, Fisher JE, Hayes SC (Eds.) *Cognitive Behavior Therapy: Applying Empirically Supported Techniques in Your Practice*. New York, NY: Wiley & Sons, 2003, 361–67.
33. Lang PJ, Melamed BG, Hart J. A psychophysiological analysis of fear modification using an automated desensitization procedure. *J Abnorm Psych* 1970; 76: 220–34.
34. Hays PA, Iwamasa GY. *Culturally Responsive Cognitive-Behavioral Therapy: Assessment, Practice, and Supervision*. Washington, DC: The American Psychological Association, 2006.
35. Organista KC. Cognitive-behavioral therapy with Latinos and Latinas. In Hays PA, Iwamasa GY (Eds.). *Culturally Responsive Cognitive-Behavioral Therapy: Assessment, Practice, and Supervision*. Washington, DC: The American Psychological Association, 2006: 73–96.
36. D'Zurilla TJ, Nezu AM. *Problem-Solving Therapy: A Social Competence Approach to Clinical Intervention, 2nd edition*. New York, NY: Springer Publishing Company, 1999.
37. Winston A. The nuts and bolts of supportive psychotherapy. *Psychiatric News (APA)*2012; 47(12): 6b-7.
38. Winston A, Goldstein M. Theory of supportive psychotherapy. In Gabbard GO, (Ed.) *Textbook of Psychotherapeutic Treatments*. Arlington, VA: American Psychiatric Publishing Inc., 2009: 393–416.
39. Hellerstein DJ, Rosenthal RN, Pinsker H. et al. A randomized prospective study comparing supportive and dynamic therapies: outcome and alliance. *J Psychother Pract Res* 1998; 7: 261–71.
40. Etkin A, Phil M, Pittenger C, Polan HJ, Kandel ER. Toward a neurobiology of psychotherapy: basic science and clinical applications. *J Neuropsychiatry Clin Neurosci* 2005; 17: 145–58.
41. Wampold B. *The Great Psychotherapy Debate: Models, Methods and Findings*. Mahwah NJ: Lawrence Erlbaum & Associates, Inc., 2001.
42. Peterson B, Boivin J, Norre J, Smith C, Thorn P, Wischmann T. An introduction to infertility counseling: a guide to mental health and medical professionals. *J Assist Reprod Genet* 2012; 29(3): 243–48.

Chapter 4

Fertility counseling for couples

Brennan D. Peterson

> Natalie (35) and Lee (37) have been married for six years and have tried unsuccessfully to start a family for the past two. After receiving a combined factor diagnosis, they attempted three cycles of intrauterine insemination (IUI) and two cycles of in vitro fertilization (IVF) – none of which resulted in pregnancy. While their marital relationship was strong at the beginning of treatment, the cumulative stresses of the infertility experience have begun to take a toll on their marital satisfaction. Their differing emotional reactions, communication styles and coping strategies have left each of them feeling alone in the struggle, and the stresses resulting from multiple treatment failures have put a strain on their personal and emotional well-being. Both feel a sense of profound loss and report decreased satisfaction in their sexual relationship. They also feel a sense of isolation from others and cannot agree upon how much information they will share with others regarding their fertility treatments. Natalie reports depressive symptoms and Lee reports a sense of personal failure in dealing with the fertility challenges. Prior to starting a third IVF cycle, they decide to talk with a counselor who specializes in working with couples experiencing the stresses of infertility.

The case presented above is typical of a couple fertility counselors are likely to see, and they present with many of the issues that will be addressed in this chapter. Couples experiencing infertility are faced with a multitude of stressors and unexpected difficulties. While some couples grow closer because of the infertility experience [1], the stress of infertility can erode the strength and stability of even the most satisfied relationship. Fortunately, there have been significant advances in the practice of fertility counseling for couples over the past decade, and counselors are more prepared than ever to deal with the specific challenges couples face when experiencing infertility [2,3].

The purpose of this chapter is to provide fertility counselors with the tools necessary to effectively assess and treat couples experiencing fertility problems so that these couples can improve their relationships, reduce psychological and infertility related distress, and regain control and direction in their lives. The chapter will outline the challenges unique to couples experiencing infertility, and will integrate several case vignettes which portray common profiles of couples who fertility counselors may encounter. Gender differences in how couples communicate and cope with infertility distress will be presented. The chapter will also examine the impact of infertility on a couple's sexual relationship, strategies to help couples best share infertility related treatment information with others and the importance of working through grief and loss. The challenges unique to couples experiencing age-related fertility decline will also be presented, as will the usefulness of mindful meditation as a method for approaching fertility related thoughts and feelings.

General assessment and treatment considerations

Over the past two decades, infertility has increasingly been conceptualized as a stressor that impacts both members of a couple. This is a critical shift in perspective as it challenges the myth that infertility is primarily a woman's issue. It is also consistent with

The addenda referred to in this chapter are available for download at www.cambridge.org/9781107643116

Fertility Counseling: Clinical Guide and Case Studies, ed. Sharon N. Covington. Published by Cambridge University Press.

the prevalence rates of infertility diagnoses which consistently indicate that one-third of the causes of infertility are attributed to female factors, one-third are attributable to male factors and one-third to a combination of male and female factors.

The emotional, physical and financial burdens of infertility and its treatment are high. It has been estimated that 15–20% of couples seeking medical treatments experience emotional distress that warrants psychological counseling [4]. Experts recommend that couple counseling be made available to all patients, at a low threshold, to encourage use and provide reassurance – even if such services are never used [4,5]. Specifically, it has been recommended that these services be available at the beginning and at the end of treatments, times that are especially important as couples are considering varying options as well as potentially coping with significant loss.

The field of fertility counseling encompasses a wide variety of services including the provision of therapeutic counseling, aimed at helping couples cope with the psychosocial challenges of infertility, as well as implications counseling that assists couples in decision-making and clarification regarding third party reproduction [6]. Regardless of the form of counseling used, a comprehensive and accurate assessment is the foundation for effective intervention. Couple counselors can use a combination of assessment measures and interview questions to determine the level of distress the couple is experiencing and inform the type of counseling they will provide.

The form of counseling provided, whether it be therapeutic counseling or implications counseling, will be determined by the needs of the couple, the timing of treatment and the couple's level of distress. Less distressed couples may require brief counseling models that emphasize education, while supportive counseling can be used when couples are more moderately distressed. Longer-term therapeutic counseling can be used when psychological stressors and symptoms are more severe, or after a failed fertility treatment cycle when stress is greatest. Implications counseling, addressing decision-making, treatment options, and third party arrangements (donor insemination, egg donation, or surrogacy), most commonly occurs before treatment begins and is especially relevant for same-sex couples as this is a mandatory element of the fertility treatment. Because the scope of the issues related to implications counseling exceeds this chapter, please refer to Chapters 7–10 and 13 of this book for a more in-depth exploration of these topics.

Assessment measures and interviews

There are several standardized measures that can be used to inform a counselor's assessment. Five that are particularly useful for fertility couple counselors are the Fertility Problem Inventory (FPI) (see Addendum 4.1), the Beck Depression Inventory II (BDI-II), The Beck Anxiety Inventory (BAI), The Fertility Quality of Life (FertilQol) tool and the Dyadic Adjustment Scale (DAS).

Counselors can use the 46-item FPI to assess the level of infertility related stress experienced by both members of the couple [7]. The FPI provides a global infertility stress score in addition to five sub-scale scores including social infertility stress, sexual infertility stress, relationship infertility stress, need for parenthood, and beliefs about living a child-free lifestyle. Counselors can use percentile ranks based on standardized norms to determine the levels of infertility stress in each domain for each member of the couple (see Addendum 4.2). The FPI is particularly useful in noting which areas should be a focus of treatment by informing the counselor of the domains that are causing the most significant stress for each member of the couple, as well as if the couple is congruent on their perceived levels of infertility related stress – a potential key indicator of the couple's depression and marital adjustment rates [8].

The BDI-II and the BAI can be used to provide a snapshot of each member of the couple's depressive and anxiety symptoms [9,10]. Both measures are brief (21 items) and can be completed by each member of the couple. The BDI-II measures depressive symptoms such as sadness, indecisiveness, self-criticism and loss of interest in pleasurable activities. The BAI measures neurophysiological anxiety (e.g., dizziness, shakiness), autonomic anxiety (e.g., sweating), subjective anxiety (e.g., inability to relax, fearing the worst, nervousness) and panic symptoms (e.g., heart racing, difficulty breathing). Both depression and anxiety play an important role in a couple's medical treatments and fertility counseling. Higher rates of patient anxiety have been linked with increased sexual stress [11], and men and women who experience severe depressive symptoms prior to undergoing fertility treatments are at risk of experiencing higher fertility stress levels when compared to those who don't [12]. Furthermore, women with severe depressive symptoms are likely to participate in fewer overall treatment cycles when compared to women who do not report severe depressive symptoms [13].

Fertility counselors can also use FertilQol to assess for the impact of fertility problems and their treatment on quality of life, and the DAS to assess the strength of the couple's relationship. FertiQoL is currently available in 31 different languages, with others in progress, and uses six sub-scales (emotional, mind/body, relational, social, treatment environment and treatment tolerability) to measure the impact of infertility on quality of life [14]. FertiQol can be accessed and scored on the Internet by patients or healthcare providers (http://www.fertistat.com/fertiqol). The DAS measures the global perception of a couple's relationship as well as their levels of satisfaction, cohesion, consensus and their demonstrations of affection [15]. Fertility couple counselors can use the scores from the DAS to determine if the couple's relationship is a resource or a stressor.

In addition to standardized measures, fertility counselors should obtain a detailed psychosocial history from each member of the couple. It is important to ask direct, yet sensitive questions to both members of the couple to obtain a comprehensive picture of the relationship and fertility history. Questions can target information including, but not limited to: the couple's relationship history; fertility treatment history; individual reactions to the fertility problem; gender differences in communication and coping patterns; physical and emotional impact of treatment; impact of infertility on the sexual relationship; current levels of familial and social support; cultural/ethnic background; religious or spiritual factors that influence support or distress; and impact of infertility on employment. Gathering such detailed information from both partners of the couple will assist the counselor in gaining a more complete understanding of the systemic and interactional nature of the couple's response to infertility. An example of a psychosocial intake, specifically designed for fertility counseling with couples, is provided in Table 4.1.

General treatment considerations

Historically, the main role of counselors in fertility clinics was to provide general support for patients in crisis and/or carry out screening before treatment.

Table 4.1 Components of couples psychosocial fertility assessment.

Purpose of Visit
Relationship History • Length of relationship • Children from current or past relationships   · If yes, conceived naturally or from fertility treatment • Length of time trying to start a family

Fertility History
• Length of infertility diagnosis
• Type of infertility (male factor/female factor/combined/unexplained)
• Fertility treatments
  · Medications/surgeries
  · IUI cycles (if yes, how many)
  · IVF treatments (if yes, how many)
• Treatment results
  · Failed treatment, miscarriage, stillbirth, live birth
• Consideration of third party reproduction and other family building options
  · Egg donation, sperm donation, surrogacy, adoption

Impact of Infertility and Treatment • Individual and relational impact of fertility problem • Individual and relational impact of treatment stress (managing medications, doctor visits, egg retrieval, 2-week waiting period) • Communication about infertility (talked about too little, too much, agreement among couple) • Coping patterns in dealing with infertility stress (gender differences) • Impact of infertility on the sexual relationship • Marital benefit (ways the relationship has been strengthened by the infertility experience) • Ways of handling the stresses of treatment failure (if applicable) • Potential concerns about future treatments impacting relationship
Family History • History of infertility in family • Quality of relationships with parents and siblings • Family reaction to infertility – pressure to have children
Employment Factors • Employer stressor or support – employer flexibility to accommodate fertility treatments • Concerns about work disruption and loss of income
Social Support/Social Networks • Friendship networks providing support or stress • Close friends or family having children – couple reactions • Impact of sharing infertility related information with family and friends
Cultural/Religious Factors • Cultural or religious factors that provide support • Cultural or religious factors that add stress or strain
Type of Counseling Needed • Therapeutic counseling • Implications/decision-making counseling
Goals for Counseling • Relational and individual

Counselors have also been called upon to develop and evaluate interventions tailored to specific challenges, such as coping with the two-week waiting period before the pregnancy test and preparing couples for treatment [16]. While these roles continue to be important, fertility counselors are also expected to provide therapeutic counseling aimed at decreasing fertility and psychological distress and improving relationship satisfaction; as well as implications counseling to guide couples through the complexities of decision-making regarding third party reproduction.

There are a variety of areas fertility counselors can target for treatment including: (1) helping the couple to more effectively manage the stresses and demands of fertility treatment; (2) improving couple communication patterns; (3) altering problematic coping patterns which cause negative relational outcomes; (4) preparing for the possibility of failed treatment cycles; (5) assisting couples to reduce sexual distress; (6) understanding social, cultural and religious factors that contextualize the infertility experience; (7) helping couples set appropriate boundaries related to sharing infertility related information with others and (8) facilitating decision-making regarding ending treatment, and considering other family building options such as adoption, third party reproduction, or child-free living.

While this chapter addresses some of these treatment issues in greater detail, it leaves other areas of treatment less defined. Fertility counselors can apply empirically supported models and therapies to these situations, such as cognitive-behavioral couple therapy interventions (e.g., cognitive restructuring) [2] and narrative approaches to working with couples (e.g., externalization) [17] in order to address issues that are only briefly mentioned in the chapter.

Gender differences and fertility counseling

It is essential that fertility counselors be aware that men and women often experience infertility differently. Nearly all studies confirm that women experience greater amounts of fertility related stress than men, and women are more likely than men to report depression and anxiety symptoms [18]. Women are also more likely to take an active role in medical treatment, to respond more poorly following treatment failure and to be more willing to seek counseling. Men, on the other hand, experience fertility stress, but appear less emotionally affected than women and are more willing to consider treatment termination. Women and men are also likely to communicate differently regarding infertility, both within the relationship and to others outside of the relationship.

Gender differences in how men and women experience impaired fertility need to be routinely attended to during the counseling process. Fertility counselors should assess if gender is playing a key role in how each member perceives treatment and how they communicate about fertility related challenges. It is common for infertile couples to become stuck in a circular pattern where partners seek connection and emotional support, yet communicate in ways that lead to emotional invalidation and interpersonal distance. The following case vignette provides a common illustration of how gender differences impact couple communication patterns.

Ian (36) and Karen (35) have been undergoing fertility treatments for one year. After two failed IUI cycles and one failed IVF attempt, the couple sought counseling because of increasing marital conflict. Karen reports high levels of sadness and discouragement regarding the treatment failures. She also reports feeling stifled from expressing these emotions, as Ian avoids infertility related conversations and won't tell her how he feels. She feels that Ian is not taking the infertility as seriously as she is and she privately wishes that it was as hard for him as it was for her. Ian feels that he is trying to make the best out of a very difficult situation. He hates seeing Karen in emotional pain and only wants to help her. He is trying to be helpful in offering solutions when Karen wants to talk about the sadness she feels – he even agrees to do more fertility treatments as soon as possible. However, Karen frequently does not appreciate his problem-solving efforts and communication, telling him he isn't helpful. He reports feeling a sense of helplessness, and he copes by withdrawing from future conversations. Both Ian and Karen report feeling emotionally unsupported and rejected by the other.

Gender-based communication

In this case, Ian and Karen provide an example of a typical couple who are doing their best to support each other, but who are inadvertently stuck in negative communication cycles. Karen is experiencing

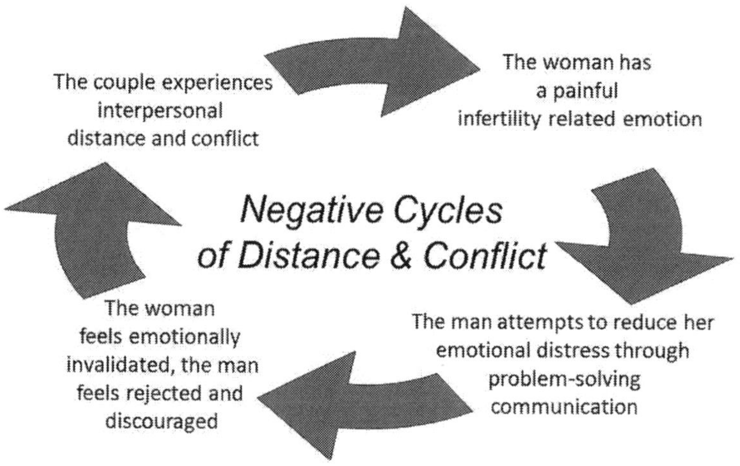

Figure 4.1 Negative gender-based communication in infertile couples.

repeated sadness and discouragement because of treatment failure and Ian is seeking to help her, using a problem-solving strategy. While Karen is seeking a place to share her sadness and receive emotional validation and support, Ian's well-meant problem-solving efforts backfire as Karen feels she has not been heard or supported. This is a challenge for men as they often try to solve the problem of infertility and the sadness it causes their partners, but they ultimately cannot fix it, nor can they fix their partner's sadness and discouragement. Because of this, Ian leaves the interactions feeling frustrated and ineffective while Karen leaves these interactions feeling emotionally invalidated and alone. Instead of experiencing connection and emotional support, the couple now likely experiences interpersonal distance and conflict. Figure 4.1 below shows this common gender-based communication pattern in couples experiencing infertility.

When confronted with this negative communication cycle, the fertility counselor can assist the couple by interrupting the cycle and seeking to create a positive interaction cycle using an intervention called "*the emotional paradox*." This intervention is aimed at helping both members of the couple change their contribution to the cycle, thus creating space for a new, more positive interaction cycle to emerge.

In this instance, the counselor helps Ian to see the limited success of his problem-solving attempts while at the same time asking about the motivations behind his problem-solving behavior. For many men, the core of their problem-solving efforts is a mixture between male-patterned problem-solving socialization, and a desire to protect their partner from experiencing emotional pain. For Ian, the counselor reframes his attempts to fix Karen's pain as protecting behavior and validates his concern for his partner. While validating his protecting behavior, the counselor then asks Ian to let go of these problem-solving communications when Karen is seeking emotional validation. In other words, rather than fix her emotional response to fertility distress, Ian is asked to be emotionally present with Karen while she is experiencing her sadness and simply give her the emotional space she needs to express the depth of her pain and stress. Thus, he paradoxically meets her needs by doing less and ultimately providing emotional support instead of solutions. For many men, implementing this idea requires a tremendous amount of trust in the counselor as it often goes against their natural instincts.

Since couple communication is always systemic, the counselor helps Karen to see her contribution to the problematic communications as well. In this case, the counselor helps Karen identify what she wants and needs from Ian during the times she communicates with him about her infertility related pain. If she is seeking emotional validation rather than a problem-solving discussion, the counselor helps her learn to clearly communicate this to Ian, prior to the discussion, thus improving the chances that both partners' needs will be met. If this intervention is done properly, Ian and Karen can create a positive, interaction cycle where Karen feels emotionally validated, understood and supported, and Ian feels connected and helpful (see Figure 4.2).

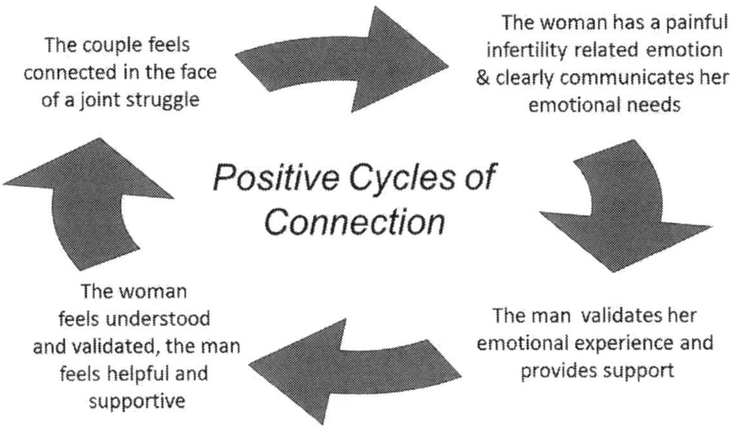

Figure 4.2 Positive gender-based communication in infertile couples.

Gender and coping with infertility

Gender differences also play a large role in the different ways men and women cope with infertility stress [19]. The most common coping strategies used when experiencing infertility stress are social support-seeking, behavioral avoidance, minimization and distancing, heightened emotional self-control, problem-solving and creating a new meaning of infertility through positive reappraisal. Women seek more social support by consulting with medical professionals and by speaking with those who have had, or are experiencing, fertility problems. However, they also use more avoidance strategies to prevent being reminded of the problem, such as avoiding pregnant women or those with young children, a coping strategy that has been consistently linked to increased psychological distress. Men, on the other hand, are more likely to distance themselves from the pain of infertility by minimizing its importance, and are more likely to use problem-solving strategies.

Over the past decade, studies on coping have begun to widen the lens for examining the impact of one partner's coping strategies on the other partner [20]. These studies have consistently found that coping is not only an individual process (i.e., how one partner copes with infertility affects how he or she feels) it is also a relational process (i.e., how one partner copes with infertility affects how his or her partner feels). While this may seem obvious at first glance, men and women often feel that they cope with fertility problems in isolation and their behaviors do not impact their partner.

When working with couples, fertility counselors must be aware that individual coping strategies have a dyadic impact. Counselors can begin to address the relational effects of coping by encouraging both partners to share their reasons behind their preferred individual coping style, and then assessing the relational implications of this coping by asking their partner how they react to that strategy. The goal for fertility counselors, as with negative fertility related communication cycles, is to identify and change coping behaviors that have a negative dyadic impact, by increasing the couple's awareness of problematic coping patterns and by interrupting these patterns and replacing them with coping strategies that have a positive individual and relational impact.

Kyle (35) and Lindsey (33) have come to counseling to address the marital distress they have been experiencing over the past six months. They have been pursuing fertility treatments for the past three years and have experienced several IUI failures and two IVF treatment failures. The couple has found the entire treatment unexpectedly stressful. At first, it was manageable because their strong relationship shielded them from the stresses they encountered. Six months ago, however, the couple began to notice that the different ways in which they coped with treatment failure were beginning to have a negative impact on their relationship. Kyle tended to distance himself from the treatment process, often refusing to talk about it or downplaying the significance of not having a family. Lindsey was hurt by Kyle's reaction; she felt alone in her strong desire for parenthood and developed depressive symptoms. Faced with unhelpful comments and suggestions by family and friends, Lindsey stopped talking to others about her emotional reactions to infertility and felt as if she had no one to turn to. When she turned to Kyle only, it led to increased conflict driven by problematic coping patterns. The couple has always viewed the infertility journey as a joint struggle they could overcome together. Now they worry they might not overcome infertility at all, and the strong, connected relationship they enjoyed before treatments may not return. The couple sought counseling to help them cope with the stresses of infertility, reduce their marital conflict and regain the strength in their relationship they once enjoyed.

This case illustrates the systemic patterns that can result when each partner engages in coping strategies that are individually adaptive, but relationally problematic. Kyle's use of distancing – which involves trying to minimize the significance or the impact of infertility – is related to Lindsey's reports of depression. This dynamic has been supported by research, which found increased female depression and decreased marital satisfaction in couples where men engage in frequent distancing and women do not [21]. While Kyle's use of distancing is helping him manage his reaction to the potential losses they may encounter, it is negatively impacting Lindsey's view of the relationship and the definition of their joint struggle. She now feels that he does not share her strong desire for parenthood and that he is not equally committed to having children, thus increasing her sense of isolation and depression, and decreasing the resourcefulness of the marital relationship. Fertility counselors can seek to improve the couple's relationship satisfaction by addressing the dyadic nature of the couple's coping patterns. By framing the coping process as one that is personally useful for Kyle, but relationally harmful, counselors can help him to use more productive and healthy coping strategies that confront the pain he feels related to treatment failure, while also promoting new, more positive systemic interactions that will allow for growth and adjustment in his partner.

Women can also use coping strategies that have a positive impact on themselves, but have a negative impact on their partner. In this case, Lindsey has begun to cope through heightened emotional self-control by keeping her feelings to herself, and attempting to keep her feelings from interfering with other things in her life. In couples where women report a high need for emotional self-control and privacy and men describe low needs for control and privacy, male partners report increased marital distress [21]. This extreme difference in approach to managing infertility stress may lead to pressure, from the woman, not to disclose infertility information to others – precluding the man from obtaining external support, while the woman simultaneously fails to receive any of the benefits associated with sharing her emotional experience. As a result of such pressure and emotional restriction, couples may encounter increased marital disagreements and conflict. Once this systemic pattern occurs, the relationship ceases to be a safe harbor against outside stressors, and each member of the couple may be less likely to communicate with their partner about their infertility stress and thus fail to receive the benefits of partner support.

Fertility counselors can help couples, such as Lindsey and Kyle, who are stuck in such patterns to see that excluding their partner from hearing about their significant emotional distress can create a potential barrier to developing emotional closeness and intimacy, which are keys to decreasing marital conflict and stress. To change the problematic coping pattern, each partner must feel heard and understood regarding their motivations behind the use of individual coping strategies, and receive validation and understanding from their partner. Once this happens, the counselor can work with the couple to stop engaging in old coping strategies and develop more productive and relationally beneficial coping patterns.

Infertility and the sexual relationship

The stresses of the infertility experience can have a powerful impact on a couple's sexual relationship, and sexual difficulties reported by couples are much more likely to be the consequence, rather than the cause, of an infertility diagnosis. Women commonly report decreased sexual desire, sexual satisfaction and sexual desirability, while men commonly report decreased sexual desire, erectile dysfunction and feelings of marginalization when the sole purpose of sex is for conception [22]. As with coping strategies, sexual stress in one partner can impact sexual stress in the other, supporting an emerging view that sexual dysfunction is a disorder of the couple as opposed to a disorder of the individual [23]. Ironically for couples, increased sexual strain in the relationship can result in reduced frequency of sexual relations which lowers the chance of achieving a pregnancy.

The specific elements of the couple's sexual relationship should be carefully examined during the counselor's assessment procedure and through an evaluation of the couples scores on the FPI's sexual-stress sub-scale, which measures the degree to which a couple's sexual relationship has changed and acts as a stressor. If one or both members of the couple is experiencing heightened levels of sexual stress, counselors should develop plans to address this issue in more detail. The counselor can assess if both members of the couples are equally or unequally distressed, and also assess if the couple recognizes the potential difference between "procreational" and "recreational" sex (e.g., sex for the sole purposes of pregnancy, compared to sex for pleasure, intimacy and connection).

One of the most basic interventions counselors can use is to normalize sexual stress by providing the couple with educational information that addresses the impact of infertility on the sexual relationship. This can normalize and reduce the impact of current sexual stress and prevent future stresses from getting worse [24]. Counselors can also inform clients that sexual stress is impacted not only by infertility, but by other health and lifestyle factors including general stress, anxiety, poor nutrition and lack of exercise [22]. Counselors can provide specific suggestions, such as paradoxically taking a break from sexual relations when they are not required to do so for medical treatments [11]. Such breaks can provide couples with time to examine why the sexual relationship has become strained, and make plans to improve it once the stresses of fertility treatment are past.

Unfortunately, for many couples, there does not seem to be an optimal time to focus on improving the sexual relationship once the infertility journey has begun. During fertility treatments, couples are commonly too focused on achieving a pregnancy to work on this issue and have little interest in recreational sex. If the couple achieves pregnancy, they are often nervous that sex may cause pregnancy complications or miscarriage. And following the birth of a child, couples are often too overwhelmed to renew their sexual relationship because they are dealing with the stresses and demands of parenting. However, if the sexual relationship is not given priority and attention by couples, there is no guarantee it will improve or return to pre-infertility levels of satisfaction. In fact, it is not uncommon for the stress on the sexual relationship to continue long after treatments end [22]. Thus, an important part of working with couples undergoing sexual stress is to help them reclaim the intimacy and closeness they once achieved through sex, prior to the infertility diagnosis.

Sharing infertility related information with family and friends

A frequent component of couple counseling involves discussing to what degree and with whom the couple shares information about their infertility related struggles. While some couples may agree on how best to do this, others may disagree, which can lead to relational strain. Counselors can help couples openly discuss these issues, promote acceptance of differences in partner disclosure patterns, and help couples find mutually agreeable strategies to disclose their infertility related struggles to family and friends.

When a couple is first diagnosed with infertility, they may find that their level of sharing with family and friends is highly open because they are seeking support and they are optimistic about their chances of success. However, if multiple treatments fail, well-intending family and friends may try to provide unrealistically positive reassurance that is not useful for the couple and inevitably promotes a more closed position in the future. Disclosing treatment failure over and over again to inquiring friends and family can be overwhelmingly painful for couples. Thus, communicating in advance about how couples might handle sharing or not sharing information in the event of a treatment failure can be an important counseling goal.

Christopher and Sara were having difficulty agreeing on the best way to share infertility related information with family and friends. Following a third failed IVF treatment, the couple realized the old strategy of telling each inquiring person was too overwhelmingly painful and emotionally exhausting. After a thoughtful discussion with their fertility counselor, they talked about how best to inform family and friends while considering the needs and disclosure preferences of each other. The couples discussed many alternatives – each posing their preferred method and why they felt most comfortable with it. They finally agreed to create a joint email to be sent to all of their friends and family that informed them of the IVF treatment failure, while also setting a boundary that they didn't want to share any more information about the fertility process unless they, themselves, brought it up.

Here, the solution of writing a joint email illustrates the mutuality of the couple's efforts to work together to support each other and communicate effectively with family and friends. In addition, the boundary setting of managing future infertility related communications can be an empowering task for the couple who feels powerless in the wake of treatment failure. An actual example of a letter written by a couple who received counseling from the author has been included in Addendum 4.3.

Loss and therapeutic rituals

The number of losses a couple can experience during the infertility journey can be overwhelming, and helping couples share and grieve these losses can be a vital component of couple counseling. In the early stages of the infertility journey, losses can range from changes in family and social support networks, to a loss of spontaneity and passion in their sexual relationship. As couples move through fertility treatments, the loss of control over their daily lives become more paramount. Losses become most profound if couples experience failed fertility treatments, or if couples experience a miscarriage or stillbirth following a successful pregnancy.

From one perspective, repeated treatment failure and miscarriage might be conceptualized as a series of losses, and couples who fail to grieve these losses are at risk for increased psychological distress. Fertility counselors can help couples verbally express the pain of their losses by asking questions that help couples make contact with previously avoided thoughts and emotions, and allow them to explore these during the counseling sessions. Experiential exercises such as letter writing, expressive art therapy and the empty chair technique can be used to encourage emotional expression and grief resolution. Counselors can caringly ask questions like, "How did you feel when you learned about the latest treatment failure?" or "Can you describe what it was like for you when you decided to stop treatments without having a child?" These questions are highly sensitive and will likely evoke powerful emotional reactions in the couple. Fertility counselors must provide adequate time for couples to emotionally process the implications of such questions. Counselors should validate the couple's emotional reactions while helping them understand that experiencing strong emotions of sadness and grief is a necessary part of the healing process.

Therapeutic rituals can also facilitate grieving for infertility related losses, such as miscarriage, stillbirth or the inability to conceive. Elements of therapeutic rituals build on existing cultural ceremonies and traditions that recognize expected and predictable life-cycle transitions such as anniversaries, graduations and funerals [25]. However, rituals for infertility are unique in that they bring to light previously invisible and stigmatized losses by providing a tangible context for mourning and grief. For example, a ritual acknowledging the anniversary of their final failed IVF attempt or decision to stop treatment can provide a context for mourning where new meaning of the infertility experience can emerge.

Counseling couples with age-related infertility

Lucas (42) and Maria (39) are experiencing infertility after trying to have children for the past two years. The doctors attributed their inability to get pregnant to age-related fertility decline. Maria has a master's degree in business (MBA) and works as a Chief Financial Officer (CFO) for a small software company. Lucas has a degree in graphic design and works as a web designer. They are in excellent health, exercise regularly, eat a balanced diet and have normal BMI ratings. Neither partner uses cigarettes or has a history of sexually transmitted diseases. They have been married for 10 years and planned to have two children. After Maria received a highly sought after promotion two years ago, they felt ready to begin trying to have a child. Maria was pregnant within the first six months, but had a miscarriage during the first trimester. After being unable to get pregnant again, they bypassed IUI treatments and underwent three unsuccessful IVF treatments. The couple was shocked to learn they might have difficulty having a child due to advanced female age. Maria has experienced regret and sadness. Lucas is struggling to keep his wife's spirits high, but he also has struggled with his own feelings of despondency as he realizes there may be no solution to the infertility and he may not become a biological father. Both Lucas and Maria are angry that they didn't realize the impact of age on her fertility, and have begun to feel guilty for not knowing this. They have also begun to fight about their previous career choices and argue over why they did not try to conceive sooner.

This case study illustrates a typical couple experiencing age-related fertility decline. This couple is usually in their late 30s or early 40s, is educated and achievement-oriented, and often has intentionally delayed childbearing to pursue other life-goals and pursuits. These couples are more likely to be found in developed countries where delayed childbearing reflects changing social norms of postponing marriage and securing education and economic stability before attempting conception. In the United States, for example, the proportion of first births to women aged 35–39 has increased 50% over the past two decades [26]. Furthermore, studies throughout the world have consistently found that educated and career-oriented men and women lack an awareness of the impact age has on fertility [27,28]. In the United States, for example, 67% of undergraduate university women and 81% of undergraduate university men inaccurately believed female fertility markedly declines after the age of 40, with one-third of women and nearly half of men believing this decline takes place after the age of 44 – an age at which a woman's fertility window is likely at an end, and she has only a 3–5% chance of delivering a live birth using the most advanced reproductive treatments [28,29].

Fertility counselors should be aware that because of decreased egg quality and quantity, female fertility begins to decline as early as 28 years of age and markedly declines at approximately age 37 [28]. In addition, advanced maternal age at first birth is also associated with increased rates of miscarriage, stillbirth and health risks for the mother and child [30]. Advanced paternal age is also a significant issue and has been associated with decreased fertility and increased incidence of miscarriage, as well as birth defects, schizophrenia and autism in a couple's offspring [31,32]. While couples dealing with age-related fertility decline will face the same challenges as other couples detailed throughout this chapter, they may also experience some unique challenges including self-blame, guilt and marital conflict revolving around how the postponement decisions were made. (See Chapter 11 on older patients seeking treatment for further information.) In the example above, a discussion with Lucas and Maria about when they planned to have children, and how their education and career circumstances played a role in their decisions, will be a vital part of the counseling process.

Lucas and Maria's goal-oriented and high-achieving personalities – which have been strengths throughout their lives – may, instead, be a liability to them during the infertility experience. Because infertility is a long-term, largely uncontrollable stressor, Lucas and Maria may struggle with the lack of control they face when dealing with it. In fact, this may be the first problem they have faced that cannot be solved by working harder. While they can work diligently in researching infertility, setting up doctor's appointments, committing to the medication regimen, and keeping medical appointments faithfully, a successful outcome is still largely out of their control. Because of this, couples such as Lucas and Maria commonly feel anger, frustration, guilt, helplessness, and ultimately question the fairness of life and the meaning and value of their past decisions.

Fertility counselors can assist couples in this situation by delicately asking questions about the process and context of prior decision-making. Both men and women need to feel heard and understood by their partner – particularly as it relates to their motivations for delaying childbearing. Were Lucas and Maria in agreement regarding how they perceived the timing of having a child, or were there times when there was disagreement when one partner wanted to delay because of a work opportunity or life situation? Helping couples share their history in this context is important. If Lucas and Maria demonstrated congruence (e.g., agreement) related to how they perceived the timing of the future childbearing decisions, they may have an easier time managing the stressful outcomes they encounter. However, if one partner encouraged a delay while the other felt strongly they should begin sooner, the couple may find themselves experiencing increased tension or conflict in the relationship until this issue is discussed and resolved.

A second, more subtle therapeutic issue that may arise is secondary infertility (when a couple with one biological child is unable to have a second). Because secondary infertility can be just as disruptive as primary infertility [33], counselors can help the couple examine their infertility distress in the context of being unable to have a second child and what this may mean for their future family. Even if Lucas and Maria have one child, they may still not be able to achieve their desired family size. In a recent study of undergraduate students in the United States, only 1% of participants wanted one child, while the strong majority of participants wanted two to three children [28]. Counselors can ask couples about their motivations to have a second child, about how they view the role and importance of a sibling in the life and development of their child, and about what their lives might look like if their future family size consists of only one child.

Secondary infertility may also occur with remarried couples who are experiencing infertility in their newly formed marital system [34]. For these couples, the secondary infertility often is the result of one's spouse's decision to have a vasectomy or a tubal ligation after having children in a prior relationship. For remarried couples, they often begin trying to have a child within the first two years of the union, while the stabilization of the blended family unit takes approximately five to seven years [34]. Thus, the overlap of this timing can take a toll on the couple's relationship, stressing a family system that is not yet cohesive and is vulnerable to disruption. In addition to helping these couples with the stresses of infertility, fertility counselors should also be aware of the challenges that arise in a newly formed blended family. Even if the couple has been together several years, counselors must help both members of the couple explore the implications of past marital relationships, prior reproductive decisions and the status of their current family unit as they relate to the stress of infertility.

Lastly, it is important for couple counselors to help men and women such as Lucas and Maria to understand the limitations of fertility treatments for those in their late 30s and early 40s (or older), as well as the possibility of family building through egg donation or third party reproduction. Fertility counselors should educate couples that even the most advanced medical treatments often cannot overcome age-related decline in fertility. For instance, when a couple delays childbearing between ages 30 and 35, reproductive technologies can compensate for only half of the births lost due to natural decreases in fertility during this time period [35,36]. Helping couples make informed decisions based on their age and treatment success rates is an important clinical responsibility for the fertility counselor. It is very likely that Lucas and Maria have unrealistic expectations about the success rates of treatments. Recent data from 54 countries around the world estimate a 22% live delivery birth rate for patients using IVF [37]. In the United States, the average live birth rate per cycle of IVF, using fresh non-donor eggs, is 30%, with a success rate of 12% for women ages 41–42, and only 5% for women ages 43–44 [29].

Mindfulness

When a couple experiences infertility stress, their minds can become dominated by negative and aversive infertility related thoughts and emotions. These are painful reminders of their losses and, as such, men and women will avoid and suppress them, which paradoxically can make them more powerful and aversive. Because of this, couples may actively avoid situations that trigger infertility related thoughts and emotions, and thus experience significant disruption to their lives in an effort to prevent increased psychological distress.

Mindfulness (i.e., mindful meditation) is a clinical intervention fertility counselors can use to help couples who feel overwhelmed by the pain of their infertility related thoughts. Mindfulness balances awareness of the present moment with nonjudgmental and compassionate acceptance of one's experience. This allows one to respond more flexibly and less literally to thoughts and emotions by creating a healthy distance between oneself and one's internal experiences. For couples experiencing infertility, this struggle is especially salient [38]. For example, instead of trying to dispute or otherwise change thoughts such as "It's unfair that we can't have a baby," or "I can't stand this infertility stress any longer," couples learn to acknowledge these thoughts as mere thoughts that can simply be observed, but that don't need to be believed or acted upon.

Emery (35) and Matthew (36) have been married for seven years and have been trying to start a family for the past four. The couple has attempted multiple cycles of clomiphene medication treatment, one IUI treatment and two IVF treatments. The couple was referred to counseling after the latest failed IVF attempt when Emery reported heightened infertility related stress levels and depressive symptoms. The last year has been particularly difficult for both members of the couple as Matthew's sister had a child and Emery found she could neither hold her niece nor spend time with her sister-in-law. Additionally, this has put a strain on Emery and Matthew's relationship as Matthew feels torn between his wife and his sister. Emery also finds it impossible to be in the presence of friends and their children, and her stress and anger about her infertility has begun to escalate. Emery and Matthew report that they cannot control nor handle the powerful negative infertility related thoughts they have both recently had.

When presented with the idea of observing painful fertility related thoughts and emotions, rather than actively avoiding them, couples such as Emery and Matthew are often skeptical. To help couples initially consider this idea, fertility counselors can have the couple participate in an experiential exercise using a Chinese finger trap. In the case of Emery and Matthew, the counselor asks the couple to put one finger in each end of the trap, and then attempt to remove their fingers. The couple inevitably finds their fingers trapped, and the more they struggle to get their fingers out, the tighter and more restrictive the finger trap becomes. To get out of the trap, the couple must do something counterintuitive – they must push their fingers towards each other, rather than pulling away. Thus, this paradoxical movement helps free them from the constraints they were experiencing. This metaphor provides a basis for approaching painful infertility related thoughts and emotions in a different manner than in the past, by helping couples see the possible effects of "moving into" the stress, rather than pulling away from it.

The concepts of mindfulness and compassionate acceptance should be introduced to Emery and Matthew early in the counseling. Basic five-minute centering exercises can be conducted at the beginning of each counseling session, and counselors can incorporate more advanced exercises during the middle and end of treatment (see Addendum 4.4 for scripted mindfulness exercises specifically adapted for infertility related stress). The counselor can also assign daily mindfulness exercises, for practice at home during the week, using a variety of easy-to-use online resources (i.e., UCLA Mindfulness Awareness Research Center http://marc.ucla.edu; fertility apps available for purchase on iTunes). The use of mindfulness as an effective component of fertility counseling has been supported by research which found that an integrative body–mind–spirit (I-BMS) intervention, which included mindfulness-based training and practice, reduced anxiety in women undergoing their first IVF treatment, and also increased patient tranquility and marital satisfaction [39].

By practicing daily mindfulness exercises that emphasize compassionate acceptance of their fertility related stress, couples such as Emery and Matthew can begin to reduce the negative influence of their thoughts and increase their flexibility in responding to these thoughts – even in the presence of powerful infertility related emotions. The use of mindfulness can also help Emery and Matthew increase the amount of self-compassion they feel about their infertility struggle, which can reduce self-blame and unneeded psychological suffering. By reducing the power of negative infertility related thoughts and emotions, they become more tolerable and manageable. When the couple realizes this, and has increased their capacity to move toward the fertility stress instead of away from it, psychological flexibility is increased. Thus, they are freed to act in different, more positive ways, which can ultimately lead to healthier cycles of interaction and communication.

Conclusion and personal reflections

The purpose of this chapter is to provide a framework for understanding the unique challenges faced by couples experiencing infertility [40]. Fertility counselors can help couples understand the impact of gender on infertility related communication patterns and coping strategies. They can also increase couples' awareness of the impact of infertility stress on their sexual relationship, help them find ways to plan for how to share infertility related treatment information with others and assist them in grieving the many losses associated with the infertility experience. Being aware of the impact of age on fertility is also of vital importance in working with couples experiencing the challenges of age-related fertility decline. Finally, fertility counselors can use mindful meditation to help couples approach stressful fertility related thoughts and feelings, thus breaking negative cycles of avoidance and emotional distress.

On a personal level, I consider it a privilege to work with couples as a fertility counselor. I have great compassion for these couples as their lives have been so unexpectedly disrupted by the multitude of stresses that accompany an infertility diagnosis. I have been privileged to witness, first-hand, the courage it takes to face the emotional suffering and psychological distress that is so common for couples during this experience. I have also learned about the power of resilience as couples work through tremendous difficulty only to discover newfound strength, fortitude and determination. It is my hope that fertility counselors will be able to use the ideas presented in this chapter to help couples regain the emotional closeness and intimacy they once enjoyed, and to help them create new meaning and connections in their lives as a result of the infertility experience.

References

1. Peterson BD, Pirritano M, Block JM, Schmidt L. Marital benefit and coping strategies in men and women undergoing unsuccessful fertility treatments over a 5-year period. *Fertil and Steril.* 2011 Apr: 95(5); 1759–63.
2. Newton CR. Counseling the infertile couple. In: Covington SN, Burns LH, editors. *Infertility Counseling: A Comprehensive Handbook for Clinicians.* 2nd edn. New York: Cambridge University Press; 2006, pp. 143–55.
3. Peterson BD, Boivin J, Norré J, Smith C, Thorn P, Wischmann T. An introduction to infertility counseling: a guide for mental health and medical professionals. *J Assist Reprod Genet.* 2012 Jan; 29(3): 243–48.
4. Boivin J, Scanlan L, Walker SM. Why are infertile couples not using psychosocial counseling?*Hum Reprod.* 1999 May; 14(5): 1384–91.
5. Wischmann T, Scherg H, Strowitzki T, Verres R. Psychosocial characteristics of women and men attending infertility counseling. *Hum Reprod.* 2009; 24(2): 378–85.
6. Canadian Fertility and Andrology Society Counselling Special Interest Group. Assisted human reproduction counselling practice guidelines. 2009.
7. Newton CR, Sherrard MA, Glavac I. The fertility problem inventory: measuring perceived infertility-related stress. *Fertil and Steril.* 1999 Jul; 72(1): 54–62.
8. Peterson BD, Newton CR, Rosen KH. Examining congruence between partners perceived infertility-related stress and its relationship to marital adjustment and depression in infertile couples. *Fam Process.* 2003 Mar; 42(1): 59–70.
9. Beck AT, Steer RA, Brown GK. *Beck Depression Inventory: Manual.* 2nd edn. San Antonio: Harcourt Brace, 1996.
10. Beck AT, Brown G, Epstein N, Steer RA. An inventory for measuring clinical anxiety: psychometric properties. *J Consult Clin Psychol.* 1988; 6: 893–7.
11. Peterson BD, Newton C, Feingold T. Anxiety and sexual stress in men and women undergoing infertility treatment. *Fertil and Steril.* 2007 Oct; 88(4): 911–14.
12. Peterson BD, Sejbaek CS, Pirritano M, Schmidt L. Are severe depressive symptoms associated with infertility-related distress in individuals and their partners? *Hum Reprod.* 2014 Jan; 29(1): 76–82.
13. Sejbaek C, Hageman I, Pinborg A, Hougaard C, Schmidt L. Incidence of depression and influence of depression on the number of treatment cycles and births in a national cohort of 42 880 women treated with ART. *Hum Reprod.* 2013 Apr; 28(4): 1100–09.
14. Boivin J, Takefman J, Braverman A. The fertility quality of life (FertiQol) tool: development and general psychometric properties. *Fertil and Steril.* 2011 Aug; 96(2): 409–15.
15. Spanier GB. Measuring dyadic adjustment: new scales for assessing the quality of marriage and similar dyads. *J Marriage Fam.* 1976 Feb; 38(1): 15–28.
16. Lancaster D; Boivin J. A feasibility study of a brief coping intervention (PRICI) for the waiting period before a pregnancy test during fertility treatment. *Hum Reprod.* 2008; 23(10): 2299–2307.
17. Diamond R, Kezur D, Meyers M, Scharf CN, Weinshel M. *Couple Therapy for Infertility.* New York: The Guilford Press; 1999.
18. Griel AL, Slausen-Belvins K, McQuillan J. The experience of infertility: a review of recent literature. *Social Health Illn.* 2010 Jan; 32(1): 140–62.
19. Peterson BD, Newton CR, Rosen KH, and Skaggs GE. Gender differences in how men and women who are referred for IVF cope with infertility stress. *Hum Reprod.* 2006 Sep; 21(9): 2443–49.
20. Peterson BD, Pirritano M, Christensen U, Boivin J, Block J, Schmidt L. The longitudinal impact of partner coping in couples following 5 years of unsuccessful fertility treatments. *Hum Reprod.* 2009 Mar; 24(7): 1656–64.
21. Peterson BD, Newton CR, Rosen KH, Schulman RS. Coping process of couples experiencing infertility. *Fam Relat.* 2006 Apr; 55(2): 227–39.
22. Daniluk JC, Frances-Fischer JE. A sensitive way to address your infertile patients' concerns. *Sex Reprod Menopause.* 2009; 7(1): 3–7.
23. Nelson CJ, Shindel A, Naughton C, Ohebshalom M, Mulhall J. Prevalence and predictors of sexual problems, relationship stress, and depression in female partners of infertile couples. *J Sex Med.* 2008; 5: 1907–14.
24. Burns LH. Sexual counseling and infertility. In: Covington SN, Burns LH, editors. *Infertility Counseling: A Comprehensive Handbook for Clinicians.* 2nd edn. New York: Cambridge University Press; 2006, pp. 212–35.
25. Imber-Black E. Creating meaningful rituals for new life cycle transitions. In: McGoldrick M, Carter B, Garcia-Preto N, editors. *The Expanded Family Life*

Cycle: Individual, Family, and Social Perspectives. 4th edn. Boston: Allyn & Bacon; 2011, pp. 429–39.

26. United States. Martin J, Hamilton B, Sutton P, Ventura S, Menacker F, Kermeyer S, Matthews TJ. Births: final data for 2006. *National Vital Statistics Reports.* Hyattsville, MD: National Center for Health Statistics; 2009.
27. Lampic C, Skoog Svanberg A, Karlstrom P, Tyden T. Fertility awareness, intentions concerning childbearing, and attitudes towards parenting among female and male academics. *Hum Reprod.* 2006 Feb; 21(2): 558–64.
28. Peterson BD, Pirritano M, Tucker L, Lampic C. Fertility awareness and parenting attitudes among American male and female undergraduate university students. *Hum Reprod.* 2012 Mar; 27(5): 1375–82.
29. United States. Centers for Disease Control and Prevention. Assisted Reproductive Technologies Report: National ART Success Rates. 2011 *National Summary.* Atlanta, GA: Centers for Disease Control and Prevention; 2011.
30. Tough S, Tofflemire K, Benzies K, Fraser-Lee N, Newburn-Cook C. Factors influencing childbearing and knowledge of prenatal risks among Canadian women and men. *Matern Child and Health J.* 2007 Mar; 11(2): 189–98.
31. Bray I, Gunnell D, Smith, GD. Advanced paternal age: how old is too old? *J Epidemiol Community Health.* 2006; 60: 851–53.
32. Hultman CM, Sandin S, Levine SZ, Lichtenstein P, Reichenberg A. Advancing paternal age and risk of autism: new evidence from a population-based study and a meta-analysis of epidemiological studies. *Mol Psychiatry.* 2011; 16: 1203–12.
33. Simons, HF. Secondary infertility. In: Burns LH, Covington SN, editors. *Infertility Counseling: A Comprehensive Handbook for Clinicians.* New York: The Parthenon Publishing Group; 2000, p. 313–22.
34. Hafkin N, Covington S. The remarried family and infertility. In: Burns LH, Covington SN, editors. *Infertility Counseling: A Comprehensive Handbook for Clinicians.* New York: The Parthenon Publishing Group; 2000, p. 297–312.
35. Leridon H. Can assisted reproduction technology compensate for the natural decline in fertility with age? A model assessment. *Hum Reprod.* 2004 Jul; 19(7): 1548–53.
36. Schmidt L, Sobotka T, Bentzen JG, Andersen AN. Demographic and medical consequences of the postponement of parenthood. *Hum Reprod Update.* 2012 Feb; 18(1): 29–43.
37. Nygren, K, Sullivan E, Zegers-Horchschild F, Mansour R, Ishihara O, Adamson D, et al. International Committee for Monitoring Assisted Reproductive Technology (ICMART) world report: assisted reproductive technology 2003. *Fertil and Steril.* 2011 Jun; 95(7): 2209–22.
38. Peterson BD, Eifert GH. Using acceptance and commitment therapy to treat infertility stress. *Cogn Behav Pract.* 2011 Nov; 18(4): 577–87.
39. Chan CH, Chan CL, Ng EH, Ho PC, Chan TH, Lee GL, et al. Incorporating spirituality in psychosocial group intervention for women undergoing in vitro fertilization: a prospective randomized controlled study. *Psychol Psychother.* 2012 Dec; 85(4): 356–73.
40. Peterson BP, Gold L, Feingold, T. The experience and influence of infertility: considerations for couple counselors. *Fam J Alex Va.* 2007 Jul; 15(3):251–57.

Chapter 5

Spirituality in fertility counseling

Eileen A. Dombo and Megan Flood

"Be fruitful and multiply"....

Genesis 1:28

The commandment to "be fruitful and multiply" is seen several times in the Old Testament. As part of the creation story in the Book of Genesis, God gives this commandment to both Adam and Eve, and Noah and his sons. This religious teaching informs much of Judeo-Christian messages on the subjects of marriage, childbirth and family. Also throughout the Old Testament are stories of infertility; of women like Rachel, Sarah and Hannah who could not have children without God's intervention. The story of Hannah is a particularly powerful one, as she is the only wife of Elkanah who could not become pregnant. Her husband wants to see that Hannah can be happy just by being married to him; that should be enough for her, but it is not. Hannah prays to God time and again to allow her to bear a son, and promises to give that son to God. She does give birth to her son Samuel, and keeps her promise to God by turning him over to the temple to become a priest. Because she keeps her promise to God, she is rewarded with three more sons and two daughters. This story of prayer, perseverance and keeping promises made to God sends a powerful message to individuals and couples facing challenges to their own fertility [1,2].

Introduction

As we see in the Old Testament as well as many other sacred texts, spirituality has been shown to be a source of comfort and support during times of distress. One's spiritual practices can help create meaning and bring strength to situations where it is normal to feel powerless and helpless, such as the struggle of infertility. Additionally, an individual's religious or spiritual traditions can influence the meaning they make of the experience of infertility, and the options they are willing to consider [3]. Given this, it is hard to believe that, until fairly recently, therapists were not encouraged to discuss religion or spirituality with clients. Integrating the spiritual dimension of the person into treatment was thought to raise difficult ethical situations and blur boundaries between mental health treatment and pastoral guidance [4]. Over the past 25 years, we have seen an increased focus on the spiritual dimension. We also are aware of the need to discuss religion and spirituality with clients in an ethical manner [5].

This chapter will explore ways to address spirituality in fertility counseling, offer clinicians guidance on how to understand the degree of spirituality or religiosity in their clients' lives, and address how or if they are related to the challenges of infertility. For the purposes of this chapter, spirituality is defined as the search for meaning, purpose and connection with self, others, the universe or a higher power outside the self. This may or may not be expressed through religious practices or formal institutions. Religion, considered one expression of spirituality, is an organized, systematic set of beliefs, practices and traditions related to spirituality, which is shared by a community or social institution [6]. These issues are explored in this chapter.

World religions and infertility

Most religious teachings speak to the significance of procreation, as well as the gender role expectations for men and women to become fathers and mothers. Through this lens, infertility can impact the self and relational identities of people wishing to become parents. Therefore, we see the risk for both a crisis of identity and of faith [7]. The relationship between religion and help-seeking for infertility is complicated [8],

Fertility Counseling: Clinical Guide and Case Studies, ed. Sharon N. Covington. Published by Cambridge University Press.

and continues to be a growing area for inquiry among doctors, therapists and others in helping roles [9]. Clinicians treating individuals and couples grappling with the challenges of infertility are advised to approach this dynamic with an "informed not knowing" stance, which will be explicated later in this chapter.

The body of scholarly literature on the subject of infertility and the role religion plays in decisions regarding intervention has been limited until recently. Layne demonstrates that, regardless of faith tradition, people who experience infertility may feel a sense of shame rooted in specific religious teachings [10]. At the same time, religious practices can help to manage and alleviate that stigma. There are several important writings that shed light on the attitudes of specific faith communities with regard to infertility and its treatment. In some cultures, childlessness may be experienced as punishment for some previous transgression [11]. Exploring the lived experience of Orthodox Jews in New York, Kahn describes the current rabbinical debates about what interventions are and are not permitted [12]. Important considerations include evaluating the suffering of the couple as they struggle with the principle of family and Jewish integrity. Assisted reproductive technologies (ART) are viewed as an aid to fulfilling the commandment to be fruitful and multiply; therefore Rabbis may permit many forms ART with certain limitations or accommodations. This is consistent with previous research showing that people of Jewish faith tend to be more approving of the use of ART than those of the Christian faiths [13].

Exploring the tension between science and religion, Roberts investigates the ways Catholic physicians in Ecuador reconcile religious teachings with scientific endeavors. The Roman Catholic Church has long held clear prohibitions against ART. The Vatican asserts that it represents human intervention in a domain that belongs to God alone. As scientists in a predominately Catholic culture, these practitioners overcome this divide through their spirituality. Many hold beliefs that God "is in the laboratory" and "is taking direct action" through science [14, p. 509]. They pray during procedures, and believe that, ultimately, God decides which procedures are successful [14].

Moving beyond Judeo-Christian religions, Hindus in India have been grappling with the Western view of infertility. Here ART is employed to assist God, and outcomes from treatment are not guaranteed. Many couples interviewed in Bharadwaj's research speak of Hindu gods and goddesses they pray to for divine intervention. They recount being told by doctors and nurses to "leave things to God" after treatments [15, p. 456]. Many clinics have icons and pictures of patron saints, gods and goddesses, and some are even named for them. Pairing spiritual practices with science is seen as a form of *parallel science*. Like the Ecuadorian Catholic practitioners, Hindu practitioners in India speak of prayer as part of their scientific process. For those unable to conceive a child, the Hindu concept of *karma* can be a source of comfort; some women see their destiny to be childless as karma, or "destiny for a higher purpose in life" [11, p. 751].

Islamic law prohibits ART that involves any third party donation, as it violates teachings of the holy Q'uran related to adultery, incest and the integrity of biological descent. However, there are attempts to address this through legislation that would allow for embryo donation [16]. This has arisen through differences in beliefs between Sunni and Shi'ite Muslims in countries such as Iran, Egypt and Lebanon. Because of the cultural value placed on paternal lineage and property inheritance, there is less support for sperm donation than embryo donation [17].

African traditional religion places a strong emphasis on interconnectedness. Infertility experienced by an individual or couple impacts the entire clan. Many believe that ancestors who are not properly respected through certain rituals are angered, and curse those family members with infertility. Therefore, there are important cultural and spiritual practices that must be carried out as part of any intervention for members of these cultures. As the majority of Africans report using traditional healing before approaching more conventional medical care, these practices should be explored when working with African clients in treatment for infertility [11,18].

It is vital for clinicians to be educated about the role of religion and spirituality in the lives of clients who are coping with infertility and considering seeking help to address it. Higher levels of religiosity have been found to be associated with lower levels of acceptance of childlessness, and higher levels of intent to seek assistance with solutions to infertility [8]. It is crucial that clinicians avoid making assumptions about infertility and spirituality that may or may not apply to their specific client system. A summary of the major world religions' positions on ART can be found in Table 5.1.

Table 5.1 World religions and views on assisted reproductive technology.

Religion	Permitted	Forbidden	Questionable
Anglican Church	Most forms of ART	None are strictly forbidden	MPR
Buddhism	Most forms of ART	MPR	SD related by blood ED SD
Eastern Orthodox	Only permits medicine and surgical interventions	All forms of ART	
Hinduism	Most forms of ART	MPR, SUR	
Islam	Any form of ART that does not include a third party ED or SD	ED SD SUR	Embryo donation to infertile spouses
Judaism	Most forms of ART that does not include a third party ED or SD		ED, SD, MPR, ZIFT
Mormonism	AI and IVF that does not include a third party ED or SD	ED SD SUR	No formal statements about other forms of ART
Protestantism*	AI, IVF	MPR	ED, SD, EMBD, GIFT, ZIFT
Roman Catholicism	GIFT	ED, EMB, IVF, MPR, SD, SUR, ZIFT	AI within married couples

* includes Baptist, Methodist, Lutheran, Presbyterian, Episcopal, United Church of Christ, Christian Science, Jehovah's Witness, and Mennonite denominations.

Abbreviations for ART (Assisted Reproductive Technologies)

AI = Artificial Insemination
ED = Egg Donation
EMBD – Embryo Donation
GIFT = Gamete Intrafallopian Transfer
IVF = In Vitro Fertilization
MPR = Multifetal Pregnancy Reduction
SD = Sperm Donation
SUR = Surrogacy
ZIFT = Zygote Intrafallopian Transfer

Sources: [24–30]

Understanding your client's specific ideology

Clinicians working with individuals and couples struggling with infertility should determine what, if any, spiritual or religious beliefs influence clients' decisions regarding medical intervention [19]. Social networks have been found to influence help-seeking behavior [20], and religion has been found to be both a resource and a burden when dealing with infertility [3]. Thus, it is useful to determine whether religious or spiritual communities are a part of the client's life, and in what way. Other variables that intersect with religion and spirituality should also be explored. For example, the role gender plays may also be a factor. For some, the pull to fulfill gender expectations of manhood and womanhood that relate to having children may override religious prohibitions against ART [21].

A thorough assessment of the significance of religion and spirituality for clients addressing infertility should include exploration of their use in making meaning, coping with psychosocial distress and the presence of faith-based strengths to support them in the process [3]. Does the client experience their religious teaching, spiritual practices and community support as helping them to bear the unbearable, as a source of judgment and set of limitations on options, or both? Do conflicting religious beliefs and spiritual practices exist within a couple? If so, how does that impact decisions about ART? Not all spiritual people adhere to one specific religion or set of teachings, and individuals who identify with a specific religion may hold beliefs and engage in practices that differ from formal teachings [6]. The careful clinician will assess for these beliefs and meanings and not make assumptions based on gender, religiosity or spirituality alone. Suggested assessment questions are presented in Table 5.2.

When assessing spirituality with clients, it is common for them to inquire about the clinician's personal views and practices. Clients may seek out a particular therapist because they assume shared religious traditions. Or they may ask specifically about beliefs

Table 5.2 Assessing the role of religion and spirituality in fertility counseling.*

Where do you turn for help in dealing with difficulties in your life?
Has some of your strength come from a religious or spiritual practice?
What is your clearest sense of the meaning of your life at this time?
How has the context of your family of origin's religious/spiritual practices shaped your own religious/spiritual beliefs?
What are your religious community's expectations regarding parenthood?
Did you have expectations about your fertility?
What have you learned about infertility from these religious or spiritual teachings?
What is the meaning of infertility to you?
Do you find comfort or support from a religious or spiritual community?
If so, how would this community support you during the experience of infertility?
How do your spiritual beliefs inform your understanding of your infertility?
Do you and your partner have conflicting beliefs about infertility and its treatment? Do these differences stem from religious beliefs or spiritual practices?
Are there ways that you disagree with your religious or spiritual community's teaching on assisted reproductive technology?
Do you have an image of God/Spirit – what is that image?
Is your God/Spirit judging you/others – if so in what way?
Has that image been challenged or changed by infertility?
Do you think God/Spirit answers prayers?
How would you know that God/Spirit is listening?
Would you make a choice to pursue ART that isn't sanctioned by your religious teachings?
Is there anything else about your religious or spiritual belief that is important for our work?

* Adapted from Griffith & Griffith [31]

and practices if this has not been assumed. Clinicians should normalize wanting to know this information as it is such an important part of life. Knowing how much of this personal information one is willing to disclose is helpful up front, to avoid awkward moments or sharing beyond what feels comfortable. This can also be a helpful moment in the engagement process, as the client is seen as unique and the clinician as wanting to understand more about what religion and spirituality means to them. Whether the clinician and client are the "same" or "different," it is helpful to have a safe and confidential place to discuss the client's specific, individual views and experiences. Some clients will feel more comfortable with someone who does not share the same religion because they will not judge them. Others will feel it is important that the clinician understands their beliefs and practices. Either way, the clinician can process the importance of religion and spirituality, thereby demonstrating openness to learning more from the client. In our experience, willingness to explore these themes outweighs the significance of the clinician's personal beliefs.

Spirituality and spiritual bypassing

In addition to determining the role that religiosity and spirituality play in decision-making, clinicians ought to be aware of the potential to use these resources as a means of avoiding deeper psychological work. The term *spiritual bypassing*, coined by John Welwood in 1984, refers to the use of spiritual ideas, practices and rituals to sidestep more psychologically painful work that may be necessary to face unresolved emotional issues [22]. When engaging in spiritual bypassing, people typically are defensive about their religious or spiritual practices and unwilling to explore them in depth. There is often an oversimplification of spiritual concepts, and an intellectualization of their spiritual practices. When clients are able to connect emotionally and spiritually to their struggles with infertility, they are not using spiritual bypassing. It is when these practices are used to remain emotionally numb and distant from the psychic pain that they are most likely attempting to pass over the psychological distress.

It can be helpful to ask clients to explore the emotions that arise when praying or meditating, and how these practices help with their struggle. Clients who resist exploring the psychological dimensions of their spirituality may be engaging in spiritual bypassing. They may make statements such as "it's all in God's hands now, and there's nothing I can do" and "I'm giving it up to God." Further assessment must be done before making a determination, as clients who are not bypassing will make these types of statements as part of their acceptance of powerlessness over their fertility. This can be a good starting point for the clinician to differentiate whether spiritual practices are being engaged as a support, or are being used to avoid difficult emotional experiences.

Spiritually based interventions for infertility

For clients who are spiritually inclined, the crisis of infertility can ignite a simultaneous crisis of faith; others draw upon their spirituality as a source of strength; still others experience mixed feelings or confusion about previously unquestioned spiritual tenets. As each client experiences infertility idiosyncratically, so too is each client's understanding of the intersection of infertility and spirituality unique. Nevertheless, common themes surrounding spirituality may emerge in clinical work with patients experiencing challenges to family building.

As clinicians who are open to attending to spirituality in our work with clients experiencing obstacles to family building, we have identified the following intervention strategies to help clients navigate these two very profound and complex dimensions of the human experience. These include:

- informed not-knowing;
- telling the story;
- naming the losses;
- speaking the unspeakable;
- grieving the losses; and
- identifying options.

These intervention strategies are not necessarily linear over the course of treatment, nor are they related to a timeline. Instead, they are thematic and intended to provide the clinician with a general guideline to treatment. In essence, they are tools to use in addition to an existing professional skill set. The client should set the pace of treatment, and feel free to return to earlier material, if necessary. The clinical vignettes presented below are fictionalized composites of case material. No identifying information is included.

Informed not-knowing

Every clinician brings his or her own professional training and personal experience to each client encounter and, at times, the circumstances of clients' lives may seem all too familiar if the therapist has a personal history of infertility or shares similar spiritual beliefs with his or her clients. By adopting a stance of informed not-knowing, therapists are reminded that knowledge and training can provide an outline or rough draft out of which clients are able to tell their version of the story. The questions therapists ask in assessment and throughout the treatment help bring diffuse feelings into sharper focus, and continue to challenge the therapist's assumptions. The therapist asks clients to define their experiences, rather than imposing the therapist's own understandings upon clients. The questions the therapist asks are informed by knowledge, training and personal experiences with spirituality and infertility, but clients are the experts about their own experiences, feelings and beliefs. The manner of the therapist's questions and interventions communicates respect, curiosity and lack of judgment about clients. Therapists are not afraid to ask for clarification if they do not understand what clients are telling them. This attitude of informed not-knowing gives clients authority to help the therapist understand their unique experiences of infertility and spirituality. (See Table 5.2 for a complete list of spiritually informed questions regarding the role of religion, spirituality and infertility.)

> Melinda and her clients, Dav and Miriam, are members of the same Orthodox Jewish community (although they worship at different synagogues). Melinda has extensive professional and personal experience with infertility; she used a donor embryo to become pregnant with her only daughter, and feels no conflict between her religious beliefs and her own treatment choice. As she works with Miriam and Dav, she finds herself feeling frustrated by what she sees as Miriam's dogmatic interpretation of Orthodox Jewish beliefs regarding ART. Melinda is aware of her feeling that were Miriam and Dav to proceed with using a donor egg, or to undergo an adoption process that resulted in adding a child to their family, Miriam would change her mind about the importance of being biologically related to the child. Melinda views her frustration as a signal that there is something she is not understanding about her clients' experience; her awareness of the differences between her viewpoint and that of her clients reminds her to adopt a stance of informed not-knowing in her work with them.

Melinda's religious background is important in her work with Miriam and Dav; in fact, the couple was referred to her because of her connections in the Jewish community. Melinda's familiarity with the couple's religious beliefs strengthens their work together, to the degree that they all "speak the same language." At the same time, Melinda's awareness of maintaining a position of informed not-knowing helps her appreciate how Miriam's and Dav's understandings and experiences differ from her own. In spite of the similarities in their backgrounds, informed not-knowing helps Melinda tune into her clients' unique interpretations and experiences.

Telling the story

The experience of infertility can be an intensely personal and isolating one. Many clients have had few, if any, opportunities to tell the story of their family building journey to a supportive listener who is patient, concerned and familiar with matters related to infertility. Moreover, many clients are unaccustomed to considering the influence of the past on present events. Some clients, overwhelmed by intense feelings or single-minded in pursuit of medical treatments, haven't paused to think about the narrative of their experience. Additionally, if a client's spiritual community has an expressed position about expectations for family building or approved intervention options for treating infertility, he or she may feel hesitant to tell his or her story for fear of disapproval or pressure from the community to adhere to its guidelines. Therapy with a clinician who is both experienced in working with infertility and open to understanding the client's spiritual orientation can provide an opportunity for the client to organize experiences, feelings and beliefs into his or her own unique story, without having to edit details for a particular audience.

Construction of a narrative can help the client understand his or her infertility as a story that has evolved over time, with characters that are influenced by a variety of life factors, including those of a spiritual nature. This is similar to Jaffe and Diamond's notion of *the reproductive story* [23]. Using this intervention, the clinician helps the client surface unconscious or conscious narratives of family building and addresses how current challenges to fertility have interrupted those stories. Weaving in spirituality, the clinician helps the client understand an additional, often powerful dimension of the story.

Saily began therapy for depression after her sister-in-law gave birth to a baby boy, the first grandchild in the family. She was puzzled by her feelings of apathy towards her nephew, who is a source of great pride to the family. The priest in Saily's Hindu temple held a ceremony for the entire community to celebrate the auspicious date of the baby's birth. Saily, the baby's Godmother and only aunt, played a special role in the ceremony. Although Saily's family and many of the members of her temple were aware of her history of infertility, no one, including Saily, considered that her depression and her infertility might be related. On the contrary, the community and Saily considered her position as Godmother an enviable one because of her special relationship to the baby and to God. Furthermore, they viewed her childlessness as karma and expressed their belief that Saily's role was to serve others. Saily's depression seemed incongruent with her community's and her own spiritual expectations of herself.

Saily's presenting problem of depression seemed inexplicable to her in the spiritual context of events in her life. She felt ashamed of her self-perception as unloving and unappreciative of her family's good fortune. Her therapist's curiosity about Saily's feelings related to her infertility experience helps her to consider that her current reactions might make sense if understood as a piece of a larger story of her life. In therapy, Saily constructs a narrative that makes sense of her depression; she is not an unappreciative Godmother, unwilling to fulfill her karmic duties. Instead, she is a mother grieving the losses of her own babies. Her lack of enthusiasm about her nephew is a logical part of a larger story, and makes sense when considered in the context of her life. Saily becomes able to see herself as worthy of empathy, which alleviates feelings of guilt about her ambivalence towards her nephew.

Naming the losses

Clients experiencing infertility, especially those who never have had a pregnancy, often feel an acute sense of grief but have not labeled their experience as such, because of the intangibility of the losses. Previously held assumptions about fertility, good health, success, masculinity, femininity and the future, many of which are reinforced by faith communities, are no longer reliable. Because these losses are amorphous and invisible, clients often feel a sense of dissonance between their personal experience and the reactions of those around them. Well-meaning friends, family and faith community members can underscore this sense of confusion by encouraging clients to "hang in there" or "be grateful for all you have." Spiritual clients are sometimes told to think of their infertility as part of God's plan, which may invoke feelings of shame if they are angry or sad about their plight. In addition to the losses infertility brings, clients may also feel the loss of connection with those around them who are unable to understand their experience. Moreover, infertile clients may feel the loss of a previously unwavering faith in a loving higher power that now seems absent. The therapist's task is to help her clients name these experiences as losses worthy of grieving, and validate the legitimacy of clients' feelings of loss where others are unable to do so.

> Karim and his wife, Laila, have suffered six miscarriages over the last four years and are contemplating pursuing IVF at the recommendation of Laila's Obstetrician. Laila is eager to begin treatment; Karim is supportive but cautious about the financial and emotional investment of fertility treatments. Karim and Laila are Muslim, but neither he nor his wife are outwardly religious. Karim notes that until his experience with infertility, he considered his Islamic faith to be an internal source of comfort and support. He describes his earlier belief that he had an ongoing internal conversation with Allah, but now he feels as though he is talking only to himself; Allah isn't listening, and maybe isn't even there. Just as Karim's assumption that he would easily become a father is being challenged by his infertility, so too is his former assumption of a loving God shaken.

As she listens to Karim's story, Karim's therapist is aware of the multiple losses he has endured over the last four years. He describes feeling uncertain about how to characterize the miscarriages; after all, he notes, it's not as though he and Laila lost an "actual child." Still, he describes feeling as though he has suffered several deaths. Like many clients, Karim is reluctant to identify the miscarriages in the same category as other less ambiguous losses. The therapist's willingness to identify Karim and Laila's miscarriages as losses worthy of grieving lends legitimacy to Karim's experiences of this very thing. Conceiving of the miscarriages as losses allows Karim to consider that he may be grieving other related losses, too. For instance, control of Laila's health and the family finances may also be felt as lost given the possibility of fertility treatments in the couple's future. In addition to the loss of the pregnancies and the losses of future financial and medical stability, Karim is wrestling with the profound existential loss of his faith in God. Any one of these losses, alone, would be difficult to endure; for clients experiencing multiple losses simultaneously, feelings of grief are intensified. In helping clients name all of the losses related to infertility, including those having to do with a shift in faith, therapists validate the intensity of the feelings and create space for grieving previously unnamed, ambiguous and powerful losses.

Speaking the unspeakable

Some may consider the feelings evoked in clients by the experience of infertility unkind, inappropriate and even blasphemous. Faith communities frequently discourage expressions of "negative" feelings such as envy, rage, hatred, frustration, fear and doubt, yet clients dealing with infertility commonly experience these feelings. Clients are often surprised when clinicians are interested in, and even encourage them to speak about, "unacceptable" thoughts and feelings out loud in sessions. The therapist is tolerant, accepting and unafraid of hearing all of the client's thoughts, fears, fantasies and feelings about infertility, pregnancy, people with children and even God. When these feelings are spoken in session and normalized by the therapist, clients often are surprised to learn that they are not alone in their negative emotional responses to infertility. Often, clients feel relieved of the pressure they experience in many other settings to deny these feelings or pretend they feel otherwise. The therapist may expect that, for some clients, speaking the unspeakable can feel alarming and shameful. It is important to allow the client to set the pace of expression of these feelings, and to attend to the experience of saying out loud and feeling in session frightening and forbidden material.

> Leah is an active member of a Christian Evangelical Church. She and her husband were raised in the tradition, met each other at church, and identify their faith as central to their lives. When Leah suffered a late miscarriage church members organized a meal-delivery schedule and an extra prayer service to provide support to Leah and her husband. Leah felt grateful for the support, but also found herself feeling envious of church families with infants and small children, many of whom visited Leah during her recovery. She found herself bristling when well-intentioned friends told her the loss was "God's plan," although she herself might have agreed with

this sentiment before the miscarriage. Leah recounts with regret an incident with a pregnant friend who told Leah that she felt blessed to be expecting a child. Leah's angry response, "Well, then, I guess I'm cursed!" was met by her friend's shock and judgment, and Leah felt exposed, ashamed and misunderstood.

Therapists working with clients like Leah are accustomed to hearing such stories. In addition to painful feelings of loss about the miscarriage, Leah is aware of her "un-Christian" feelings of jealousy and rage, but notes that she does not believe she should have them, let alone express them. The therapist's suggestion that Leah can say anything at all in the privacy of therapy at first feels foreign to Leah. However, as Leah begins to experience the therapist as receptive to hearing all of her feelings, even the unkind ones, Leah begins to feel more tolerant of these feelings in herself. This tolerance allows Leah to examine the "bad" feelings and decide how she would like to manage them, should they arise again. Moreover, by sharing these feelings with a supportive therapist, Leah finds that she is also able to experience loving and concerned feelings towards her pregnant friend.

Grieving the losses

As clients are able to identify their infertility related losses, including those having to do with issues of faith, and articulate the unspeakable fears and feelings related to these losses, the task of treatment becomes helping clients engage in the grieving process. Clients are given space to express feelings of grief, and the therapist assists in the mourning process by staying with the sadness in sessions. There is no rush to solve the problem, "look on the bright side," or deny any part of the reality of the experience for the patient. The therapist allows the client to take the time he or she needs to feel feelings, without rushing to move away from the pain. Spiritually sensitive clinicians are attuned to ways in which clients' spirituality may serve as a source of support in the grieving process.

For some clients part of the grief and healing process may include the practice of a ritual to formally acknowledge a loss. Rituals may be established practices through formal religions, such as funerals, burials or the Christian practice of Baptism of miscarried or stillborn babies. Clients may also choose to create their own ritual to remember the loss.

Melia and Lou suffered a late-term stillbirth when Melia was 36 weeks pregnant with a baby girl who was to be named Sara. The couple had prepared a nursery and had a collection of ultrasound images of the baby taken throughout their problem-free pregnancy. There was also a photograph taken of Melia holding Sara after the delivery, which Melia reported to the therapist after several sessions. The therapist expressed an interest in seeing the picture, if Melia and Lou wanted to share it. The couple brought the photograph and other items such as infant clothing and stuffed animals to subsequent sessions. The therapist's expression of interest, admiration and sadness provided space and permission for the couple to begin the work of grieving the loss of their baby. The couple subsequently decided to hold a memorial service for Sara in their garden, and invited close family and friends to share memories of the pregnancy, reflections about the photograph, and wishes and dreams for the couple.

The therapist's interest in the photograph of Sara communicates her willingness to see and hear every part of Melia and Lou's experience, and honors them in their role as parents to Sara. The couple's work with the therapist helps them construct a ritual to recognize Sara as a part of their family, and to include important people in their lives in their grieving process. Couples may ritualize any part of the infertility process; for example, attending religious services before an IVF cycle, saving ultrasound images of embryos, or planting seeds in the ground after a miscarriage.

Identifying options

Clients experiencing infertility usually are eager to identify solutions that will put an end to what is most always a very stressful and disappointing life chapter. Often, clients are better able to identify options and create plans after they have spent time in therapy exploring their feelings about infertility, parenthood, faith and their dreams of how their future family might look. Certain paths, such as ART, adoption, or living child-free, which once felt incomprehensible, may feel more viable after this exploration in therapy. If clients are spiritual, the therapist can assist them in clarifying how spiritual beliefs may inform their decisions about parenthood, moving forward. For some clients facing infertility, spiritual tenets provide guidelines that are reassuring and helpful in making choices about treatment. Making decisions that are consonant with their religious beliefs may mitigate, for these clients, accompanying feelings of loss or disappointment if parenthood is not the result of their treatment decisions. Other clients discover that they are willing to make choices that are not sanctioned by their faith communities. Sometimes clients are able to find a way to remain connected to their spiritual beliefs even if their choice departs from what is permissible by their religions. And some clients choose to forsake their faith communities if they feel unsupported in their decisions about how to address their infertility.

After several years of infertility, including six rounds of IVF and nine months of individual therapy, Jessica informs her therapist that she would like to consider other medical interventions to achieve pregnancy. As a devout Mormon, Jessica is aware that her church does not approve of third party sperm, egg or embryo donations. It is important to Jessica to adhere to the teachings of her church, but she also is aware of her very strong desire to be pregnant, and feels that she will deeply grieve the loss of that experience in her life. With the help of her therapist, Jessica considers how it might feel to go against the beliefs of her faith in order to achieve pregnancy using donor gametes or embryos. Ultimately, Jessica decides to pursue adoption, but agrees with her husband to keep trying to get pregnant each month without medical assistance. This compromise helps Jessica to feel that she is not giving up her dream of experiencing pregnancy, and also is remaining adherent to the religious beliefs that are important to her.

In therapy, Jessica is given permission to imagine a variety of options. She is able to acknowledge that she has a *choice* in how she will proceed, and finds that her choice includes adhering to the teachings of her church. Jessica's decision to pursue adoption while continuing to try to conceive naturally accommodates the three desires that are most important to her: her faith, becoming a parent and trying to achieve pregnancy.

Spirituality as a source of strength

For many clients wrestling with infertility, spirituality is a main source of strength. It is critical for therapists to encourage clients to identify and draw upon this resource if it seems appropriate. Often, clients have built-in support systems in their faith communities and can call upon fellow believers or spiritual leaders for help.

Leslie and Jack are devout Catholics who have been unable to get pregnant after three years. The couple is committed to adhering to church guidelines regarding treatment for infertility and have decided to continue their attempts without medical assistance. In therapy, Leslie and Jack acknowledge the emotional pain of this decision. Although their struggle is painful, they find the weekly ritual of Communion reaffirming of God's presence in their lives; the miracle of Communion reminds them of God's power. Biblical stories of suffering and modern examples of saints such as Mother Teresa help the couple endure their infertility, and experience their own suffering as a legitimate response to their situation. They are close with their parish priest, and often meet with him privately to pray. Leslie and Jack volunteer to teach Sunday School and have developed relationships with many of the children and families in the parish. Both Leslie and Jack believe that God will decide how children will be part of their lives, and they feel comforted knowing that if they are unable to have children of their own God will provide other opportunities for them to have meaningful relationships with youngsters.

Therapists can help clients identify non-traditional expressions of spirituality in their lives that provide hope and strength while they are coping with infertility. Non-religious clients may nevertheless engage in spiritual rituals that provide a sense of meaning and connection during the often isolating experience of infertility.

While traveling abroad after Lisa's failed IVF cycle using Laura's egg and donor sperm, the couple learn of a religious shrine in Greece for childless women at the top of a steep mountain with many steps. At the top, pilgrims light candles and pray to Greek goddesses and the Virgin Mary to become pregnant. Although Lisa and Laura are not religious and do not identify as believers in a traditional sense, they are moved by the idea that they are not alone in their sadness, and decide to climb the mountain to feel part of a timeless community of people yearning to become parents. The experience is profound for the couple, and they now remember it when they feel alone in their struggle.

While this couple might not have identified this experience as religious or spiritual, the therapist understands that it was meaningful and that it helped Lisa and Laura feel connected to something greater than their infertility. It is not necessary to label such an experience as spiritual or religious to the client if the client does not consider it as such. Nevertheless, the therapist may consider clients' search for meaning, purpose and connection to something greater than their own experiences in the same vein as other more traditional expressions of spirituality or religiosity.

Countertransference

Infertility is an experience fraught with complex emotions of grief, loss, anger, ambivalence, jealousy and more. Clients often present for treatment in the midst of a crisis, such as an unexpected diagnosis, a failed IVF cycle, or a pregnancy loss. Therapists working with these clients must have an awareness of how these powerful experiences can elicit a variety of emotional responses in the clinician. If the clinician is also undergoing infertility, or has a personal experience with infertility, as do many therapists who choose this specialty, the potential for experiencing overwhelming countertransference is great. The subjects of spirituality and religion often are laden with myriad emotional material. Clinicians are not exempt from this. Therapists working with these aspects of human experience simultaneously must be aware, as much as possible, of their own personal attitudes and unresolved feelings to understand the influence of these in the clinical work.

We have found that it is critical to be aware of our own views about family building and spirituality or religion in providing fertility counseling. Our personal spiritual or religious ideologies, views of family, parenthood and child-free lifestyles, attitudes towards ART, personal experience with infertility and loss, feelings towards authority (as may be represented by certain religious organizations or medical professionals, for instance) will surface when working with clients. It is imperative, though often very difficult, to keep in check our own desires and wishes for clients that are based in our own histories of family and spirituality, and to remain always in touch with what clients wish for themselves, which may be very different from choices we might make. We sometimes experience a sense of loss when clients choose options that we ourselves would not choose, or become invested in particular outcomes that may resonate with our own experiences. We have found that our own clinical supervision, peer support, and personal therapy are essential to remaining aware of our countertransference and finding ways to use it to help us better understand our clients.

Conclusion

Fertility counseling can be greatly enhanced by attending to the religious beliefs and spiritual practices of clients. A general understanding of the major religions of the world provides the clinician with a good framework, but it is not adequate on its own. Practitioners who utilize an informed not-knowing stance can understand each client's unique experience of religious teachings and the influence those teachings may or may not have with regards to what they are willing to do to have a child. In addition, working with spiritual practices and rituals to support clients in the midst of fertility counseling can greatly enhance the work and provide comfort and support for the clients. Along with supporting client strengths and resilience in the face of infertility, spirituality and religion can be used to avoid deeper psychological work. An ability to identify the signs of spiritual bypassing can help practitioners address this, or work collaboratively with a supportive person from within that spiritual community.

The case vignettes presented in this chapter are designed to give clinicians a sense of how themes of spirituality can be present with clients experiencing infertility, and to outline concrete interventions. The case illustrations demonstrate the ways in which a thorough assessment of the client's spirituality can be vital to understanding the meaning made of infertility. It is also critical for the therapist to pay attention to countertransference when providing counseling for infertility with clients who raise themes around spirituality. In order to meet clients where they are, and be most effective in helping them reach family building decisions that are best for them, therapists must attend to the spiritual dimensions they present.

References

1. Dake, C. L. *Infertility: A Survival Guide for Couples and Those who Love Them*. Birmingham, AL: New Hope Publishers; 2002.
2. Stein, G. Hannah: A case of infertility and depression – psychiatry in the Old Testament. *The British Journal of Psychiatry*, 2010; 197(6): 492.

3. Roudsari, R. L., & Allan, H. T. Women's experiences and preferences in relation to infertility counselling: A multifaith dialogue. *International Journal of Fertility Sterility*, 2011; 5(3): 158–67.
4. Sheridan, M. Ethical issues in the use of spiritually based interventions in social work practice: What are we doing and why? *Journal of Religion & Spirituality in Social Work: Social Thought*, 2009; 28: 99–126.
5. Hoge, D. R. Using spiritual interventions in practice: Developing some guidelines from evidence-based practice. *Social Work*, 2011; 56(2): 149–58.
6. Kvarfordt, C. L., & Sheridan, M. J. The role of religion and spirituality in working with children and adolescents. *Journal of Religion and Spirituality in Social Work: Social Thought*, 2007; 26(3): 1–23.
7. Burnett, J. A., & Panchal, K. Incorporating ideological context in counseling couples experiencing infertility. *Journal of Humanistic Counseling, Education and Development*, 2008; 47: 187–211.
8. Griel, A., McQuillan, J., Benjamins, M., Johnson, D. R., Johson, K. M., & Heinze, C. R. Specifiying the effects of religion on medical help-seeking. *Social Science & Medicine*, 2010; 71: 734–42.
9. Gaydos, L. M., Smith, A., Hogue, C. J., & Blevins, J. An emerging field in religion and reproductive health. *Journal of Religion and Health*, 2010; 49(4): 473–84.
10. Layne, L. L. Pregnancy loss, stigma, irony, and masculinities: Reflections on and future directions for research on religion in the global practice of IVF. *Culture, Medicine, and Psychiatry*, 2006; 30: 537–45.
11. Sewpaul, V. Culture, religion, and infertility: A South African perspective. *British Journal of Social Work*, 1999; 29: 741–54.
12. Kahn, S. M. Making technology familiar: Orthodox Jews and infertility support, advice, and inspiration. *Culture, Medicine, and Psychiatry*, 2006; 30: 467–80.
13. Lasker, J. N., & Murray, D. Jews, non-Jews, and attitudes toward reproductive technologies. *Contemporary Jewry*, 2001; 22(1): 80–97.
14. Roberts, E. F. God's laboratory: Religious rationalities and modernity in Ecuadorian in vitro fertilization. *Culture, Medicine, and Psychiatry*, 2006; 30: 507–36.
15. Bharadwaj, A. Sacred conceptions: Clinical theodicies, uncertain science, and technologies of procreation in India. *Culture, Medicine, and Psychiatry*, 2006; 30: 451–65.
16. Larijani, B., & Zahedi, F. Ethical and religious aspects of gamete and embryo donation and legislation in Iran. *Journal of Religion and Health*, 2007; 46: 399–408.
17. Inhorn, M. C. Making Muslim babies: IVF and gamete donation in Sunni versus Shi'a Islam. *Culture, Medicine, and Psychiatry*, 2006; 30: 427–50.
18. Seybold, D. Choosing therapies: A Senegalese woman's experience with infertility. *Health Care for Women International*, 2002; 23: 540–49.
19. Connor, J., Sauer, C., & Doll, K. Assisted reproductive technologies and world religions: Implications for couples therapy. *Journal of Family Psychotherapy*, 2012; 23: 83–98.
20. White, L., McQuillan, J., Greil, A. L., & Johnson, D. R. Infertility: Testing a helpseeking model. *Social Sciences & Medicine*, 2006; 62, 1031–41.
21. Jennnings, P. K. "God had something else in mind": Family, religion, and infertility. *Journal of Contemporary Ethnography*, 2010; 39(2): 215–37.
22. Welwood, J. *Toward a Psychology of Awakening*. Boston, MA: Shambhala; 2000.
23. Jaffe, J., & Diamond, M. O. *Reproductive Trauma: Psychotherapy with Infertility and Pregnancy Loss Clients*. Washington, DC: American Psychological Association; 2011.
24. Alvare, H. M. Catholic teaching and the law concerning the new reproductive technologies. *Fordham Urban Law Journal*, 2002; 30: 107–34.
25. Cohen, C. Protestant perspectives on the uses of the new reproductive technologies. *Fordham Urban Law Journal*, 2002; 30: 135–45.
26. Dutney, A. Religion, infertility, and assisted reproductive technology. *Best Practice & Research Clinical Obstetrics & Gynaecology*. 2007; 21(1): 169–80.
27. Ott, K. *A Time to be Born: A Faith-based Guide to Assisted Reproductive Technologies*. Westport, CT: Religious Institute; 2009.
28. Schenker, J. G. Assisted reproductive practice: Religious perspectives. *Reproductive BioMedicine Online*, 2005; 10(3): 310–19.
29. Simpson, B. Managing potential in assisted reproductive technologies: Reflections on gifts, kinship, and the process of vernacularization. *Current Anthropology*, 2013: 54(7), 87–96.
30. Proctor, M. Bodies, babies, and birth control. *Journal of Mormon Thought*, 2000; 159–76.
31. Griffith, J., & Griffith, M. *Encountering the Sacred in Psychotherapy*. New York, NY: Guilford Press; 2002.

Chapter 6

Reproductive psychiatry and fertility counseling

Katherine Williams

Ms. G. is a 42-year-old woman who has had three pregnancies and one birth, who presents to the mental health specialist with complaints of depression and anxiety that have been increasing over the past five years. Ms. G. explains that she has been trying to have a second child, but she has been unsuccessful. Her only child, Nicholas, is now 9 years old. She says that she and her husband started trying to conceive a second child when her son was 3 years old. She had conceived Nicholas without difficulty within four months after discontinuing oral contraceptives. Her pregnancy and delivery were uncomplicated, and Nicholas was developing normally and "the love of her life." Since she was only 33 years old at the time that she first tried to conceive, she and her husband did not seek infertility evaluation and treatment until after her first miscarriage at six weeks pregnancy, when she was 35 years old. Ms. G. was encouraged to continue trying "naturally," but she did not conceive for two more years, so she again sought infertility treatment. Infertility work up has so far been negative for both Ms. G. and her husband and they have continued to try to conceive without assisted reproductive technologies (ART).

Ms. G.'s second miscarriage occurred ten months ago, at ten weeks pregnancy. She and her husband had been very excited and hopeful because they had seen a heartbeat on ultrasound at seven weeks. She began to spot at eight weeks and was found to have no fetal heartbeat, and so she underwent a dilation and curettage (D&C). Ms. G. describes increasing depression since the miscarriage, with intense feelings of sadness, difficulty concentrating, decreased motivation, onset and middle insomnia, guilty ruminations, low energy and decreased appetite. The week before the onset of her menstrual cycle she feels much worse. Her symptoms include irritability, depressed mood, alternating hypersomnia and insomnia, carbohydrate craving and severe, debilitating headaches. Ms. G. says that her premenstrual syndrome symptoms began after the birth of her baby, but they were never as intense as they have been recently.

Ms. G. and her husband have decided to pursue a "last ditch" effort for pregnancy with in vitro fertilization (IVF). She is worried about the "hormonal emotional roller coaster" that she has heard about with IVF. She will undergo the "flare procedure" – one month of oral contraceptives followed by 1–2 weeks of a GnRH agonist Lupron, followed by FSH/LH recombinant injections, followed by progesterone supplementation (100–200 mg/day).

Ms. G. has never seen a mental health professional before, and she is wondering, "How can you help me?"

Introduction

The close relationship between the experience of infertility and psychological distress, mood and anxiety disorders has been recognized for centuries. The loss of control, grief and interpersonal stress associated with infertility increase the risk for new onset or recurrence of mood or anxiety disorders in both women and their partners. Infertility treatments themselves may also have central nervous effects that are associated with mood symptoms. While psychotherapy – individual, group and couples – remains the first-line treatment of these conditions [1], at times women will present with depression and anxiety symptoms that have been resistant to psychotherapy, and psychopharmacological treatment will be considered. This treatment is complicated by a number of factors, including the potential interaction of the infertility treatments with psychiatric medications, the potential perinatal

Fertility Counseling: Clinical Guide and Case Studies, ed. Sharon N. Covington. Published by Cambridge University Press.

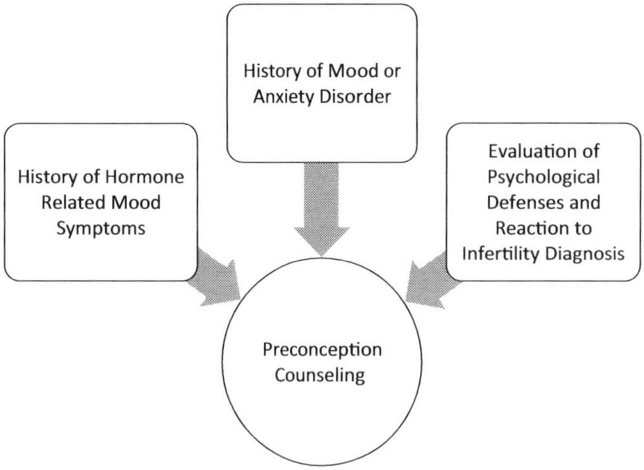

Figure 6.1 Preconception counseling components.

risks of the use these medications and the limited number of long-term developmental follow-up studies of children exposed to psychiatric medications in pregnancy.

Consequently the fertility counselor has several important roles while working with the patient undergoing infertility evaluation and treatment. First, the mental health professional (MHP) has a role in preconception counseling. In this role, the MHP evaluates the patient's risk for onset or recurrence of mood or anxiety disorder during the process of treatment. Second, the fertility counselor will have a role in evaluation and treatment of infertility medication-associated psychiatric symptoms. When a patient's anxiety and depression symptoms do not remit with the intervention of psychotherapy, the reproductive psychiatrist can work with the infertility treatment team to provide recommendations regarding psychopharmacological treatments.

The goals of this chapter are to provide an overview for fertility counselors of the following issues in reproductive psychiatry:

1. preconception counseling;
2. infertility medication-emergent side effects; and
3. psychopharmacology considerations for infertility patients, before, during and after treatment.

These issues are part of the larger new field of reproductive psychiatry, which is a specialty that focuses upon the unique role of hormones and female reproductive life events in women's mental health. This field focuses on the evaluation and treatment of such disorders as premenstrual dysphoric disorder, antenatal and postpartum depression, perimenopausal mood and anxiety disorders, and infertility treatment-related mood and anxiety disorders.

Preconception counseling: how the fertility counselor can help the patient and medical team

Preconception counseling refers to the important opportunity that mental health specialists have to help patients identify issues that may affect their transition to parenthood. The counseling session focuses on the unique biological psychological and social factors in the patient's mental health that are potentially modifiable or which will need special treatment during the perinatal period. See Figure 6.1.

Evaluation of psychological defensive functioning and psychological reactions to the infertility diagnosis

The fertility counselor has a unique role in the infertility treatment team, as this clinician can help identify patients who may be at risk for psychological disturbances as well as mood and anxiety disorders during infertility treatment. While studies have not shown higher rates of personality disorders in women with infertility [2], the stress of the infertility process may lead to psychological problems in women with personality disorders, and even women without personality disorders may demonstrate psychological defenses that will interfere with their treatment. Consequently, preconception counseling should include an evaluation of psychological functioning to clarify for both the patient and the treatment team whether the complex and stressful process of infertility treatment will be associated with extreme distress. For example, patients with personality disorders can be especially challenging for medical staff and could be identified in preconception counseling sessions, particularly borderline personality disorder, narcissistic personality disorder and histrionic personality disorder. Patients with these disorders may be at a greater risk for creating "drama" during the treatment process, including setting up "splitting" between infertility doctors and nurses, excessive phone calls due to fears of abandonment or lack of compliance due to devaluation of members of the treatment team. Patients with obsessive-compulsive personality disorder, or strong traits, will be at risk for perseveration over the details of the infertility treatments, and extreme indecisiveness regarding future treatment planning. Recognition of these personality disorders and traits early on will help all members of the treatment team continue to work collaboratively. For instance, psychoeducation about personality styles and support from the fertility counselor on the treatment will enable the team to plan which patients might be best seen at the end of the clinic, so as not to disrupt the flow of other patients; which patients will need more frequent scheduled follow-up phone calls, or which patients may need extra instruction in procedures.

The fertility counselor also plays an important role in evaluating the patient's psychological reaction to the infertility diagnosis. Recent research has demonstrated that infertility patients often suffer from profound feelings of external shame, a sense that others are judging them harshly as inadequate, as well as internal shame, the sense of negative self-judgment, often based on past events, such as a previous abortion, or desire to delay childbearing [3]. Since shame has been found to be risk factor for the development of mood and anxiety disorders [4,5], and the character trait of neuroticism has been found to predict depression and anxiety in infertility patients [6], exploration of the patient's reaction to the infertility diagnosis and treatment during the preconception counseling session will help identify patients who may need to be followed more closely by the fertility counselor, or referred for more in-depth therapy.

Evaluation of hormonal sensitivity

The preconception counseling session should include an in-depth review of the patient's history of hormonal sensitivity. No large prospective studies have yet been completed that compare rates of new onset or recurrence of major depression or anxiety disorders in women in infertility treatment with or without a history of mood and anxiety symptoms. Nonetheless, it is recommended that clinicians determine a baseline understanding of reproductive hormone sensitivity prior to infertility treatment, as some women do appear to be especially sensitive to the effects of hormones. One example of a reproductive-cycle-oriented interview is the Composite International Diagnostic Interview for Women, which focuses upon the interaction of psychiatric symptoms and reproductive events and stages [7]. At the very minimum, the preconception therapy session should include:

1. Psychiatric history – special attention to history of affective and anxiety disorders, including bipolar disorders.
2. Review of psychological symptoms at the following times:

   puberty
   oral contraceptive pills
   ovulation and luteal phase
   pregnancy and postpartum.
3. Family history of reproductive-related psychiatric symptoms:

   premenstrual dysphoric disorder
   postpartum depression
   perimenopausal depression.
4. Family history of major depression and bipolar disorder.

Evaluation and treatment of behaviors with potential effects on fertility/pregnancy

The fertility counselor is poised to be a very helpful member of the infertility treatment team for the evaluation and treatment of conditions that may affect fertility and pregnancy, such as eating disorders, smoking and alcohol cessation, healthy eating habits in both men and women (see Figure 6.2). The gynecologist or reproductive endocrinologist may identify these problems in the history and physical examination, but it is the MHP who can provide a

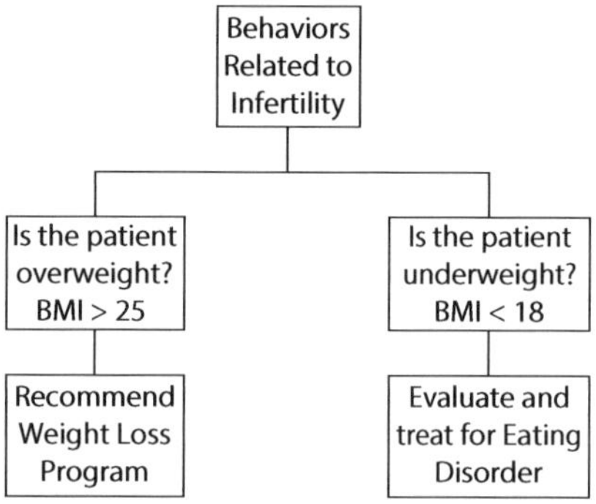

Figure 6.2 Example of options for behavior related to infertility.

more complex and nuanced evaluation and treatment plan. To date, there are no specific evidence-based treatments for eating disorders or substance use disorders in infertility patients, and treatment guidelines are usually based on treatments for patients in the general population [8]. Motivational interviewing will be an extremely important component of treatment for this population as it is in the general population [9]. Overweight and obese patients should be educated about studies that have shown increased rates of fertility in women and men who have been able to reduce their BMI through diet and exercise [10,11].

Cigarette smoking has been shown to have deleterious affects on both male and female fertility. In women, cigarette smoking may have multiple routes of fertility disruption, including altered hormonal milieu, disruption of ovarian transport in the fallopian tubes, and negative effects on the uterine environment, as women undergoing ovum donor assisted ART who smoke more than ten cigarettes per day have lower pregnancy rates than women who do not smoke [10]. In men, cigarette smoking is associated with reduced sperm motility, sperm count and fertilizing capacity; and it may be associated with an increased risk of sex chromosome abnormalities and disomies. Cessation of smoking for three months was associated with improvement in sperm concentration, motility and vitality in one study [10]. Because of this increasing research that cigarette smoking has negative effects on both male and female reproductive health, fertility counselors should identify this modifiable fertility factor, provide education about its effects on infertility treatment and aid patients in choosing and implementing a smoking cessation treatment plan.

Infertility medication-emergent side effects

For many infertility patients, review of potential medication-emergent side effects of treatment should be a standard part of the preconception counseling. Patients with prior history of hormonal sensitivity will be especially concerned about the potential central nervous effects of infertility medications, and they should be counseled regarding the current research, the implications of this research for their personal story and current gaps in knowledge.

Oral contraceptives

Many women are concerned about taking oral contraceptives (OCPs), a standard phase of early infertility treatment, because of the common belief that oral contraceptives are associated with mood changes. However, while earlier studies with higher dose estrogen and progesterone preparations suggested increased depressive symptoms in normal women [12] more recent studies evaluating pills with lower doses show most women do not experience mood changes with OCPs [13,14]. One side effect of OCPs that may occur in all women, though, is decreased libido. Oral contraceptives increase sex hormone-binding globulin that decrease free testosterone levels, which is associated with decreased libido in some women [14].

Gonadotropin releasing hormone agonists

Gonadotropin Releasing Hormone Agonists (GnRH agonists) are used frequently at the beginning of an infertility cycle. These medications lead to decreases in luteinizing (LH) and follicular stimulating (FSH) by negative feedback, and this hypogonadal state is similar to the hormonal milieu of menopause. Consequently, women taking GnRH agonists will frequently complain of hot flashes and sleep disturbance [15]. To date, studies of psychiatric symptoms with GnRH agonists have been small and involved women without mood disorders [16,17]. In general these medications have the potential to cause the side effects of irritability, depressed mood, anxiety, problems with memory and concentration [18]. Women in infertility treatment are likely to only be exposed to these medications for a few weeks, at most. A recent study of short-term GnRH use in healthy women failed to confirm early reports of significant memory and concentration changes [19] and another showed that depression and anxiety increased in women exposed to GnRH agonists not in the hypogonadal phase (i.e., the follicular phase), but later in the IVF cycle [20]. If these medications are required for extended period of time for treatment of fibroids, for instance, and if major depression emerges, sertraline (Zoloft) has been found to be a useful treatment [21].

Clomiphene citrate (Clomid)

Women with unexplained subfertility or polycystic ovarian syndrome (PCOS) are frequently prescribed clomiphene citrate as an infertility treatment. Clomiphene citrate is a synthetic estrogen receptor modulator with mixed agonist–antagonist properties. It is taken orally days 3–7 of menstrual cycle and creates a central perception of low estradiol [22]. Many women and their partners have reported that clomiphene citrate is associated with mood lability, often characterized as "super]PMS" [23,24]. While these symptoms appear to be most pronounced during the time that the medication is taken, it also has a long half-life, so these symptoms could theoretically persist beyond the time of oral intake.

Clomiphene citrate has even been associated with case reports of psychosis, occurring in patients with and without previous psychiatric history. In these case reports, there is a forewarning of sleeplessness and agitation progressing to auditory hallucinations, paranoia, delusions and ideas of reference. Notably, the onset of symptoms was within 48 hours of initiation of medication and neuroleptics and/or ECT resolved the symptoms [25–29].

Human menopausal gonadotropins

Women who are undergoing IVF (or in some cases intrauterine insemination) will use human menopausal gonadotropins, which are synthetic peptides similar in structure to GnRH that are delivered via injection.

These medications increase the number of ovarian follicles and are associated with extremely high serum estradiol levels. As in the case of clomiphene citrate, women exposed to these medications frequently describe mood lability [24].

In summary, detailed studies of women undergoing IVF with gonadotropins and progesterone supplementation showed increased depressive symptoms as they moved from the estrogen dominant phase (follicular) to the progesterone dominant phase (luteal phase), suggesting that changing levels of estrogen, rather than absolute levels of estrogen, were associated with changing symptoms [30]. Furthermore, women who had a previous Axis I diagnosis of anxiety or depression had even greater elevations in mood symptoms [31].

Psychopharmacology considerations for infertility patients

Infertility patients represent a unique population when psychiatric medications are being considered. As described in other chapters of this book, psychotherapy, with both individuals and couples, remains the first-line treatment of depression and anxiety disorders. If patients do require the addition of psychotropic medications to their psychotherapy, several important issues must be addressed, including impact of psychiatric medications on the menstrual cycle and ovulatory function, risk of spontaneous abortion, risk of congenital malformations and other perinatal complications.

Impact of antidepressants on the menstrual cycle

In general, antidepressants have not been commonly associated with menstrual cycle dysfunction. While typical and atypical antipsychotics are most commonly associated with increased prolactin levels, SSRIs have been associated with moderate increases as well, and hyperprolactinemia is associated with menstrual cycle abnormalities, including amenorrhea and oligomenorrhea [32]. Antidepressants that do not affect serotonin levels, such as Bupropion, are not associated with increases in prolactin. If a patient describes significantly increased breast size or pain, or nipple discharge or change in menstrual cycle length after initiation of an SSRI, they should be evaluated for elevated prolactin levels and consideration should be made to switch to another antidepressant if possible, such as Bupropion, and prolactin level rechecked.

Impact of antidepressants on spermatogenesis

The impact of SSRIs on sperm concentration, morphology and mobility remains controversial. Only a few small studies have been completed to investigate this question, but all have shown that treatment with SSRIs is associated with decreased sperm concentration and mobility, and increased DNA fragmentation

[33,34]. Men who are taking SSRIs for premature ejaculation should be referred to behavior therapy for this problem since it has been shown to be effective in several studies and is without the potential risks to sperm [35].

Impact of antidepressants on IVF outcome

To date, there are only three small studies comparing reproductive outcome in women undergoing IVF who are either on or not on SSRIs. One study randomized women who had normal anxiety levels at baseline to either Fluoxetine (Prozac) or folic acid during the IVF cycle. In both groups, anxiety increased significantly over the IVF cycle, and Fluoxetine was no more effective than placebo in treating the anxiety. There was no significant difference in IVF outcome between the two groups – no difference in quality of embryos, number of embryos transferred, pregnancy rate, spontaneous abortion rate or live birth rate [36]. Two retrospective chart reviews comparing women taking SSRIs to women not taking antidepressants also did not find significant differences in IVF outcomes [37,38]; although one study did report that women on antidepressants had a lower ongoing pregnancy rate [38]. In summary, to date, antidepressant exposure does not appear to affect egg quality or embryo development, but it is still not clear whether it has an effect on risk of spontaneous abortion.

Antidepressants and miscarriage

All antidepressants, regardless of class, have been associated with an increased rate of spontaneous abortion in individual studies and meta-analyses [39–41]. The causes of this possible increased rate of miscarriage remain unclear. Most studies have compared women with depression on antidepressants to women without depression not on antidepressants; consequently, the increased rate of spontaneous abortion may be due to the underlying condition of depression. To date, the studies examining antidepressants and the risk of spontaneous abortion are limited by methodological problems. When discussing this finding with patients, it is important to point out this limitation in the studies, as well as other confounding variables, such as the fact that no studies controlled for Body Weight Index (BMI), occult thyroid or medical illnesses commonly associated with infertility, or ovarian reserve. Furthermore, in several of the studies the significantly higher rate of miscarriage was still within the general population background rate, for instance 13% spontaneous abortion rate in antidepressant users, compared to 8% in nonusers [42]. Nevertheless, all fertility patients should be counseled about the potential increased risk of spontaneous abortion with use of antidepressants immediately prior to and during pregnancy because this is such an important consideration for this group.

Antidepressants and congenital malformation risks

All patients who are attempting to become pregnant will be concerned about whether antidepressants are associated with an increased risk of major congenital malformations. After several decades of research and thousands of children exposed worldwide to antidepressants, general consensus is that commonly used antidepressants, including serotonin reuptake inhibitors (SSRIs), serotonin norepinephrine reuptake inhibitors (SNRIs), tricyclic antidepressants (TCAs) and Bupropion are not major teratogens, that is adversely affecting the embryo [42]. To date, the associations between individual antidepressants and congenital malformations are based on very small numbers of cases, and no consistent, single type of malformation has been found across all classes of antidepressants, so currently it appears that the risk of a unifying teratogenicity is low. However, patients should be counseled about the conflicting reports of increased risk of cardiac defects with Paroxetine (Paxil) and it is not currently considered a first choice SSRI in perinatal patients [42].

Antidepressants and perinatal complications

While antidepressants do not appear to be highly associated with an increased risk of congenital malformations, they may be associated with perinatal complications such as persistent pulmonary hypertension, increased rates of preterm labor, neonatal adaptation syndrome and unknown long-term neurodevelopmental outcomes.

Persistent pulmonary hypertension

Persistent pulmonary hypertension (PPHN) is a rare condition occurring in term or near-term newborns associated with severe respiratory failure. It occurs when there is failure of the newborn to move from a high pulmonary vascular resistance to low pulmonary vascular resistance state at birth. The most recent, largest study of PPHN, a multinational cohort study ($n = 1\ 618\ 255$) of 17 053 SSRI exposed infants in early pregnancy and 11 014 later than week 20, found that exposure to SSRIs in late pregnancy was associated with approximately twice the rate of PPHN in newborns. Since PPHN is very rare, occurring in 1–3/1000 births, the highest rate in SSRI-exposed infants would be 1–6/1000 [43]. Other known risk factors for PPHN include Caesarian section and use of nonsteroidal anti-inflammatory agents (NSAIDs) [44], so patients who are likely to need these interventions should be counseled about possible additive risks.

Preterm labor and delivery

Preterm labor and delivery are defined as labor and delivery before 37 weeks. Some studies have reported higher rates of preterm delivery in women with depression on antidepressants in pregnancy compared to those who are not [42]. Currently, the relationship between antidepressant use and preterm labor and delivery remains controversial, but patients should be counseled that medication may confer additional risk and, consequently, patients should be even more conscientious about modifying other known risk factors for preterm labor, such as smoking, drinking and illicit drug use.

Neonatal adaptation syndrome

Maternal use of SSRIs and SNRIs in the third trimester of pregnancy has been associated with neonatal adaptation syndrome. This syndrome has included both signs of serotonin withdrawal and serotonin toxicity. The most common symptoms include restlessness, autonomic nervous system disturbances, respiratory distress, tremors, myoclonus and rarely seizures. The syndrome is common, affecting up to 30% of infants exposed to SSRIs and SNRIs in the last trimester, but to do date is not associated with mortality. All women taking SSRIs or SNRIs in pregnancy should be warned about this potential perinatal complication, and since it may be dose related it is yet another reason to encourage that all pregnant patients on antidepressants be treated with the lowest effective dose [42].

Long-term neurodevelopment

The long-term neurodevelopmental effects of antidepressant exposure in utero remain unknown. Infertility patients should be cautioned that SSRIs have been associated with developmental differences in fine and gross motor development, but the clinical significance of these differences is not yet known. For instance, in one of the earliest follow-up studies of infants of depressed mothers, infants exposed to depression during pregnancy and antidepressants had subtle fine motor abnormalities, including tremor [45]. These children have not been re-evaluated, so it is not known whether these were lasting changes beyond the age of 3 and if they were clinically significant. These neurodevelopmental follow-up studies have many methodological problems, and several have not controlled for critical confounding variables, such as familial history of neurodevelopmental problems [46]. While an early study of children exposed to SSRIs in utero reported a higher rate of autism spectrum disorders in exposed children [47], a later study, which controlled for autism in siblings, failed to find this association [48].

While antidepressants in pregnancy have been associated with the risks described above, it is important to point out that untreated major depression and anxiety disorders in pregnancy have also been associated with increased risk of perinatal complications, such as preterm labor and delivery, small for gestational age infants and newborn irritability [49].

Case discussion

Ms. G. underwent preconception counseling, following the guidelines outlined in this chapter. She was found to have strong personality traits of obsessionality, but she did not meet criteria for obsessive-compulsive personality disorder, or obsessive-compulsive disorder. She did have perfectionistic tendencies, and desire for her schedule to be predictable and all her "ducks in a row." When things were out of order, or unexpected, it caused a great deal of distress and anxiety. The fertility counselor helped Ms. G. and the treatment team identify ways that she could feel more in control and less anxious about her upcoming IVF procedure. She was given a detailed printed schedule of the medications, including a daily calendar. She was given the opportunity to attend as many injection-teaching classes as she needed, and the MHP normalized this process. Ms. G.'s husband was provided education as well, and he agreed to talk with his supervisor about decreasing his work schedule during the IVF cycle in order to provide extra household and emotional support. This intervention was extremely important to Ms. G., because she was also working outside the home, and it enabled her to have "fewer loose ends to worry about" and a predictable time for the injections.

Ms. G.'s depressive symptoms did meet criteria for major depression, moderate. She had no suicidal ideation and, at first, she said she was too busy to begin psychotherapy. Ms. G. confided to the fertility counselor that she felt she should "snap out of it," and that she should be grateful that she had at least one child, since many women in the infertility clinic had none. The MHP educated her about the increased risk of major depression in women after a miscarriage, and that women with recurrent miscarriages are at even greater risk [50]. The fertility counselor educated Ms. G. that her current symptoms were like other medical illnesses, and that major depression has well-established treatments, which include evidence-based psychotherapies, such as cognitive-behavioral therapy (CBT), interpersonal psychotherapy and brief dynamic psychotherapies. She explained to Ms. G. that therapy is the first-line approach to the treatment of anxiety and depression in infertility patients, but that at times medications may be needed as well.

She was advised to begin psychotherapy and be followed closely through the IVF cycle, because recent research has suggested that women with current or past anxiety and depressive symptoms do in fact have greater psychiatric distress during the complex hormonal manipulations of IVF, compared to women who are not currently depressed or anxious and who have no such history [31]. The fertility counselor explained that currently there is very little literature comparing antidepressants and psychotherapy in patients with infertility and depression, such as Ms. G., but that the available evidence suggested that either one alone or in combination could be very helpful [51,52]. Ms. G. was not currently suicidal, and was functioning well despite the distress, and she was very concerned about the safety of antidepressants in pregnancy. Since she was not in any sort of current treatment, and appeared to be an insightful, motivated and an excellent psychotherapy candidate, the fertility counselor and she chose to begin weekly psychotherapy. The MHP also referred Ms. G. to a mindfulness-based group therapy (MBSR) that was offered at night at the infertility clinic, since there is emerging evidence that MBSR is also effective in decreasing psychological distress associated with infertility diagnosis and treatment [53].

Ms. G. began weekly cognitive-behavioral psychotherapy with the fertility counselor, as well as MBSR group on Tuesday nights. Ms. G.'s husband followed through on his commitment to change his schedule, and he was home each night at 6:30 pm, which enabled Ms. G. to attend all MBSR meetings, to rely on him for her injections and to feel a greater sense of predictability in the nightly routine. Despite these interventions, Ms. G. experienced increased anxiety, irritability and obsessionality during the week after embryo transfer. She had noted increasing anxiety and insomnia as her estradiol levels increased during the cycle, but after the transfer, she felt even worse. Ms. G.'s depression had been clearly improving over the 8 weeks since the initial consult with the fertility counselor, despite the exposure to oral contraceptive for a month, and the week of GnRH flare. Ms. G. was referred to a cognitive-behavior therapy for insomnia therapist (CBT-I) and she was confused by the referral because she "thought she already was in CBT." The fertility counselor explained that CBTI-I is a specialized form of CBT. Ms. G. agreed to begin CBT-I because, she admitted, she had suffered on and off from insomnia throughout her life, but she insisted on a medication for immediate relief because she was so agitated, anxious and distressed at night because of inability to fall asleep or sustain sleep. Given the overall clear improvement in depression and anxiety and the acute onset of her symptoms, it was decided to treat her insomnia and anxiety symptomatically for a few days, with an antihistamine for sleep and a benzodiazepine on an as-needed basis.

Psychopharmacology with the perinatal patient

Insomnia and anxiety

Many patients with infertility will complain of insomnia and it is very important for the fertility counselor to clarify whether this insomnia is associated with the stress of the infertility process, whether it is associated with infertility medications and therefore likely time-limited, or whether it is due to an underlying primary psychiatric illness, such as major depression or an anxiety disorder. To date, there are no studies of evaluation and treatment of insomnia in infertility patients, and the clinician must base treatment decisions on the perinatal literature. Cognitive-behavior therapy for insomnia (CBT-I) is the first-line approach to insomnia in pregnant women, once other causes such as restless leg syndrome and obstructive sleep apnea have been ruled out by clinical history [54]. For patients for whom an acute treatment for insomnia is needed, many clinicians will begin with a trial of an antihistamine, such as diphenhydramine 25–50 mg at night because, to date, the use of antihistamines in pregnancy for a wide range of conditions, including allergies, hyperemesis and insomnia has not been associated with an increased rate of congenital malformations [55]. If diphenhydramine is not effective, hypnotic benzodiazepine agonists, such as Zolpidem, can be tried on a very limited basis as they too, to date, have not been associated with congenital malformations in the limited available studies [56].

Benzodiazepine use in pregnancy is very controversial, since the early case control studies of benzodiazepines reported increased risk of cleft lip and cleft palate. More recent prospective studies and case control studies have not found such a strong association, yet, in general, these medications should be used sparingly in the perinatal population, and if the patient has persistent anxiety and depression, despite improved sleep and psychotherapy, then an SSRI would be the next step for ongoing anxiety.

Postpartum depression

Depression and anxiety during pregnancy increase the risk for postpartum depression [57]. To date, there are very few studies investigating rates of postpartum depression in infertility patients. While some studies have found lower rates of depressive symptoms in pregnant women who conceive through IVF [58,59], others have reported depressive symptom rates as high as 25% [60], although have used differing measures and have not consistently confirmed a major depressive episode, but rather reported symptoms. Higher numbers of IVF cycles, Caesarian section and poor social support may increase the risk for postpartum depression depression [60] in women who have undergone IVF. For some women, the stress of infertility diagnosis and treatment may be associated with some symptoms of trauma, especially if the infertility journey has included miscarriage or stillbirth. All women should be screened by their healthcare providers for anxiety and depression during pregnancy and postpartum, and women who have experienced infertility and now delivered a healthy child should be screened as well, as it should not be assumed that they are immune to the development of depression.

Even if the woman is not depressed or anxious during pregnancy, women with a past history of major depression, perinatal medical complications, low social support, marital/partner problems and personality characteristics of perfectionism should be carefully followed and assessed after giving birth because these are common risk factors for postpartum depression.

Women with a history of bipolar disorder are at an especially high risk for the development of postpartum depression and postpartum psychosis, with some studies suggesting rates as high as 50% [61]. Treatment of women with bipolar disorder during pregnancy and the postpartum period should be reserved for a perinatal psychiatrist who specializes in this area, since assessment of the risks and benefits of continuing or discontinuing mood stabilizers and antipsychotics in pregnancy is a rapidly changing, extremely challenging clinical specialty [62,63].

Conclusion

Infertility patients are a high-risk group for anxiety and depressive disorders, and infertility medications themselves may have neuropsychiatric effects. Consequently, the fertility counselor has an extremely important role in the infertility treatment team. Early evaluation and treatment of psychological distress in infertility patients will improve their quality of life, enhance compliance and facilitate care during a complex and challenging time. MHPs specializing in this area must be constantly reviewing the literature regarding emerging therapies, and the safety of psychopharmacological interventions in the perinatal population, as the field is constantly changing. To date, the literature strongly supports the use of psychotherapy as a first-line treatment of mood and anxiety symptoms in infertility patients [1], but if psychopharmacologic intervention is required, a very careful review of up-to-date literature is needed in order to help the patient, her partner and involved family members and friends feel as comfortable as possible with the choice of medication. The reader is referred to the following websites, which are routinely updated, for more information:

MotherToBaby: https://www.mothertobaby.org.

MotherRisk Program: http://www.motherisk.org.

Reflections from the reproductive psychiatrist

Over the past 20 years, there has been a growing awareness and appreciation for the emotional and physical stress involved in the diagnosis and treatment of infertility. As I reflect on my 20 years in the field of perinatal psychiatry, it has been a great relief to see that the psychological and psychiatric complaints and concerns of patients are being taken seriously both by the clinician and the researcher. While early reports of side effects from the infertility medications were initially overlooked, recently these complaints have been the subject of careful studies [20]. Women are finally being screened for mood and anxiety disorders during treatment and for risk factors for medication emergent side effects. It is exciting to see that mental healthcare has become an integral part of the infertility treatment process.

References

1. Domar AD, Moragianni VA, Ryley DA, Urato AC. The risks of serotonin reuptake inhibitor use in infertile women: a review of the impact on fertility, pregnancy, neonatal health and beyond. *Hum Reprod.* 2013 Jan; 28(1): 160–71.
2. Mazure C, Greenfeld DA. Psychological studies of in vitro fertilization/embryo transfer participants. *J In Vitro Fertil Emb Transfer.* 1989; 6: 242–56.
3. Galhardo A, Pinto-Gouvela J, Cunha M, Matos M. The impact of shame and self-judgment on psychopathology in infertile patients. *Human Reprod.* 2011; 26(9): 2408–14.
4. Andrews B, Qian M, Valentine J. Predicting depressive symptoms with a new measure of shame: the experience of shame scale. *Br J Clin Psychol.* 2002; 41: 29–42.
5. Tangney J, Wagner P, Gramzow R. Proneness to shame, proneness to guilt and psychopathology. *J Abnor Psychol.* 1992; 101: 469–78.
6. Volgsten H, Ekselius H, Poromaa L, Sundstrom I, Svanbert AS. Personality traits associated with depressive and anxiety disorders in infertile women and men undergoing in vitro fertilization treatment. *Acta Obstet gynecol Scand.* 2010; 89: 27–34.
7. Martini J, Wittchen HU, Soares CN, Rieder A, Steiner M. New women-specific diagnostic modules: the Composite International Diagnostic Interview for Women (CIDI-VENUS) *Arch Womens Ment Health* 2009; 12: 281–9.
8. American Psychiatric Association, ed. *American Psychiatric Association Practice Guidelines for the Treatment of Psychiatric Disorders: Compendium 2006.* American Psychiatric Pub, 2006.
9. Lundahl B, Moleni T, Burke BL, Butters R, Tollefson D, Butler C, Rollnick S. Motivational interviewing in medical care settings: a systematic review and meta-anlysis of randomized controlled trials. *Patient Educ Couns.* 2013; 93(2): 157–68.
10. Campagne DM. Can male fertility be improved prior to assisted reproduction through the control of uncommonly considered factors? *Int J Fertil Steril.* 2013; 6(4): 214–23.
11. Sharma R, Biedenharn KR, Fedor JM, Agarwal A. Lifestyle factors and reproductive health: taking control of your fertility. *Reprod Biol Endocrinol.* 2013; 11: 66.
12. Oinonen KA and Mazmonian D. To what extent do oral contraceptives influence mood and affect? *J Affect Disord.* 2002; 20: 229–40, review.
13. Rapkin A, et al. Decreased neuroactive steroids induced by combined oral contraceptives are not associated with mood changes. *Fertil Med Steril.* 2006; 85: 1371–8.
14. Graham CA, Bancroft J, Doll HA, Greco T, Tanner A. Does oral contraceptive-induced reduction in free testosterone adversely affect the sexuality or mood of women? *Psychoendocrinology* 2007; 32: 245–55.
15. Jogge H, White DP, Crawford SL, McCurnin KE, Economou N, Connors S, Hall JE. Adverse effects of induced hot flashes objectively recorded and subjectively reported sleep: results of a gonadotropin-releasing hormone agonist experimental protocol. *Menopause* 2013; 20(9): 905–14.
16. Warnock JK, Bundren JC. Anxiety and mood disorders associated with gonadotropin-releasing hormone agonist therapy. *Psychopharmacol Bull.* 1997; 33: 311–16.
17. Toren P, Dor J, Mester R, Mester R, Mozes T, Blumnesohn R, Rehavi W, Weizman A. Depression in women treated with a gonadotropin-releasing hormone agonist. *Biol Psychiatry* 1996; 39: 378–82.
18. Varney NR, Syrop C, Kubu CS, et al. Neuropsychologic dysfunction in women following leuprolide acetate induction of hypoestrogenism. *J Assist Reprod Genet.* 1993; 10: 53–7.
19. Schmidt PJ, Keenan PA, Schenkel LA, Berlin K, Gibson C, Rubinow DR. Cognitive performance in healthy women during induced hypogonadism and ovarian steroid addback. *Arch Womens Ment Health* 2013 Feb; 16(1): 47–58.
20. Bloch FM, Azem F, Aharonov I, Avi B, Yagil Y, Schreiber S, Amit A, Weizman A. GnRH induced

depressive and anxiety symptoms during in vitro fertilization-embryo transfers. *Fertil Steril.* 2011; 95: 307–9.

21. Warnock JK, Bundren JC, Morris. Sertraline in the treatment of depression associated with gonadotropin releasing hormone agonist therapy. *Biol Psychiatry* 1998; 43: 464–5.
22. Martikainen H, Ronnberg L, Ruokonen A, Kauppila A. Gonadotropin pulsatility in a stimulated cycle: Clomiphene cit rate increases pulse amplitudes of both luteinizing hormone and follicle stimulating hormone. *Fertil Steril.* 1991; 56: 641–5.
23. Brenner JL. Clomiphene-induced mood swings. *J Obstet Gynecol Neonatal Nurs.* 1991; 20: 321–7.
24. Choi SH, Shapiro H, Robinson GE, Irvine J, Neuman J, Rosen B, Murphy J, Steward D. Psychological side-effects of clomiphene citrate and human. *J Psychosom Obstet Gynaecol.* 2005; 26: 93–100.
25. Cashman FE. Clomiphene citrate as a possible cause of psychosis. *Can Med Assoc.* 1982; 15: 118.
26. Oyffe I, Lerner A, Isaacs G, Harel Y, Sigal M. Clomiphene-induced psychosis. *Am J Psychiatry* 1997; 154: 1169–70.
27. Altmark D, Tomaer R, Sigal M. Psychotic episode induced by ovulation-initiating treatment. *Isr J Med Sci.* 1987; 23: 1156–7.
28. Siedntopf F, Horskamp B, Stief G, et al. Clomiphene citrate as a possible cause of a psychotic reaction during infertility treatment. *Human Reprod.* 1997; 12: 706–7.
29. Parikh AR, Kiskow BI. Manic delirium associated with clomiphene induced ovulation. *Psychosomatics* 2007; 48(1): 65–6.
30. Bloch M et al. Gonadal steroids and affective symptoms during in vitro fertilization: implications for reproductive mood disorders. *Psychoneuroend.* 2011; 36(6): 790–6.
31. Zaig I, Azem F, Schreiber S, Amit A, Litvin YG, Bloch M. Psychological response and cortisol reactivity to in vitro fertilization treatment in women with a lifetime anxiety or unipolar mood disorder diagnosis. *J Clin Psychiatry* 2013; 74(4): 386–92.
32. Ajmal A, Joffe H, Nachtigall LB. Psychotropic-induced hyperprolactinemia: a clinical review. *Psychosomatics* 2014; 5(1): 37–44.
33. Koyuncu H, Serefoglu EC, Yencilek E, Atalay H, Akbas NB, Sarica K. Escitalopram treatment for premature ejaculation has a negative effect on semen parameters. *Int J Impot Res.* 2011; 23(6): 251–61.
34. Tanrikut, Feldman AS, Altemus M, Paduch DA, Schlegel PN. Adverse effect of paroxetine on sperm. *Fertil Steril.* 2010; 94(3): 1021–6.
35. Melnik T, Althof S, Atallah AN, Puga ME, Glina S, Riera R. Psychosocial interventions for premature ejaculation. *Cochrane Database Syst Rev.* 2011; 10(8): 1–22.
36. Serafini P, Lobo DS, Grosman A, Seibel D, Rocha AM, Motta EL. Fluoxetine treatment for anxiety in women undergoing in vitro fertilization. *Int J Gynaecol Obstet.* 2009 May; 105(2): 136–9.
37. Friedman BE, Rogers JL, Shahine LK, Westphal LM, Lathi RB Effect of selective serotonin inhibitors on in vitro fertilization outcome. *Fertil Steril.* 2009; 92: 1312–14.
38. Klock SC, Sheinin S, Kazer R, Zhang X. A pilot study of the relationship between selective serotonin reuptake inhibitors and in vitro fertilization outcome. *Fertil Steril.* 2004; 82: 968–9.
39. Hemels ME, Einarson A, Koren G, Lanctot KL, Einarson TR. Antidepressant use during pregnancy and the rates of spontaneous abortions: a meta-analysis. *Ann Pharmacother.* 2005; 39: 803–9.
40. Broy P, Bérard A. Gestational exposure to antidepressants and the risk of spontaneous abortion: a review. *Curr Drug Delivery* 2010; 7(1): 76–92.
41. Einarson A, Choi J, Einarson TR, Koren G. Rates of spontaneous and therapeutic abortions following use of antidepressants in pregnancy: results from a large prospective database. *J Obstet Gynaecol Can.* 2009 May; 31(5): 452–6.
42. Byatt N, Deligiannidis KM, Freeman MP. Antidepressant use in pregnancy: a critical review focused on risks and controversies. *Acta Psychiatrica Scand.* 2013; 127(2): 94–114.
43. Kieler H, Artama M, Engeland A, Ericsson O, Furu K, Gissler M et al. Selective serotonin reuptake inhibitors during pregnancy and risk of persistent pulmonary hypertension in the newborn: population based cohort study from the five Nordic countires. *BMJ* 2012; 12: 1–19.
44. Grigoriadis S, Vonderporten EH, Mamisashvili L, Tomlinson G, Dennis CL, Koren G, Steiner M, Mousmanis P, Cheung A, Ross LE. Prenatal exposure to antidepressants and persistent pulmonary hypertension of the newborn: systematic review and meta-analysis. *BMJ* 2014:348.
45. Casper RC, Fleisher BE, Lee-Ancajas JC, Gilles A, Gaylor E, DeBattista A, Hoyme HE. Follow up of children of depressed mothers exposed or not exposed to antidepressant drugs during pregnancy. *J Pediatr.* 2003; 142(4): 402–8.
46. Gentile S, Galbally M. Prenatal exposure to antidepressant medications and neurodevelopmental outcomes: a systematic review. *J Affect Disord.* 2011; 128: 1–9.

47. Croen LA, Grether JK, Yoshida CK, Odouli R, Hendrick V. Antidepressant use during pregnancy and childhood autism spectrum disorders. *Arch Gen Psychiatry* 2011 Nov; 68(11): 1104–12.

48. Sørensen MJ, Grønborg TK, Christensen J, Parner ET, Vestergaard M, Schendel D, Pedersen LH. Antidepressant exposure in pregnancy and risk of autism spectrum disorders. *Clin Epidemiol.* 2013 Nov 15; 5: 449–59.

49. Hanley GE, Oberlander TF. The effect of perinatal exposures on the infant: depression and antidepressants. *Best Pract Res Clin Obstet Gynecol.* 2014; 28(1): 37–48.

50. Lok IH, Neugerbauer R. Psychological morbidity following miscarriage. *Best Pract Res Clin Obstet Gynaecol.* 2007 Apr; 21(2): 229–47.

51. Pasha H, Faramarzi M, Esmailzadeh S, Kheirkhah F, Salmalian H. Comparison of pharmacological and nonpharmacological treatment strategies in promotion of infertility self-efficacy scale in infertile women: a randomized controlled trial. *Iran J Reprod Med.* 2013; 11(6): 495–502.

52. Faramarzi M, Pasha H, Esmailzadeh S, Kheirkhah F, Heidary S, Afshar Z. The effect of the cognitive behavioral therapy and pharmacotherapy on infertility stress: a randomized controlled trial. *Int J Fertil Steril.* 2013; 7(3): 199–206.

53. Galhardo A, Cunha M, Pinto-Gouveia J. Mindfulness based program for infertility: efficacy study. *Fertil Steril.* 2013; 100(4): 1059–67

54. Jones CR. Diagnostic and management approach to common sleep disorders during pregnancy. *Clin Obstet Gynecol.* 2013; 56(2): 360–7.

55. Mitchell AA, Werler MM, Yau W, Hernández-Díaz S. Assessment of antihistamine use in early pregnancy and birth defects. *J Allergy Clin Immunol.* 2013; 1(6): 666–74.

56. Wikner BN, Kallen B. Are hypnotic benzodiazepine receptor agonists teratogenic in humans? *J Clin Psychopharmacol.* 2011; 31(3): 356–9.

57. Siu BW, Leung SS, Ip, P, Hung SF, O'Hara MW. Antenatal risk factors for postnatal depression: A prospective study of chinese women at maternal and child health centres. *BMC Psychiatry* 2012; 12: 22.

58. Fisher JR, Hammarberg K, Baker GH. Antenatal mood and fetal attachment after assisted conception. *Fertil Steril.* 2008; 89(5): 1103–12.

59. Harf-Kashdaei E, Kaitz M. Antenatal moods regarding self and baby and spouse among women who conceived by IVF. *Fertil Steril.* 2007; 87(6): 1306–13.

60. Lee SH, Lin LC, Kuo PC, Lee MS. Postpartum depression and correlated risk factors in women who received in vitro fertilization treatment. *J Midwifery Womens Health* 2011; 56(4): 347–52.

61. Di Florio A, Forty L, Gordon-Smith K, Heron J, Jones L, Craddock N, Jones I. Perinatal episodes across the mood disorder spectrum. *JAMA Psychiatry* 2013 Feb; 70(2): 168–75.

62. Vemuri M, Williams, KE. Treating bipolar disorder during pregnancy. *Curr Psychiatry* 2011; 10(9): 59–66.

63. Robakis TK, Williams KE. Atypical antipsychotics during pregnancy. *Curr Psychiatry* 2013; 12(7): 12–18.

Chapter 7

Counseling recipients of anonymous donor gametes

Patricia L. Sachs and Carol B. Toll

"Welcome to the Waiting Room."

Our waiting room is full, shared by people with many different stories. Their eyes focus on anything but those seated around them and many look serious, uncomfortable, and anxious. As fertility counselors, we often hear from patients what a lonely place the waiting room can be; rarely will they reach out to one another. However, we know that if they are recipients of anonymous donor gametes they share the common loss and pain of not being able to conceive a child genetically connected to them: the woman who is "aging out" of being able to use her own eggs; the man who is shocked to learn that he has no sperm; the single woman who finds she must now use both a sperm donor and an egg donor; and the same-sex couple who are using donor gametes to create their family – all of them can be found in the waiting room. Wishing to feel hopeful, they may sometimes also feel confused, worried, perhaps ashamed, and possibly alone. As you read through this chapter you will learn more about them and the role played by the fertility counselor in their journeys as anonymous donor gamete recipients.

In this chapter, we will take you into the waiting room, presenting the psychosocial aspects of family building using anonymous egg donation, sperm donation and embryo creation, and the clinical issues that arise. The role of the fertility counselor providing preparation, support, education and evaluation as an integral member of the reproductive treatment team will be explored. This will include how to prepare for and conduct the recipient interview, helping patients to identify issues unique to their situation, including decision-making, informed consent, donor selection and disclosure. We will use vignettes to illustrate these stories related to the use of donor gametes, and will share reflections on our experiences of counseling recipients of donor gametes.

The addenda referred to in this chapter are available for download at www.cambridge.org/9781107643116. Password: AX164BKR7.

Introduction

The use of donated oocytes (OD) has become an option for family building since the 1980s, with the first egg donor pregnancy occurring in Australia in 1984 [1]. Though initially used for women with Primary Ovarian Insufficiency (POI), egg donation is now used successfully to treat a wide range of conditions including women who have survived cancer, experienced multiple pregnancy losses, carry genetic diseases and have poor egg quality due to advanced maternal age. Donation prior to this time had been centered on insemination with donated sperm for severe male factor infertility, which for over 100 years was the only option. However, with the advent of ICSI (intracytoplasmic sperm injection) in 1990, men with even extremely low sperm counts are able to father a child through the use of even one healthy sperm. Since the sperm may need to be obtained surgically or still result in unhealthy embryos, recipient couples also need to be prepared, through counseling, for the possibility of using donor sperm as "back up." Furthermore, reproductive technology now also allows for the use of not only donated eggs, but both donated eggs and donor sperm chosen before treatment, referred to here as embryo creation (EC). (EC differs from embryo donation, where embryos previously created during infertility treatment, cryopreserved, and no longer needed, are donated by one individual/couple to another, which will not be addressed in this

Fertility Counseling: Clinical Guide and Case Studies, ed. Sharon N. Covington. Published by Cambridge University Press.

chapter.) This broadens the ability to conceive a child not only genetically unrelated to one parent, but to neither.

There is almost universal consensus by professional organizations and legislative bodies worldwide that counseling for patients considering third party reproduction (i.e., recipients of donated gametes or surrogacy) is important. The first country to establish oversight of assisted reproductive technologies was the United Kingdom in 1990 with The Human Fertilisation and Embryology Act [2], which required that counseling be offered to all potential donor gamete recipients for psychoeducational, but not evaluative, purposes. The HFE Act was amended in 2004 and 2008 to require that donor identity be made available to donor-conceived offspring. Some Australian states have followed with mandated fertility counseling for all gamete recipients as well as donors, and both Victoria and Western Australia have legislated the right of donor-conceived offspring to learn the identity of their donors [3]. In addition, the Mental Health Professional Group (MHPG) in collaboration with the Practice Committee of the American Society of Reproductive Medicine (ASRM) [4] and the Psychological Special Interest Group of the European Society of Human Reproduction and Embryology (PSIG/ESHRE) have developed guidelines for psychological counseling for all parties involved in sperm and oocyte donation [5].

While there is strong international consensus on the importance of counseling in third party reproduction, there is diverse opinion about allowing anonymity in gamete donation. In Australia, the Netherlands and the UK, for example, a donor must provide identifying information, and a child in the UK can find their donor in a national registry. However, in both Spain and the USA anonymous donation is allowed, though channels for getting information for reasons of medical urgency do exist. There are those who believe strongly that it is in the best interests of the child and family that the donor's identity be accessible. However, the discussion continues and evokes strong feelings on the part of donors who feel that their identity should be protected, as well as recipients who prefer to keep these matters private. In Spain, for example, where the importance of the traditional family remains strong and where outsider knowledge of donor conception is perceived as potentially stigmatizing, there is an argument for maintaining anonymity in gamete donation. Therefore, it is unlikely that in countries like Spain or the USA anonymity will disappear anytime in the near future [6], which necessitates a chapter such as this.

Psychosocial impact

Receiving the diagnosis that egg donation, sperm donation or both are needed in order to conceive is distressing for anyone to experience. A range of feelings, including loss, sadness, anger, shame and betrayal may create a deep sense of grief over the inability to have a genetically linked child.

Donor egg

The use of an egg donor is rarely a first choice, and there may be gender differences in how men and women react to this information. For women, being told that their eggs are "too old" may be devastating. They may feel defective or damaged, their very sense of being a woman threatened, including feeling "less than" female. Women may worry about attachment to a baby conceived through the use of an anonymous woman's eggs. Men may experience the loss equally, and feel helpless in easing their partner's pain. Men will have the genetic connection to a child and may be pleased that one parent will still be genetically related, but feel guilty at the same time. For women, the ability to be biologically (if not genetically) attached to their baby through pregnancy, the strong desire to nurture the unborn child and the ability to have their baby be genetically connected to their male partner, are all strong motivating factors in a woman's/couple's ultimate decision to pursue egg donation [7].

Sue, 40, and Adam, 42, have been married for three years. Sue has been pursuing an academic career and could not take time off for marriage and a baby until achieving tenure. Now, they are ready to have a family but have had no success trying on their own. Adam has a busy technical career and also felt waiting was the right thing. However, they are both beginning to doubt the wisdom of their choices. Sue wonders why she was uninformed about age and fertility and is blaming herself and "society" for putting women in a bind between career and parenthood. Learning that egg donation is an option, Sue is initially uninterested, still reeling from shock and grief. Adam, although distraught at first, quickly accepts egg donation as a practical and viable solution. Sue wonders how he can possibly give up the thought of their genetic child and feels angry that he does not seem to be as distressed as she is. Sue and Adam agree that they need time to learn more about the process and the long-term implications.

The fertility counselor often meets with donor egg recipients at different points in the egg donation process. Early on in this case, Sue needs the chance to express her feelings of loss. Labeling this as a grieving process can give her the chance to normalize the emotions she has and give her time to process all that has happened to her dreams. Adam, accomplishing this process more quickly, may also have the same deep feelings Sue has, but wants to move to a solution to make it better for her. One partner may focus on positive statistics and financial options, while the other is slower to embrace this path. Normalizing that it takes time for acceptance and that the process itself is lengthy can give them permission to move forward at their own pace.

Donor sperm

For men, getting the news that they are azoospermic can be an enormous shock, particularly if there is no clear cause and no known family history of male factor infertility. For men raised in families/cultures where masculinity is especially prized, it may feel particularly embarrassing or humiliating to not be able to "get their wives pregnant." Men may feel less masculine, as they may associate fertility with virility. Research has shown that men's attitudes towards the use of donor sperm are more negative than towards the use of donor eggs [8]. They may also grieve the end of their "family line" if they are the only male child in their family of origin. They may fear rejection of their child by the family as well as rejection of themselves by the child. Unlike women using a donor egg, who can still be connected to their baby through pregnancy, men using donor sperm lose a vital connection to the potential child and may wonder how they will feel a sense of attachment.

George, age 29, and Cindy, age 27, have been married for three years, and been trying to conceive for the past year. Surprised that she wasn't getting pregnant despite being relatively young, Cindy thought it was time that the couple consult a fertility specialist. They were shocked to learn that while Cindy's testing was normal, George had no sperm. The couple was unfamiliar with male factor infertility and felt surprised, because there was no apparent cause. The diagnosis and lack of treatment options left George with feelings of confusion, sadness, anger and guilt. He began pulling away emotionally from Cindy, though he worried that she might reject him for being "the problem" and might want to look for a fertile partner. He was ashamed at having this "defect" which made him feel like less of a man. Coming from many generations of sons, he felt like a failure at being "the end of the line," and wondered if his family could ever accept a child conceived with donor sperm as being truly "theirs." He also wondered how he could bond with a child that was not genetically his. For her part, Cindy felt confused, sad, and, silently, angry at George for their situation, though rationally she knew he was not to blame.

As a fertility counselor working with this couple, it is important to give both George and Cindy the time and space to identify and grieve the many losses that accompany this diagnosis. Additionally, the counselor can help them to see that though the medical problem lies with George, this really is an issue shared by the couple. Going beyond shame and blame to the commonality of their feelings can help them move towards acceptance of the situation, and assessment of whether the use of donor sperm is a viable option for them.

Embryo creation (EC)

When faced with the need for both donor egg and sperm, recipients may choose this option because of the ability to select each of the donors, experience a pregnancy and have some control over the process. While some recipients may question the idea of creating embryos when children needing adoptive families already exist, others prefer to take charge and create a child of their own by selecting each of the donors. The idea of creating a child not genetically connected to either parent may raise spiritual, ethical and social concerns that will need to be addressed in counseling. In addition, a child created from two donors may potentially feel a sense of genetic bewilderment, with no genetic link to a parent. The fertility counselor can be helpful in guiding recipients to understand these issues.

Heather, a 42-year-old single woman, has been attempting unsuccessfully to become pregnant through the use of donor sperm for the past two years. It appears that due to her advancing age, her best chance for a pregnancy now would be to create embryos through the use of donor eggs and donor sperm. While she feels that she had successfully grieved the loss of being able to have a baby with a partner/father for her child, the idea now of giving up the ability to be the genetic mother is much more challenging for her. She worries about how a child will feel about having been created in this way, (i.e., in effect, "related to no one") and what characteristics she would use to select each of the donors. She also wonders how she would tell the child about its donor origins, since the decision to use an egg donor is such an emotional one for her. Heather herself was adopted as an infant and says that this will enable her to have more empathy for the child, whose situation will be "sort of the flip" of hers – related not genetically but biologically. She wants the experience of pregnancy, yet she feels it would have been "healing" in some way to be able to see another person who might look like her.

The fertility counselor can empathize with Heather's need to give birth and experience a biological connection with another human being as well as being in a unique position to understand how the child might feel, being unrelated genetically to his/her parent. The fertility counselor has an opportunity to prepare future parents like Heather by helping her to process her background and how it relates to parenting a child created in this way. As Heather feels more confident in her role as a mother, she will in turn transmit these feelings of comfort, security and acceptance to her child about his/her means of creation.

Same-sex recipients

Gay and lesbian couples come for treatment knowing that they will need to use a sperm/egg donor to have a child and face different issues than heterosexual couples. For gay male couples using an egg donor (and gestational carrier), a first step may be to become more familiar with the female reproductive system in the context of fertility treatment. Gay couples will need to decide whose sperm will be used, and whether they will be looking for characteristics in an egg donor that will somehow replicate the appearance, talents, and so on of the non-genetic father. Lesbian couples using a sperm donor will need to make corresponding decisions as well. When same-sex couples use an anonymous donor, many are also concerned about having access to donor information to share with their child in the future. Many sperm banks offer an "open identity" donor, which enables couples to select a donor willing to make himself known/available to a potential child upon reaching the age of 18, if the child initiates contact. Lesbian couples may sometimes find this a favorable option as a means of leaving the door open for their child to obtain more information or even perhaps a relationship with the donor, as they may not otherwise have a "father figure" in their lives. In addition, some egg donor agencies have various layers of openness with donor information and access. For gay couples, the chance to be able to provide more information about a donor to a potential child can also be desirable and a consideration in donor selection. (For more information on counseling same-sex couples, please refer to Chapter 13.)

Kevin and Mario have been together for five years and recently married. Prior to their marriage both had discussed the desire for children together, as Kevin has a son, 12, from a previous relationship who will be living with them. Mario is getting adjusted to the idea of day-to-day parenting as well as feeling stressed about all that needs to be managed in the process of finding an egg donor and gestational carrier. They are working with a supportive agency but the logistics and finances are daunting. Because Kevin already has a child, he wants Mario to be the genetic father and to choose the egg donor. Mario is looking for an egg donor who shares Kevin's traits and hopes a child will look like Kevin's son. Mario spends considerable time reading donor profiles without seeing a match. He begins to worry that he will never find "the one."

Kevin and Mario are experiencing several life changes. Many donor recipients find themselves starting treatment during times of transition and often one member of a couple will "take charge" of the fertility process. This can sometimes become overwhelming, leading to stress and "getting stuck" in the process. Mario may feel there is an ideal donor for them and is growing frustrated and worried when that perfect candidate has not emerged. The fertility counselor can help them understand the emotional as well as practical issues that arise with donor selection and talk through their options. Couples may benefit from working as a team to review candidates as well as to make a final choice. Mario may be relieved that he will not have to carry all of the responsibility in making decisions that will affect both of them, as well as their future child. Further acknowledgment of their changes and adjustments may also relieve stress and help them have realistic expectations of themselves and the process.

Making the decision to use a donor

The decision to use a donor(s) can be complex and involve emotional, physical and practical considerations uniquely configured for each recipient. Understanding what is involved in this decision can help recipients feel more engaged and able to appreciate what they can still experience or control in a positive way, as what they have lost is usually readily apparent. For many, the goal of becoming parents can still be achieved. One parent may have a genetic connection to the child or be able to participate in the selection of both donors as in EC. The often longed for experience of pregnancy, physically and socially, can be a reality. When age is a factor, using a donor can reduce the genetic risks associated with age or relieve anxiety over concerns about their own genetic history. Yet by selecting donor characteristics that are similar to the recipient's own, a child may still look as if they "fit in" a family, alleviating fears that others would see a child as "not like" the parents. If recipients have already gone through fertility treatment they may feel comfortable or at least familiar with being a fertility patient. They may continue to take advantage of fertility treatment insurance benefits or financial programs such as "shared risk" options, to help manage treatment costs. Sharing donors increases the possibility of other "genetically related" children and opens the idea of using a registry established for donor siblings. Adoption, while an acceptable option for many, involves learning the complexities of a new system and requirements that may limit options due to age or situation. Using donation to build a family seems to help recipients feel more in control and the increased chances of success bring "new hope" to those who choose this path.

With time and the resolution of the grieving process, most recipients are able to adjust to the reality of their medical situation and grow to see egg and/or sperm donation as a good, albeit different way to form a family. They may strive to create a child who resembles them in some way. Most recipients will try to select their donors on the basis of a healthy, medical/genetic family history that is a good match with their own, as well as considering similarity in appearance, race/ethnicity, educational level and personality [9]. In reality, however, donor selection may well be dictated by available options rather than idealized characteristics.

Recipient counseling interview: purpose and process

The role of the counselor

Patients and those who provide medical care acknowledge the importance of emotional preparation before treatment through counseling. Research supports the idea that there is benefit not only at the time of treatment, but that it imparts a positive impact for the future of families created through egg donation, sperm donation and embryo creation [10].

There is debate among mental health professionals and fertility counseling organizations over the role of the fertility counselor, with some believing that the counselor's role should be evaluative, while others see it more as a matter of preparing the recipients for treatment, providing education on donor-related issues, and offering support at the time of treatment and into the future. These two roles can conflict, if recipients view the counselor as a potential "gatekeeper" who is evaluating their suitability to be parents and whether or not they should be permitted to continue with treatment.

It is important that the counselor be clear with the recipients as to the scope of his/her role. When counseling is required as part of a clinic's protocol, it is natural for recipients to experience some anxiety while wondering if they are being assessed or might possibly even be denied treatment. In the initial contact, the counselor should inform the recipients that the primary purpose of the interview is psychoeducational in nature, that is to consider the implications of donor reproductive assistance as well as to give information and resources. The counselor will ask about the infertility history of the recipients, how they made the decision to proceed with donor gametes, provide information, explore current thinking about major issues and how to handle these issues with others, as well as a future child. However, if the counseling is evaluating the patient's appropriateness for treatment, this should be clearly stated before the consultation begins.

Studies have shown that most infertile people are emotionally healthy and not significantly different than others [11]. Thus, the expectation should be that these are healthy individuals trying to cope with an abnormal, highly stressful event in their lives, and attempting to make the best possible decisions in dealing with it [12]. However, circumstances may come to light that indicate significant issues that need to be addressed before treatment is recommended. There may be significant disagreement about the desire to have a child, have a child through donor procedures, or about the impact of this decision on future family functioning. One partner may feel pressured or resistant to moving forward. Recipients may also exhibit significant relationship problems or find themselves at odds over life goals and financial choices. Communication may have become strained. Instead of being on their "best behavior" as is usually seen, patients may "fight" in front of the counselor, possibly as a way of expressing their distress. Untreated or unacknowledged mental health problems may impair their ability to complete treatment, make decisions, or give consent. There may be emotional ramifications if changes in medication are needed due to pregnancy. Drug or alcohol abuse issues may surface and need to be addressed. Recipients may be reluctant to acknowledge their unique needs as a family created through donation. For example, they may be noncompliant with future children's rights to information where legally mandated. Recipients may also have consistent and unusual difficulty in selecting a donor(s), unrelated to donor candidate options and availability. It is expected that donor selection may be stressful and time-consuming for many. However there are instances when no donor characteristics meet recipient expectations. This reluctance to choose a donor may indicate issues that once identified can be resolved.

The role of the fertility counselor is to bring the concern to the attention of the medical team and work together with the recipients to find solutions. This might include making recommendations for referral for treatment, such as marital counseling, drug/alcohol treatment or evaluation for psychiatric care/medication. The counselor may also recommend to the medical team that treatment be deferred until the issue(s) are resolved.

Melinda, age 42, and Pauline, age 50, a same-sex couple together for many years, met with their fertility counselor for their required recipient counseling session prior to proceeding with the use of donor egg and donor sperm. They had already attempted unsuccessfully several IUI cycles with Melinda having been inseminated with donor sperm. Due to Melinda's apparent low ovarian reserve, the doctor was now recommending IVF with donor egg and sperm. Though sad about giving up the use of her own eggs, Melinda felt ready to move along to a treatment that she hoped would finally result in a baby. However, in the session, much to Melinda's surprise, Pauline stated that she really did not think she could "love a baby that was not related to Melinda," that is not created through the use of her eggs. Melinda replied that she really "didn't know what that would mean in terms of their relationship." The counselor recommended that they defer treatment rather than make any rash decisions.

Several months later the couple returned for a follow-up session. Pauline stated that though she had been a bit upset with the counselor at the time for recommending that they put things on hold, she now realized that this had been a good decision. She had researched egg donation, and now felt that a baby "would be Melinda's since it would grow in her." Counseling had helped them to recommit to each other and recognize their desire to have a baby together.

By taking a "defer not deny" attitude towards treatment, the fertility counselor was able to give this couple permission to think things through in a way that felt supportive rather than threatening to them as a couple. Ultimately this helped them to make an informed decision about a matter with lifelong implications.

The recipient interview

Broadly speaking, the interview strives to weave the goals of psychoeducation, preparation, assessment and support into a discussion with patients facing a challenging situation often experienced as a life crisis. Table 7.1 identifies the issues to be covered during the interview. (Addendum 7.1 contains an example of questions to be asked during a psychosocial interview and Addendum 7.2 is an example of a psychosocial consultation record notation.)

Table 7.1 Issues covered in anonymous recipient consultation.

- Relationship history
- Infertility history
- Family background
- Feelings about egg/sperm donation and mourning the loss of genetic contribution
- Concerns about donor egg/sperm and bonding
- Donor sibling issues
- Disclosure issues/resources
- Feelings about and risk factors associated with multiples
- Feelings about selective reduction and cryopreservation
- Issues pertaining to donor screening/preferences/selection/consanguinity
- Future contact issues: anonymity/legal changes
- Other family building options
- Availability of mental health professional for future support
- Support groups/resources

Appointment preparation

Recipients often have questions/concerns prior to the interview and can benefit from receiving information to review before the appointment. An appointment confirmation email with appointment time, address, costs and directions, including attached reading materials is an efficient way to provide resources. The resources could include internet sites, book lists, articles and support sources related to talking to children about these issues. By having access to this information ahead of time, the recipients can come to the session prepared to engage in an informed discussion, having had time to talk about the material as a couple beforehand. (Examples of handouts we use in our practice of reading materials and internet support resources are included in Addenda 7.3 and 7.4.)

Goals of the interview

The primary goal is to establish a positive relationship with the recipients, providing a safe and confidential place to discuss their current situation as donor recipients now and in the future. Unexpected circumstances may arise where support could make the difference in navigating the treatment process successfully. Counseling helps to identify psychosocial issues related to third party reproduction and address concerns or problem areas. Helping to identify and address any unresolved feelings or hesitations before treatment can allow participants to feel prepared and "ready" to proceed with confidence. Having established a relationship, recipients know where to find ongoing support.

Patient education is also a vital part of the recipient interview. Materials sent in advance may be supplemented with additional resources relevant to recipient specific needs. Books for children can be displayed helping recipients to feel they have help with the telling of a child's story. It can be reassuring to know that the counselor can be a resource regarding openness if feelings change or if questions arise in the future. Informing recipients about support groups, educational workshops or online groups also help recipients connect with others to explore feelings or concerns.

Informed consent and release of information

The first part of the interview includes a discussion of the intent of the meeting, the relationship of and interactions between the fertility counselor and the medical treatment team, and review and completion of consents and release of information forms. The recipients are made aware of how the information from the interview will be used and if it will be shared with the medical team. Whether written reports are kept separate from the medical record or available to the recipient and the fact that any recommendations from the session will be shared with the patient and the medical treatment team should be discussed. Recipients may also consider seeking additional legal, ethical or religious counsel. (Please see examples of consents and record releases in the Addendum section from Chapter 21, Legal Issues.)

Recipient(s) history

The clinical interview should be comprehensive, beginning with taking a reproductive history of fertility issues, pregnancy, children, losses and any relevant genetic history and treatment attempts. This will include a discussion of the decision to use gamete donation to build a family and include the emotional implications of that decision. A psychiatric history should include any history of counseling, use of psychotropic medication and effect on treatment and pregnancy, coordination with other medical providers, and any substance abuse, or current emotional issues, for example depression or anxiety.

A further history of marital/relationship status, including relevant sexual history, should also be taken including any stresses on the relationship or ambivalence about treatment. The impact of the use of a donor on each person, as well as any concern over bonding issues should be addressed. Discovering how potential recipients are coping with donor issues as well as other stresses and disappointments is important. Integrating the idea of treatment with a donor into their lives helps develop a sense of optimism and hope for the future. The Comprehensive Psychosocial History of Infertility can be used as a reference [13].

Disclosure/openness

The early days of sperm donation were shrouded in secrecy, and it was thought to be better that no one ever knew for sure whether the baby was conceived with the father's or the donor's sperm. Often couples were told to go home after the insemination and have intercourse, and not have testing to determine the true genetics of the baby. This led to psychological confusion for all parties. Today, fertility counselors, who understand the problems that can occur around "family secrets," generally agree that it is best to be clear about whose gametes are being used for conception. In fact there has been a movement away from the language of "secrecy" in favor of use of the term "privacy," thereby highlighting the idea that the use of donor gametes is not shameful, but rather a loving and positive choice.

With this evolution in attitude has come the dilemma for recipients of whether and how to handle information about their use of a donor with family, friends and ultimately with a child. For heterosexual couples using donor eggs or donor sperm, a pregnancy looks like any other, with no readily apparent reason to disclose. By contrast single women, single men, and lesbian and gay couples may be faced early on with questions, particularly from a potential child, about their identity. Asking recipients about how open they have been is a good start to a discussion of their thoughts on if, when and how to tell potential children about their donor history. The fertility counselor can discover whether there are any moral, religious, or ethical concerns of their own or their family/support network and how to handle these. Many recipients have elected to defer a decision about openness until a child is born or until any difference of opinion between recipients has been resolved. Recipients should be encouraged to explore their feelings and be reassured that although they have time to make these decisions, it is helpful to open the discussion now.

There are, however, reasons why recipients may choose not to disclose donor origins to a child, and the role of the counselor is to explore and discuss, but not to judge or persuade. Recipients may feel that within their particular family or culture the idea of donor gametes would not be well accepted and a child might in fact face discrimination or rejection. Additionally, recipients might feel that a child would gain little from learning about the existence of a donor who they can never meet or learn more about. The counselor's role is to present the pros and cons of disclosure, but ultimately to understand and respect the autonomy of the recipients to make their own decisions, helping them understand that these opinions may change over time. (Please refer to Chapter 18 for more information on disclosure.)

Donor selection

Some programs "match" anonymous recipients and donors, while many others allow the recipient to choose their donor. When given the opportunity, recipients are often eager to discuss the donor selection process. Most recipients are inclined to pick a donor with physical characteristics, interests and talents matching the partner whose gametes are not being used [9]. The goal is to enable this partner to see some of his/her attributes represented in the child, as well as to help the child to "fit in" with the family. The recipients may have many choices before them: fresh vs. frozen eggs; eggs shared between other recipients during the cycle; clinic vs. private agency egg donors; anonymous vs. known; and closed vs. open identity sperm donors. They will have to determine how much information they wish to have in order to be able to select a donor, as these various options may provide differing degrees of anonymity. On the one hand recipients may feel that knowing as much as they possibly can about their donor will enable them to make the best possible choice; on the other hand, they may feel that personalizing the donor too much feels threatening to their legitimacy as a parent, and they may prefer keeping the donor as a more distant figure. The role of the counselor in donor selection may involve helping the recipients to grieve the loss of the genetic connection to a child by one of the partners, and to accept the limitations of the donor pool and what this means in terms of the loss of their "fantasy" child. However in discussing the thoroughness of the donor-screening process, the counselor can also help recipients to feel more confident in the fact that they are giving their child the best possible start in life through choosing a healthy donor, and to understand that there is not just one "perfect" donor who can help them achieve this goal of a healthy baby.

In EC, the issue of donor selection becomes more complex, involving the combination of two unknown genetic quantities to produce a child who most likely will resemble no one in the recipients' families. The recipient couple/individual will need to explore this issue of resemblance/genetic similarity and determine how important it is to them in choosing their donors, or whether perhaps the goal is first and foremost to have a healthy baby. Recipients will have the opportunity to process how they anticipate addressing these issues with their future child.

Group counseling

Group counseling in the form of support groups and educational workshops can be an effective adjunct to individual recipient counseling. Attending a group can normalize and validate the recipient experience. Having an opportunity to share feelings and experiences with others may create relationships that extend well after group participation. Educational workshops can provide recipients with specific knowledge and resources, building hope and confidence in their decision to create a family through gamete donation.

Support groups

> The Donor Recipient Support Group gathers once a month with both couples and single recipients in attendance. Around the circle, introductions and updates begin with the announcement of two new pregnancies. Congratulations follow, but caution remains due to previous disappointments and losses. One participant discusses the search for a donor match, while another couple describes their struggle to decide whom to tell about their decision to use a donor, including their child conceived by egg donation. Lastly, a recent unsuccessful cycle challenges the determination of a single woman, who tearfully wonders if she should continue treatment. As the group closes, email addresses are exchanged, linking the supportive new relationships that are formed that evening and sustaining participants through the month to come.

Support groups provide a safe place to talk with other recipients of donor egg, donor sperm or both, normalizing their experiences. A trained fertility counselor is the ideal leader providing education and appropriate leadership to establish an environment in which group members can feel comfortable and open. The attendees should agree to confidentiality, sharing only their own feelings outside the group. Recipients may come to a group for the first time "just to listen" but often find themselves drawn into the discussion. Recipients may be at the beginning stages of treatment with donation and wonder how others made their decisions. Patients may also be in the midst of treatment, awaiting news of results or experiencing an unexpected complication. Often, recipients have told no one about their use of donation, and find it an enormous relief to share joys and disappointments with those who "get it." Group members may benefit from hearing about the varied cultural and ethnic perspectives of members that may have implications for donor selection, openness, family support and religious issues. The shared experiences of group participation can cushion losses, preserving emotional energy for patients to persevere after a setback. The group will need to decide if recipients who are successful can continue to attend while pregnant. It can be helpful to follow the experiences from "trying" to "pregnancy" to "parenthood." A further positive outcome of group participation is to create and maintain friendships with families created similarly. Sharing an email list and encouraging contact outside the group promotes the beginning of what could become long-term relationships, continuing a safety net for newly created families for years to come. (For more information on fertility group counseling, see [14].)

Educational workshops

> The Educational Workshop "Talking and Telling" is being held on a Saturday morning for three hours co-led by two fertility counselors. Recipients had requested more in-depth information on this topic and an agenda was developed using discussion, videos, group time and written materials. Attendees have come as couples, singles, with family members, and some are parents through gamete donation. During the morning they have seen videos, explored developmental issues, research findings, attitudes, concerns and resources. They leave the workshop with an array of new tools and greater confidence about telling their own "Family Story."

In addition to support groups, patients often indicate a desire to explore specific aspects of forming a family through donation on a deeper level. There are models of educationally based groups run successfully in Germany [15] using a seminar approach. Professionals from related fields such as a physician, a lawyer, and mental health professional all contribute their expertise. Additionally, time is scheduled for patients to interact, providing the support element.

There are many educational topics that may interest recipients. The development of an educational group should include assessing the need for a group, reaching patients/advertising the group, developing the content and deciding on the format. Keeping in mind that there may be a limit to resources for groups, the fertility counselor should note the concerns that are raised most often by recipients. A brief survey can be useful as well and avoid duplication of existing groups. Once the topic is established, multiple ways to reach appropriate participants can be used. Developing and distributing informational flyers, posting on appropriate websites and social media, informing associated relevant organizations, such as RESOLVE, informing existing support group members and asking medical staff to promote the group can help get the word out.

Using a pre-workshop and post-workshop questionnaire is a quick way to gather information on the impact of the group experience. This exercise provides immediate feedback to patients about any changes in attitude and thinking about openness and also proves useful to couples in comparing their responses. Group facilitators can learn about successful aspects and overall effectiveness of the presentation. Table 7.2 provides an example of an educational group framework for the "Talking and Telling" workshop. (Examples of pre-workshop and post-workshop questionnaires are included in the Addendum 7.5 and 7.6.)

Table 7.2 Example framework for an educational group: "talking and telling."

1. Introduction a. Describe the interactive workshop as exploring issues around talking to children about their donor conception. b. Providing information and tools to assist parents with the disclosure process
2. Pre-workshop questionnaire a. Current thoughts/plans on telling b. Confidence and comfort in talking
3. Small-group exercise: Fears and Positives a. Identify concerns/fears about disclosure b. Identify positive beliefs about disclosure
4. Presentations a. Developmental stages of children b. Approaching disclosure during these stages c. Research on impact of disclosure for donor-conceived families
5. Small-group exercise: Creating a Family Story a. Descriptions of how the family came together b. The help that was needed to be a family c. Pictures, books and family rituals unique to this child d. Lovingly told and in greater detail over time
6. Books and resources a. MHPG Book list at www.asrm.org b. The American Fertility Association articles at www.theafa.org c. Donor Conception Network resources at www.dcnetwork.org
7. Audiovisual presentation a. YouTube video clips of donor-conceived parents and children talking b. Discuss participants' reactions
8. Post-workshop questionnaire a. Shift in thinking about disclosure after the workshop b. Comfort and confidence in being able to talk to their children

Cross-border reproductive services

Cross-border reproductive services (CBRS), or the travel of infertility patients across geographical borders in order to obtain treatment, not only exists, but is a growing trend due to both the unavailability/illegality of anonymous donation in some countries, or the enormous costs associated with it in others. In Canada and the UK, for example, where anonymous donation is not available, recipients are traveling to the USA for treatment with anonymous donor eggs [16]. Europeans seeking anonymous donors may also travel to Spain, where perhaps they can find donors with greater physical resemblance. Additionally, due to the typically high costs of egg donation treatment in the USA and the general lack of insurance coverage, Americans may seek treatment abroad as well.

When counseling recipients who have crossed borders for gamete donation, the fertility counselor must be sensitive to the attitude that their culture is likely to hold towards reproductive technology in general and the use of gamete donation in particular. It may in fact be immoral or even illegal in a particular society and the ramifications of using donor gametes can range from stigma to punishment [16]. When counseling recipients about disclosing their use of donor gametes, for example, it is important to consider with them how a potential child would be regarded within their individual family, as well as within the larger society, if this fact were known. (Please refer to Chapter 22 for further discussion of CBRS.)

What might the future hold?

Changes in the field of reproductive medicine may have important implications for gamete donation. With the growing availability and popularity of using fertility preservation technology for social, as well as medical, reasons, the need for egg donation may decrease. There is also a growing trend toward openness with donor registries in use worldwide. The availability of donors may decline as donors realize it may be difficult to remain anonymous forever [17,18]. Growth of "facial recognition" software as well as easy and inexpensive genetic testing may also cause anonymity to disappear, and with it the desire to be a donor. Ultimately there may no longer be a need for a chapter, in books such as this one, on the use of anonymous donor gametes.

Reflections of the fertility counselors

Back to the waiting room ...

What is it like to enter into the family building dreams of recipients of donor gametes? As stated earlier, one of the goals of our counseling is to establish a positive relationship. Often we become one of only a few people to know of their plans to use gamete donation. Many do not share this information even with close family members. This can feel like a privilege for us and be a relief for them: a chance to explore and process this important life-long decision in a "safe" and confidential setting. We are here for the beginning of the story, we work with them through decision-making, wait for treatment results and share their joy or sadness at the outcome. At other times we may only be present for an initial contact and wonder about how things turned out. We may also share the joy of recipients returning to show us their babies.

As fertility counselors, we may not always share the views of the recipients with whom we sit in terms of what may ultimately be in the best interests of their child/family. However, we must respect their autonomy to make their own decisions. We hope that we will be seen as a safe resource if needed now or in the future, as we consider options and ramifications together.

PS: I will never forget a woman from Southeast Asia who came to our clinic needing egg donation. She arrived in my office attired in a striking gown, headdress and jewelry, saying almost desperately that she "needed a baby or [she] will die." I initially felt overwhelmed by the intensity of her emotions, while also wondering if our cultural differences might be a barrier to my understanding her needs. However, she did undergo treatment and became pregnant through egg donation, but sadly had an early miscarriage, which was devastating to her. Just as she had deeply touched me after only a brief time, she endeared herself to everyone, so much so that she was able to raise funds through her friends and community to try treatment again. Ultimately she had a baby, who she clearly adores, and has maintained close contact with our staff through calls, visits and sending regular photo updates. I continue to look forward to the pleasure of following her child's growth for years to come. What I saw in this woman was her incredible strength in continuing to go forward towards her goal, despite difficult obstacles. I learned about respecting our cultural differences and that ultimately, all she wanted was a baby. Finally, I learned that deep connection may develop when you least expect it.

CT: I have been running an open-ended support group for anonymous gamete recipients for many years. Once a month the patients participating have a bit of fun rearranging the waiting room, to "make it their own" when we gather. To be able to manipulate the physical aspects of a place in which they often feel little control is surprisingly empowering. This action then sets the tone for the group, where they can own their feelings and contributions. One of the most satisfying things for me as the facilitator is to bear witness to their experiences. While preparing to write this, I searched through a collage of memories of group meetings for that perfect example to highlight. What I realized stays with me, however, is not so much their individual stories, but the expressions of genuine kindness and caring that these group members, relative strangers, offer to one another. The power of shared stories, then, is really the example I want to share. Although month after month, year after year, there are different people rearranging the waiting room, what does not change is the spirit of generosity displayed. Their creation of a hopeful environment in the waiting room at night is sustaining. It is what allows them to persevere and generates the strength needed for them to face that same waiting room by the light of day.

References

1. Lutjen P, Trouson A, Leeton J, et al. The establishment and maintenance of pregnancy using in vitro fertilization and embryo donation in a patient with primary ovarian failure. *Nature* 1984; 307: 174–75.
2. Glennon T. UK and US perspectives on the regulation of gamete donation. In Richards M, Pennings G, Appleby JB, eds. *Reproductive Donation: Practice, Policy and Bioethics*. Cambridge: Cambridge University Press, 2012; 90–111.
3. Haase JM, Blyth E. Global perspectives in infertility counseling. In Covington SN, Burns LH, eds. *Infertility Counseling: A Comprehensive Handbook for Clinicians, Second Edition*. Cambridge: Cambridge University Press, 2006; 544–57.
4. American Society for Reproductive Medicine. Recommendations for gamete and embryo donation: a committee opinion. *Fertil Steril* 2013; 99: 47–62.
5. Boivin J, Kentenich H, eds. *ESHRE Monograph: Guidelines for Counseling in Infertility*. Oxford: Oxford University Press, 2002.
6. Garcia-Ruiz Y, Guerra-Diaz D. Gamete and embryo donation: a legal view from Spain. In Richards M, Pennings G, Appleby JB, eds. *Reproductive Donation: Practice, Policy and Bioethics*. Cambridge: Cambridge University Press, 2012; 112–29.
7. Hershberger P. Recipients of oocyte donation: an integrative review. *J Obstet Gynecol Neonatal Nurs* 2004; 33: 610–21.
8. Eisenberg ML, Smith JF, Millstein SG, et al. Perceived negative consequences of donor gametes from male and female members of infertile couples. *Fertil Steril* 2010; 94: 921–6.
9. Lindeim SR, Kavi S, Sauer M. Understanding differences in the perception of anonymous parties: a comparison between gamete donors and their recipients. *J Assist Reprod Genetics* 2000; 17: 127–30.
10. Tarlatzis BC, Pakos G. Oocyte donation: Clinical and practical aspects. *Moll Cell Endocrinol* 2000; 161: 99–102.
11. Greil A, Slauson-Blevins K, McQuillan J. The experience of infertility: a review of recent literature. *Sociol Health Illn* 2010; 32: 140–62.
12. Sachs PL, Burns LH. Recipient counseling for oocyte donation. In Covington SN, Burns LH, eds. *Infertility Counseling: A Comprehensive Handbook for Clinicians. Second Edition*. Cambridge: Cambridge University Press, 2006; 319–38.
13. Burns LH, Greenfeld DA. CPHI: Comprehensive psychosocial history for infertility. In Covington SN, Burns LH, eds. *Infertility Counseling: A Comprehensive Handbook for Clinicians. Second Edition*. Cambridge: Cambridge University Press, 2006; 563–64.
14. Covington SN. Group approaches to infertility counseling. In Covington SN, Burns LH, eds. *Infertility Counseling: A Comprehensive Handbook for Clinicians. Second Edition*. Cambridge: Cambridge University Press, 2006; 157–68.
15. Thorn P, Daniels KR. A group-work approach in family building by donor insemination: empowering the marginalized. *Hum Fert* 2003; 6: 46–50.
16. Pennings G, Gurtin ZB. The legal and ethical regulation of transnational donation. In Richards M, Pennings G, Appleby JB, eds. *Reproductive Donation: Practice, Policy and Bioethics*. Cambridge: Cambridge University Press, 2006; 130–49.
17. Hammarberg K, Johnson L, Bourne K, et al. Proposed legislative change mandating retrospective release of identifying information: consultation with donors and Government response. *Hum Reprod* 2013 Dec 6. [Epub ahead of print].
18. Bratt S, Sacrannie RR, Thomas GE, et al. Can we improve recruitment of oocyte donors with loss of donor anonymity? A hospital-based survey. *Hum Fertil* 2008; 11: 101–7.

Chapter 8

Counseling anonymous gamete donors

Laura Josephs and Uschi Van den Broeck

Meet our donor applicants…

Hallie, age 23, has been accepted as an egg donor at a donor egg (DE) program which practices anonymity. During a blood draw, she mentions to the nurse that she is hoping that she can someday meet her genetic offspring. The nurse shares the conversation with the program's mental health professional.

Eva, age 28, meets with a psychologist for an egg donor evaluation. She describes a relatively problem-free life as a well-functioning graduate student with a close circle of friends. She denies psychological problems, psychotherapy and psychiatric medication usage, past and present. But the MMPI-2 psychological testing, taken later that day, reveals a likelihood of clinical depression.

Jeff, age 28, applies for the sperm donor program after a report in the news about the shortage of sperm donors. He tells the mental health professional that he's currently not in a relationship or in a phase of life where he cares much about children. He has not thought much about potential offspring and seems not to care either way. However, he's enthusiastic about getting thoroughly screened and learning more about his own fertile status. The laboratory technician who goes over the paperwork with him notices that Jeff seems extremely interested in his sperm count and his genetic screening.

Kaitlyn, age 25, is enthusiastic about anonymously donating her eggs and feels comfortable with the prospect that her donation will result in the creation of one or more children who are genetically related to her but not her children. During the course of her psychological evaluation, she reveals that she does not plan to tell her boyfriend about the prospective donation. She explains that she was brought up in a highly progressive family but that he was raised in a very traditional culture and "wouldn't understand" her desire to help another woman in this way.

James, age 35, meets the psychologist who does the counseling for the sperm donor program. He is motivated to donate sperm as he's experienced his best friend Sam struggling with not being able to conceive naturally. After discussing his idea of becoming a donor with his wife, the couple decides that they would prefer an anonymous system so as not to interfere too much with their own family life with their two sons. James is a well-functioning lawyer without a history of psychological problems. His family history, however, reveals several cases of bipolar disorder.

Barbara, age 24, tells the reproductive medicine program's social worker that she is highly motivated to donate her eggs because she wants to help childless couples. However, she is strongly against abortion and wants to be assured that a pregnancy she could help to create could not potentially end up being terminated.

Introduction

"It's a very important decision in my life to donate sperm. It fits into my life and into my way of thinking. I'm a bone marrow donor, I'm registered as an organ donor in case I have an accident or something. I'm just saying, donating sperm is a very personal issue. It defines me."

The egg donor or sperm donor plays a very important role in the reproductive medicine practice. The donor is both a patient and not a patient. He or she is a patient in that s/he must be taken care of both physically and psychologically. He or she is not a patient, in that the

Fertility Counseling: Clinical Guide and Case Studies, ed. Sharon N. Covington. Published by Cambridge University Press.

donor is not presenting for his/her own treatment. In fact, especially for the egg donor, who is undergoing medical risk in order to provide her oocytes to another woman who wishes to have a child, treatment goals for the patient (i.e., the donor egg recipient) may be in conflict with the interests of the donor [1]. One could argue that, when it comes to psychological aspects of gamete donation, the interests of either the sperm or the egg donor could conflict with the interests of those receiving donated gametes. For example, a parent's wish for his/her child to someday know the identity of the egg or sperm donor, whose gametes helped to create this child, may conflict with a donor's desire to not be known and/or contacted by any genetic offspring.

Anonymous gamete donation: history and current practice

Though isolated cases of donor insemination were reported at various points in the early and mid twentieth century, it was in the 1970s and 1980s that improved methods of sperm collection led to the creation of sperm banks [2]. Contrary to popular belief, sperm donation is not the result of a casual impulse that leads a young man to pay a quick visit or two to a sperm bank, make a few dollars, and rapidly move on. Rather, most sperm banks in the United States require the donor to make a relatively time-intensive and long-term commitment of at least one donation weekly for a period of one year [3].

Oocyte donation requires the technology of in vitro fertilization, which was pioneered in 1978. In 1983, oocyte donation was introduced when Australian physicians provided an egg from one patient to another fertility patient with ovarian failure [2].

Though sperm cryopreservation has been practiced for over 60 years, oocyte cryopreservation has been a more challenging endeavor for scientists. Oocyte cryopreservation is only recently a promising technology due to medical and laboratory advances, in particular the use of a freezing technique known as vitrification. As of 2012, the American Society for Reproductive Medicine (ASRM) no longer considers oocyte cryopreservation to be an experimental procedure [4]. Though egg donation with fresh oocytes (i.e., synchronization of donor egg recipient and donor in their cycles, retrieval of eggs from the donor, fertilization by recipient's partner or sperm source, and consequent creation of an embryo or embryos which are then transferred into the uterus of the recipient) remains prevalent, egg "banks" of cryopreserved donor oocytes clearly represent a growing trend in the world of egg donation.

Worldwide, gamete donation is by no means a homogenous entity. In some countries, gamete donation is legally prohibited. The International Federation of Fertility Societies (IFFS) 2013 survey found that sperm donation for use in non-IVF infertility is not allowed in 22% of the countries surveyed, it is permitted in 51% of the cases, it is not specifically mentioned in roughly 20% (suggesting that it is used in about 70% of countries), and the status is unknown in 4% [5]. Respondents reported that sperm donation is not allowed in Egypt, Libya, Senegal, Tunisia, Saudi Arabia and Turkey, and in other African countries it is not addressed (Uganda, Togo, Ivory Coast, and Democratic Republic of the Congo). These prohibitions stem from religious, moral and/or cultural traditions. In most countries that follow Islamic law, gamete donation is disallowed or restricted. With respect to egg donation, a similar trend is recognized from the survey, with 73% of the countries reportedly performing the procedure, 12% reporting it is "not mentioned" in the guidelines and 14% not performing egg donation [5]. Most European countries reportedly allow egg donation, with the exceptions of Austria, Germany, Norway and Switzerland.

For countries that do allow gamete donation, policies and practices vary, most notably in terms of the issues of donor anonymity and monetary donor compensation. A donor who begins in the context of anonymity, meaning that he or she is unknown to the donor sperm or egg recipients, may remain anonymous or, alternatively, at some point his or identity may be revealed to the recipients or, more likely, to the adult (18-year-old) offspring of the gamete donation. In the United Kingdom, in 2005, the Human Fertilisation and Embryology Authority (HFEA) eliminated all donor anonymity and monetary compensation (other than minimal expenses) and established a central donor registry; all gamete donors must agree to be contacted in the future by genetic offspring [6]. In Australia, the state of Victoria has a mandatory donor registry [7]. Canada established the Assisted Human Reproduction Agency in 2004. Canada moved to prohibit donor anonymity through the Assisted

Human Reproduction Act, but legal challenges to the Act have left the anonymity question under the jurisdiction of the individual provinces, and Canada allows for both anonymous and identity release donation. Donor compensation is prohibited [8].

When countries have implemented regulations to eliminate donor anonymity and/or to eliminate or drastically reduce donor compensation, these countries have often seen significant drops in individuals donating their eggs or sperm. According to a review in 2011 by HFEA of changes in gamete donation in the UK since the 2005 removal of donor anonymity and donor compensation, there are reported waiting times of up to five years for donor oocytes. The number of patients receiving donor gametes has dropped, and unlicensed donor/recipient matching websites are on the rise [9]. In Canada, del Valle and associates [10] attempted to recruit sperm donors based on altruistic rather than economic motivation, but the vast majority of prospective donors either withdrew their applications or were disqualified, and the recruitment effort had little success. Ekerhovd and colleagues [11] note that in Sweden, where legislation requires that sperm donors be identifiable to offspring, there is a "shortage of sperm donors." Swedish healthcare providers are willing to assist in treatment abroad and more than 250 Swedish donor sperm recipients travel to Denmark each year for reproductive purposes. A study of Danish sperm donors [12] concluded, "few [donors] would continue if they did not receive financial compensation" and also that "to maintain anonymity is still important for the majority of the donors."

At the same time, it has been posited that, although the initial response of prospective donors is a negative attitude to a legislative change of removing anonymity, the way in which donors are recruited and the current societal legislation, practices or beliefs about anonymity or openness seem to play a very important role in donors' attitudes and perhaps in their behavior, meaning their decision to donate or to continue donating [13]. Demographics also seem to matter: sperm donors who are older and married with children tend to donate even when anonymity is not assured. Daniels [14], in reviewing the research regarding sperm donors' views on anonymity, has hypothesized that identity release donors will need to be recruited via a different model than has been used to attract anonymous donors.

Gamete donation and the role of the fertility counselor

"I think it's important to be able to see a professional counselor because, you know, it needs to be a conscious decision. You have to be sure you know what you're getting into."

The fertility counselor is a mental health professional (MHP) with specialized training who, in the context of gamete donation, often serves multiple functions. One important function is consulting with the gamete donor for evaluation and counseling. Within this function, the fertility counselor plays multiple critical roles, from "assessing the suitability of the donor, to facilitating the donor's understanding of the implications of donating one's genetic material to another person, and in providing long-term support and education" [2]. It is important that the fertility counselor recognize the complex nuances of his/her clinical relationship with the donor.

The fertility counselor's primary goal is assessing the donor in order to determine his/her suitability as a provider of gametes/genetic material to others (the recipients of the genetic material). The aim of the session is not to tackle the donating individual's general psychological concerns or difficulties, nor to enhance the donor's psychological well-being, as would occur in counseling or psychotherapy. Specifically, the fertility counselor is addressing these broad questions:

1) Is there reasonable certainty that the donor is without significant psychological difficulties that could potentially indicate problematic genetic susceptibilities that could be passed on to prospective genetic offspring?
2) Is there reasonable certainty that the life experience of donating would be psychologically tolerable for the donor, that there are neither inherent psychological susceptibilities nor specific emotions/psychological conflicts about donating gametes that could render the experience of donation emotionally harmful or destabilizing for the donor?
3) Is there reasonable certainty that the donor can comply with donation requirements in a responsible manner and, for the egg donor, can psychologically withstand the physical burdens of

oocyte donation in order to complete the donation process?

It is important for the fertility counselor to recognize the nature of his/her clinical relationship with the donor; and gamete donor candidates need to be made aware that the fertility counselor is meeting with them for assessment rather than therapeutic purposes. At the same time, the fertility counselor must prioritize the psychological well-being of the egg or sperm donor in the counselor's dealings with the donor and with the medical team.

The ASRM recommends psychological screening of oocyte and sperm donors in their Practice Committee opinion and outlines guidelines for psychological care in gamete donation [15]. In 2002, the Psychological Special Interest Group (PSIG) of the European Society of Human Reproduction and Embryology (ESHRE) published the Guidelines for Counselling Infertility, a comprehensive document outlining fertility counseling issues with specific recommendations on sperm and oocyte donation [16]. Additionally, ESHRE has issued a wide array of Task Force reports including one on gamete donation [17]. Included in the ESHRE guidelines are recommendations that the psychological evaluation include an assessment "of the general abilities and intellectual capacity of the donor candidates," along with "minimal information about the donor concerning appearance, education, profession, social background and motivation for donating" [17, p. 1408].

Over the years, worldwide, fresh egg donation cycles have generally taken place within a reproductive medicine practice or program. Often, per ASRM and IFFS recommendations, egg donors are evaluated by a fertility counselor, frequently one who practices within the reproductive medicine program or has an ongoing affiliation with the program. In sharp contrast, in the USA and throughout the world, sperm donors are typically not offered fertility counseling for gamete donation or meet with a MHP. Donation cycles generally take place in physicians' offices and reproductive medicine programs with sperm banks supplying the frozen sperm and, while anonymous sperm donors are evaluated medically by the banks, they rarely meet with a MHP for counseling or assessment.

Assessment of the gamete donor

The psychological evaluation of the gamete donor and the attention to the donor's well-being go hand in hand, and do not entail separate or distinct approaches in the fertility counselor's interactions with the donor. Evaluation of the donor involves a psychological assessment of the donor's childhood and life history, his/her psychological functioning both as a child and as an adult, and the assessment for any psychopathology, including possible mental health and substance abuse issues. Table 8.1 contains a detailed list of areas to be addressed in the psychological assessment of the gamete donor.

Psychological evaluation of the donor also includes a detailed effort to understand the donor's relationship to his/her donation: motivation for and feelings about donating gametes, feelings about the prospective genetic offspring, and implications of the donation in terms of anonymity vs. identity release. Table 8.2 details important areas to cover in speaking with donors about the psychological meaning and implications of donating one's gametes.

Table 8.1 Donor interview: psychological assessment.

A) Current/Adult Life Situation
1) Job/career
2) Educational background
3) Relative stability of life situation vs. current/ongoing stresses
4) Marital/relationship status & relationship history
5) Interpersonal/social relationships
6) High and low points of donor's adult life
B) Childhood/Family History
1) Family constellation/family life
2) Donor's personality/experience of self as a child
3) Donor's experience of parents
4) Parents' relationship with each other
5) Donor's experience of siblings
6) Significant family problems – physical or mental illness of parent or other family member, alcoholism/substance abuse in family member, abuse within or outside family, sexual abuse within or outside the family
7) High and low points of donor's childhood
C) Psychological Assessment
1) Mood and affect of donor
2) Content and process of thought
3) Donor's communication with interviewer
4) Assessment of possible mood disorder
5) Assessment of possible anxiety disorder
6) Assessment of possible eating disorder
7) Assessment of possible alcohol/substance use/abuse
8) Assessment of psychosis
D) Psychological History
1) History of psychological difficulties
2) History of psychotherapy
3) Psychiatric medication usage past or present
4) Alcohol/substance abuse history
5) Family history of psychological and/or substance problems

Table 8.2 Donor interview: implications of donation.

A) Motivation
1) Stated motivation for donating eggs or sperm
2) Altruistic and/or economic motives, or other motives (personal/psychological motives)
3) Need for money, plan for using money earned through donating
4) Any coercion/pressure from others (e.g., for financial reasons)
5) History of reproductive/pregnancy loss or pregnancy termination
6) Donor's relationship to his/her own children

B) Donation of Genes/Genetic Connection with Prospective Child
1) Perceived connection to recipient(s); feelings about person(s) receiving gametes
2) Relinquishment of control/dominion over gametes
3) Feelings about genetic connection with child "out there" who is not one's own
4) Thinking about prospective genetic connection in the shorter and longer term
5) Relationship to/feelings about own's gametes/DNA

C) Anonymity vs. Identity Release Issues
1) Clarity of donor regarding anonymous vs. non-anonymous nature of gamete donation
2) Comfort of donor with anonymity (or non-anonymity) plan
3) Limits of anonymity
4) Implications of anonymity or identity release over the long term
5) Willingness to be contact in the future if there is medical need of donor-conceived offspring.

D) Physical/Medical Aspects
1) Comfort with medical setting
2) For egg donors, comfort with medical procedures and medications
3) For egg donors, appreciation of risks of donation process
4) Restrictive aspects of serving as a gamete donor

E) Social Support
1) If donor has an intimate partner, has he/she discussed the donation with the partner?
2) Is donating likely to introduce any difficulties into the donor's primary relationship?
3) Has donor discussed prospective donation with others in social network?
4) Does donor have good sources of social support?

During the course of the psychological assessment process, the fertility counselor may uncover aspects of the donor's emotional status, which could indicate that either: (1) s/he might not be suitable as a provider of gametes/genetic material, or (2) s/he might be adversely impacted by serving as a gamete donor. In some instances, both might apply: unsuitability as a donor and adverse impact on the prospective donor. Applegarth and Kingsberg [2] have described psychological indicators for acceptance or rejection of gamete donors. Donors should be without significant psychopathology and without significant current stress, including significant economic instability. They should be able to provide informed consent. Their standardized psychological testing should be within normal limits. Current use of psychotropic medications, positive history of major psychiatric disorders or substance use disorders, or history of legal problems/sociopathy would warrant exclusion of the prospective donor, and family history of psychiatric disorders or substance abuse would also potentially rule out the prospective donor.

Recall our donor applicants at the beginning. Eva, whose psychological testing indicated the likely presence of clinical depression, was reassessed and ultimately excluded as a donor for the combined reason that her depression was both a risk factor in terms of possibly passing on an inherent susceptibility to genetic offspring, along with the concern that donating oocytes, an elective process, could add stress to her daily life and negatively impact her mental health. Hallie, who was poised to donate anonymously but had a desire to meet her genetic offspring, was brought in for a follow-up meeting with the DE program's fertility counselor and was excluded as an anonymous donor, because it was deemed not in her personal psychological interests to make an anonymous donation about which she could likely feel regret. In this case, the prospective donation did not conflict with the DE program's or the recipient's interests but rather with the donor's potential interests. In contrast, there are prospective egg donation cases that are halted due to program/recipient interests, as opposed to the donor's interests. A case where the donor herself is without significant psychological problems, yet has a family member (or members) with psychological and/or substance abuse problems, would be an example of the latter.

> *"The fact that it's anonymous does make you wonder though, what if my daughter ever comes home with a man who could be her half-brother? I might know because he could look like me and maybe I would wonder about that... But still my own child is my own – there's a difference and that's where I draw the line. I hope of course that these children end up in decent families. But in the end that's not within my control and I can only hope and have confidence in that you screen potential parents really well."*
>
> (Anonymous Sperm Donor)

It is important for fertility counselors to discuss with the prospective donor his or her motivations and his or her sense of the implications, now and in the future, of making a donation. For donors who are compensated monetarily, it is to be expected that economic motives will be present. However, if the fertility counselor perceives that the donor desperately needs money, this will compromise the prospective donor's ability to evaluate his/her comfort with donation with reasonable objectivity. For donors who are donating in a system/country without monetary compensation, it is to be expected that more altruistic motives, as well as more personal and psychological motives, may play an important role in the decision to donate. In these cases, the fertility counselors should ascertain if these motives are balanced in a healthy way and that the prospective donor is aware of the short- and long-term implications of donating gametes. Remember Jeff, who was mostly concerned with his own fertility, which seemed the primary reason for him to donate? If after thorough implications counseling, this still remains his primary motivator, it is questionable whether sperm donation is a good decision for him at this point in his life and he would be excluded from the program.

Because donating gametes often offers a monetary gain for the donor but no other direct benefit, obtaining informed consent may not be a straightforward process. Skillern and colleagues [18] point out that, for the egg donor, financial compensation "may limit information seeking and impair decision making," and, parallel to this, the physician or donor recruiter "may be eager to have a potential donor agree to proceed" (p. 1737). Skillern and associates have developed the Egg Donor Informed Consent Tool (EDICT) in order to better assess prospective donors' understanding of the process of egg donation and its risks, especially the physical risks. Beyond an appreciation of the physical risks, it is vital that the fertility counselor ascertain that the gamete donor understands as much as possible about the short-term and long-term emotional implications of donation.

If the (male or female) donor is married, and the spouse opposes the donation, the fertility counselor should exclude the donor, given the weight of foreseeable harm to the donor's committed relationship and thus to his/her day-to-day life and future. However, many gamete donors evince a less clear-cut version of this dynamic. In the example of Kaitlyn, whose boyfriend "wouldn't understand" her desire to be an egg donor, but who nonetheless wanted to donate, the prospective donor was brought in to discuss the nature/level of commitment of her relationship with her boyfriend and to talk through the potential emotional risks of the planned donation to her relationship and hence her own well-being. For a prospective donor who is not at all certain about the future of his/her current intimate relationship and who makes life decisions very independently of the partner, donation might proceed so long as the donor understands the potential implications. The donor's relationship is important, but so is his/her autonomy. Arguably, it makes sense for the fertility counselor to err on the side of protecting the donor's relationship, in that his/her making a decision to donate also serves the interests of the reproductive medicine program.

Worldwide, some gamete donation programs require that a donor's significant other be included in the assessment and/or consent process; other programs do not have this requirement. Though the impact of gamete donation on the partner's current and future relationship is equally important for sperm donors as for egg donors, this is usually not reflected in clinical practice. In the case of sperm donors, many fertility centers or sperm banks don't even offer psychological counseling for the donor himself, nor do they seek the input of a current partner or spouse.

And what of informed consent in terms of anonymity or identity release? For men or women who are "anonymous" donors, is there an appreciation of the various ways in which such anonymity is limited? What if, in the future, a donor gamete recipient or donor-conceived individual successfully petitioned a court of law to order the opening of closed donation records? What if laws are written in the future which affect donor anonymity, and the change were to be applied retroactively to past donations? What of certain genealogy testing protocols that are already available to the public, which can potentially link up individuals (with their agreement) who are genetically related to each other, whereby a donor-conceived individual could be linked to a close relative of the donor, even if the donor him/herself did not participate in such testing? [19].

For gamete donors who at the time of donation have agreed to identity release, it may be difficult to appreciate the potential impact of being known to genetic offspring some 18 or more years into the future, when the donor's life situation will undoubtedly be different than at the time of donation. For example, how will the introduction of genetic offspring into one's life affect the family that one may have almost two decades later, but not at present? In fact, one model of anonymity/non-anonymity (practiced, for example at the California Cryobank) [20] entails that the donor can make a decision about identity release at the time the genetic offspring reach adulthood, if any such offspring after the age of 18 requests that the donor be contacted. Thus, the donor does not have to give consent for releasing his identity or anticipate his own needs, feelings and wishes until the far future.

Experience of the gamete donor

> *"I'm comfortable being an egg donor. I'm not using these eggs right now. They're just getting flushed away every month. I might as well give them to someone who really needs them."*

As with many things in life, practice makes perfect. Fertility counselors performing assessments and providing counseling for prospective gamete donors learn best about the specifics and pitfalls of gamete donation by seeing as many different donors as they possibly can. However, today a growing body of evidence in the literature [13,21] can help us gain insight into donor characteristics and experiences that should be taken into account when meeting with a prospective egg or sperm donor.

Motivation of gamete donors

> *"The older I got, the more I felt that 'I need to leave "something" behind.' It's reassuring in a way that I can still procreate, well... maybe that's a very Darwinian approach (laughs...) but I think it's important that everyone procreates. And for me the idea that these kids have my genes... well I don't think that's a bad thing for society, you know? It sounds a bit like showing off maybe and that's why I would never say it like that to people, but still..."*
>
> (Sperm Donor)

In general, studies have distinguished between four different types of motivation: altruism, financial compensation, procreation or genetic fatherhood, and finally questions or concerns about the donor's own fertility. It seems evident that a gamete donor's motivation is multifaceted. However, in practice, the focus is mostly on either financial or altruistic motives and these are frequently thought of as being diametrically opposed to one another. Other factors, such as legal and institutional aspects (e.g., the system a country or center uses to recruit donors) or the way in which the donor is asked about his/her motivation, can influence what a donor will reveal about his/her primary incentive. Though financial or altruistic motives may be seen as primary motives, a number of secondary motives may be just as, or even more, important to potential donors as they are of a more intrinsic nature but perhaps not perceived by the donor as socially acceptable. Secondary motives frequently mentioned in studies include procreation, passing on their own genes and investigating their own fertility status. Interestingly, egg and sperm donors' primary motivations seem similar. Sperm donors seem to indicate more secondary motivations (such as procreating and investigating their fertility status in their decision to donate sperm [22]), but these motivations are also evident among egg donors.

> *"I'd love to give my genes to other people. I don't want to sound egotistical but I think I'm a wonderful person. Why not pass on a couple of my genes to the rest of the world?"*
>
> (Egg Donor)

Recruitment strategies

As mentioned, the way in which donors are recruited can influence the type of donor a center may attract. The literature clearly shows that the media, advertisements and word-of-mouth advertising are good ways to inform and attract potential donors. Both potential and actual donors are influenced by their social environment or because they know infertile couples, but this seems to have less of an impact for sperm donors compared with egg donors [23,24].

Anonymity and contact with offspring

It is current practice to counsel prospective gamete recipients concerning issues such as donor anonymity and the possibilities of future knowledge and/or contact with their donor. This practice is largely based on considerations of future well-being of possible offspring, as well as the gamete recipients' family system. However, these issues are much less standard practice in counseling prospective gamete donors. As mentioned previously, most countries and fertility centers have regulations and guidelines concerning the psychological assessment and counseling of egg donors. However, generally sperm donors are neglected in this area and have to make do with information from the medical practitioners, their sperm bank or fertility center, or even the Internet. Nevertheless, in ascertaining whether or not gamete donation is harmful for the (current and future) emotional and psychological health of the donor, topics such as the donor's views and information concerning donor anonymity and future contact with offspring are of vital importance.

There is some evidence to show that the demographic profile of recruited sperm donors, in particular their marital status and age, can have a profound impact on their attitude towards anonymity and contact with offspring [13]. Younger, single donors are often students largely motivated by financial gains and compensation, are less likely to continue donating without the guarantee of anonymity, and are less likely to want or seek contact with offspring. They are, however, open to revealing non-identifying information to offspring. It has been suggested (both by researchers and actual donors) that donors of this type may benefit from implications counseling, as they may not fully be aware of the future implications of their current sperm donation.

On the other hand, older, married donors who often have children of their own are largely motivated by altruism related to the positive experience of fathering a child. Most of them would continue donating even when anonymity could not be guaranteed. This type of donor feels comfortable disclosing non-identifying information, but the point of view on contact and disclosure to offspring varies: some of these donors are more open to contact with offspring because they take into account offspring's feelings and curiosity about their conception; others do not wish contact with offspring.

Another, smaller sub-group emerges from the research: single men and/or homosexual men may be more strongly motivated by procreation and passing along their genes. Homosexual men are, compared with both single and married heterosexual donors, more open to contact with offspring and feel comfortable providing identifying information to offspring and, furthermore, some of them would even like a "father" role with offspring. Mostly, both types of donors are interested in the outcome of their donation, though this does not always have a clear association with their attitudes towards anonymity or disclosure towards offspring.

The literature reveals an important distinction between potential donors' openness towards anonymity and the release of non-identifying information, and their openness towards providing the recipients and offspring with identifying information. In a study by Godmand and others [25], almost 40% of potential sperm donors would not donate without a guarantee of anonymity. However, more than 75% of these potential donors felt positively towards releasing non-identifying information to offspring, such as physical characteristics and level of education. Half of the donors felt that offspring should be permitted access to identifying information at the age of 18 years [25]. Other studies seem to confirm these findings [11,26]. Both Godman and associates [25] and Riggs and Russell [27] report that single or homosexual men are significantly more inclined to release their identity than married, heterosexual men, indicating that psychosocial and demographic differences may influence attitudes towards anonymity and disclosure.

Studies that have measured women's intentions to potentially donate eggs before, during or after the removal of donor anonymity (in countries such as Sweden and the UK) do not provide a clear picture because of many methodological issues. Some of these studies report intentions versus actual behavior, which may of course differ. The literature on egg donors' attitudes concerning anonymity reveals some inconsistencies [21]. Although volunteer egg donors reported they did not want any contact with the egg recipients or any involvement with the upbringing of donor egg offspring, they were nonetheless very curious about the recipients, wished to know the outcome of the donation and cared about the recipients' treatment, believed they would not be able to forget about their donation, and also reported that donor offspring should be informed of their genetic origins.

Though few studies have investigated the impact of donor counseling on donor attitudes, there is some evidence to suggest that attitudes towards disclosure changed after a counseling session: before counseling 64% of potential donors felt that offspring had the right to information about their conception, whereas after counseling almost all donors felt offspring had the right to information [28].

Impact of legislation on gamete donors

There is some indication that country of residence (and regulations and laws that are country specific) may influence the type of motivation. Studies with potential donor populations from the USA often report higher percentages of (sperm donor) men with a financial motivation, which is not surprising considering the number of commercial centers in the USA [23,26]. Studies performed in Sweden and Australia report higher percentages of altruistic motivation [11].

Psychosocial needs of the donor

Whatever the motivation a potential egg or sperm donor may have in starting the donation process, it is clear that some of the donor's attitudes (e.g., anonymity, donor payment, contact with offspring) may shift during the donation process. For example, potential donors are often more unclear about anonymity and disclosure to offspring compared with actual donors. However, a considerable number of donors feel very uncertain and undecided about both anonymity and future contact with offspring. This implies that counseling pre- and post-donation might be beneficial to donors. Considering the cultural shift towards more openness in third party reproduction and disclosure of using donated eggs or sperm to offspring, clinicians and researchers alike should start to focus on follow-up of donors. Research should take into account their life issues relating to the donation as well as their (changing) attitudes concerning offspring.

Zweifel and colleagues [29] have suggested that donor egg programs are ethically obligated to follow-up with prospective donors who have been rejected. Although little research has been done that focuses on follow-up of these would-be gamete donors, this is certainly an important clinical issue. Follow-up should address the reason for exclusion from a program, whether it be medical or psychological, and should attempt to ensure that the exclusion does not destabilize the donor's (current and future) emotional health. In these cases, the rejected donor's self-esteem may be affected and/or s/he may have questions regarding the impact on his/her own current or future children. The fertility counselor can provide reassurance in terms of the very strict guidelines for gamete donors and offer a platform for the rejected donor to discuss the implications of his/her exclusion from the program.

Sometimes egg donors are excluded due to results of psychological testing, most often Minnesota Multiphasic Personality Inventory (MMPI-2) or the Personality Assessment Inventory (PAI), as occurred earlier with Eva. Psychological testing in screening gamete donors is useful in that such testing may reveal the possibility of hidden psychopathology. If testing indicates the presence of significant psychopathology such as a substance use disorder, psychosis, mood or anxiety disorder, or a personality disorder, then the candidate would not be allowed to proceed as a donor. Psychological testing can also indicate if the donor is approaching the process in an open, forthright manner. Both the MMPI-2 and PAI contain validity scales, which reflect subjects' defensiveness. It is expected that donor applicants, who are being evaluated, will attempt to present well and will therefore show a degree of defensiveness. However, significant defensiveness will diminish the validity of a test's clinical scales, and may be evidence of a lack of honesty and candidness to the process.

Screening out the possibility of psychopathology is an important goal for a gamete donation program. However, for the individual donor candidate herself, psychological testing is but one important piece of data. Should a prospective donor be excluded due to psychological testing results, it is important to clarify with the candidate that no single psychological test is diagnostic, and the testing should not be taken by her as definitive evidence of a particular pathology. After discussing with the candidate the need for the donor egg program to "err on the side of caution" in not accepting donors who may have underlying psychological problems, the meaning and possible implications of her test results, for her personally, should be discussed. If she identifies at all with the problems that the testing shows, then referral for appropriate treatment is indicated. Finally, though psychological testing is routine and often mandatory in egg donation programs throughout the USA, this practice is not applied globally. Many countries and centers prefer relying on the clinical impression and experience of the fertility counselor and the self-report of the donor candidate in screening for psychopathology.

In another of the opening examples, James was rejected from the sperm donor program due to his negative family history. He was offered a follow-up session with the fertility counselor of the clinic and was very thankful for the opportunity to discuss his worries. Though he'd known about the occurrence of bipolar disorder in his family, he had never specifically thought about the genetic impact on his own children. His sperm donor application started out with good intentions but now turned into a very ambivalent experience: on the one hand, he understood why he was rejected from the program and the rationale of the strict exclusion rules, but on the other hand he felt more responsible for the future mental health of his two sons. If it was not okay for his sperm to help other couples get pregnant, then how could it be okay for his own family? Didn't they deserve the same high standard? Should he have been aware of the genetic impact before starting a family with his wife? As a fertility counselor, I (UV) could reassure him in his own family building choices and point out what he could do with this new information that came from the donor screening. He would at least know and be aware of some of the early symptoms and could understand their familial component. Finally, James also found it helpful to discuss the differences between genetic and social parenthood when dealing with "family tree" issues. It is a given that gamete donors will be held to a different and more exacting "standard" in terms of procreation than we would hold ourselves or our partners. Further, for most people with the ability to use their own genes, the desire to use those genes will be stronger than the wish for a possibly "cleaner" or more problem-free family medical history.

In the last case, Barbara, the donor applicant who felt uncomfortable with the idea that a pregnancy to which she had contributed could end in a termination, was counseled out of the donor egg program. There was no realistic way that the assurances she sought could be carried out; clearly, donating her oocytes and relinquishing control over the path of any potential pregnancy would be a source of emotional conflict/psychological distress for her.

The experience of gamete donation

On the whole, there is consistent evidence demonstrating that the oocyte donation procedure is well tolerated and most donors of all donation types report high levels of satisfaction with the quality of medical care [21]. An important feature in a donor's experiences of donation was the opportunity to meet with the fertility counselor. Studies have found that the majority of donors of all donor groups questioned found counseling invaluable [30], and also helpful in making disclosure decisions in known donation [31,32]. It is striking that the literature documenting the experience of the process of sperm donation remains largely absent. It seems that the sperm donor as a person and as a stakeholder has been widely neglected in both medical and psychosocial research on this topic. Rather the sperm donor is "a means to an end," especially in studies evaluating institutional factors pertaining to legislation, recruitment strategies and attitudes influencing donor recruitment and participation.

As the process of gamete donation entails many other different stakeholders, the role and status of the gamete donor may become obscured or forgotten. What complicates gamete donations is that all of the stakeholders have different interests: *the donor* in terms of his rights, responsibilities, motives and attitudes; *the intended parents* and their rights, responsibilities, opportunity for access to information, social parenthood versus genetic parenthood; *the child* and his/her right and access to information about his/her origin; *the professionals* in terms of their (legal and/or medical) responsibility in screening potential donors and parents, as well as their responsibilities towards the resulting child; and finally *society* with its legal, religious, cultural and ethical frameworks that guide third party reproduction practices.

Reflections of the fertility counselors

> *"It is always advisable to perceive clearly our ignorance."*
>
> *"The very essence of instinct is that it's followed independently of reason."*
>
> – Charles Darwin

UV: I remember vividly the first assessment I ever did of a donor egg candidate. I can't recall what she looked like exactly but I remember that she was young and pretty. I'd researched a bit about donor egg counseling but was baffled in that first interview by one central thought: "Why would a young woman like that donate her eggs?" Over the years I've learned that there are many reasons and none of them are completely straightforward. There are those donors who are truly altruistic – they want to give and expect nothing in return. There are those who are driven by a touching story or a close experience with the consequences of infertility in their daily lives. And there are those who come upon the idea by coincidence because they saw an advertisement or heard something in the media. Each prospective donor has a story to tell about his or her motivation to be here, in this specific place, at this specific time in their lives. However, sometimes their stories are not so very clear and that very first instinctual question I have when seeing a donor remains unanswered. In these cases, I've learned to listen to my instincts and ask more questions, not just for my sake – to get a better picture of the whole, but also for the donor's sake. It's an important decision to part with some of your own genetic material and no matter how comfortable some candidates are with this idea, it's certainly not something that you do every day.

My country (Belgium) does not allow monetary compensation for gamete donors and my center uses an anonymous cross-donation system (i.e., each egg recipient couple needs to provide an egg donor, whose gametes then cross over to a different recipient couple). So sometimes recipients push a donor, emotionally or financially, because they're not getting her eggs and will only be able to move forward with the program if they provide a donor. Sometimes egg or sperm donors actually want a child of their own but their partners don't agree. Sometimes egg donors feel that they have to "make up" for a previous abortion or a miscarriage. Sometimes egg donors put themselves through a number of cycles such that it is questionable whether or not this altruistic motivation is still in the best interest of the donor and her family. Sometimes sperm donors come in and explain that they are gay and this is their way to still have a child even though they're not planning to pursue the often very wanted parenting experience. Sometimes donors come with a story that's just a little bit too much "by the book" and I'm left wondering: What are they not telling me?

In all of these cases, I try to be as transparent as I can be and communicate my doubts. I've had cases where I've been rebuffed and met with a wall of resistance. These are the most difficult cases in which to balance the donor's best interest, that of the recipient and that of the fertility center. When I'm in doubt, I've learned to trust my instincts and give people the benefit of the doubt. I've also had cases where my questions regarding a donor's motivation have been the starting point for a donor's introspection (and in many cases also my own). This is when I feel that I've done a good job and have dared to voice questions and uncertainties that would have surfaced in the long run anyway. This is, for me, what donor assessment and counseling does at its best: It makes sure that everyone involved knows what they're doing, head and heart.

LJ: Rarely, I find that a young woman's donation is completed and she presents back to me as not being happy. Though I have not had the experience of a donor coming in and saying she regrets her donation or was psychologically harmed by the process, over the years I have had a couple of donors who, following donation, have shown a decline in mood or other emotional difficulties. Lena, age 25, came to see me shortly after her egg retrieval and said that she had been feeling unhappy and stressed. Unfortunately, during the time of the cycle, she was also experiencing problems with her roommates and was likely going to need to move. Countertransferentially, I was aware of not wanting to feel that the egg donation – the donation that I had psychologically approved – had been an undue stress for her, of not wanting to feel that the donation had harmed her emotionally. Of course, one of our important functions as fertility counselors is to assure that donating is not likely to be emotionally harmful. For that reason, it was especially important in the aftermath of the donation that I try as much as possible to hear her out, in terms of her experience of donating her eggs, and to be open to the idea that donating was in fact a significant stressor for her. Although she herself denied this, it was important to underline this idea as a possibility for her to consider, and also to make a recommendation against donating again in the future.

This brings about another crucial issue that I (UV) became conscious of throughout that very first interview and in many more to follow: my responsibilities as a fertility counselor and what I later learned to recognize as a strange ambivalence in doing this job. During that first egg donor session, I wanted to make sure that this donation was right for the prospective donor but at the same time I realized her eggs or, for the male donor, his sperm, would help make a baby for some couple who'd been waiting for a long time. On top of it all, I felt I owed it to my colleagues at the fertility center to do a thorough assessment. I was caught up in the multiple perspectives and the multiplicity of relationships involved in gamete donation. I've learned that sometimes you can't please everyone and the "best" decision given the circumstance is often not the easiest one to make. I've learned to be brave and to voice my concerns in the best interest of my patients and, if necessary, my team. I've been surprised by donors commenting on my job and saying that they understand and agree with a thorough assessment, and that they hope the recipients are equally well counseled because they want their eggs or their sperm to do well and be well, wherever they are. In the end, we owe it to the future children to do the best job we can with the information that we have at that time.

References

1. Cholst I. Oocyte donation and the therapeutic misconception. *Fertil Steril* 2013; 99: 1561–2.
2. Applegarth LD, Kingsberg SA. The donor as patient: assessment and support. In: Covington SN, Burns LH, Eds. *Infertility Counseling: A Handbook for Clinicians, 2nd edition*. New York: Cambridge University Press; 2006; 339–55.
3. Almeling R. *Sex Cells: The Medical Market for Eggs and Sperm*. Berkeley and Los Angeles: University of California Press, 2011.
4. The Practice Committees of the American Society for Reproductive Medicine and the Society for Assisted Reproductive Technology. Mature oocyte cryopreservation: a guideline. *Fertil Steril* 2013; 99: 37–43.
5. Ory SJ, Ed. International Federation of Fertility Societies Surveillance (IFFS) 2013. http://c.ymcdn.com/sites/www.iffs-reproduction.org/resource/resmgr/iffs_surveillance_09-19-13.pdf. (Accessed May 25, 2014.)
6. Donors: donating for treatment and research [Online]. Available from: URL: http://www.hfea.gov.uk.
7. Fertility Society of Australia: Reproductive Technology Accreditation Committee. Code of practice for assisted reproductive technology [Online]. 2010 October. Available from: URL: http://www.fertilitysociety.com.au/rtac.
8. Assisted human reproduction act [Online]. Available from: URL: http://www.hc-sc.gc.ca/index-eng.php.
9. A review of the HFEA's sperm and egg donation policies – 2011 [Online]. Available from: URL: http://www.hfea.gov.uk/donationreview.
10. Del Valle A, Bradley L, Said, T. Anonymous semen donor recruitment without reimbursement in Canada. *Repro BioMedicine* 2008; 17: 15–20.
11. Ekerhovd E, Faurskov A, Werner C. Swedish sperm donors are driven by altruism, but shortage of sperm donors leads to reproductive traveling. *Ups J Med Sci* 2008; 113: 305–13.
12. Ernst E, Ingerslev HJ, Schou O, Stoltenberg M. Attitudes among sperm donors in 1992 and 2002: a Danish questionnaire survey. *Acta Obstet Gynecol Scand* 2007; 86: 327–33.
13. Van den Broeck U, Vandermeeren M, Vanderschueren D, Enzlin P, Demyttenaere K, D'Hooghe T. A systematic review of sperm donors: demographic characteristics, attitudes, motives and experiences of the process of sperm donation. *Hum Reprod Update* 2013; 0: 1–15.
14. Daniels K. Anonymity and openness and the recruitment of gamete donors. Part I: semen donors. *Hum Fertil (Camb)* 2007; 10: 151–8.
15. Practice Committee of the American Society for Reproductive Medicine and the Practice Committee of the Society for Assisted Reproductive Technology: Recommendations for gamete and embryo donation: a committee opinion. *Fertil Steril* 2013; 99: 47–62.
16. Guidelines for counseling in infertility [Online]. Available from: URL: http://www.eshre.eu.
17. ESHRE: Task Force on Ethics and Law. Gamete and embryo donation. *Hum Reprod* 2002; 17: 1407–8.
18. Skillern A, Cedars M, Huddleston H. Egg donor informed consent tool (EDICT): development and validation of a new informed consent tool for oocyte donors. *Fert Steril* 2013; 99: 1733–8.
19. Distant, Daniel, Christian Post Reporter: Sperm Bank Mix-Up in Utah: Convicted Felon Fathered 21-Year- Old Girl, Possibly Hundreds of Others. www.christianpost.com/news/sperm-bank-mixup-in-utah-convicted-felon-fathered-21-year-old-girl-possibly-hundreds-of-others-113219. January 23, 2014.
20. California cryobank [Online]. Available from: URL: http://www.californiacryobank.com.
21. Purewal S, van den Akker OBA. Systematic review of oocyte donation: investigating attitudes, motivations and experiences. *Hum Reprod Update* 2009; 15: 499–515.
22. Jadva V, Freeman T, Kramer W, Golombok S. Sperm and oocyte donors' experiences of anonymous donation and subsequent contact with donor offspring. *Hum Reprod* 2011; 26: 638–46.
23. Schover LR, Rothmann SA, Colllins RL. The personality and motivation of semen donors: a comparison with oocyte donors. *Hum Reprod* 1992; 7: 575–9.
24. Sydjo G, Svanberg AS, Lampic C, Jablonowska B. Relationships in IVF couples 20 years after treatment. *Hum Reprod* 2011; 20: 1952–7.
25. Godmand KM, Sanders K, Rosenberg M, Burton P. Potential sperm donors', recipients and their partners' opinions towards the release of identifying

information in Western Australia. *Hum Reprod* 2006; 22: 3022–6.

26. Mahlstadt PP, Probasco KA. Sperm donors: their attitudes toward providing medical and psychosocial information for recipient couples and donor offspring. *Fertil Steril* 1991; 56: 747–53.

27. Riggs DW, Russell L. Characteristics of men willing to act as sperm donors in the context of identity release legislation. *Hum Reprod* 2011; 26: 266–72.

28. Hammarburg K, Carmichael M, Tinney L, Mulder A. Gamete donors' and recipients' evaluation of donor counseling: a prospective longitudinal cohort study. *Aust N Z J Gynaecol* 2008; 48: 601–6.

29. Zweifel JE, Biaggio B, Schouweiler C, Lindheim SR. Follow-up assessment of excluded oocyte donor candidates. *J Obstet Gynaecol Res* 2009; 35: 320–5.

30. Jordan CB, Belar CD, Williams RS. Anonymous oocyte donation: a follow-up analysis of donors' experiences. *J Psychosom Obstet Gynaecol* 2004; 25: 145–51.

31. Winter A, Daniluk J. A gift from the heart: the experiences of women whose egg donations helped their sisters become mothers. *J Couns Dev* 2004; 82: 483–95.

32. Yee S, Hitkari JA, Greenblatt EM. A follow-up study of women who donated oocytes to known recipient couples for altruistic reasons. *Human Reprod* 2007; 22(7): 2040–50.

Chapter 9

Counseling surrogate carrier participants

Tara H. Simpson and Hilary Hanafin

Katrina is a 45-year-old law professional, married to David, a 46-year-old chemical engineer. The couple currently resides in Sweden. Katrina is a Swedish citizen and David has dual citizenship in Sweden and the United States. They have been married 15 years and report a "strong relationship" despite the many years of assisted reproductive treatment and numerous pregnancy losses. Last year, Katrina and David had previously selected an agency in the Ukraine with a gestational carrier, but it "fell through" when the potential carrier did not clear the medical screen. The intended parent (IP) couple has decided to move forward with an arrangement facilitated by a surrogacy agency in the United States that they found online, researched, and reached out to for assistance.

Jennifer, a 30-year-old dental hygienist, applied to be a gestational carrier (GC) with a regional surrogacy agency approximately six months ago. Her husband, Joe, is 31 years old and is self-employed in the construction industry. The couple and their children live in a suburb of an urban area on the East Coast of the United States. She and her husband started discussing the possibility of her being a carrier approximately a year ago after she met a dental patient who was struggling with infertility and considering having to involve a carrier in her family building plans.

Katrina and David have been matched by the agency with Jennifer as their carrier, and the two couples will begin the process of counseling and assessment required by the clinic where treatment will take place. The GC, her husband, and the IP couple have spoken on the phone via conference call with an agency staff person facilitating the discussion. Following the phone call, all parties have begun to make arrangements to meet in person.

The addenda referred to in this chapter are available for download at www.cambridge.org/9781107643116. Password: AX164BKR7.

Introduction

Perhaps in no other arrangement in the world of fertility are the legal, medical and psychological complexities of reproduction as fraught with issues as in traditional surrogacy and gestational carrier arrangements. Although the practice of surrogacy dates back before the Old Testament, as a method through which one woman carries a child for another as a means to assist a couple in achieving their family building goals, it was not practiced in contemporary society formally until the 1970s. With technological advances in assisted reproductive technologies (ART), specifically in vitro fertilization (IVF) and egg donation, it became possible for a woman to gestate and give birth to a child that was not genetically related to her.

An early dilemma of surrogacy was the adoption and use of the appropriate terminology for the various parties involved in this type of third party reproduction. In this chapter, the term traditional surrogate (TS) will be used for a woman who carries a pregnancy to which she is genetically related as a result of contributing her oocytes at conception. The term gestational carrier (GC) will be used to describe a woman who carries a pregnancy to which she is *not* genetically related. In this arrangement, the egg(s) are from the intended biological mother, who generally for medical reasons cannot carry a pregnancy herself, or are from an egg donor. The use of a GC accounts for the majority of all surrogate pregnancies in the United States [1].

Fertility Counseling: Clinical Guide and Case Studies, ed. Sharon N. Covington. Published by Cambridge University Press.

The term intended parents (IP) is used for individuals or couples who are the contracting, prospective parent(s). The use of a GC has also allowed the possibility for gay male couples as well as single men and women to have a child. An increasing number of GCs conceive with both sperm and egg donor gametes for IPs. Women acting as TS and GC may be commercially recruited and paid for their service (the most common) or may be altruistic, or compassionate, as when a family member or friend volunteers pro bono.

Due to the increasing use and availability of surrogacy as a form of alternative family building, an entire industry has developed that identifies and brings potential GCs and IPs together from all over the world. At times, IPs may try to find a GC on their own, either through the Internet, print advertising or word of mouth, yet this may place potential IPs at risk for exploitation, and working with a reputable surrogacy agency or agent can alleviate many potential problems. The motivation to become a TS or GC, also, may involve vulnerabilities and risks to the woman and her family pursuing this arrangement. Thus, how these arrangements and relationships are facilitated becomes crucial in their success.

There is wide variation in screening and services offered by surrogacy agencies and reproductive health lawyers. Some act as a "matchmaking" service only, while others provide full legal and psychological services throughout the process. In 1986, there were at least six agencies in the United States and one in Europe that arranged for potential TS and GC to meet infertile couples and individuals. By 2010, the number of agencies in the United States grew to more than 23, with a total of 7000 births by surrogate mothers/gestational carriers occurring in the United States and more than 300 births in Great Britain. (Synesiou K. Personal conversation. Encino, CA. 25 November, 2013.) Since there is no central reporting of such contractual arrangements, the actual number is unknown and assumed to be far higher. There are virtually no statistics on how many women and families are involved in the gestational carrier market. Nevertheless, the available reports from the CDC and the Society for Assisted Reproductive Technology (SART) clearly show that the number of infants born to gestational surrogates almost doubled from 2004 to 2008, from 738 babies born to nearly 1400 [2].

International travel has proliferated for IPs requiring the service of carriers or surrogates. The growing interest in "cross-border reproductive services" (CBRS) has generated both legal and ethical concerns [3]. Surrogate parenting arrangements occur primarily in the United States, Asia and Eastern Europe. There are a number of factors that may promote such cross-border surrogacy arrangements within these three geographical areas. Internationally, the rules determining gestational surrogacy have progressed in some places and are still evolving in others. In many countries, governing bodies have taken on the task of deciding the legalities of surrogacy. Most often they address financial compensation, restrictions on who is allowed to contract with a surrogate, and mandated involvement by professionals and legal determination of parentage. Such locations are particularly appealing to CBRS participants from countries with stringent anti-surrogacy laws.

Furthermore, countries that have strong religious or cultural influences in their governing bodies prohibit surrogacy on the basis of religious tenets (e.g., Roman Catholic or Muslim) that do not condone the concept of an outside party involving herself in the creation of a couple's child. In addition, some countries may not have the specific service available because of lack of expertise, lack of affordability and/or limited numbers of donors and surrogates. For other countries, the service may be unavailable because it is not considered sufficiently safe or the service is not available for certain categories of individuals, especially at public expense, on the basis of age, marital status or sexual orientation; while other individuals and patients may fear lack of medical privacy and confidentiality, and thus travel abroad. Finally, services may simply be cheaper in other countries [4,5].

The United States has no national policy on reproductive technologies like surrogacy and gestational parenting. Issues of family law are routinely decided by individual states. Some states have determined protocols, the enforceability of a contract, and have restricted payments to TS and GC. The state laws and regulations determining gestational surrogacy are still evolving. Some states ban surrogacy outright, some ban paid surrogacy but allow a woman to offer her services as a volunteer while others are permissive of paid gestational carrier arrangements [6].

Legal consultation is imperative and will help clients make informed decisions, provide accurate information and create a basis for an informed consent. Most gestational carrier arrangements involve a contract that outlines the responsibilities, confidentiality, medical insurance coverage, financial reimbursements (including lack of), embryo transfer limits, pregnancy termination, prenatal care, lost wages and childcare costs, post-birth contact between parties, social media preferences and so on. The risks of CBRS need to be addressed. It is important for clients to know the laws in the place of the birth, laws in the parents' home state or country and the laws to any area a pregnant GC may travel [7].

The European Society of Human Reproduction and Embryology (ESHRE) and the American Society of Reproductive Medicine (ASRM), have published guidelines for professionals with recommendations for practices with gestational carriers. Both approaches have included the provision of counseling as part of patient care for all participants in TS and GC family building arrangements. ESHRE has professional guidelines on surrogacy and intrafamilial surrogacy, both of which provide specific recommendations on psychological counseling of all participants, education, assessment and support as well as provisions for rejection or denial [8]. After a long review process, the ASRM Practice Committee Guidelines were published in 2012 and outline the physicians' protocol and criteria for treating GC and IP, as well as identifying the need for psychological counseling, education and assessment (including psychological testing, "where appropriate") of IP and GC by a qualified mental health professional. It also outlines the circumstances and/or contraindications warranting disqualification or rejection of the IP or GC [9]. The publication by the ASRM Ethics Committee, entitled *Protecting the Gestational Carrier,* provides critical steps involved in the evaluation and treatment of TS and GC [10]. It outlines a standard practice of care, highlighting the importance of informed consent, legal counsel and psychological support so that all parties involved are protected.

Given the legal risk that exists with these arrangements and the ability to be sure all participants are in a good place to move forward with treatment, withstanding the uncertainties ahead, counseling becomes an important part of medical care and should occur before treatment begins. In order to minimize risks and maximize the positive outcome for both families, fertility counselors can provide valuable and thoughtful guidance and education, and assist in clarifying and exploring roles, expectations and potential outcomes for all parties involved. Fertility counselors traditionally meet separately with the IPs; separately with the GC for psychological assessment and consultation (with husband/significant other, if applicable); and finally with both the IPs and GC in a group session. Each of these sessions has different purposes and goals, yet all are components in building, planning and navigating the family building process with a gestational carrier.

As a facilitator with all parties involved, fertility counselors are presented with two sets of clients, each with their own agendas, concerns, perspectives and need for confidentiality. The control of information – who is entitled to know what – can be tenuous and difficult when conducting evaluations. It is recommended that fertility counselors address these issues early in the consultations, as well as the fertility counselor's role and who is entitled to the results of the psychological testing and assessment, so that they are acting ethically and legally. In addition, practitioners can provide ongoing support to the IPs and GC as the relationship unfolds during fertility treatment, pregnancy and postpartum. This is a set of relationships that, one could make a case, needs just as much attention and tending to during the pregnancy, following delivery and across time as the child(ren) grow up and the families – both of them – develop and mature.

Assessing and educating the intended parent(s)

Katrina and David have experienced many years of assisted reproductive treatment, using her own and then donor eggs, which resulted in three pregnancy losses in the second trimester. David indicates that while he is excited at the prospect of gestational surrogacy providing them with the family they desire, he does worry for his wife's stress level as they embark on this next type of treatment arrangement since "she has just been through so much." Due to previous losses, Katrina prefers to not terminate pregnancies unless under very serious health circumstances. She states that she feels it would be "hard to imagine having to make that decision." Despite her ambivalent feelings about selective reduction, she indicates that she and David agree that they do not desire more than a twin pregnancy or that they do not wish to carry a child with a genetic anomaly to term. Katrina prefers to transfer two embryos due to her eagerness for "treatment to work this time and for us to bring home a baby – even if there are two," while David reports, "I think we should defer to the doctor's opinion."

Katrina says that she feels cautious about getting her hopes up with Jennifer as a potential GC because of disappointments in the past with another agency. Katrina is curious to meet Jennifer in person, but states she wants to make sure that all the medical and psychological components of the prescreening are completed first.

The intended mother reveals that they are not planning to tell anyone that they will be using an egg donor, so explaining twins or triplets at her age of 45 is a stressor. Katrina originally felt that she would prefer not disclosing to the GC that the baby being carried is a result of anonymous egg donation as "it feels like it makes the baby even less mine. I would like to keep that just between my husband and I – and the child in the future if we tell it."

While she has high expectations of the GC in terms of prenatal care, activity level and communicating all the facts about the pregnancy, Katrina is not sure how she much wants a relationship with the GC after the pregnancy. "I can't see past the delivery because a pregnancy has never been sustained and it's hard to imagine a baby ever being born." The couple plans to tell the child that they were carried about a gestational carrier who was "a really nice lady in the US." It is important to note that Katrina and David will return with the child to Europe and plan to continue to reside overseas.

Psychological screening and preparation of IP(s) attempt to assess each person's readiness and ability to work with a woman who will have total care of the unborn child for the 40 weeks of pregnancy. For Katrina and David, the loss of their prior pregnancies and now the loss of control over the care for their unborn child can become a source of fear and insecurity. For the GC arrangement to be successful, it is ideal that IPs be empathic, adaptive and resilient. Participants who are overly intrusive or controlling, who are not comfortable with the concept of surrogacy (and potentially coupled with donated gametes), or who have personality or active mental health disorders, put the gestational carrier at risk. The ability to trust, contain anxieties and being generous in spirit serves IPs well. As shown in Table 9.1, the clinical interview focuses on the IPs' expectations and preferences of the surrogacy arrangement during and after pregnancy, on their decision-making processes, on the couple's coping abilities and on their marital adjustment. (Addendum 9.1 provides a detailed IP interview and group session format to follow.)

Table 9.1 Topics to review in intended parent interview.

Infertility history of IPs
Relationship history of IPs
IPs psychosocial history (mental health and substance use)
Decision-making and agreement in participation
Exploration of religious and cultural differences
If intrafamily arrangement, roles/relationships of all parties involved
Confidentiality concerns and use of social media
Communication preferences
Reactions of family and friends
IPs existing children, if any
Prenatal care preferences
Prenatal diagnostic testing
Belief and concerns about multi-pregnancy reduction
Beliefs and concerns about pregnancy termination for fetal anomaly
Preferences of disclosure to child(ren) about GC and her identity
Preferences of disclosure to child(ren) about utilization of donated gametes (if utilized)
Contact expection between the two families during the pregnancy
Contact expection between the two families after the birth
Preferences regarding delivery and hospital stay
Management of financial issues
Legal process for transfer of parentage
Fears about and wishes for their experience with surrogacy

Revealing information also comes from the IPs' perception of the gestational carrier and their comfort level for contact with her and her family. A fertility counselor needs to determine if Katrina's reluctance to envision establishing a relationship, as well as imagining a future connection for her and her child with Jennifer, is due to their personalities or due to their disappointments and lack of experience with surrogacy. They will have a long-term relationship with the carrier (and her family), lasting 13–18 months prior to the birth of the child. The ambiguous process of choosing a carrier, the intense and complicated means of conceiving, the long pregnancy and the years ahead of parenting all require comfort with the process and ideally with the carrier. Conflicts are less likely to be exacerbated if the parents have the ability not to be overly intrusive or controlling, can empathize with the carrier's situation and keep communication open. If the IPs cannot envision themselves having some contact with the surrogate or carrier, then they should not proceed since it may reveal a discomfort with their decisions and with the child's history.

The assessment of the couple needs to be culturally sensitive. There are cultural differences in perceptions of privacy, pregnancy, gift giving, family ties, parenting, disclosure, infertility and revealing feelings, to name but a few. The fertility counselor should ask the IPs to educate the GC about their religious and cultural background, as well as discuss the IPs' assumptions about the GC's culture, as a proactive step to avoid hurt feelings and minimize incorrect ideas.

A discussion of privacy, secrecy and disclosure needs to be explored as these may reflect cultural differences. Katrina's plan to keep the egg donation a secret, or perhaps not tell others about the surrogate mother, may reflect her unresolved issues; however, it may also reflect her culture. It is important to consider the culture of where the child(ren) will be raised, not just the culture of where the child(ren) will be born. Keeping the egg donation contribution secret from Jennifer is neither practical nor respectful, as they are trusting Jennifer to carry their child(ren) yet somehow feel she cannot be trusted in knowing this information. Perhaps if David and Katrina discuss their dilemma with Jennifer, their relationship may be enhanced and hurtful misunderstandings may be minimized. It is also essential that Jennifer and Joe be able to consider their own feelings about the use of donated gametes in the pregnancy and their moral, religious and ethical framework surrounding the topic. Furthermore, technology, advances in science and the Internet, may make genetic and birth secrets obsolete in the generations to come. Again, then, Katrina and David need to be resolved that the child may come to know the non-genetic variable and that Jennifer will know the origins of the children's conception.

Understanding the medical practices and prenatal care of the GC's home country is important. It is common for IP couples undergoing IVF to be in the clinic's city for two weeks prior to embryo transfer, visit the carrier's country at least once during pregnancy, and remain in that country again for a minimum of two weeks after the birth. Some countries require longer stays of four to six weeks. If children are born prematurely, new parents can be displaced for months. Having a professional interpreter available is a necessity if there is a language barrier, so that discussions of sensitive medical, psychological and legal issues are understood as thoroughly as possible. Finally, the issue of payment for medical costs of the newborn child needs to be explored prior to conception. When the IPs are not citizens of the country where the birth takes place, payment for the pediatrician and hospitalization care may be stressful and very costly. It is helpful to highlight the costs and risks of a multiple gestation. Premature birth can cause extreme financial hardship and months of displacement for the parents.

Evaluation of the gestational carrier

> Joe and Jennifer have been married for six years. The couple both describe having a "good" marriage built on friendship and similar interests. Both Jennifer and Joe have immediate family nearby and both sets of parents are aware of Jennifer's interest in being a GC.
>
> Jennifer reports three pregnancies in the past resulting in two sons (2 and 4 years old, respectively). Her first pregnancy at 24 years of age was unplanned (and not desired) and she was very sick with hyperemesis. She and Joe mutually decided to terminate the pregnancy. Jennifer has a history of pregnancy related sickness during the first trimester but states that the illness was manageable with her two sons because "I had more support, resources, and was better prepared – they were also planned and wanted by my husband and I."
>
> Jennifer indicates that her concerns in being a GC center around the potential for triplets, since she feels as if carrying twins would be enough. In addition, she reports that she is nervous about the relationship with the IPs and hopes it is a positive one. She understands that selective reduction may have to occur because of multiples or genetic anomaly. Joe is supportive of Jennifer's decision to be a GC but states he does worry about her physical health during the pregnancy, due to previous bouts of sickness, as well as the impact that the pregnancy will have on her ability to fulfill her roles and obligations on the job and within their family.
>
> As customary in the evaluation of GCs, Jennifer was given a personality inventory. The results of Jennifer's psychological testing were valid and within normal limits in clinical and content scales. She approached the inventory in an open and forthright manner, which is a positive indicator of her commitment to participating as a GC.

A significant goal of preconception counseling with a potential GC is helping her decide if being a carrier will serve a positive, satisfying purpose, or have a negative, dysfunctional impact on her life. She needs to be able

Table 9.2 Considerations for participation as a gestational carrier.

History of healthy full-term pregnancy and birth
Experience and competence with motherhood
Motivations that reveal obtainable goals
Motivations that reflect empathy
Spousal family support
Stable lifestyle
No major conflicts or major transitions in the next two years
Cognitive ability to provide informed consent and conceptualize risks
Absence of psychopathology
History of making successful decisions for herself
Financial stability
Demonstrates tolerance for ambiguous and unclear situations
Realistic expectations regarding time involved
Lack of anti-authority behavior and rigidity in thinking
Ability to communicate in her native language with medical professionals

to provide informed consent, be able to relinquish the child, and exit the experience whole and unharmed. In an effort to serve both parties, the fertility counselor must assess the candidate's motivations, her ability to accurately perceive situations, her personality and her intellectual competency. Table 9.2 identifies considerations for participation as a GC and Table 9.3 describes issues to be covered in a GC interview. Assessing decision-making processes, social and family relationships, manner of resolving problems and ability to take care of herself and others (e.g., her own children) is important. Special consideration needs to be given to issues of loss and trauma in her history, such as family of origin conflicts, history of sexual assault or physical/sexual/emotional abuse, abandonment and death of family members or significant others, as well as any unresolved pregnancy termination or loss. (Addendum 9.2 provides a detailed GC interview format to follow.)

It is recommended that a GC has previously given birth, in large part so that she can provide informed consent. A woman with no childbirth experience may encounter unknown medical risks and will not be able to fully understand the physical demands that she is undertaking. A woman with no parenting experience may not be as able to predict her own behavior and emotions as they relate to the intended child. Excluding women with risky medical conditions, or who have

Table 9.3 Topics for intake interview with surrogate/gestational carrier [11, with permission].

Discussion of motivations and her decision to pursue surrogacy
Expectations about the benefits of serving as a surrogate/gestational carrier
Description of marriage, family life and support system
Review of potential stressor or changes
History of pregnancy and postpartum recovery
Reproductive history, including abortions
Childhood family, events and traumas
Resolution status of any trauma and loss in adulthood
History of drug/alcohol abuse
History of depression and psychiatric history
Discussion of coping skills when life is difficult
History of lawsuits and difficulty with the law
Discussion of her children and assessment of how she will tell them
History of her own children's lives as it pertains to instability and loss
Expectations about relationship with the IPs
Expectations about relationship with the potential child
Beliefs about abortion due to birth anomaly
Facts about multi-fetal reduction and risks of multiples, bed rest, hospitalization,
Fantasies and predictions of her behavior and needs at time of birth

mental health or substance abuse histories, is also recommended. It is crucial to assess for any significant current stressors or anticipated life transitions, such as unemployment, divorce, or deployment of a spouse. If her participation is strictly due to acute financial need, then confounded, compromised decision-making may be present. GCs who are receiving public assistance or heavily in debt may be financially, physically and socially vulnerable during a pregnancy. Finally, lack of marital/social support, lack of empathy and unrealistic expectations about the time and process are also all negative indicators in a woman's potential role as a GC.

Motivations

Assessment questions may vary depending on whether the GC is already known to the recipients and whether the contract is altruistic surrogacy or fee-based surrogacy. Some countries, as well as specific states in the USA, only permit altruistic surrogacy, resulting in more known GC arrangements in which the participants have a preexisting relationship, whether family, friends or acquaintances. Due to this dynamic, a potential motivator is the GC's perception of coercion to participate, such as feeling overt or covert pressure from a family member or friend to assist an IP. The history of the relationship, perceived differences of the power amongst participants, and the anticipated impact between all parties should be included in the assessment.

Ideally, a GC will benefit from the experience beyond financial remuneration. Although not often definable, there needs to be a meaningful aspect of the role and/or compelling motivation for the GC. Research on GCs found results that were strikingly similar in their conclusions about the motivations and the demographics of GCs. These studies revealed that GCs in the USA were motivated by the desire to do something important in their lives; empathy for the childless couple; desire to experience pregnancy again; financial gain; and less often, an opportunity to undo or fix something in their past. Typically the participants were in their late 20s, most often married and having an average of two children, raised in the Christian/Protestant faith, and with two years of post-secondary education. Most importantly, none of the research found psychopathology in the participants [11–14].

Being a GC involves a wide array of ambiguity and potentially emotionally stressful situations. Predicting how a carrier will respond to and resolve such issues is key to protecting her and all parties involved. A personality that is resilient, adaptable, empathic and intellectually competent with good ego-strength is ideal.

Psychological testing

Psychological testing is recommended and often employed to assess potential participants, both as a means of corroborating the clinical interview and as a method of identifying personality characteristics that may negatively impact the candidate's participation. Psychological testing is useful in identifying any number of factors including personality style, psychopathology and/or potential behavioral problems (e.g., chemical abuse/addiction, hostility toward authority figures, or stress at work). It can also be helpful in identifying the potential candidate's ability to be truthful and forthcoming.

As mentioned earlier, The ASRM Practice Committee has issued guidelines in the psychological assessment of GCs, which identifies the use of standard psychological testing as part of the screening process. The common measures used for personality assessment of GCs are the Minnesota Multiphasic Personality Inventory-2 (MMPI-2 or MMPI-2RF) and the Personality Assessment Inventory (PAI). For over 70 years, the MMPI-2 has been the most widely utilized and researched psychometric test, having been translated into more than 25 languages and used as a clinical instrument in psychiatric, forensic and employment settings. The PAI is also a self-administered test that assesses personality and psychopathology. Developed in 1991, it measures 22 non-overlapping scales based on constructs that correlate with the DSM (*Diagnostic and Statistical Manual*) [15].

Research on the use of MMPI-2 with GCs has found that the majority of applicants are within normal clinical limits yet score higher on validity scales that indicate, not surprisingly, a positive presentation of high personal standards and values [16]. GCs showed significantly higher scores on the scale that measures for a presentation of goodness, contentment, patience and high morality [17]. These are all desirable qualities for a woman who is willing to gestate a pregnancy for another person(s). The use of the validity scales when interpreting test results assist in deciphering how much positive impression management is within normal limits or whether the GC is attempting to deny problems or psychopathology. In the case of an invalid psychological test during screening, fertility counselors may consider giving another personality test to the GC. However, if a candidate produces another invalid test, she is presenting herself consistently in a deceptive fashion and should be excluded from participation. Without a valid inventory, the fertility counselor cannot trust that what GC is self-reporting is true or accurate.

Understanding the social, medical and cultural context

The evaluation of a GC's social and familial support system, daily living circumstances and their available resources such as transportation and finances are important. It is standard to interview a potential GC's partner, if she has one, and in some cases consider giving the partner psychological testing if there are concerns. It is anticipated that the partner will make many sacrifices during the process and will be thrust into vague and tenuous circumstances. The strength of the relationship and the motivation for supporting the carrier should be assessed. Furthermore, her children are of utmost concern. How a candidate plans to explain the situation can reveal her own understanding of and empathy for her children's perspective and needs. Fertility counselors have a responsibility to protect children psychologically, and proceed more cautiously if the interview reveals painful histories for the candidate and/or her children. It is important to weigh the ethical and psychosocial complications of reproductive technologies on the children who already exist. Putting GCs at medical risk, housing them away from their children, and not safeguarding their financial interests need to be avoided.

It is imperative that a candidate be educated about the IVF protocols and other liabilities associated with pregnancy that she may encounter. A fertility counselor can support the carrier in determining if she is agreeable to a multiple birth and understands the increased risks due to utilizing IVF. The risks of bed rest, hospitalization, Caesarean delivery, neonatal death, financial hardships and trauma suggest that singleton pregnancies are the preferred result.

The potential GC's cultural and religious environment and belief systems should be considered during the evaluation, particularly around the issues of pregnancy termination and multi-fetal pregnancy reduction. Beyond explaining the medical issues related to termination, the fertility counselor must understand how the candidate's way of thinking is tied to her religious and moral decision-making process on these issues. In addition, culture plays a role in knowing how comfortable a carrier is with helping a couple from a different culture, race or religion. Some carriers are attracted to and comfortable with differences and can manage the potential miscommunications or ambiguities that occur, while other carriers are best served to work with IPs from a similar socio-cultural background.

Related to a GC's motivations and goals are a woman's expectations and concerns about her relationship with the IPs. A discussion of Jennifer's wishes surrounding the relationship with the couple during and after pregnancy, and with the future child, will reveal her dynamics and needs. It will also help ensure that she works with IPs who have similar wishes and expectations of the relationship. Unrealistic expectations, such as using surrogacy to fill an emotional or social void, and a lack of clarity about boundaries should be carefully assessed. Katrina's inability to imagine the relationship after the birth puts Jennifer at risk for envisioning more post-birth contact than Katrina may be able to tolerate.

The preconception joint session

Both women have spoken on the telephone and via email (beyond the initial phone consult with the agency) over the few weeks leading up to the preconception group meeting. The IP mother, despite her initial reservations of opening herself up to becoming attached, quickly finds herself becoming connected with Jennifer.

Jennifer has sent Katrina a link to her blog that she is currently writing on her experience as a GC, and as has also initiated an online relationship via social media so they can get to know each other better. During their conversations, Jennifer tells Katrina about her doctor close to her home who delivered her children and expressed a desire for the IPs to eventually meet her children. Finally, Jennifer offers to pump breast milk and Katrina is grateful that she cares to provide for the baby beyond what she had even envisioned.

At the preconception meeting, when all members are able to meet in person for the first time, the session is utilized to discuss the logistics and details of pregnancy, current and future management of the relationships of all parties, the dissemination of information, and addressing concerns and expectations.

All participants are excited and eager for treatment to begin and are pleased to find similarities in all of their perspectives about the impending experience. The IPs express their current struggle with the topic of selective reduction, but they conclude that they will follow doctor's advice on selection reduction, if triplets occur and/or if there is a genetic anomaly. Jennifer appreciates this viewpoint and underscores her agreement that any multiples more than twins would be difficult for her physically. After discussing and exploring Katrina's hesitance to divulge the use of donated gametes in the IP meeting, the IP mother decides it is best to be open about the donor egg component with Jennifer and Joe, which is appreciated by the GC and her husband. Jennifer and Joe inform the IPs that they respect their decisions about any prenatal testing, as well as any subsequent decisions that are made based upon those tests.

The IPs express their wish for a healthy diet, particularly that Jennifer not consume too much processed food and to eat organic, when possible. The birth is envisioned and the only requests that Jennifer has is that David stay by her shoulders as the baby is born, that no photos are taken, and that the baby get handed to the IPs first. In addition, the concept and concerns surrounding relinquishment are discussed, with none of the parties expressing any foreseeable problems in the ending to that particular chapter of the relationship. The notion of how conflicts will be resolved as they arise is carefully addressed. Finally, the desired contact between the two families is talked about and Jennifer underscores the importance of hearing from the intended couple during the holidays, about their family and the child, following the delivery.

The preconception meeting between the prospective parent(s) and the gestational carrier and her partner serves many different functions. It provides an opportunity to facilitate an exchange of information that protects both parties, minimizes potential conflicts, identifies any contraindications and anticipates problems. Common problems usually involve struggles with medical issues, the relationship and with logistical surprises. In addition, it allows a forum for all parties to share motivations, reactions of others and express concerns regarding the impending relationship. (See Table 9.4 covering discussion topics.)

The joint session provides an opportunity for the participants to discuss any concerns or preferences about prenatal care (e.g., diet, lifestyle, caffeine, medical care and travel). Of particular importance are medical issues, such as choice of doctor or hospital, use of medication, bed-rest, prenatal testing and what to do in the event there are negative pregnancy outcomes (e.g., miscarriage, diagnosis of a fetal anomaly, conception of multiples, pregnancy termination and reduction). It is not uncommon for IPs with a history of painful losses to be vigilant (even hyper-vigilant) about medical care.

One of the most trying problems for all the families is the challenges and failures of Mother Nature to safely bring healthy children into the world, despite everyone's best efforts. Miscarriages, high-risk complicated pregnancies, birth defects, premature births and illness all intrude, despite the best-laid plans. Mother Nature's failure raises the counseling issue of the dissimilar life experiences with reproduction. The IPs and the GC have different views of success with fertility and what is "normal." GCs tend to feel positive and invincible, while the prospective parents may feel anxious, worried, cautious and hyper-vigilant. The IPs may interpret the GC's relaxed approach to the pregnancy as disrespectful and non-caring. Once the GC becomes pregnant, the IP has to potentially deal with feelings of inadequacy, annoyance and jealousy as she watches another woman carry her baby and may have to defer to the GC's familiarity with pregnancy and motherhood – something the IP mother has never been able to achieve. Another common error includes a carrier misinterpretation of an IP's behavior, seeing only anxiety or aloofness. The dynamic of "*my body, your baby*" or "*my baby, your body*" exemplifies the different focus that the GC couple and the IP parents may have during the experience. The dissemination of information is different during the IVF cycle when the infertile couple is a patient than during the later stages of pregnancy when just the carrier is the patient. It can be helpful to identify and anticipate where some of the "normal" challenges and problem areas are during a GC pregnancy, despite the tendency for the participants to resist considering these difficulties.

Table 9.4 Issues to review prior to conception in joint session [11, with permission].

Pregnancy history of gestational carrier
Infertility history of IPs
Motivations for participation
Reactions of family and friends
Children of carrier and IPs existing children, if any
Prenatal care preferences
Prenatal diagnostic testing
Belief and concerns about multi-pregnancy reduction
Beliefs and concerns about pregnancy termination for fetal anomaly
Contact between the two families during the pregnancy
Contact between the two families after the birth
Preferences regarding delivery and hospital stay
Exploration of religious and cultural differences
Confidentiality concerns, social media
Management of financial issues
Legal process for transfer of parentage
Fears about and wishes for their experience with surrogacy

All parties will have to express their preferences in regards to how parties will communicate. Setting expectations about staying in contact, without the sense of feeling burdened or smothered, is essential. Who tells who, what and when can be a sensitive topic when the lives of IPs and GCs overlap. A discussion with the parents about who owns and controls the information about their child's beginnings is helpful. This also provides a great opportunity for preferences regarding information shared on social media since this forum allows a greater breadth and depth of information exchange that some find a breach of their personal privacy. As in any relationship, especially one in which trust is a primary component, providing accurate information, increasing empathy for the other's perspective, and making confrontations and requests wisely, is fundamental for any problem-solving of conflicts. IPs and GCs need each other to make this work, and they need to create a positive legacy for the children.

Also during the joint session, preferences about the birth itself are shared. The GC may have a strong preference for a medical provider she feels comfortable with, but this may be complicated by the laws of state where the birth facility is, by the hospital policy regarding GC births and with the specific needs of the delivery (high-risk maternal factors, such as multiples or other health issues). In terms of the birth itself, the following issues need to be discussed: who will be in attendance; will it be filmed; who can witness the delivery; who is expected to hold the baby first and when the GC holds the baby. Delivery methods and use of pain medication are discussed with all parties' preferences stated, and the topic of pumping breast milk can be brought up at this time.

A joint session should also include a walk-through of the relationship that each participant envisions during the pregnancy and following the birth. The desire for contact is part of the criteria on which they choose to work together. It is sad, stressful and hurtful when two families have dramatically different agendas. GCs benefit from the IPs responding like parents throughout the pregnancy. Their reward and comfort with relinquishing the baby are significantly increased if they know that the IPs are preparing for the baby as well as being interested in the carrier's well-being. Achieving some clarity about contact during and after the delivery prevents psychological stress and harm. Postbirth research on surrogates concludes a benefit when GCs see and/or hear about the happiness to which they have contributed [18].

The fertility counselor can help by providing structure and definition in the relationship before and after birth. Addressing participants' assumptions about how the other party feels can help to reduce ambiguities and misinterpretations. It is advisable for the parties to have mental health professional guidance during the pregnancy and, if possible, following the birth. (Fertility counselors should consider offering this service as a separate part of their contract, after the evaluation is completed. Please see Chapter 21 on legal aspects for more information.) Issues related to the transfer of the infant(s), decision-making at the hospital, how to say goodbye, respect for closure and specifics about contact should be addressed. It is commonly recommended that the surrogate's children meet the IPs, visit with the parents and the baby shortly after birth, and participate in some closure so as to minimize any confusion or anxiety about their mother or the new baby [19].

Guidance should be provided regarding future considerations with the intended child(ren), even though the issues may remain ambiguous, evolving and hard to predict. Will the child be told about the unique circumstances of his or her birth? How will the role of the carrier be explained? Will the parents or the carrier permit contact with the carrier, if the child desires it? What are each person's fears and concerns about the future? A discussion of possible actions that might minimize long-term issues is useful. These actions may include, for example, writing keepsake letters or photos, assigning an intermediary for contact or emergency issues, and documentation of history. An important variable for the child's long-term well-being is likely to be the degree of respect, warmth and integrity between the two families.

The conception and pregnancy

Shortly after learning the treatment was successful, Jennifer finds out she is pregnant with triplets. The GC and IPs had all agreed to the transfer of two embryos created by anonymous egg donation. One of the embryos has split into identical twins. Jennifer is exhausted, nervous, excited and naive about what the pregnancy will look like. The prenatal vitamins make her ill and she is growing tired of the IVF medication. She had hoped to stay with her usual obstetrician and deliver at the hospital closest to her home. However, a multiple birth will most likely demand highly sophisticated medical care for

> potentially premature births and the medical center is an hour away across state lines. She describes on her social media page how hard she worked to achieve this pregnancy and posts several ultrasounds of the babies for her friends and family to see. Jennifer is missing more time from her workplace than anticipated and worries that her job performance is being negatively impacted.
>
> Katrina and David are understandably anxious and baffled by their good news after a decade of attempts to conceive. Katrina and David want to reduce to a twin pregnancy but feel emotionally conflicted with the decision now that they are faced with it, particularly knowing that all three fetus are seemingly healthy and without any abnormalities.
>
> They appreciate Jennifer greatly, but find her already needier and more demanding than they had anticipated. Their overseas status does not provide for insurance for newborns, which heightens the concerns regarding premature birth. However, they want the best prenatal care and medical expertise possible during delivery, which appears to be in a neighboring state. Choosing this type of care in a less surrogate-friendly neighboring state has several implications including that in order for them to be able to return home, it is imperative that both of their names are on the original birth certificate, which only occurs in legally surrogate friendly states.

Jennifer, Joe, David and Katrina seemed to have done a good job of exploring possible issues and dynamics in the preconception session. Unexpected events that unfold are only best handled by having discussed how conflicts, of either interpersonal or ideological nature, are handled prior to them arising. Neither the GC nor the IPs can truly appreciate the stressors that are relevant to each without having explained or expressed them, such as stressors of a new doctor for a GC, the financial implications of CBRS for the IPs, or the repercussions of a demanding pregnancy on a GC's overall mood, daily functioning and livelihood. The fertility counselor can aid in the sharing of each party's particular experiences prior to, during and after the pregnancy as well as have each person envision how they would communicate and handle (as well as how each would like to be approached about) any personal conflicts or feelings that arise during the relationship.

A major dilemma discussed in theory in the meeting is revealed with the surprise of a triplet pregnancy for Katrina and David. The legal contract should outline what the parties agree to in regards to pregnancy termination. However, the contract is not enforceable on the issue of termination/reduction, as the GC is the medical patient and has the right to make decisions with regards to her body and any medical interventions. Leaving the decision to varying medical opinions about multiple fetal pregnancy reduction, as was agreed upon in the group interview, is not usually helpful. The medical reasons for a reduction at 12 weeks can be debated, as can other reasons for pregnancy termination. Additionally, by the time the GC is asked to agree to a termination she, like the IPs, has invested months in caring for the pregnancy and has seen many ultrasounds. This difficult decision needs to addressed up front, and not deferred to doctors in the future. The complexities of having four individuals (GC, GC's husband and the IPs) now invested in such a difficult decision makes a tough choice even more difficult. Further, the dissemination of this information on social media sites creates a hotbed for increased difficulty in making such a decision.

After confirmation of a triplet pregnancy, Katrina, David, Joe and Jennifer reached out to the fertility counselor for a follow-up session, to evaluate choices that could be made and all agreed that the pregnancy would be reduced to twins. While it may not be an ideal choice for any of the members, previous discussion surrounding respective thoughts, feelings and plans about termination and reduction served as an anchor and guide.

The group meeting allows a platform for all involved individuals to begin the discussion of all current and future unique aspects of their relationship with each other. The fertility counselor can underscore the importance of the evolving discussion and evaluation of the process by offering continued professional consultation throughout the pregnancy, as well as following the birth. The occurrence of such follow-up appointments can be built into the legal contract and the circumstances for additional meetings can be discussed (communication difficulties, medical/social stressors arise, or emotional distress occurs).

The ending/closure

> Katrina and David are quite overwhelmed and absorbed with their twin newborns. They believe that the delivery and birth were a positive experience for all parties and, except for the premature birth of

the babies by several weeks, the process went as planned. They would have liked to be more prepared with a gift for Jennifer at the time she was discharged, but they plan to take the babies to see her and Joe again, as well as meet her children, once they are medically stabilized and able to leave the hospital. Katrina wonders how Jennifer is doing, but finds that every time she thinks about reaching out to her, it is too late to call her and cell phone reception is limited in the hospital.

Jennifer visits the new parents and the babies at the hospital while the newborns are in the NICU. She finds herself not on a list to visit. The nurses are not allowed to tell her anything about the babies because she is not the mother. The breast milk she dutifully is pumping is evidently not being used. Her children have yet to see the babies. The hospital social worker suggests that perhaps Jennifer should not call and visit so often, to let the babies and parents bond. Jennifer wonders if the busy holiday activities and her work schedule make it appear that perhaps she did not do all she could to remain pregnant.

Once the IPs become acclimated to parenthood and the twins stabilize, Katrina is able to reach out to Jennifer more. Both women check in on the well-being of the other and several of the misperceptions and miscommunications are clarified with all parties feeling more reassured. Shortly after their departure from the hospital, but prior to their return to their home country, David and Katrina spent the afternoon at Joe and Jennifer's new home with the GC's children and the babies. The IPs arrived with a housewarming gift of a dogwood tree to which Katrina had attached a card that said: "For you to watch grow, as the babies grow." In addition, pictures were taken of all parties together with the babies, as well as of Jennifer with the twins. David and Katrina have started a baby book for each of the newborns, and want to document the relationship with the GC and her family as much as possible, to provide for a cohesive and thorough story for them as they grow.

Katrina and David returned to Sweden with the twins. Jennifer and Katrina have managed to maintain a robust online relationship with each other, which has allowed both women to feel connected to the surrogacy experience in their own unique way. Jennifer has been able to see pictures of the twins as they grow and Katrina, to her surprise, has taken the opportunity to elicit feedback and advice about motherhood from her GC. David and Joe, through their wives, stay abreast of the well-being of all, and Jennifer's children seem to value the connection that the continued correspondence allows to their unique role in the surrogacy process. And as agreed upon, Katrina and David send a holiday card each December.

The ending can have a profound effect on how the parties feel and the long-term impact of the participation. The ongoing research available to date, primarily from Great Britain, does reveal that the families and the surrogates overall feel positively about their experience. One study evaluated 34 surrogates who had delivered a year earlier and found no significant problems in their relationship with the parents or in their relinquishment of the baby [20]. Additional multifaceted in-depth research studies examined families created through surrogacy at regular intervals [21]. These on going follow-up studies describe a harmonious relationship with the surrogate and a perception of their experience as generally positive.

One role professionals can take in helping families obtain a positive experience is to address issues of closure. Mental health professionals understand the importance of good goodbyes and good endings. Given the understandable awkwardness, exhaustion and anxieties inherent in surrogacy, it is helpful to clearly plan the birth, hospital stay and postpartum contact. Jennifer, Joe, Katrina and David have now changed roles. The parents are in charge of the baby and the hospital may be playing a role in determining dynamics. Jennifer wants to be reassured that the babies are doing well and that she is not being disregarded. The parents are struggling with a new environment and new roles. Miscommunications are common during the final days around the birth. A lack of clarity about contact, lack of communication and not knowing when, and if, they will see each other makes for hurt feelings.

Giving attention to each family's needs and to simple rituals can be critical in assisting the families in leaving whole and happy. GCs need to feel validated, valuable and trusted. A GC and her family should not feel rushed and pushed aside or disposable. IPs need to have closure so they feel safe and clear about the psychological dynamics of their child's birthing mother. The postbirth exchange of keepsake or symbolic gifts and thank you letters is helpful. Setting aside time prior to the parent's departure when the carrier/surrogate and her family can visit with the new parents and baby, enjoy the ending, take photographs and exchange thank yous is highly recommended. A respectful, warm and appreciative closure minimizes feelings of exploitation and emptiness for a GC. Attention to closure with their surrogate does help the new parents feel secure in the relinquishment and provides a positive story to tell their child. Positive closure is in everyone's best interest, especially the child(ren), who all have helped create.

In considering the surrogacy relationship, the birth of the child(ren) is often seen as the end goal. While this is true in some respects, the birth of the child(ren) is also often a beginning. The parties part and go their separate ways, forming two distinct family units. However, the growth and management of the relationships with each other and with the child is only the beginning.

Reflections of the fertility counselors

TS: As the daughter of a nurse midwife, I have grown up seeing my mother assist other women during the pregnancy and the delivery of several thousand babies. It has been in the fabric of my life to see how another person can transform and assist individuals and couples in achieving a family. While my initial interest in fertility counseling stemmed from experience and interest in assisting with the difficulty and complexity of not achieving or maintaining a pregnancy, I think it is because of my background that I find the consultation and evaluation of all parties involved in surrogacy arrangements to be the most meaningful. While it has the inherent potential of being transformative for all parties – the GC, the GC's partner, and the IPs – the surrogacy relationship and the number of parties involved also hold great complexities and the potential for complications.

When I explain the number of sessions and the purpose of the different types of appointments, as well as psychological assessment of the GC, with the parties involved, I often use the following sentiment: "I would rather frontload all the potential dilemmas and difficulties that could occur rather than have to attempt to diffuse a large problem at the backend of the relationship." I also say, "We want you to come out of this the same, if not better – just with the family you are helping to create as an added bonus." I find myself to be honored to assist the intended parent families and the carrier families as they traverse through a process that, while complex, provides such joy.

HH: I have been providing psychological services for surrogate mothers and intended parents since 1983. In the early years, the concept of surrogacy was in and of itself an ethical debate. I did not imagine that the ethical dilemmas would so dramatically increase with time; I naively thought they would become clearer. For example, with the ever-increasing array of people seeking the help of a surrogate comes a continued challenge to reconsider my purpose to help both the surrogate and intended parent. The other unforeseen challenge is the unusually high number of high-risk pregnancies in surrogacy, leaving parents, children and surrogates at high risk for trauma and grief. What has not changed is that often our best guide is what is best for the children. Surrogacy, and egg donation, in the USA is in its second generation. Keeping foremost what is in the best interest of children continues to provide the clearest insights. Lastly, I am still continuously impressed, and even still moved to tears occasionally, when honored to witness the beauty of two families coming together with such kindness, respect and integrity to create a child.

References

1. Covington SN, Patrizio P. Gestational carriers and surrogates. In: Sauer MV, editor. *Principles of Oocyte and Embryo Donation*. 2nd edn. London: Springer Press, 2013.
2. Gugucheva M. *Surrogacy in America Report*. Boston (MA): Council for Responsible Genetics (US); 2010; 1–40.
3. Crockin SL. Gestational surrogacy. Legal conceptions, the evolving law and policy of ART. In: Crockin SL and Jones HW, editors. *Legal Conceptions: The Evolving Land and Policy of Assisted Reproductive Technologies*. Baltimore, Johns Hopkins University Press, 2010.
4. Inhorn MC, Patrizio P. Rethinking reproductive "tourism" as reproductive "exile." *Fertil Steril* 2009, 92 (3): 904–6.
5. Inhorn M, Patrizio P. The global landscape of cross-border reproductive care: twenty key findings in the new millennium. *Curr Opin Obstet Gyn* 2012, 24(3): 158–63.
6. Hinson D. States-by-State surrogacy law. [Internet] 2013. Available from: http://www.creativefamilyconnections.com/state-map-surroagcy-law-practices. Accessed October 2014.
7. Haberman C. Baby M and the Question of Surrogate Motherhood. *The New York Times* [Internet]. 2014

March 23 [cited March 23]; Available from: http://www.nytimes.com/2014/03/24/us/baby-m-and-the-question-of-surrogate motherhood.html?module=Search&mabReward=relbias%3Aw. Accessed October 2014.

8. Shenfield F, Pennings G, Cohen J. ESHRE Task Force on Ethics and Law 10: Surrogacy. *Hum Reprod* 2005; 10: 2705.
9. Ethics Committee of the American Society of Reproductive Medicine. Consideration of the gestational carrier: a committee opinion. *Fertil Ster* 2013; 19: 1838–41.
10. Practice Committee of the Society for Assisted Reproductive Technology. Recommendations for practices utilizing gestational carriers: an ASRM practice committee guideline. *Fertil Steril* 2012; 97: 301–8.
11. Hanafin H. Surrogacy and gestational carrier participants. In Covington SN, Burns LH, editors. *Infertility Counseling: A Comprehensive Handbook for Clinicians*. 2nd edn. Cambridge, Cambridge University Press, 2006.
12. Franks D. Psychiatric evaluation of women in a surrogate mother program. *Am J Psychiat* 1981; 138: 1378–9.
13. Parker JP. Motivation of surrogate mothers: initial findings. *Am J Psychiat* 1983; 140: 117.
14. Reame N, Parker JP. Surrogate parenting: clinical features of forty-four cases. *Am J Obstet Gyn* 1990; 162: 1220–5.
15. Mechanick-Braverman A, Corson SL. Characteristics of participants in a gestational carrier program. *J Assist Repro Gen* 1992; 9: 353–7.
16. Sims JA, Thomas KM, Hopwood CJ, Chen SH, Pascale C. Psychometric properties and norms for the Personality Assessment Inventory in egg donors and gestational carriers. *J Pers Assess* 2013; 95(5): 495–9.
17. Simpson TS, Bogedan TR, Mindes E, Toll C, Richter K, Covington SN. Minnesota Multiphasic Personality Inventory 2 (MMPI-2) supplementary score profiles of applicants to a gestational carrier (GC) program. *Fertil Steril* 2010; 94: S66.
18. Mindes E, Sachs TH, Simpson TS, Raque-Bogdan TL, Richter KS, Covington SN. Minnesota Multiphasic Personality Inventory 2 (MMPI-2) profiles of applicants to a gestational carrier (GC) program. *Fertil Steril* 2009; 92: S35.
19. Jadva V, Murray C, Lycett E. Surrogacy: the experiences of surrogate mothers. *Hum Reprod* 2003 Oct; 18: 2196–2204.
20. Golombok S, Reading J, Blake L, Casey P, Marks A, Jadva V. Families created through surrogacy; mother–child relationship and children's psychological adjustment at age 7. *Dev Psychol* 2011 Nov; 47(6): 1579–88.
21. Jadva V, Blake I, Casey P, Golombak S. Surrogacy families 10 years on: relationship with the surrogate, decisions over disclosure and children's understanding of their surrogacy. *Hum Reprod* 2012 Oct; 10: 3008–14.

Chapter 10

Counseling known participants in third party reproduction

Erica J. Mindes and Laura S. Covington

Maria, age 40, is diagnosed with Stage 4 chronic kidney disease (CKD). She and her husband Aaron, age 41, have wanted to start a family since they were married two years ago, but her nephrologist "put the brakes" on her carrying a pregnancy. Her sister, Rita, age 35, who has watched for the past 10 years as Maria has dealt with health problems, came forth and volunteered to be a gestational carrier (GC) for Maria and Aaron. Not wanting to delay their plans to create a family any longer, Maria and Aaron immediately sought treatment at a fertility clinic. Following the initial consult and blood work, the reproductive endocrinologist (RE) informed them there was only a 20% chance for pregnancy using her sister as a GC and Maria's eggs, and recommended they consider using an egg donor. Aaron and Maria were distressed by this news. Besides now having to grieve the loss of having a child who is genetically related to both of them, they had multiple concerns about using an anonymous egg donor including: the limited availability of Hispanic donors at the practice (Maria is Hispanic and it was important to both Aaron and her that the egg donor also be of Hispanic origin); an increased waiting time to begin treatment due to the restricted donor pool; and given Maria's own evolving health issues over the past 10 years, they were worried about the accuracy of the donor's family medical history. Maria and Aaron decided to take a few months off from treatment to process their feelings of loss and consider next steps. Maria's extended family is aware of her diagnosis of CKD and the havoc it has wreaked on her health, as well as the plans she and Aaron have to create a family. Word soon spread to family members about the couple's most recent setback and their need to use an egg donor. During their break from treatment, Maria and Aaron began to talk about their wish that Maria's younger cousin would offer to be their egg donor.

To be continued ...

The addenda referred to in this chapter are available for download at www.cambridge.org/9781107643116. Password: AX164BKR7.

Introduction

Psychosocial issues are inherent for individuals involved in any form of third party reproduction, be it gamete donation or gestational surrogacy. However, when participants have a relationship that existed prior to becoming partners in the collaborative reproduction process, the potential psychosocial issues become more complex. The role of the fertility counselor is to provide education, counseling and assessment regarding the potential psychosocial risks and benefits for each of the parties involved in treatment, as well as for the relationship that already exists between them, the broader family and/or social network and any children, whether they are born from the treatment process or are children of the gamete donor or GC.

This chapter presents practical information to aid the fertility counselor in preparing for and conducting the psychosocial counseling and assessment of known participants in third party reproduction. Topics covered in the chapter will include: (1) reasons fertility patients may wish to use a known gamete donor or GC; (2) a brief overview of professional guidelines for the counseling and assessment of known participants in third party reproduction; (3) the counseling and evaluation process for known gamete donation and gestational surrogacy; and (4) other situations that may arise in known collaborative arrangements. Case vignettes are integrated throughout the chapter

Fertility Counseling: Clinical Guide and Case Studies, ed. Sharon N. Covington. Published by Cambridge University Press.

and provide examples of issues that may develop during the counseling and evaluation process.

Definition of terms

For the purpose of this chapter, we define a known gamete donor or GC (where the pregnancy is established via in vitro fertilization [IVF] and embryos are created using oocytes from the intended mother or an egg donor) as a family member, friend or acquaintance, that is, an individual with whom the recipients or intended parents (IPs) have some type of preexisting relationship. To further clarify, while it is standard practice for IPs and GCs to meet prior to the initiation of treatment, this chapter only addresses GC arrangements where the previous relationship between parties was independent of the IPs' fertility treatment. The known gamete donor or GC may have either volunteered or been asked by the fertility patient(s) to collaborate in the third party reproduction arrangement. Please also note that for the sake of consistency throughout this chapter, the term "recipients" is used to indicate individuals or couples who receive donated gametes, and the term "intended parents" refers to individuals or couples using a GC to create their family.

Reasons for choosing a known collaborator

There are multiple reasons why an individual or couple pursuing treatment with third party reproduction may choose to use a known donor or GC. In the case of intrafamilial gamete donation, there is the assurance that some type of genetic connection will be maintained between the infertile individual and a child born from the process [1,2]. In addition, a significant physical resemblance between the donor and recipient may be a motivation [3]. In a same-sex couple, intrafamilial gamete donation can also allow for a genetic link to both members of the couple. For some individuals, the comfort with a family connection includes broader kinship ties, such as the use of a brother-in-law as a sperm donor, or a sister-in-law as the oocyte donor or GC [4]. Utilizing a general definition of a known gamete donor or GC that incorporates friends and acquaintances, as well as family members, the preference for a known arrangement may also include the more immediate availability of the third party participant and thus a shorter waiting period to treatment. Known gamete donors and GCs are often perceived by recipients and IPs to provide greater and more reliable medical, educational and social history, and to be more accessible throughout the treatment process [3–6]. In countries and jurisdictions where commercial gamete donation and gestational surrogacy is permitted, the use of a known gamete donor or GC can also decrease the costs or treatment, and for some people it is the only financially viable option to create a family. Finally, a potential advantage is that the donor or GC has the opportunity to be known to the child, develop some form of a relationship with the child, and be available, in the case of gamete donation, to provide updated health information about themselves and their families [1,5].

Professional guidelines

It is the responsibility of the fertility counselor to become familiar with and follow any guidelines created by the professional societies (e.g., American Society for Reproductive Medicine [ASRM], European Society for Human Reproduction and Embryology [ESHRE]) or government regulatory agencies that establish standards of care in the countries or regions where they work. This section is not meant to be a thorough review of all ethics, practice and counseling guidelines that address known arrangements in third party reproduction. Rather, we have attempted to highlight some areas of consensus in selected professional society and government agency guidelines.

Acceptable intrafamilial collaborations

The ESHRE Task Force on Ethics and Law [1] and The Ethics Committee of the ASRM [2] have each published reports that address the use of family members as gamete donors and surrogates. Both reports recommend against arrangements that replicate first- and second-degree consanguineous relationships. The ASRM and ESHRE documents also address collaborative reproductive arrangements that give the impression of incest or consanguinity. This may include, for example, a sister serving as a GC for her brother and his spouse, or a brother donating sperm to his sister, who will be creating embryos with an ovum donor. Neither situation is necessarily unacceptable, as genetically related individuals do not provide the gametes. However, the appearance of incest may have psychosocial implications for the participants, other family members and any children born from the process and both reports suggest this is explored carefully in counseling. Some guidelines are more restrictive than those put forth by ASRM and ESHRE with regard to the known arrangements considered permissible. For example, New Zealand's Advisory Committee on Assisted Reproductive Technology (ACART) published the "Guidelines on Donation of Eggs or Sperm between Certain Family Members" [7] in 2007. These guidelines establish that all intrafamilial donations other than sister-to-sister, brother-to-brother, or cousin-to-cousin will need to be reviewed by the Ethics Committee on Assisted Reproductive Technology.

Possibility of undue pressure or coercion

Numerous ethics, practice and counseling guidelines address the need to assess for evidence of coercion or undue influence among known participants in collaborative arrangements [1,2,7–11]. Intergenerational familial arrangements may be particularly subject to undue pressure between the parties [1,2] and the ASRM recommends that some of these arrangements should be discouraged (e.g., daughter to mother ovum donation, in which mother is remarried and thus, the embryos were not created from gametes belonging to two genetically related persons) [2]. The Assisted Human Reproduction Counselling Practice Guidelines of the Canadian Fertility and Andrology Society's Counseling Special Interest Group (CSIG) defines coercion as "influencing the actions of another, either implicitly or explicitly, by taking advantage of a weakness (exploitation), or unduly exerting power or influence" [10, p. 31]. To discern proof of coercion, the CSIG guidelines suggest fertility counselors question collaborative participants regarding: motivation for participation in the known arrangement; financial compensation; influence of others in making the decision to proceed with treatment; and anticipation of any negative consequences that could result from pulling out of the arrangement. The ASRM Ethics Committee report specifically states that prospective known gamete donors and GCs should be provided with the option to be excluded, without the IPs or recipients being informed of their hesitancy to participate [2].

Counseling and evaluation

Most professional guidelines that address known collaborative arrangements recommend independent counseling for recipients/IPs and gamete donors/GCs, including the spouse/partner of the gamete donor or GC [1,2,7–11]. A number of guidelines also suggest a group or joint counseling session that includes all of the participants [1,7–11]. The ESHRE document [1] responds to the question of whether separate counselors should be available to work with each party and concludes that counselors with an expertise in this fertility counseling ought to be able to provide appropriate services to all parties involved in the collaborative arrangement. Psychological testing of gamete donors and GCs is recommended by the ASRM [8,12] and is considered a standard of care in the United States [13–15].

Unique aspects of psychosocial counseling and evaluation for known participants

Issues to address in clinical interviews with all donors, recipients, GCs and IPs, whether known or anonymous, are addressed in Chapters 7, 8 and 9 of this book. As indicated above, best practices for the psychosocial counseling and evaluation process among known participants involves three components: (1) a counseling session with the recipients or IPs; (2) a clinical interview with the known gamete donor or GC and their spouse/partner, and psychological testing, if applicable; and (3) a group interview in which all of the parties meet together. This chapter will focus on the unique issues that need to be explored and assessed in the psychosocial counseling and evaluation process with known participants including:

- any evidence of coercion (assessed by asking about motivation for participation in the arrangement; financial compensation; influence of others in making the decision to proceed with treatment; and anticipation of any negative consequences that could result from cessation of participation);
- current status and history of the relationship and relationship dynamics between all parties, as well as the broader family or social network;
- potential effects of the arrangement on the relationship between all parties;
- implications of and responses to the collaboration in the context of the broader family or social network;
- expectations each party has regarding treatment (e.g., number of treatment cycles, disposition of embryos for known gamete donation, number of

embryos transferred for known GC arrangement, etc.);
- how participants anticipate they will cope with an unsuccessful treatment outcome (e.g., unsuccessful treatment cycle, pregnancy loss, etc.);
- expectations and boundaries pertaining to the future role of the known gamete donor or GC in the life of a child born from the process;
- whether, when and how a child born from this process will be informed of the means of their conception and the identity of the known donor or GC;
- any potential effects on the current or future children of the known gamete donor or GC; and
- plans the recipients or IPs may have to "thank" the donor or GC (e.g., writing a note, some form of a gift, or some type of symbolic thank you ritual), as a means to create a sense of closure for all parties when the process is completed.

Throughout the psychosocial counseling and evaluation process, the fertility counselor should help the known collaborators understand the need for consensus between all parties on treatment and life-long issues, and the potential negative effects that disagreement could have on the relationship between the participants, as well as the broader dynamic of the extended family or social network.

Patient preparation

The case of Maria and Aaron continues ...

After taking a three-month break from treatment that included many conversations regarding the best way to proceed, Maria and Aaron decided they would ask Maria's cousin, Sofia, if she would consider being their egg donor. When Sofia said she would be "honored to help" them, Maria and Aaron let their RE know they were ready to move forward. The RE explained that the first step was for them to contact the fertility counselor who works with the practice. Maria called the fertility counselor, who described the psychosocial counseling and evaluation process for participants in known gestational surrogacy and egg donation arrangements. Maria expressed her confusion and frustration to the fertility counselor, "These are my family members. We are very close and already know everything about one another. Why must we go through this process? It only slows things down even more."

Known collaborations may result from the gamete donor or GC either volunteering or being asked for their participation. It can be easier and less anxiety provoking for recipients and IPs when the family member or friend comes forward with an offer to help. The prospect of having to ask for such an important gift, and the potential for rejection, may be experienced by patients as an additional insult to the existing psychological injury of infertility. A fertility counselor can provide support and help educate patients on how to ask a potential gamete donor or GC to collaborate. For example, writing the proposed donor or GC a letter or email allows them and their spouse/partner to process the request without feeling the pressure of some type of immediate response. The letter should make it easy for the potential donor or GC to decline and may include statements such as, "you don't even need to respond to this if you don't want to," or "we understand if this is not something you are interested in pursuing and we just appreciate you taking the time to think about it." The letter may also incorporate the option for a potential collaborator to speak with an RE or fertility counselor and obtain more information prior to making a decision.

The fertility counselor should prepare the patient for the real possibility that the individual they ask or that person's spouse/partner may say "no," either initially or after they have had the chance to ask questions of medical or mental health personnel. The counselor can aid the patient in positively reframing what they may perceive to be another setback to creating a family. For fertility counselors who are embedded in or work closely with fertility clinics, it can be helpful to create written materials that are easily accessed by the patient and cover issues to consider when choosing a known collaborator, as well as guidance regarding how to ask a family member or friend to participate as a gamete donor or GC. (See Addendum 10.1.)

Once the fertility patient has identified their known collaborators and is referred to the fertility counselor for the psychosocial counseling and evaluation process, it is important for the fertility counselor to clearly outline the components of the process and the extent of their role. For example, the known gamete recipient or IP counseling session is usually psychoeducational in nature; it is an opportunity for the recipients or IPs to explore treatment and life-long issues specific to using a known collaborator. However, the clinical interview with the known gamete donor/GC and their husband/partner and psychological testing is

Table 10.1 Known recipients and intended parents: questions for the clinical interviews.

- How did you each arrive at the decision to use a known donor/GC?
- Who asked whom?
- Do either of you have any concerns about using a known donor/GC?
- What is the history of your relationship with the donor/GC and their spouse/partner?
- *FOR SIBLING-TO-SIBLING ARRANGEMENTS*: What has been the role, if any, of your parents? What has been or what do you anticipate to be the response of your parents?
- What has been or what do you anticipate will be the response of other family or friends?
- How would you feel if the donor/GC were not allowed to proceed with the arrangement for either medical or psychological reasons?
- How might this arrangement affect your future relationship with the donor/GC and their spouse/partner? How might a negative treatment outcome affect the relationship?
- How many treatment cycles do you expect the donor/GC to complete?
- What are your expectations of the donor/GC's role in the life of your child(ren)?
- Do you have any expectations of the donor/GC and their spouse/partner regarding custody arrangements for your child(ren) in the event of death?
- What are your thoughts about disclosure to your child(ren)? To the donor's child(ren)/future children? To family and friends?
- Have you discussed your plans for disclosure with the donor/GC and their spouse/partner?
- If you are NOT planning to disclose to your child(ren), or are planning to disclose at an older age, have you thought about how you will manage the information so your children do not find out accidentally?
- Have you thought about how you may wish to thank the donor/GC?
- *FOR RECIPIENTS*: Have you discussed with the donor and their spouse/partner their expectations for cryopreservation and the disposition of excess embryos created using their gametes, selective reduction, or termination for a fetal anomaly?
- *FOR IPs*: How many embryos do you anticipate wanting to transfer? Have you considered whether the GC and her spouse/partner are comfortable with carrying multiples? What are your feelings about selective reduction? Termination for a fetal anomaly? Have you discussed this with the GC?

an assessment of whether the donor or GC is an appropriate candidate, as well as psycho-educational about the process and implications of participation. The purpose of the group interview is to facilitate an exchange of information between all parties and identify each person's expectations regarding treatment and future relationships, including the degree of openness with family, friends and children born from the process.

As exemplified in the vignette above, it is not uncommon for fertility patients involved in known arrangements to express that they do not understand the need for a family member or close friend to undergo a counseling and evaluation process, or why all parties must participate in a group interview when "we already know everything about one another." They may also communicate the sentiment that the process is an undue burden on someone who has agreed or volunteered to provide them with this precious gift. We usually respond to these patient concerns with statements such as, "you have very close relationship (or "you are dear friends") and that's wonderful, and we want to help you to stay that way as you proceed through this process and once you have created a family."

Psychosocial counseling and evaluation process in known arrangements

Tables 10.1 and 10.2 provide examples of questions to be included in clinical interviews with known recipients/IPs and gamete donors/GCs, respectively. Please note that these questions are in addition to the standard questions asked in recipient, IP, donor and GC interviews (see Chapters 7, 8 and 9 of this book). In the sub-sections below we will return to the case of Maria and Aaron and highlight some common issues that arise during the counseling and evaluation process with known participants in third party reproduction.

The intended parent/known gamete donor recipient counseling session

During the IP/recipient counseling session, the fertility counselor explored with Maria and Aaron their attitudes and feelings about disclosure to a child born from this process. There was no question whether they would disclose the role of Maria's sister, "Auntie Rita," in their child's birth. They had already been speaking with Rita and her husband, Mike, about this issue, including disclosure to Rita and Mike's children and everyone seemed to be "on the same page." Thus, the fertility counselor was surprised when Maria and Aaron expressed their reluctance to disclose to their child the use of a donor egg or the identity of the donor. When asked about their reasons for a partial disclosure, that is, disclosure of the use of GC but not an egg donor, Maria said she thought it would too confusing for the child and

Table 10.2 Known donors and gestational carriers: questions for the clinical interviews.

- What is your motivation for being a known donor/GC?
- Who asked whom?
- Did you experience any pressure or feel an obligation to be a donor/GC because of your relationship with the recipients/IPs? Do you feel you can say "no" to the recipients/IPs? Do you wish there was a medical or psychological reason that would exclude you from being a donor/GC?
- What is the history of your relationship with recipient/IPs?
- *FOR SIBLING-TO-SIBLING ARRANGEMENTS*: What has been the role, if any, of your parents in the process? What has been or what do you anticipate to be the response of your parents?
- Who have you told about your plans to be a known donor/GC? What has been or what do you anticipate will be the response of other family or friends? Do you know how the recipients/IPs feel about others knowing?
- How would you feel if you were unable to be a donor/GC for either medical or psychological reasons?
- How many treatment cycles are you willing to participate in?
- How would you feel if treatment was not successful (e.g., treatment did not result in a pregnancy)?
- How would you feel if the child(ren) was born with a medical problem?
- Would you perceive a child(ren) born from this process as your own?
- What are your expectations regarding your role in the child(ren)'s life?
- If the recipients/IPs died, would you expect to receive custody of a child born from this process?
- What are your thoughts about identity disclosure to a child(ren) born from this process? To your own children/future children? How would you feel if the recipients/IPs felt differently about disclosure?
- *FOR DONOR*: What are your wishes regarding cryopreservation and disposition of embryos created using your gametes? Thoughts about termination for fetal anomaly? Selective reduction? Have you discussed these issues with the recipient(s)?
- *FOR GC*: Have you considered how many embryos you are willing to have transferred? Are you comfortable carrying a multiple pregnancy? Are you aware of the risks associated with carrying a multiple pregnancy? What are your feelings about selective reduction? Termination for a fetal anomaly? Have you discussed these issues with the IPs?

there was no reason s/he would need to know. The fertility counselor asked, as she had earlier in the interview, how many family and friends are aware of the couple's need to use an egg donor or that Maria's cousin, Sofia, will be the donor. Maria and Aaron acknowledged that their struggles to create a family were well known to members of their extended families, as well as to a few close friends. In addition, both of their immediate families and spouses, as well as Sofia's immediate family, and her fiancé were aware of the plan for Sofia to be the egg donor; they had not thought to request secrecy, and thus it was possible that other extended family members were aware of Sofia's donation. The counselor aided Maria and Aaron in examining whether it was practical to think that this information could successfully be kept secret from their child. Was there a possibility their child could hear this information, inadvertently, from someone other than themselves, and were Maria and Aaron comfortable with that scenario? The fertility counselor also provided education and resources about the disclosure process. Finally, the fertility counselor noted that it is important to consider how Sofia and her fiancé, Sam, feel about disclosure, and the mental health professional can help them raise this issue in the group interview.

Research has shown that most IPs plan to disclose the use of a surrogate to their children [16] and a majority of families follow through on such plans [17]. However, parents who create their families with the assistance of both surrogacy and gamete donation may be less likely to disclose the use of a gamete donor to their child, employing a strategy of partial disclosure. This partial disclosure approach may be influenced by parents' perceptions of their children's ability to understand all of the information, as well as parents' personal level of comfort with gamete donation [18]. When a recipient couple uses a known gamete donor, the disclosure decision becomes more complex due to the web of relationships that connect the collaborators. The fertility counselor should assess how many people in the family or social network are aware of the recipient's need to use a gamete donor and know the identity of the donor. Have they considered whether the donor has disclosed to anyone? If numerous people are aware of the known arrangement, the counselor can aid the recipients in determining the risks of inadvertent disclosure to the child. In addition, have the recipients thought about the donor and donor's spouse/partner's preference regarding disclosure, both to a child born from the process and the donor's current and/or future children? Could disagreement between the known participants on the issue of disclosure negatively affect their relationship with each other or the dynamic of the extended family or social network? The psychosocial counseling process provides an opportunity for known collaborators to contemplate, discuss and come to an agreement regarding an initial plan for disclosure [19]. Disclosure is often an evolutionary process and during the group interview participants should also identify a general plan to discuss disclosure issues in the future. (Please see Chapter 18 for more guidance on disclosure issues.)

The gestational carrier clinical interview

> Maria's sister, Rita, is 35 years old and has been married to her husband, Mike, age 36, for seven years. The couple has two sons, ages 2 and 4. None of the information gathered through psychological testing or from the collection of her psychosocial history during the first part of the clinical interview suggested that Rita should be excluded as a GC candidate. There was no evidence of coercion. When Rita's husband, Mike, joined the clinical interview, he indicated he was supportive of Rita serving as a GC for her sister, and there were no issues of concern in his psychosocial history. However, when the counselor asked Rita and Mike if they had thought about how many treatment cycles they would be willing to participate in, Mike responded, "How long are we talking about here?" Rita then explained that they want to have another child. She said she had initially volunteered to be a GC for her sister almost a year ago, and both she and Mike thought that by now she would be pregnant, carrying Maria and Aaron's child. She added that at this point, there would likely be at least four years difference between her younger son and a third child, "if everything went smoothly"; and she acknowledged the possibility that it may be more difficult for Mike and her to conceive when she was 37 or 38, versus 32, when she became pregnant with her youngest son. Rita said, "I feel guilty even mentioning this because we're lucky enough to already have two healthy, wonderful boys." Mike emphasized that they "really want to help Maria and Aaron, but we just didn't expect the process to take this long."

The known GC often enters the world of assisted reproductive technologies blind to the complexities and time involved in preparation, evaluation and treatment. She sees an opportunity to help her family member or friend, and may not have fully thought through the multiple ways the process could impact her, or the life of her spouse/partner and children. However, there are numerous scenarios in which the needs of the GC and her family may not be congruent with needs of the IPs. In the vignette above, Rita and Mike express that their desire to help Maria and Aaron create a family may now be in conflict with their own family building goals. Rita's feelings of guilt may have prohibited her from discussing her concerns with her sister. She is questioning whose needs come first: those of herself, Mike, and their children; or that of her sister and brother-in-law? The fertility counselor can provide positive feedback regarding Rita and Mike's willingness to help, but validate their desire to place some limits on treatment. The counselor can assist Rita and Mike in identifying the amount of time they want to devote to the treatment process. However, it is also important to explore with them how they would feel if Rita were to become infertile as a result of serving as a GC for her sister, or as Rita alluded to, the couple developed a fertility problem that inhibited their ability to expand their family after the GC process was completed. Do they anticipate they would regret Rita's decision to volunteer to be a GC for her sister, and how would this affect their future relationship with Maria and Aaron? How might this influence other decisions made about treatment? The group interview provides a forum for the GC and her spouse/partner to discuss with the IPs all aspects of the treatment plan.

The known gamete donor clinical interview

> The known ovum donor (KOD) interview with Maria's cousin, Sofia, age 30, began with an exploration of her motivation to be an egg donor. Sofia reported that her mother and Maria's mother are sisters. She said most of their extended family is aware of the severity of Maria's kidney disease, the fertility problems that have resulted, and the plans for Maria's sister to be the GC. A few months ago Sofia's mother mentioned that Maria must now use an egg donor, too, and asked Sofia if she would ever think about donating her eggs to Maria. Sofia and Maria do not have a particularly close relationship, but when Sofia was in elementary school, Maria would often babysit her. Sofia noted she has wonderful memories of the times spent with Maria and thus, when her mother brought up the idea of being an egg donor, she thought it might be nice to help Maria. Sofia said a couple of days after the conversation with her mother she accepted a new job and her boyfriend, Sam, proposed. Sofia stated, "in the midst of all of these changes, I just forgot about the egg donation." Thus, when she received an email from Maria a few weeks ago asking if she would consider being her egg donor, she was not completely surprised. Sofia felt she had been "blessed" with good fortune in recent months and thought she should share some of her luck with Maria. Within 15 minutes she wrote

back to Maria, "I would be honored to help you and Aaron." Sofia said she would "never accept payment" from her cousin. When asked if her fiancé, Sam, was supportive, Sofia responded, "at first he seemed fine, but yesterday he said he's been reading some stories on the internet and is worried my egg donation might effect our ability to have children." Sofia understands the risks are low, but does not want to proceed if Sam is not comfortable. On the other hand, she also noted her concern that if she changes her mind now, "it could create tension in the family, especially between my aunt and my mother, and we have our wedding in the next year."

This vignette highlights a couple of areas of concern. First, for a known collaborative arrangement to move forward, there needs to be "four yeses." In this vignette, Sofia's fiancé, Sam, has not been appropriately informed of the treatment process and risks. The fertility counselor may emphasize that it is reasonable and not unusual for a spouse/partner to have questions or concerns about treatment. The counselor can also recommend or help facilitate an opportunity for the spouse/partner to speak with a member of the medical team; often this may alleviate concerns. Ultimately, however, all parties, including a donor or GC's spouse/partner must be "on board," and thus the "four yeses."

A second issue underscored is that elements of potential coercion may not necessarily be overt. Although Sofia was asked by the recipients to be their egg donor, there was no initial evidence of coercion. Similar to most KODs, Sofia seems motivated to be a donor because of her relationship with the recipient, her cousin Maria, and her empathy for the difficulties Maria has had in achieving motherhood [20]. Sofia indicated there is no financial compensation arranged or expected. Although Sofia's mother asked her if she would consider donating her eggs to Maria, it does not appear her mother exerted any pressure. Nor was there any indication Sofia felt pressed to donate as a result of receiving Maria's email. However, by the time Sofia realizes her fiancé may not feel comfortable with her egg donation, the process has begun to move forward, and she perceives the potential for some negative consequences should she decide to withdraw from the arrangement. In this type of situation the fertility counselor can hypothetically ask the gamete donor (or GC) how she would feel if there was a medical reason that would exclude her from participating. The counselor can also directly inform the donor (or GC) that if she does not want to proceed with the donation (arrangement), a reason can be found for her to be excluded, without the recipients being made aware of the donor's hesitancy to participate.

Table 10.3 Group interview questions with known participants.

- How might the process impact the relationship between each of you?
- How might an unsuccessful treatment outcome or miscarriage affect your relationships with one another?
- What are the expectations of all parties regarding the number of treatment cycles?
- What do each of you anticipate the relationship will be between donor/GC and the child? Is everyone in agreement?
- What are the recipients'/IPs' plans for disclosure to a child born from the process? Are the donor/GC and their spouse comfortable with that plan?
- What does the donor/GC plan to tell their children about the donation/GC pregnancy? How do the recipients/IPs feel about this?
- Who else have each of you already told about this arrangement? What is the plan for disclosure to family/friends? Is everyone in agreement?
- How do you all plan to handle issues that may arise in the future (e.g., treatment/pregnancy/delivery issues, relationship between the GC/donor and child, disclosure)?
- Is there a plan for seeking counseling as a group, in the future, if necessary?
- *FOR DONOR ARRANGEMENTS:* What are the expectations of all parties regarding cryopreservation and disposition of excess embryos created with the donor's gametes? Selective reduction? Termination for a fetal anomaly?
- *FOR GC ARRANGEMENTS:* What are everyone's feelings about the number of embryos transferred? Selective reduction? Termination for a fetal anomaly? How do you plan to handle these situations?

The group interview

During the counseling sessions and clinical interviews with recipients, IPs, known donors and GCs, respectively, the fertility counselor should review the topics that will be covered in the group interview and ask all participants if there are any other issues they would like the counselor to put forth. We often describe the group interview as a "working session." It provides an opportunity to create consensus, develop a plan and identify a means by which the parties can discuss potential changes to the plan. The group interview allows each of the known participants to start out with the same basic "road map." Table 10.3 provides examples of questions to be included in the group interview with known participants.

Other situations that may arise in known collaborations

The impression of incest or consanguinity

> Approximately three years ago, Karen, a 42-year old physician, initiated fertility treatment as a single mother by choice, using anonymous donor sperm. After four unsuccessful cycles of IVF, her RE recommended she consider egg donation. Karen felt strongly that she wanted to maintain a genetic connection to her child. She decided to ask her brother, Jeff, and his wife, Gayle, also physicians, if they were open to the possibility of Jeff being the sperm donor, as she continued to pursue treatment using an anonymous donor egg. During the counseling and evaluation process, the fertility counselor was struck by the purely scientific approach that Karen, as well as Jeff and Gayle, took in discussing the arrangement. Karen said she had always planned to disclose to her child the use of anonymous donor sperm in his/her conception. She noted that a "family story" that reflected this new arrangement would be "a bit trickier to craft," but she never considered secrecy as an option. During their clinical interview, Jeff and Gayle indicated they are comfortable with Karen disclosing to her child Jeff's identity as the sperm donor. However, when the fertility counselor asked Jeff and Gayle about their plans to disclose to their own 10- and 12-year-old daughters, there were a few seconds of silence before Gayle responded, "we don't keep secrets in our family, but I am concerned that given our girls' ages, their first response may be 'ewwww'. And it may take them a while to get past that reaction."

In the scenario described above, the collaborative arrangement is considered acceptable because no genetic connection exists between the gamete donors. However, there is a social perception of consanguinity or incest. Karen, Jeff and Gayle appear to view the sperm donation through a clinical or scientific lens. The information provided suggests they will likely create clear relationship boundaries between the donor and a child conceived through the sperm donation, thatis Jeff would maintain his role as Uncle to Karen's child. The concern in this situation is the potential for adverse emotional or psychosocial effects on other family members, specifically the donor's children. A pre-adolescent or adolescent child may not perceive their father's sperm donation in the same scientific manner as the adults involved in the collaboration. Karen, as well as Jeff and Gayle, seem to place a greater moral value on openness, versus secrecy, in their relationships with their children. Yet, it is possible that disclosure could temporarily disturb the understanding and meaning of familial relationships for a preadolescent or adolescent child [21]. For example, how might Jeff and Gayle's children process the information that their soon-to-be-born cousin is the genetic offspring of their father, but the social roles remain that of uncle and nephew or niece; or that their cousin is also their genetic half-sibling?

By its very nature, intrafamilial assisted reproduction disrupts conventional schema of family relations. Arrangements that create an impression of incest or consanguinity may be perceived negatively by the larger society and thus, carry the potential for greater psychological risk for collaborators and their families [4]. The role of the fertility counselor is to highlight and encourage participants to consider the potential emotional impact of the arrangement on themselves, as well as other members of the family, especially any children born from the process and existing children. The counselor can reinforce general strategies to reduce the psychological risk for participants and their families including: (1) the need for clear boundaries in the social, versus genetic or gestational, relationships between family members; (2) providing guidance to participants as they create a framework and language for disclosure; (3) reminding collaborators of the importance of sensitivity to the individual needs of family members, especially children; and (4) normalizing additional counseling for collaborators and their families, as issues arise over the years.

When a known gamete donor or GC is not an appropriate candidate

> Nikki, age 31, has volunteered to be a GC for her close friend, Patti, with whom she has been friends since freshman year of college. During the interview Nikki reported she separated from her husband approximately two years ago, and her divorce was finalized within the past six months. She stated that she has full custody of her 4-year-old son, although her ex-husband recently initiated proceedings to try to obtain joint custody. Nikki noted her husband had been emotionally abusive throughout their marriage, calling her names, controlling the finances, and so

on. She also reported one incident of physical abuse that was the impetus for her to finally separate from him and end the marriage. Nikki said that she would not have had the courage to leave her husband if Patti and her husband, Will, had not offered for her and her son to move into a small carriage house apartment in their backyard. Nikki stated, "I'm so thankful to Patti and Will. They helped me get out of a very bad situation, and now I want to return the favor. My pregnancy and delivery were very easy. It's something I'm really good at and there's not much in life that I can say I'm good at." Nikki noted that Patti and Will have refused to let her pay rent on the carriage house, although she acknowledged she could not afford the "going rate." Nikki also reported to the counselor a history of multiple incidents of childhood sexual abuse by an older male cousin, when she was 13 and the cousin was 16. She said she had never previously told anyone else about the abuse and has "just tried to forget about it." She stated she avoids family events when she knows that her cousin will be in attendance. Nikki denied any history of participating in counseling to address her history of childhood sexual abuse, the emotional or physical abuse by her ex-husband, or any other issues. Psychological testing results were not within normal limits and suggested that Nikki may have learned to adjust to a chronic level of depression.

Psychosocial considerations for exclusion of gamete donors and GCs are discussed in Chapters 8 and 9 of this book. Fertility counselors should also refer to guidelines created by the professional societies [e.g., 8,10,12] and government regulatory agencies in the countries or regions where they work. In the vignette above, there are multiple reasons why Nikki is not an appropriate candidate to serve as a GC for her friend Patti. These reasons include: (1) Nikki's history of untreated and unresolved abuse; (2) a living situation in which she is dependent upon the IPs; (3) the stress associated with a possible legal battle with her husband as he seeks joint custody of their son; and (4) abnormal psychological testing results that suggest Nikki may experience some chronic level of untreated depression. Regardless of how obvious it may be to the fertility counselor that Nikki should be excluded from proceeding as a GC, Nikki likely does not perceive her situation in the same manner. For example, while she might acknowledge some issues related to her history of childhood sexual abuse or the emotional and physical abuse by her husband, she may feel she has coped "just fine," sees no need for counseling, and cannot imagine that any aspect of being a GC for her good friend could recapitulate her previous experiences of trauma. In addition, Nikki may view the fact that she lives in a carriage house apartment in Patti's backyard as an opportunity for Patti and Will to "be more involved in the pregnancy" and the free rent as a "gift." It is important to be respectful of the GC/gamete donor's perspective. Ultimately, however, the decision to exclude a known GC or gamete donor comes down to a clinical judgment on the part of the fertility counselor regarding the potential for harm to any of the parties directly involved in the collaborative arrangement, as well as current or future children.

One of the most difficult aspects of our role as fertility counselors has been when we have had to inform known participants we are making the recommendation that they do not proceed with the current collaborative arrangement. In each case we have wondered, is there the potential for any of the known participants to experience emotional harm as a result of the GC/gamete donor being excluded? How do we explain this in a way such that the known GC or gamete donor does not feel we are passing judgment on their life? Will excluding the GC or gamete donor negatively impact the relationship between all of the parties in the known arrangement? We have found it can be helpful to prepare known participants, upfront, for all the possible outcomes of the evaluation process. For example, during interviews with the known IPs/recipients and GC/donor we say, "although it is not frequent, sometimes we obtain information through either the interview process or psychological testing, that indicates a known GC or gamete donor does not meet necessary criteria. This could be for psychosocial reasons or testing results." If participants ask for more information, we emphasize that these situations are not common and that the guiding principle is to minimize the risk of harm to all parties.

When it has been determined that a known GC or donor is not an appropriate candidate, it is ideal to meet face-to-face with each of the parties to discuss the reasons for exclusion. Unfortunately, this is not always possible and sometimes the conversations must occur over the telephone. Regardless, it is important to stress the positive. Focus on the GC/gamete donor's motivation to help the IPs/recipients, versus the fact that the arrangement did not work out. For example, with GCs/gamete donors the fertility counselor may say, "it was such a great thing for you to even propose to do this"; or with IPs/recipients, "it is wonderful that someone cares about you so much that they would offer you this gift."

When reviewing the reasons for exclusion, the fertility counselor should reiterate that the decision was not taken lightly and made after careful consideration of the potential psychosocial risks to the GC/donor, their spouse/partner/children, IPs/recipients, and the relationship that exists between all of the participants. Some statements we commonly use are, "sometimes the best way to preserve the relationship is by not moving forward," or "you only have one family and you don't want to do anything to harm those relationships." If the evaluation process has revealed the known GC or gamete donor may be experiencing significant psychological symptoms, then a referral for treatment should be provided. In some cases, known participants will either appeal to the RE or medical staff to override the fertility counselor's recommendation, obtain a second opinion on the psychosocial evaluation, or seek treatment at another RE practice, with the end result being the arrangement moves forward. This is a scenario the fertility counselor cannot control. All we are able to do is conduct a thorough evaluation and know our recommendation was made based on our best clinical judgment, given the information available at that time. Finally, the exclusion process is never easy and can be emotional for the mental health professional. The fertility counselor should remain aware of how they are feeling and seek consultation and support when necessary.

When treatment is not successful

Laila, age 34, had volunteered to be an egg donor for her dear friend, Jada. The RE had told Laila, she was "older that we usually like to see for an egg donor," but Laila was not concerned. She had three daughters, ages 6, 4 and 3, and with each child she became pregnant the first month she and her husband tried to conceive. Laila also knew she was Jada's only option, as Jada and her husband could not afford treatment using an anonymous or agency egg donor. Laila was surprised by how physically and emotionally drained she felt during the treatment process. This may have been due to the time involved in attending medical appointments, her compulsivity regarding administering her injections properly, or just from adding egg donation on to her already full plate of a career and parenting three young girls. Jada and Anthony ended up going through one fresh and one frozen transfer cycle with embryos created as a result of Laila's egg donation. Neither treatment cycle resulted in a pregnancy for Jada. Laila had never let herself consider the possibility that treatment might fail. She felt more than just disappointed for her friend, she felt extremely sad and a personal sense of failure that her efforts did not result in Jada becoming a mother.

As described in the vignette above, the known gamete donor or GC invests time and emotional energy, as well as incurring inconvenience and disruption of their family life, to help friends or loved ones achieve parenthood. Often based upon their own experiences of conception, pregnancy and delivery, they assume treatment will be successful. A medical work-up in which gamete donors and GCs meet necessary physical criteria also reinforces a sense of optimism. A failed treatment cycle can have a negative psychological impact [4,22]. Preparing the known gamete donor and GC for the possibility that treatment will not be successful is part of the counseling process and occurs throughout the interview. For example, when the fertility counselor asks about the individual's motivation to be a known donor or GC, the response usually includes a statement indicating they want to help their friend or family member create a family. At this point the counselor can stress that the donor or GCs participation does not guarantee that an embryo will be created, a pregnancy will be achieved, or a child will be born alive and healthy. We will often say, "This process has many moving parts, and a fault or break down can occur in a part that has nothing to do with your contribution. The gift you are giving the recipients/IPs is an opportunity that they otherwise wouldn't have had to create a family. It is not a guarantee." We have found that when we ask a known donor or GC how they will feel if treatment is not successful, they will often respond by saying "I will be disappointed for [e.g., my sister]." At this point the fertility counselor can explain that sometimes, when treatment fails, the known donor or GC may feel particularly sad, and the counselor is available to meet with them or can provide a referral to another mental health professional. By addressing these issues during the evaluation and counseling process, the known donor or GC is less likely to be blind-sided by treatment failure or any concomitant psychological responses. The aim is to reduce the possible risk of emotional harm to the donor or GC.

Issues that may arise between participants after a child is born

> Bridget, age 30, and Bree, age 35, are sisters who were initially referred for a KOD assessment. Bree was diagnosed with Primary Ovarian Insufficiency (POI) when she was age 20, and despite ongoing attempts to get pregnant, Bree and her husband had decided to move forward with Bridget as a KOD. Bridget, newly married, was eager to help her sister. Bridget knew that she wanted to have her own family but decided to wait, in part to help her sister. After an assessment, Bree, Bridget and their husbands felt positive about moving forward. Bridget successfully donated to Bree, who gave birth to a healthy girl. Bridget returned to the reproductive medical practice and counseling about a year after the donation, because she was now trying to conceive, unsuccessfully. It was learned that her husband, Ian, had low sperm motility. Bridget came in feeling anger towards her sister. She tearfully reported, "I keep feeling like I gave my sister my chance at having a child. I decided to delay having children because of her, and I never thought I would have problems with getting pregnant. However, here I am on the other side." Bridget continued on about how she had been avoiding her sister and her niece because of her feelings of regret and grief.

There is no way of predicting the future or knowing all the issues that will arise when going through a known donation process. Ideally, the known donor and recipients' family form a special bond with explicit and clear boundaries about dealing with each other and the child, and the KOD would have already finished having children. However, sometimes issues may arise after treatment has been completed. When recipients and the KOD and their spouse/partner come into the psychosocial assessment, everyone is on their best behavior [23], and they often only see the positives and do not want to think about any negative issues that could arise. In approaching the assessment, it is important to discuss the use of the sessions to help all parties have the best experiences that can be anticipated. This requires discussion of all the potential possibilities and problems that could occur in the future, and how they might be experienced and handled. Extensive predonation preparation done through the assessment is important, and while not always possible, ongoing support is recommended [24]. It is better to go in prepared than to have to address the issues after the fact.

When Bridget came in for counseling following her infertility diagnosis, the purpose of the meeting focused on forming a therapeutic alliance and not on psychosocial assessment as occurred previously [24]. The counseling should allow a safe place for Bridget to begin to explore her conflicted emotions around her own infertility and the grief she is experiencing. The job of the fertility counselor is to offer an open and supportive environment in which Bridget can discuss her feelings around being a donor to her sister as well as feelings around seeing her sister as a mother.

When a KOD is going through the process with her sister, she might often expend energy into her sister's process because she is invested in the outcome [24]. In the therapy session with Bridget, it might be worth considering the process and energy expended during her sister's pregnancy journey and how this impacts her current experience. Empathetic listening and reflection can help Bridget explore these many issues in the context of her own experience.

Reflections of the fertility counselors

Although we entered the field of fertility counseling at different times, we both initially had a level of discomfort with the counseling and assessment of known participants in third party reproduction. The issues seemed far more complex than in anonymous or previously unknown arrangements and the potential pitfalls appeared to carry more weight. After all, we are working with a group of people who not only bring their individual baggage to the arrangement, but also a suitcase filled with the history, and potential future, of their relationships with one another and their broader family or social networks (including any current or future children). Perhaps our respective unease had to do with the importance we place on our own family relationships and friendships. We each sought more information, but there was not a lot written on the counseling and assessment process in known arrangements; only small sections or paragraphs within general chapters or articles on GCs, IPs, donors and recipients (although that has begun to change [e.g., 4]). Over time, however, each of our initial feelings of discomfort dissipated. We developed an appreciation of our role in preparing participants, and providing a safe space for them to explore their thoughts and feelings on the multitude of issues involved, as well as reminding them to consider the welfare of the children born from the process and any existing children. We continue to learn from the clients we counsel, and are often struck by the capacity of all participants for empathy, generosity, selflessness and love. Finally, we now sit more comfortably with the fact that our work is guided by the information provided by the collaborators and our impressions at the time of the counseling and assessment process. There is no crystal ball to predict the future of a family's story.

References

1. De Wert G, Dondorp W, Pennings G, Shenfield F, Devroey P, Tarlatzis B, et al. Intrafamilial medically assisted reproduction. *Hum Reprod* 2011; 26: 504–9.
2. American Society for Reproductive Medicine Ethics Committee. Using family members as gamete donors or surrogates. *Fertil Steril* 2012; 98: 797–803.
3. Baetens P, Devroey P, Camus M, Steirteghem ACV, Ponjaert-Kristoffersen I. Counselling couples and donors for oocyte donation: the decision to use either known or anonymous oocytes. *Hum Reprod* 2000; 15: 476–84.
4. Vayena E, Golombok S. Challenges in intra-family donation. In: Richards M, Pennings G, Appleby J, eds. *Reproductive Donation: Practice, Policy and Bioethics.* New York: Cambridge University Press; 2012; 168–88.
5. Sachs P, Burns LH. Recipient counseling for oocyte donation. In: Covington SN, Burns LH, eds. *Infertility Counseling: A Comprehensive Handbook for Clinicians.* 2nd edn. New York: Cambridge University Press; 2006; 319–38.
6. Jaffe J, Diamond MO. *Reproductive Trauma: Psychotherapy with Infertility and Pregnancy Loss Clients.* Washington, DC: American Psychological Association, 2011.
7. Advisory Committee on Assisted Reproductive Technology (ACART). Guidelines on Donation of Eggs or Sperm between Certain Family Members. 2013.
8. American Society for Reproductive Medicine and the Society for Assisted Reproductive Technology. The Practice Committees.Recommendations for gamete and embryo donation: A committee opinion. *Fertil Steril* 2013; 99: 47–62.
9. German Society for Fertility Counseling. Guidelines for psychosocial counseling in the area of gamete donation. *BKiD* 2008.
10. Canadian Fertility and Andrology Society. Counselling Special Interest Group (CSIG). *Assisted Human Reproduction Counselling Practice Guidelines.* 2009.
11. Australian & New Zealand Infertility Counsellors Association (ANZICA). Guidelines for Professional Standards of Practice Infertility Counselling, 2003.
12. American Society for Reproductive Medicine and Society for Assisted Reproductive Technology. The Practice Committee. Recommendations for practices utilizing gestational carriers: An ASRM practice committee guideline. *Fertil Steril* 2012; 97: 1301–08.
13. Applegarth LD, Kingsberg SA. The donor as patient: assessment and support. In: Covington SN, Burns LH, eds. *Infertility Counseling: A Comprehensive Handbook for Clinicians.* 2nd edn. New York: Cambridge University Press; 2006; 339–55.
14. Covington SN, Patrizio P. Gestational carriers and surrogacy. In: Sauer MV, ed. *Principles of Oocyte and Embryo Donation.* 2nd edn. New York: Springer; 2013; 277–88.
15. Hanafin H. Surrogacy and gestational carrier participants. In: Covington SN, Burns LH, eds. *Infertility Counseling: A Comprehensive Handbook for Clinicians.* 2nd edn. New York: Cambridge University Press; 2006; 370–86.
16. MacCallum F, Lycett E, Murray C, Jadva V, Golombok S. Surrogacy: the experience of commissioning couples. *Hum Reprod* 2003; 18: 1334–42.
17. Jadva V, Blake L, Casey P, Golombok S. Surrogacy families 10 years on: relationship with the surrogate, decisions over disclosure and children's understanding of their surrogacy origins. *Hum Reprod* 2012; 27: 3008–14.
18. Readings J, Blake L, Casey P, Jadva V, Golombok S. Secrecy, disclosure and everything in-between: decisions of parents of children conceived by donor insemination, egg donation and surrogacy. *Reprod Biomed Online* 2011; 22: 485–95.
19. Klock SC. Disclosure decisions among known and anonymous egg donor recipients. In: Sauer MV, ed. *Principles of Oocyte and Embryo Donation.* 2nd edn. New York: Springer; 2013; 195–276.
20. Purewal S, van den Akker OBA. Systematic review of oocyte donation: investigating attitudes, motivations and experiences. *Hum Reprod Update* 2009; 15: 499–515.
21. Yee S, Blyth E, Tsang AKT. Views of donors and recipients regarding disclosure to children following altruistic known oocyte donation. *Reprod Biomed Online* 2011; 23: 851–9.
22. Yee S, Hitkari JA, Greenblattt EM. A follow-up study of women who donated oocytes to known recipient

couples for altruistic reasons. *Hum Reprod* 2007; 22: 2040–50.

23. Josephs LS, Grill E, Crone K, Applegarth L, Cholst I, Rosenwaks Z. Sister ovum donation: psychological outcomes. *Fertil Steril* 2004; 82: S102.

24. Winter A, Daniluk J. A gift from the heart: the experiences of women whose egg donation helped their sisters become mothers. *JCD* 2004; 82: 483–95.

Chapter 11

Last chance or too late? Counseling prospective older parents

Julianne E. Zweifel

Older parenting is oddly controversial in that, to many, it is an unquestionably bad idea fraught with medical, social and emotional hazards for both parent and child. But there are two sides to the coin. Many proffer the advantages of mature parents and the practical impediments to earlier family building.

Counseling older prospective parents is an exceptionally delicate endeavor influenced by the circumstance of the presenting patients, societal influences, fertility clinic policies, medical providers' views and the fertility counselor's own views and experiences as a child and parent. It is a tough knot to untie. Consider the following vignette:

> Michael and Susan are mired in conflict over the prospect of having children. Michael, age 55, has two children, ages 16 and 20, from his first marriage. Susan, age 46, avoided pregnancy in her first marriage due to her husband's alcoholism and unsuccessful attempts at sobriety.
>
> Michael and Susan met through a bicycling club. Prior to marriage, they discussed their ages and the thought of children. At that time, Michael was enjoying their active lifestyle and shared his philosophy that "age is just a state of mind." He thought it could be exciting to have kids again.
>
> Shortly after the wedding Susan broached the topic of having children but was shocked, angry and heart broken when he said he was having second thoughts. He was already going to be 61 years-old when his youngest graduated college and he couldn't imagine being in his late 70s when a new child graduated. Further, he was not far from 64, the age at which his own father died after an exhausting battle with cancer.
>
> He recalled being an active father with his children and felt that, despite the divorce, he'd been able to provide them with a stable and rewarding childhood. He was also beginning to enjoy relating to them at a new level as they emerged as adults. He was worried that he would not be able to provide this kind of experience for a future child. In short, Michael was deeply concerned about how a new child would be impacted by having an older father.
>
> Susan was overwhelmed with feelings of betrayal and panic that Michael would not agree to have a child together. She protested that he had already committed to having a child and that it was unfair to go back on his word. She had some appreciation for his concerns but was confident that the child would be fine. She did not envision Michael losing his health or dying anytime soon but even if he did, she was certain that she could help a child through the loss of a father and effectively single parent. Susan discussed years of containing envy as friends had children. She felt punished for being responsible and not having children in her first marriage. Susan dismissed age concerns asserting that she was healthy and looked young for her age. She brushed off the idea that her child might struggle claiming that, "all kids think their parents are old and embarrassing" and "any one of us can die at any age!" Overall, she just wanted to have a child and felt powerless in that struggle.

This vignette is rich with complexities of older parenting. It is emotionally and practically challenging to help a couple like this. The "easy" portion of counseling is helping the couple consider their various motivations and concerns about older parenting. The tough side of this work, which many may avoid, is sharing research and clinical data on potential negative consequences of older parenting for the resulting child. Parents may be motivated to discredit the concerns or the counselor. It is even harder and more tempting to avoid the toughest part of this counseling,

Fertility Counseling: Clinical Guide and Case Studies, ed. Sharon N. Covington. Published by Cambridge University Press.

which is frank discussion about the fact that someone's needs must prevail in the eventual decision (e.g., the needs/concerns related to the child or the needs of the prospective parents). In short, although very uncomfortable to broach, the question must be asked whether these adults should forego parenting in order to prevent harm to a hoped-for-child.

The goal of this chapter is to provide a foundation for those who counsel prospective older parents. The chapter will examine the impact of older parenting beginning with a review of age and childbearing trends with and without medical intervention. Theoretical perspectives and research related to patients' pursuit of delayed parenting will be considered as will medical risks of delayed parenting. Parental and child perspectives on the advantages, disadvantages and experiences of delayed parenting will be discussed. Rights and ethics associated with reproductive care of older prospective parents will be considered and followed by a discussion of age restrictions in treatment. Finally, the chapter will highlight the role of the fertility counselor in work with patients and reproductive health clinicians on the issue of delayed parenting, and discuss counseling patients like Michael and Susan.

The history of older mothers

Baby boomers, those born post World War II between 1946 and 1964, are a powerful group known for challenging societal expectations in many realms including family building. The preceding generation, the baby boomers' parents, was typified by families of four or more children, where mothers started having children around age 20 and wrapped up family building by their mid-30s [1]. This mold is now clearly being cracked if not broken. The baby boomer generation has been having fewer children, starting childbearing later and pushing back the age boundaries for having children. While it was once rare to see a 45-year-old mother with an infant, this is no longer uncommon. Indeed, we now see examples of 50, 55 and even 65-year-old "new" mothers.

Certainly, there have always been "older new mothers," however, over time the actual age associated with the term "older" has changed considerably. The term "elderly gravida" dates back to the 1940s and was used in discussions of obstetric risks for mothers aged 35 and beyond [2]. The term "elderly gravida" has fallen out of favor and is now replaced by "advanced maternal age." Advanced maternal age typically refers to women 35 years or older whereas "extreme advanced maternal age," refers to women 45 years or older [3].

Naturally occurring advanced maternal age

There are many reports of women naturally conceiving and bearing children in their 50s and even 60s, although it has been suggested that in truth the oldest naturally conceived pregnancy was in a 57-year-old woman [2]. A more representative picture of age and reproduction can be found by examining birth rates in populations that proscribe contraception and encourage reproduction until menopause. Researchers have looked at the rates of reproduction for women 45 years and beyond in two such populations: the Bedouins and those in ultra-orthodox Jewish communities. Births to this older group of women accounted for only 0.2 to 0.38% of all deliveries at the medical centers that serve these communities [4,5].

This data suggests that unassisted conception above the age range of 45–50 is exceptionally rare. Academically, these occurrences may be viewed as "outliers." One may conclude that without medical intervention, only a very small minority (perhaps less than 0.38%) of births would be to women 45 and beyond.

Changes in reproduction patterns

The median age of menopause is 51.4 years and there is some scant evidence that women with higher educational attainment, higher socio-economic status and physical activity may experience menopause a few months later than women of prior generations [6]. While further data would be helpful in clarifying whether women are experiencing later menopause, substantial data confirms that women are having children later in life. Data from the United States National Center for Health Statistics indicates that, across the country, the average age at which women had their first child increased from 21.4 to 25.0 years (a 3.6 year increase) from 1970 to 2006 [7]. This increase varied geographically; women in more central states showed a comparatively modest increase in age at first birth by having their children 2.0 to 2.6 years later in 2006 compared to 1970, whereas women in the northeast had their first child 4.3–5.5 years later in the same time frame. This trend towards later parenting, especially pronounced in more urban areas, has also been found in other developed countries [8].

Further data from the National Center for Health Statistics allows a closer look at the increased incidence of women having children later in life [9]. From 1996 to 2008, the overall birth rate in the United States rose 9.15%. In this same time frame, the birth rate to women aged 40–44 years rose 47.6% from 72 000 births to 106 000 births. The birth rate to women aged 45–49 rose 133% from 3000 births to 7000 births. Finally, although the absolute number of births in the 50–55 year maternal age bracket has remained small, the increase from 114 births in 1997 to 541 in 2008 represents an increase of 276%. Further, as women delay childbearing and age at first birth increases, the total number of children born to each woman decreases [2].

While it is possible that the average age of menopause may be increasing slightly, it would be folly to attribute the rise of births to older women to this potential marginal increase in childbearing years. Rather, it is clear that the increase in births to women 45 years and above is due to the rise in oocyte donation and IVF.

Factors contributing to older parenthood

The incidence rate of older parenting is increasing and eventually many fertility clinics and counselors will be approached by older patients wishing to pursue pregnancy. It's to the clinician's advantage to understand factors contributing to older parenting.

Older reproduction possible with the advent of IVF and oocyte donation

Those in the field of assisted reproduction are well acquainted with the fact that Louise Brown, born in 1978, was the first child born via in vitro fertilization (IVF). Six short years later in 1984, the world welcomed the first children born via egg donation [10]. Initially, premature ovarian failure, gonadal dysgenesis, cancer treatments and oophorectomy were the indications for oocyte donation; however, this treatment now extends to women of advanced maternal age who have experienced menopause.

Psychological and emotional contributors to older parenthood

Certainly, it's reasonable to presume that older prospective parents are looking forward to parenting for the same reasons as their younger counterparts. They may be anticipating "Happiness" (expected feelings of affection and happiness in the relationship with a child); "Well-being" (an expected positive impact on the individual's life); "Motherhood/Fatherhood" (an expectation of enjoying and being satisfied by parental activities); "Identity" (a means of enhancing one's self-concept and attaining adulthood); "Continuity" (opportunity to live on through children, have a relationship with children in old age, and pass on family names and traditions); "Social Control" (implied or explicit pressure from outside the couple to procreate); and "Marital Completion" (children are the reason for marriage and children are important for a happy marriage) [11].

These potential parents differ from their younger counterparts, however, in that they have postponed parenting. Many factors may explain this postponement. Usually the first step to parenting is having a suitable partner who is ready and willing to have a child. A recent study found that the combined concerns of partner suitability and partner interest in having a child were second only to concerns of financial preparedness in regards to factors influencing decisions to have a child [12]. Another partner-related issue is second marriages. As noted in the opening case, many feel that having a child adds to marital completion; thus, those entering into a second union may be motivated to have a child, which will occur later in life.

It is also clear that the need to be "prepared" to have a child is contributing to the postponement of childbearing. Financial preparedness has been found to be the primary factor influencing readiness for childbearing [13]. There is an interesting paradox about preparedness, especially for women, the prospective parents who are most likely to experience reduced income due to leaving the workforce or working fewer hours because of children's needs. In short, researchers have found that attainment of higher education and income can actually act as a disincentive for women to have children. The explanation is simple in that, as women attain higher wages, they stand to lose more by decreased work hours relative to when they had lower hourly wages; higher wage earners simply lose more money by having children than lower wage earners. It can be theorized then, that as women work to prepare themselves for children, they will perceive a greater economic disadvantage to having a child and further postpone childbearing until they have reached a point of perceived economic security.

Table 11.1 Live expectancy at birth by race and sex 1930–2007.

	White			Black		
Year	Both Sexes	Male	Female	Both Sexes	Male	Female
2007	78.4	75.9	80.8	73.6	70.0	76.8
2000	77.6	74.9	80.1	71.9	68.3	75.2
1990	76.1	72.7	79.4	69.1	64.5	73.6
1980	74.4	70.7	78.1	68.1	63.8	72.5
1970	71.7	68.0	75.6	64.1	60.0	68.3
1960	70.6	67.4	74.1	---	---	---
1950	69.1	66.5	72.2	---	---	---
1940	64.2	62.1	66.6	---	---	---
1930	61.4	59.7	63.5	48.1	47.3	49.2

--- Data Not Available
Data From National Center for Health Statistics National Vital Statistics Reports, Vol. 54, no. 19, June 28, 2006 www.cdc.gov/nchs

It has also been asserted that men and women are postponing childbearing because they believe they have an ample number of years left in their lives to provide sufficient and effective parenting [14]. Two factors contribute to this thinking. The first fact is that people are living longer. Table 11.1 illustrates this: in comparison to their counterparts born in the 1930s, white men and women born in 2007 can expect an additional 17 years of life [15]. Black males and females can anticipate an additional 25 years of life. The second issue is that people tend to "feel younger" than they are. In a 2009 Pew Research Center survey, nearly half of 50-year-olds reported "feeling" at least 10 years younger than their age. Those who were 65–74 years old reported feeling 10–19 years younger than their age [16]. The experience of feeling younger than one's age, coupled with the expectation of a lengthy additional life expectancy, may lead individuals to conclude that they can safely embark on parenting late in life.

Finally, some instances of late parenting are prompted by the death of another child within the family [17]. Although there may be some instances in which this new child can be seen as a "replacement child," other times a new child is brought into a grieving family to create a new sense of hope and happiness.

Social acceptance of older childbearing

As in developing countries, Western cultures are often described as "pronatalist" in that there is a social dictate to have children, but with limits. Indeed, Western societies have proscriptions about engaging in childbearing either too early or too late [18]. A European study of nearly 22 000 men and 22 000 women across 25 countries demonstrated that society has firm ideas about when it is no longer appropriate for men and women to have children [18]. When asked, "After what age would you say a woman [or man] is generally too old to consider having any more children?" over 96% of respondents cited a mean maternal age limit of 41.7 years with 57% suggesting a deadline of less than 40 years for potential mothers. The data was slightly more permissive for potential fathers with over 90% of respondents citing a mean paternal age limit of 47.3 years and nearly half suggesting a deadline of 45 years for potential fathers.

A similar Australian survey asked respondents at what age a woman is too old to have a child using another woman's eggs [19]. Only a minority, 37.9%, of respondents agreed that a postmenopausal woman should be able to use another woman's eggs to have a child. Interestingly, older respondents were significantly *less* accepting of postmenopausal women receiving donated eggs.

Psychological theories and older parenting

Psychological theories can be helpful in understanding why older adults may consider having children.

Strategic social comparison process

Weiss has noted that, like gender and ethnicity, age is a fundamental social category to which an individual belongs, unfortunately however, as one grows older, chronological age becomes a less desirable or even an undesirable characteristic. Thus, growing older is a challenge in that one is confronted with a possible worsening of one's self-concept. Individuals are motivated to maintain a positive view of themselves, and thus they will try to evade threats to their positive self-concept. One proposed mechanism for diminishing the threat of a worsening age-associated self-concept is to differentiate or contrast one's self from same-age peers [20]. Individuals may judge themselves to be "atypical" for their age. They may conclude that, "I am better than my age group." As older adults differentiate themselves from their age-mates, they perceive themselves as being similar to and a part of a younger age group. Weiss describes this as a "strategic social comparison process."

It is interesting to view older parenting within the "strategic social comparison process" concept. It may be that as older adults assimilate to younger age cohorts, they may consider enacting life choices that are characteristic of that younger cohort. They may engage in late reproduction to demonstrate that they still retain the qualities of youth and productivity, which are valued in our society.

Egocentrism

Egocentrism is a theory originally put forth by Piaget that refers to an individual's difficulty in considering and understanding another's point of view. The individual's self-perspective interferes with the ability to fully appreciate the perspective of another. As Piaget described, the individual with egocentrism has not yet discovered the multiplicity of possible perspectives and remains blind to all but his own as if that were the only one possible [21]. While initially applied to children, the theory of egocentrism is also applicable to adults.

An older individual's decision to have a child late in life may be viewed within the context of egocentrism. As an older individual considers having a child, possibly due to a tendency to see themselves as atypical for their age group and more like younger adults, they may be making the decision based on their own psychological needs. It is certainly true that research on motivations for having children suggests that most, perhaps all, adults anticipate personal benefit to having children (e.g., it's fun, someone to be with in my old age, etc.), and thus perhaps all individuals have some degree of egocentrism impacting their desire to have children. It can be argued, however, that older adults may neglect or not fully appreciate the child's experience of being parented by older adults as they contemplate having children.

Clinical issues to consider in older parenting

Medical risk associated with delayed parenting

Even with the use of donated eggs, women of advanced maternal age face increased risks during pregnancy and delivery. Older women are more likely to experience pregnancy induced hypertension, gestational diabetes, placenta previa and Caesarean section [2,22]. Older women are also more likely to present with pre-existing hypertension, diabetes, obesity and chronic disease; these pre-existing factors result in a 2- to 3-fold increased rate of hospitalization, Caesarean section, and pregnancy related complications relative to younger, healthier women [2]. The risk of maternal death also increases with age although the overall risk of dying during childbirth is very low in developed countries [2]. Finally, some studies have suggested an increased risk of low birth weight and fetal mortality in pregnancies occurring in women over 50 [22].

Advanced paternal age has been defined as a paternal age $\geq$ 45 [23]. Decreased fertility associated with advanced paternal age has a number of causative factors including decreased coital frequency, reduced sexual function and poorer semen quality [2]. Advanced paternal age is associated with increased risk of Down syndrome, Klinefelter syndrome, achondroplasia and some forms of childhood cancer [2,22]. Autism, schizophrenia, bi-polar disorders, attention deficit disorder, suicide attempts, substance use problems and lower academic achievement are more common in children of older fathers and, strikingly, a dose–response relationship has been found between paternal age and incidence of these disorders [23]. More specifically, comparisons of siblings born to the same father reveal that children born later in that same father's life are more likely than their older siblings to demonstrate these difficulties. Paternal age is

Table 11.2 Child's expected age at time of father's death.

Father's Age at Child's Birth	Father's Expected Age at Death, at Time of Child's Birth	Child's Expected Age at Father's Death	Father's Probability of Death by Child Age 5	Father's Probability of Death by Child Age 10	Father's Probability of Death by Child Age 15	Father's Probability of Death by Child Age 20
20	76	56	0.74%	1.45%	2.19%	3.10%
25	77	52	0.71%	1.46%	2.38%	3.77%
30	77	47	0.75%	1.68%	3.08%	5.17%
35	77	42	0.94%	2.34%	4.45%	7.56%
40	78	38	1.42%	3.54%	6.69%	10.91%
45	78	33	2.16%	5.34%	9.63%	15.69%
50	79	29	3.26%	7.63%	13.83%	22.19%
55	80	25	4.52%	10.93%	19.57%	31.46%
60	81	21	6.71%	15.76%	28.21%	44.91%
65	82	17	9.70%	23.05%	40.94%	61.72%
70	84	14	14.79%	34.60%	57.61%	79.02%
75	85	10	23.25%	50.26%	75.38%	91.98%

Source: Life Tables, United States, 2006, National Vital Statistics Reports, June 2010

also associated with cleft lip and cleft palate independently of maternal age [24]. An additional, perhaps surprising, finding is that advanced paternal age may also be associated with increased risk of Caesarean section independent of maternal age [25]. It is often concluded that the individual increased risk to the offspring attributable to advanced paternal age is low. However, as the incidence of advanced paternal age increases, the impact of these well-documented disadvantages may become more apparent [24].

Impact on the parenting experience

Researchers have examined the perceived benefits and detriments for those embarking on later parenting [26]. In interviews with men and women who had their children when the woman was 40 or older, reported benefits of delayed parenting included maturity, emotional readiness, financial security and strong co-parenting relationships. Older parents also reported that having children later in life helped them to feel young longer and motivated them to stay physically fit.

Disadvantages were also reported. Beyond the need for fertility treatment, the most commonly cited drawback for delayed parenting was a lack of physical energy. Another significant concern was fewer life years with their children and awareness that, due to their age, parents were more likely to become ill and die while their children were still comparatively young. The authors of this study note that *parental concerns over the risk of illness and death only emerged after their children were born*. These parents also noted that, despite initial desires for larger family sizes, the demands of parenting at an older age ultimately led them to have just one child. Finally, older parents reported concerns that their child would experience social stigma related to having parents who were visibly older than other parents.

A concern regarding fewer years with children is supported by actuarial data. Analysis of data from the United States Life Tables (2006) allows for the prediction of years of parenting and a child's age at the time of the mother and father's expected deaths (see Tables 11.2 and 11.3) [27]. Looking at the data within Table 11.2 it is clear that nearly 10% of children fathered by 45-year-old men will lose their fathers by the time they turn 15 and nearly 16% will lose their fathers by the time they are 20. In contrast, when fathered by a man of 35, less than 5% of 15-year-olds will have lost their fathers and less than 8% of 20-year-olds will have lost their fathers. For children fathered by 55-year-olds, nearly 20% will lose their father by age 15 and more than 30% will lose him by age 20. In short, *the risk of losing one's father by age 15 or 20 doubles when the father is 45 versus 55; and the risk increases*

Table 11.3 Child's expected age at time of mother's death.

Mother's Age at Child's Birth	Mother's Expected Age at Death, at Time of Child's Birth	Child's Expected Age at Mother's Death	Mother's Probability of Death by Child Age 5	Mother's Probability of Death by Child Age 10	Mother's Probability of Death by Child Age 15	Mother's Probability of Death by Child Age 20
20	81	61	0.24%	0.53%	0.89%	1.42%
25	81	56	0.28%	0.64%	1.18%	2.03%
30	81	51	0.36%	0.90%	1.75%	3.03%
35	81	46	0.54%	1.39%	2.68%	4.51%
40	82	42	0.86%	2.15%	4.00%	6.62%
45	82	37	1.30%	3.16%	5.81%	9.86%
50	82	32	1.88%	4.57%	8.67%	14.47%
55	83	28	2.73%	6.92%	12.83%	21.60%
60	84	24	4.30%	10.38%	19.39%	32.86%
65	85	20	6.35%	15.77%	29.85%	48.76%
70	86	16	10.06%	25.09%	45.28%	67.94%
75	87	12	16.71%	39.16%	64.35%	85.45%

Source: Life Tables, United States, 2006, National Vital Statistics Reports, June 2010

more than 4-fold when comparing risk of paternal loss when the father is 35 versus 55 at the time of birth.

Similar data is found regarding maternal age, although women's life expectancy is a bit greater than men's. Looking at the data in Table 11.3 for 45-year-old mothers, it is evident that approximately 6% of 15-year-olds and nearly 10% of 20-year-olds will have experienced the death of their mother. In contrast, for children whose mothers were 35 at their birth, less than 3% of 15-year-olds and less than 5% of 20-year-olds would be expected to experience the loss of their mother. If the age of the mother is 55 at the time of birth, nearly 13% of 15-year-olds and nearly 22% of 20-year-olds would be expected to have lost their mother. Thus, *the risk of losing one's mother by age 15 or 20 doubles when the mother is 45 versus 55; and the risk increases nearly 5-fold when comparing risk of maternal loss when the mother is 35 versus 55 at the time of birth.*

In sum, there are advantages and disadvantages to delayed parenting. It is interesting to note, however, that in the above study of older parents, nearly two-thirds of men and women stated that they wished they would have had their children 5 to 10 years earlier than they had, most reported the optimal age for parenting was in the early to mid 30s, and only 10% reported that the optimal age for parenting was over 40 [26].

Childhood experience with older parents

Given that oocyte donation only became available in 1984, it is not yet possible to meaningfully discuss the full life impact for children who have been born to women who had them postmenopausally. Before oocyte donation was available, the concept of late parenting was applied to individuals or couples between the ages of 35 and 40. Two writer/researchers published books, in 1988 and 1991, examining the impact on the child when parented by these 35- to 40-year-old "older parents" [28,29]. Together, these writers conducted extensive interviews with approximately 100 adults who were born when their parents were 35 or beyond. A few themes emerged within these interviews. Positive themes included parents being mature, stable in their relationships, financially secure, patient and giving of their time and attention [28].

Several disadvantages were also noted by these adult children of older parents [28,29]. These adult children recalled feeling that they were not as child-like as their peers. More precisely, they recalled feeling like little adults at an early age, not engaging in as much active play as peers, and being viewed as "old-fogeys" by other children. They also reported feeling as if their youth was foreshortened by entering into the world of old-age experiences and issues before their time.

Another concern was the increased age discrepancy between pa[illegible]ents and child. This resulted in children feeling as i[illegible]ey lived in a "different world" than their parents. It [illegible] also noted that older parents had lost touch wi[illegible]hild inside them and were less involved in li[illegible]ies. Lastly, respondents felt that the extensi[illegible]mpaired their ability to view their paren[illegible]odels.

A po[illegible] concer[illegible]s intense fear of parental d[illegible]d that many children [illegible]ese adult children [illegible]s concern. M[illegible]arental death by[illegible] those who are [illegible]en a child alre[illegible]ay not be aw[illegible]ve, but they *are* [illegible]re closer to death[illegible]

A final ther[illegible]il-dren of older paren[illegible]d opportunity for the[illegible]r life and, because ma[illegible] *only* children, they also re[illegible]riences due to the lack of si[illegible]t opportunity to relate to thei[illegible] adult perspective and to enjoy pa[illegible]r midlife years. Demographers have no[illegible]r-rent life expectancies, most individuals w[illegible]eir parents available to them well into their own [illegible]dle age [30]. More specifically, a large majority of 50-[illegible]ear-old adults now have a living mother. Children of older parents stand in strong contrast to this current norm. As noted earlier in Tables 11.2 and 11.3, a sizeable percentage of children whose parents were 45 or older when they were born will lose their parents by the time they are 20. Thus, while most young adults can rely on the support and guidance of their parents for quite a number of years after reaching adulthood, the children of older parents will forfeit this benefit much earlier in life.

Certainly there are many struggles that may be inherent in being the child of older parents. It is important to note, however, that many of these children are quick to affirm that they love and appreciate their parents greatly. They simply would have preferred to have been born to those same parents years earlier.

Children as caretakers

It has been noted that most individuals can expect to be in a situation where their parents will depend on them emotionally, practically and perhaps also financially [30]. While the care of one's parents may be an experience common to many adults, it is not common to face this care-taking role at an early age. By being thrust into a care-giving role early in life, children of older parents may face an unusually high dose of responsibility in relation to their same-age peers.

As noted previously, life expectancy has increased and adults can now hope to live more than 15 years longer than counterparts born a generation or so earlier. Not all of these years will be ones of good health. Table 11.4 [31] presents data from the Healthy People 2010 report (National Center for Health Statistics) on continued life expectancy and the number of additional years of good or better health that one may anticipate given a particular age and sex. A comparison of expected number of additional life years to the expected number of years of good or better health suggests that for those age 45 and beyond, more than 20% of additional life years will *not* be ones of good or better health. Those who are 65 would expect that more than 30% of their additional life years *will not* be characterized by good or better health. These data are important in the discussion of children taking care of older parents. When a child is born to a parent age 45 or beyond, it can be anticipated that 20% of that child's time with a parent will be impacted by the parent's declining health. This data highlights both a loss experience for the child and the child-as-care-taker experience. In terms of loss, in contrast to peers parented by younger parents, these children of older parents will enjoy fewer years of healthy active parenting and will begin to witness the health decline of their parents earlier in their lives. In regards to child-as-care-taker, these children are apt to take on a care-taker role much earlier in life than their peers.

Table 11.4 Life expectancies and expected years in good or better health for selected ages of the white and black population, by sex: United States 1995.

Sex and age	Expected years of life	Expected years in good or better health	Years in good or better health as a % of life expectancy	Expected years in excellent health	Years in excellent health as a % of life expectancy
Male					
Birth	72.8	64.6	88.7	27.1	37.3
20 years	54.0	46.2	85.5	17.2	31.9
30 years	44.9	37.3	83.1	13.0	29.0
45 years	31.5	24.6	78.1	7.4	23.3
65 years	15.9	11.2	70.4	2.4	14.9
70 years	12.8	8.8	68.9	1.7	13.6
75 years	10.1	6.7	66.5	1.2	11.8
80 years	7.7	4.9	64.2	0.8	10.8
Female					
Birth	78.8	68.4	86.8	25.7	32.6
20 years	59.8	49.8	83.3	15.8	26.4
30 years	50.1	40.6	81.2	12.3	24.6
45 years	35.9	27.6	76.9	7.3	20.2
65 years	18.8	13.4	71.3	2.8	14.8
70 years	15.1	10.6	70.1	2.1	14.0
75 years	11.7	8.0	67.9	1.6	13.7
80 years	8.7	5.7	65.9	1.2	14.2

Children engaged in care-giving roles with their parents help with household tasks such as shopping, cooking and cleaning, personal care such as dressing and bathing, medical care such as changing bandages and giving medication, and entertainment such as playing games, reading to the parent and general visiting [32]. Higher rates of depression, anxiety and behavioral problems are reported for young care-givers [33].

Although care-giving can be challenging, especially for young care-givers, there may be positive aspects to the experience. In a retrospective study of 51 young care-givers' experiences, the now adult respondents recalled that early care-giving (beginning at a mean age of 11.6 years) was "hard yet gratifying." It taught them responsibility and useful skills, allowed them to feel needed, brought them closer to their families, and allowed them to grow up faster [32]. Difficulties recalled included less time for homework and extra-curricular activities, also the need to miss special school-related events. Four of the 51 respondents reported that they dropped out of high school because of their care-giving responsibilities. Respondents also recalled having less time for friends, dating and leisure activities. Some recalled being reluctant to bring friends home or tell friends about their care-giver responsibilities. Finally, respondents reported difficulty with watching their parent deteriorate, be sick, or be in pain. Some reported being fearful of finding their parent dead.

Care-giving children may also have difficulty emancipating from the home and may delay higher education, dating and marriage due to a care-giving commitment to their parents [14]. The term "overload" describes a situation in which an adult, generally a woman, is simultaneously in a care-giving role towards her parents or in-laws and her own children. It has been suggested that women who provide care to parents may delay having children and/or have fewer children in an attempt to limit the number of years and intensity of the "overload" situation [30]. Thus, although few children of older parents report wanting to have their children late in life [28,29], they may find themselves "needing" to delay having children of their own as a consequence of being born to older parents.

The impact of early parental death

Although parental death is certainly difficult, if not traumatic, at any point in life, research suggests that when parental death happens too early in a person's life, the trauma can be particularly intense and disruptive to life and further development. Parents are generally the central attachment figures for children and provide a basis of emotional security as well as practical support. A parent's role as an attachment figure and care-giver lessens as the child ages such that, by the time a child has entered into adulthood, other relationships begin to be the primary source of emotional support. The shifting of support beyond parents results in the adult child being less vulnerable to the potential trauma inherent in parental death. Children, however, remain dependent on their parents and the loss of parental support through death can result in an increased risk for emotional and behavioral problems, social withdrawal, social skills deficits, lowered self-esteem, separation stress and psychiatric disorders [34]. Both sons and daughters experience greater distress at the loss of a mother compared to the loss of a father. Indeed, adults recalling the early loss of their mother describe it as the end of childhood [34].

Parentally bereaved children are also apt to experience collateral losses that are difficult. Collateral losses can include losing the family home and/or moving, changing school systems and friendship networks, loss of familiar community support and functions (athletic activities, art and dance classes, etc.), and reduced family income [34].

While grief as marked by weeping, sadness, anger and withdrawal may be expected following parental death, clinical depression is not an inevitable experience. Research in the area of childhood grief suggests that children are more able to experience "healthy mourning" if they experience strong emotional and psychological support from the surviving parent and feel free to share feelings, thoughts and questions about their deceased parent including discussions of the version of life and future experiences they lost when their parent died [34].

Healthy mourning is a life-long process rather than a discrete period of time. Parentally bereaved children will re-experience the loss of their parent at successive developmental stages and salient life experiences [34]. The child-like desire for the parent may never truly end. As they age, they rework their formulations of the death and the hypothetical life that they would have had if their parent had survived. This cyclical grief process is a primary context within which their development progresses. In short, parental death is a core element of the bereaved child and impacts the child for a lifetime [34].

Age restriction considerations

Review of age-related restrictions on fertility care

Many Western countries subsidize in vitro fertilization. Commonly, this subsidy is limited in some way such as the number of cycles funded, the number of children already born to the woman (and sometimes the number of children fathered by the man) and the age of the woman pursuing treatment. While women may be legally free to pursue and fund their own fertility care, once beyond a set age point they are no longer eligible for subsidized IVF. Age limits associated with subsidized treatment vary considerably. Comparatively low age cutoffs of 37, 38 and 39 can be found in northern Swedish countries, Scotland, and Northern Ireland, respectively [35,36]. Several countries extend the age of subsidized IVF up through the 40–45 age bracket including Wales, England, Israel, Denmark, France, Germany, Belgium and some Swedish countries [35–41]. Greece has a limit of 50 years for subsidized fertility care [42] while Italian law requires that those receiving fertility care must be "potentially fertile," which has generally been interpreted to mean premenopausal [17]. Finland, Australia, Canada, the United States and Spain do not have an age limit [16,43–45]. In countries with no established age limit, many clinics set clinic-specific age limits for fertility care.

Male-specific age restrictions to fertility care are less common but do exist. In Austria, fertility care is restricted to men 50 and younger [46] while in Sweden it is restricted to men 55 and younger. In a discussion of male age restrictions in Sweden, the National Board of Health and Welfare "recommends that the age of the prospective father be at a level where one can expect that he could take care of the future child through all its childhood"; this is interpreted to be a limit of 55 [35].

Setting limits: ethical issues and rights

It is important to distinguish between positive rights and negative rights before discussing reproductive rights. *Positive rights* require others to provide an individual with goods or services; restated, they are the right to claim entitlement to a service or means to obtain something. Alternatively, *negative rights* refer to the right to pursue something without interference [17].

It is also important to examine the *Right to Reproduce.* The United Nations Universal Declaration of Human Rights and the 14th Amendment to the US Constitution both discuss the right to have children. Examination of these documents, however, reveals that they refer to negative rights rather than positive rights [17,47]. A similar analysis regarding rights in reproduction can be found in the American Society for Reproductive Medicine (ASRM) Ethics Committee report on childrearing ability and provision of fertility services; "Reproductive rights protected under the United States and state constitutions are rights *against* state interference, not rights *to have* physicians or the state provide requested services." The report further notes, "It is also important to recognize that constitutional rights to reproduce are, like all rights, not absolute and they can be restricted or limited for good cause" [47, p. 866]. In sum, there is not an absolute right to have a child.

Professional autonomy is another salient consideration. Professional autonomy is the freedom to determine the conditions or limits of practice. ASRM has noted that professional autonomy entitles physicians to choose *not to treat* persons if there are concerns regarding parenting and the well-being the resulting child. The same professional autonomy also entitles the provider *to treat* such patients [46].

Provider, or professional autonomy coupled with the absence of an absolute right to have a child sets the stage for individual clinicians and clinics grappling with the question of supporting, tolerating, or disallowing fertility treatment with older patients. A review of ethical principles may provide guidance in this task.

Those who support patients having children late in life reference the concept of *reproductive autonomy.* Reproductive autonomy suggests that personal reproductive decisions should be free from interference unless it is clear that others will incur serious harm [48]. Under this concept, those who would seek to restrict reproductive autonomy would be charged with providing proof of serious harm to another. In this instance, one would need to provide substantial proof that children are seriously harmed by being born to older parents.

It is undebatable that others will be affected by the choice of older parents to have a child. As others have asserted, "unlike other actions that could have little effect on others, reproductive choice *always affects others, and in particular affects any child who is brought into existence*" [48, p. 43]. It is difficult, however, to proffer compelling proof that children are seriously harmed by their parents' choice to have them late in life. Compelling proof is often obtained through scientific study; however, as noted previously, it is not yet possible to rigorously study the full impact on a child when it is born to older parents.

Since it has not been empirically established that children are harmed by being born to older parents, it may seem that reproductive autonomy would then justify provision of fertility services to older individuals. However, there is a flaw to this argument relating to the difference between positive and negative rights. Reproductive autonomy refers to a negative right; the right to make reproductive decisions free from the influence of others. Older parents, however, are *seeking the assistance of others* in the conception of their child. Further, when they seek the assistance of a clinician to attain a pregnancy, they are implicating that clinician in the outcome [47]. Any older individual asserting the right to treatment is proposing a positive right to fertility care; however, reproduction is a negative right, not a positive one. In sum, *although older individuals enjoy reproductive freedom when they reproduce without the assistance of others, they do not have the right to demand fertility treatment.*

There are additional ethical concerns related to age limits in fertility care. Many claim that age-based restrictions in fertility care are sexist and ageist. Those who claim age-based limitations are sexist note that, historically, men have been fathering children late in life and have never faced age-based reproductive restrictions. It is argued that to impose age-based restrictions on women's reproduction is therefore sexist [49]. Although it is certainly meritorious to avoid sexism in fertility care, this argument fails to take into account the fact that, prior to the introduction of oocyte donation, when men had children late in life the child's mother was in her reproductive years and therefore able to provide more years of parenting. The child was therefore not likely to experience the death or health decline of both parents at a young age. Having a younger mother reduces the child's psychological risk whereas having a set of older parents or a single older parent potentiates risk [50].

The ageist argument posits that age-based restrictions presume that older individuals have a reduced capacity to parent effectively. The argument notes that many grandparents have been effective in taking on a parenting role for grandchildren and that establishing age-based limits to fertility care disrespects the childrearing provided by grandparents. A counter-argument concedes that grandparents may successfully fill the role of the parent when there is a breakdown in the original family, but asserts that this is not justification for deliberately using medical technology to place a child at risk for psychological harm [22,50].

The ageist argument often expands to suggest that if reduced capacity to parent and fewer years of parenting are the basis for curtailing reproductive care to older prospective parents, similar restrictions should be applied to individuals with disabilities and also to individuals with health-related reduced life spans [51]. These assertions have been effectively countered by noting that the attempt to equate age-related limitations with limitations due to disability "only considers physical limitations and fails to consider that young physically disabled parents are not cognitively and psychologically different from their able-bodied counterparts" [50, p. 59]. In response to the suggestion that individuals with medically related decreased life expectancy should face restrictions, it has been noted that cases such as these are generally considered based on pertinent individual health and social circumstances, not the least of which is the individual's social support network. The support network commonly includes a partner and that partner's ability to provide parenting for the child is integral in reproductive decisions.

Counseling the prospective older parent

Assisted reproduction programs may refer older prospective parents like Michael and Susan for a psychological consult. Individual factors will impact the precise content of this consult; however, several key factors are important to address. These factors are considered below and applied to the case of Michael and Susan.

Identifying psychological factors

Susan and Michael's story exemplifies many psychological factors discussed above. Susan's view of herself as young for her age demonstrates the strategic comparison process whereas her dismissal of social/emotional difficulties for children of older parents, including coping with parental death, is suggestive of egocentrism. Alternatively, Michael exemplifies the finding that adults are more concerned about children once they have them. Further, he presents a personal testimonial to the benefits of comparatively young parenting as well as the impact of caring for parents through illness and death.

Anticipate further aging and declining health

Presumably, most prospective older parents will feel that they are in good health and vigorous at the time they request treatment. It is important to encourage them to look beyond the next 10 years, a time of presumed good health, and anticipate their physical condition 20 or 30 years out and to consider their ability to meet the needs of their child who will still benefit from support in early adulthood.

Clearly Michael *is* anticipating the impact of age, decline and death. Susan, however, sees these as distant worries. It may be helpful to have her imagine specific parent–child experiences, such as physical play/sports/dance, visiting prospective colleges, planning weddings, and welcoming their children's children into the world and consider how their ages and health may impact these experiences for their child. It may also be helpful for her to consider at what age she was truly ready to lose her parents and to review actuarial tables to see the likelihood of their child losing a parent at a young age.

Understand the child's experience with older parents

While prospective parents generally feel young, it is important for them to recognize that their children will be fully aware that they are older than peer's parents. The children may be embarrassed of their parents' age and experience teasing by peers. They may also experience intense worry over parental death. It is psychologically difficult to simultaneously respect these worries yet go forward with decisions that may set these problems in motion. Therefore, patients, such as Susan, may be motivated to view these concerns as minor. The fertility counselor needs to encourage a patient like Susan to consider whether and why they are engaging in this type of self-deception. Still, patients may go forward with treatment. In this outcome, patients should be educated on the importance of supporting their child's social struggles and openly discussing fears of parental death or decline. Further, given that most children of older parents are only children and will have limited or no experience with grandparents, parents need to be aware of their child's potential feelings of lost opportunities and loneliness [14]. Alternatively, in a case such as Michael and Susan's, there may be siblings who are significantly older than the hoped-for child. The fertility counselor can help such parents consider assumptions that they, or the older existing children, may have regarding older siblings assuming care of younger sibling in the case of parental death.

Ramifications of having older parents

It is difficult but important to discuss the probability of a child assuming a care-giver role in the parent–child relationship including the associated emotional toll and how it may impede the child's ability to pursue educational goals, career goals, independence, intimate relationships and parenting of their own. It is also important to acknowledge that the child is very likely to experience parental death comparatively early in life which may have life-long emotional and developmental impact. The fertility counselor can help Michael and Susan consider their views on children's responsibility to older parents and develop a plan for how they can proactively discuss this with their child. They should also be advised to establish plans for guardianship and financial security of their child.

Work with clinic staff

Countertransference

As discussed previously, adults tend to view themselves as younger than they are and are also apt to consider engaging in activities or lifestyles more consistent with their younger peers [16,20]. These tendencies apply to clinic staff, not just prospective patients. Countertransference is a term common to those in the field of mental health and refers to the feelings or reactions that a provider may experience in response to clinical work with a patient. Providers vary in their awareness of countertransference and the same provider's awareness can vary across interactions.

Clinician's individual feelings about aging may influence their receptivity to working with older patients. Clinicians invested in seeing themselves as young and spared the impact of aging may be inclined to devalue concerns associated with late parenting. The fertility counselor working with reproductive health clinics can raise the issue of countertransference and help clinicians disentangle their own feelings from their clinical judgment and, hopefully, dispassionately consider the potential concerns.

Theory of mind and empathy

Theory of mind refers to the ability to understand another's perspective. Many clinicians report experiencing empathy, an aspect of theory of mind, towards older prospective parents. This empathy leads them to appreciate the prospective older parents' desire for a child and to conclude that they would make loving parents. Theory of mind in general and empathy in particular increases in relation to the similarities between individuals and also in relation to the amount of interaction between individuals. This leads to a situation in which a clinician is more apt to understand and empathize with the perspective of the older prospective patient, whom she/he has met and can relate to, than to the concerns of the potential child, whom she/he has never met. In short, this leads to a propensity for the older parents' desires to overshadow the concerns of the potential child. The fertility counselor working with reproductive health clinics can highlight this potential imbalance and help reproductive health clinicians realistically appraise the potential experience for the child as they make decisions about providing treatment.

Susan's predicament is likely to evoke empathy from clinic staff. Her decision to not have children with her addicted ex-husband is an admirable decision that has had the unfortunate consequence of delaying and possibly jeopardizing her goal to have children. Staff may feel that life is unfairly punishing her for making good decisions. As such, they may be motivated to put aside concerns for the child and support her going forward with treatment. Here the fertility counselor needs to help staff recognize how empathy is impacting judgment and underscore the fact that unfairness in the parent's life does not justify increasing risk of psychological harm to a potential child.

Implementing treatment limits

As noted above, professional autonomy permits clinics and clinicians to set limits to their practice. Any clinic that implements an age restriction for treatment will, of course, need to be forthright with prospective patients about their precise policies. Certainly, it may be difficult to inform older prospective patients that they exceed the clinic's age limit. It may be more difficult, however, to enforce age limits with patients who were younger than the cut-off when they initiated treatment but are now approaching/exceeding the age cut-off while pursuing continued treatment. Thus, age restrictions, whether for autologous IVF or with donor egg, should be clearly stated and repeated as treatment limitations near.

Reflections on a difficult clinical role

Increasingly, good-hearted people with a myriad of motivations want to have a child late in life. Their personal circumstances are often moving and even I have a hard time not being taken in by their stories and wishing for them the happiness of a child and dreading the heart break of that dream unfulfilled. Yet still, the child, and likelihood of all the difficulties discussed above, must not be lost in clinical judgment. It is an unhappy role that the fertility counselor takes on when he/she discusses all of these concerns with prospective parents and clinic staff, yet ethics and responsibility demand it. An honest review of risks and benefits must be completed and the question must be asked whether it's reasonable to satisfy the needs of a parent at potential cost to the resulting child.

In closing, consider the real-world case of John and Elizabeth Edwards, highly visible figures in American politics in the presidential elections of 2004 and 2008. Elizabeth was 28 years old when she married John in 1977. They had their son Wade in 1979 and daughter Cate in 1982. Wade was tragically killed in a car accident in 1996 at age 17. Devastated but determined to create a new sense of hope and happiness, Elizabeth and John underwent fertility treatment. Emma Claire was born in 1998 and Jack was born in 2000. Elizabeth was 49 and 51 years old at the time of Emma Claire and Jack's births, respectively, while John was 45 and 47 years old at the time of the children's arrivals. Elizabeth and John likely anticipated many healthy years together to raise their two new children. Sadly, Elizabeth went on to be diagnosed with cancer and died in 2010 at the age of 61; Emma Claire was 12 and Jack was 10. While it is easy to understand the impulse to bring the happiness of new children into a home where there is sadness and longing, in cases such as this, the "happiness-bringers," that is to say, the children, are the one's ultimately shouldering the sadness and loss.

References

1. Kirmeyer SE, Hamilton BE. Childbearing differences among three generations of U.S. women. *National Center for Health Statistics Data Brief no.68:* Hyattsville, MD; 2011. Available at http://www.cdc.gov/nchs/data/databriefs/db68.pdf. Accessed March 10, 2014.
2. Johnson J, Tough S. SOGC Committee Opinion. Delayed child-bearing. *JOCG* 2012; 34(1): 80–93.
3. Yogev Y, Melamed N, Bardin R et al. Pregnancy outcome at extremely advanced maternal age. *Am J Obstet Gynecol* 2010; 203(6): 558 e1–7.
4. Laufner N, Simon A, Samueloff A, et al. Successful spontaneous pregnancies in women older than 45 years. *Fertil Steril* 2004; 81: 1328–32.
5. Gielchinsky Y, Mazor M, Simon A, et al. Natural conception after 45 in Bedouin women, a uniquely fertile population. *J Assist Reprod Gen* 2006; 23: 305–9.
6. Dratva J, Gomez Real F, Schinder C, et al. Is age at menopause increasing across Europe? Results on age at menopause and determinants from two population-based studies. *Menopause* 2009; 16(2): 385–94.
7. Matthews TJ, Hamilton BE. Delayed childbearing: more women are having their first child later in life. *NCHS Data Brief, Number* 21, August 2009. Available at: http://www.cdc.gov/nchs/data/databriefs/db21.pdf. Accessed March 10, 2014.
8. Vranes HS, Gall V. Secular trends in parental age in Croatia from 1985–2009. *Anthropol Anz* 2013; 70(3): 347–55.
9. Martin JA, Hamilton BE, Sutton PD, et al. *Births: Final Data for 2008. National Vital Statistics Reports; Volume 59, Number 1.* Hyattsville, MD: National Center for Health Statistics. 2010. Available at: www.cdc.gov/nchs/data/nvsr/nvsr59/nvsr59_01.pdf. Accessed March 10, 2014.
10. Buster J. The first live birth donation. *Sex Reprod Menopause* 2008; 6(4): 23–8.
11. van Balen F, Trimbos-Kemper TCM. Involuntarily childless couples: their desire to have children and their motives. *J Psychosom Obstet Gynaecol* 1995; 16(3): 137–44.

12. Tough S, Tofflemire K, Benzies K, et al. Factors influencing childbearing decisions and knowledge of perinatal risks among Canadian men and women. *Matern Child Health J* 2007; 11(2): 189–98.
13. Benzies K, Tough S, Tofflemire K, et al. Factors influencing women's decisions about timing of motherhood. *J Obstet Gynecol Neonat Nurs* 2006; 35(5): 625–33.
14. Zweifel JE, Covington SN, Applegarth LD. "Last-chance kids": a good deal for older parents – but what about the children? *Sex Reprod Menopause* 2012; 10(2): 4–12.
15. Minino AM, Heron MP, Smith BL. *Deaths: Preliminary Data from 2004. National Vital Statistics Reports; Volume 54, Number 19.* Hyattsville, MD: National Center for Health Statistics. 2006. Available at: http://www.cdc.gov/nchs/data/nvsr/nvsr54/nvsr54_19.pdf. Accessed March 10, 2014.
16. Pew Research Center. Growing older in America: expectations v reality. June 29, 2009. Available at: http://pewresearch.org/pubs/1269/aging-survey-expectations-versus-reality. Accessed March 10, 2014.
17. Caplan, AL, Patrizio P. Are you ever too old to have a baby? The ethical challenges of older women using infertility services. *Semin Reprod Med* 2010; 28(4): 281–86.
18. Billari FC, Goisis A, Liefbroer AC, et al. Social age deadlines for the childbearing of women and men. *Hum Reprod* 2011; 26(3): 616–22.
19. Bowman MC, Saunders DM. Community attitudes to maternal age and pregnancy after assisted reproductive technology: too old at 50 years? *Hum Reprod* 1994; 9(1): 176–71.
20. Weiss D, Freund AM. Still young at heart: Negative age-related information motivates distancing from same-aged people. *Psychol Aging* 2012; 27(1): 173–180.
21. Piaget J. *The Child's Conception of the World.* London: Kegan Paul Trench Trubner; 1929.
22. Ethics Committee of the American Society for Reproductive Medicine. Oocyte or embryo donation to women of advanced age: a committee opinion. *Fertil Steril* 2013; 100(2): 337–40.
23. D'Onofrio BM, Rickert ME, Frans E, et al. Paternal age at childbearing and offspring psychiatric and academic morbidity. *JAMA Psychiatry* 2014; Published online February 26, 2014.
24. Bray I, Grunell D, Smith GD. Advanced paternal age: how old is too old? *J Epidemiol Community Health* 2006; 60(10): 851–53.
25. Faro R, Santolaya-Forgas J, Canterino JC, et al. Paternal age and risk for cesarean delivery. *J Matern Fetal and Neonatal Med* 2012; 25(12): 2713–16.
26. MacDougall, K, Beyene Y, Nachtigall RD. 'Inconvenient biology': advantages and disadvantages of first-time parenting after age 40 using in vitro fertilization. *Hum Reprod* 2012; 27(4): 1058–65.
27. Arias E. United States life tables, 2006. *National Vital Statistics Reports*; vol 58, no 21. Hyattsville, MD: National Center for Health Statistics. 2010. (Tables 11.2, 11.3). Available at: http://www.cdc.gov/nchs/data/nvsr/nvsr58/nvsr58_21.pdf. Accessed March 10, 2014.
28. Morris M. *Last-chance Children: Growing Up with Older Parents.* New York, NY: Columbia University Press; 1988.
29. Yarrow A. *Latecomers: Children of Parents over 35.* New York, NY: Free Press, MacMillian; 1991.
30. Menken J. Age and fertility: How late can you wait? *Demography* 1985; 22(4): 469–483.
31. Molla MT, Madans JH, Wagner DK, Crimmins EM. *Healthy People 2010. Summary Measures of population Health: Report of Findings on Methodologic and Data Issues.* National Center for Health Statistics: Hyattsville, MD; 2003. Available at: www.cdc.gov/nchs/data/misc/pophealth.pdf. Accessed March 10, 2014.
32. Lackey NR, Gates MF. Adults' recollections of their experiences as young caregivers of family members with chronic physical illnesses. *J Adv Nurs* 2001; 34 (3): 320–8.
33. Bauman LJ, Foster G, Silver EJ, et al. Children caring for their ill parents with HIV/AIDS. *Vulnerable Child Youth Stud* 2006; 1(1): 56–70.
34. Biank NM, Werner-Lin A. Growing up with grief: revisiting the death of a parent over the life course. *Omega* 2011; 63(3): 271–90.
35. http://politiskfilosofi.com/2006/06/08/financing-policies-of-ivf-in-sweden/ Retrieved from the website March 10, 2014.
36. http://www.hfea.gov.uk/fertility-treatment-cost-nhs.html. Retrieved from the website March 10, 2014.
37. http://www.haaretz.com/news/national/israeli-health-ministry-considers-cutting-fertility-treatment-subsidies-for-older-women-1.434194. Retrieved from the website March 10, 2014.
38. http://www.touchpoint.dk/xdoc/wss/74/docs/289/Infertility_lecture_2003.pdf. Retrieved from the website March 10, 2014.
39. LeRay C, Scherier S, Anselem O, et al. Association between oocyte donation and maternal and perinatal outcomes in women aged 43 years or older. *Hum Reprod* 2012; 27: 896–901.

40. http://www.dailymail.co.uk/news/article-1385185/Baby-vacuum-Germany-start-paying-families-IVF-reverse-dwindling-birthrate.html. Retrieved from the website March 10, 2014.

41. http://www.children.gov.on.ca/htdocs/English/infertility/report/caretoproceed.aspx. Retrieved March 10, 2014.

42. http://www.embryoland.gr/en/pages/ivf-abroad-greece/Legal-Issues-IVF-Greece.asp. Retrieved from website March 10, 2014.

43. http://www.ivf.net/ivf/finland-passes-new-fertility-legislation-o2315.html. Retrieved from the website March 10, 2014.

44. http://www.theaustralian.com.au/news/opinion/ivf-is-not-a-treatment-but-provision-of-a-commodity/story-fn562txd-1226249710890. Retrieved from website March 10, 2014.

45. http://www.ivf.net/ivf/world%92s-oldest-ivf-mother-dies-from-cancer-two-years-after-giving-birth-o4339.html. Retrieved from website March 10, 2014.

46. http://www.ivf-worldwide.com/Education/policy-of-reimbursement.html. Retrieved from website March 10, 2014.

47. Ethics Committee of the American Society for Reproductive Medicine. ASRM Ethics Committee report: child-rearing ability and the provision of fertility services. *Fertil Steril* 2009; 92(3): 864–867.

48. Blyth E, Frith L, Crawashaw M. Ethical objections to sex selection for non-medical reasons. *Reprod Biomed Online* 2008; 16 Suppl 1: 41–45.

49. Appel JM. Motherhood: Is it ever too late? Huffington Post Healthy Living. July 15, 2009. Available at: http://www.huffingtonpost.com/jacob-m-appel/motherhood-is-it-ever-too-late_b_233916.html. Accessed March 10, 2014.

50. Landau R. The promise of post-menopausal pregnancy (PMP). *Soc Work Health Care*. 2004; 40(1): 53–69.

51. Paulson RJ, Sauer MV. Pregnancies in post-menopausal women. Oocyte donation to women of advanced reproductive age: "How old is too old?" 1994; *Hum Reprod* 9(4): 571–2.

Chapter 12

Counseling single women and single men choosing parenthood

Lauri A. Pasch and Sarah R. Holley

"I never really was into the dating thing when I was younger. At 37, I'd had few years of looking for the 'right' man to start a family with, and I'd come to realize I probably didn't have the time I needed anymore to grow to trust a man enough, and that I didn't know if I really needed one. I read Single Mothers by Choice by Jane Mattes which made me realize that there were other people out there just like me: Women who were willing to do this motherhood thing alone. Because of my background (I was raised by a single mother), I did not doubt my ability to bring up a child on my own. I felt I was in a good place. I had a good paying job and I was healthy. It was time."

"It took a great deal to come to a place where I realized I simply had to choose between trying to find love or trying to have a baby. To give up on finding love was a horrible choice to be forced to make, so it took me a long time. I did not start to actively and seriously look into fertility options until I was 41. I had many concerns. But for years, I always said that if I never found the guy, I'd still have a child."

This chapter provides the background needed for counseling single women and men who choose to become parents on their own, a group often referred to as *single mothers or fathers by choice*. The term single mothers or fathers by choice refers to any individual who elects to have child without a partner and without the intent to have a co-parent, distinguishing them from individuals who become single parents as a result of relationship dissolution, divorce, death of a spouse, or unintended pregnancy. For women, parenthood in this context is most commonly achieved via the use of sperm donation or adoption, whereas for men, parenthood options include adoption or having a baby with the help of egg donation and a gestational carrier. This chapter provides an overview of single parenting by choice, discussion of the relevant psychological and social issues, and a framework for therapists to guide counseling sessions with prospective single parents by choice.

This chapter focuses on single women and men who actively seek to become single parents through fertility treatment, as these are the types of patients likely to be seen by fertility counselors. As the vignettes above illustrate, just as there is no typical mother, there is no typical single mother by choice. Selections from the actual words of single mothers by choice appear throughout the chapter to highlight the range of experiences single mothers by choice face as they navigate through the family building process. Because the idea that single men might choose to become parents is relatively new, the chapter is largely focused on women. Although many issues for men may be similar, we don't yet know enough about them to draw firm conclusions. Specific information associated with single men is noted when available.

Historical background

The societal context in which single individuals seek fertility care to have their own child has undergone dramatic change. References to the idea of single women requesting donor insemination (DI) first appeared in legal commentaries in the 1940s. Under the assumption that procreation should be strictly the domain of the "traditional family unit" (i.e.,

The addenda referred to in this chapter are available for download at www.cambridge.org/9781107643116. Password: AX164BKR7.

Fertility Counseling: Clinical Guide and Case Studies, ed. Sharon N. Covington. Published by Cambridge University Press.

heterosexual married couples), a US legislative ban on single women using DI was suggested, along with arguments that children born to single women using DI would be considered illegitimate [1]. In the 1970s, most providers refused to inseminate single women [2]. Some argued that such services should not be offered because the resulting child would be raised with limited financial resources, experience stigmatization for lack of a father, suffer poor psychological development due to lack of a male role model, and might not develop normal gender identity [3]. Some contended that single women requesting DI should be offered treatment, but only as long as they met various criteria such as evidence of adequate financial security and emotional adjustment [4–6]. Others argued that there was no sound legal or ethical reason to prohibit single women from using DI [7]. A significant shift began in the late 1980–90s toward more acceptance of patient autonomy with respect to fertility services. In 2006, the American Society for Reproductive Medicine's (ASRM) Ethics Committee published a powerful statement declaring that "denial of access to fertility services on the basis of marital status or sexual orientation cannot be justified" [8, p. 1333]. Similarly, in 2008, the United Kingdom Human Fertilisation and Embryology Act (HFEA) was revised to remove the clause that required clinics to consider the child's need for a father in decisions about whether to provide treatment [9]. These changes paved the way for more women to achieve single parenthood using DI. Internationally, there is a general shift toward many more countries allowing single women to use fertility services in recent years, although restrictions persist in many parts of Asia and the Middle East [10]. In many countries from the USA to the UK to China, there appears to be an increase in recent years in the number of women who choose to become single mothers [11–14].

It is difficult to assess precisely where "single mothers by choice" fit demographically within the broader category of "single mothers" because demographic research has generally not been able to distinguish the two groups. Although the negative consequences for children of being raised in single parent families (e.g., lower educational attainment, child behavioral problems) have consistently been highlighted, it has been argued that these findings do not fully apply to single mothers by choice because they have distinct characteristics as compared to single mothers via divorce, widowhood, or unintended pregnancy. Specifically, single mothers by choice tend to be older, successfully employed, have considered their decisions carefully, and intentionally planned to get pregnant [15–19].

The existing research on child adjustment further shows that family structural variables such as divorce, single parenthood, parent gender, parent sexual orientation and genetic relatedness between parents and children are less important factors than the quality of parenting, parent–child relationships, and the economic and social resources available to the family [20,21]. This suggests there is nothing inherently less optimal about being raised by a single parent by choice, provided the parenting quality and access to resources is adequate. Reflecting this equivalence, an emerging research literature on child and family adjustment indicates that families created by single mothers by choice are generally not different from other types of families; where differences appeared, they were in the direction of more positive functioning in single mother by choice families [22–25]. It should be noted, however, that the cultural context in which family structures operate may impact perceived acceptance and support, and affect parental functioning for single parents by choice. For example, in Israel, research has shown that single mothers by choice reported higher parental stress and lower general well-being than other family constellations, possibly because they felt less support. It may be that the cultural context in Israel, where traditional concepts of family structure dominate, could make it more likely that single mothers feel stigmatized or marginalized [26].

Although the discussion above concerned single women choosing parenthood, it is reasonable to hypothesize that similar conclusions could be drawn regarding the functioning and outcomes of single men choosing parenthood. Some evidence that single fatherhood by choice is on the rise can be inferred from media references. For example, popular media stories about the concept of single men by choice have appeared recently, describing unpartnered men deciding to become parents on their own. These stories further indicate that surrogacy and adoption agencies, as well as men's support groups, are reporting many more single gay and heterosexual men seeking to be parents than ever before [27,28].

Major considerations for prospective single parents by choice

Choosing single parenthood

Few people grow up thinking they will become single parents at all, much less single parents by choice. Rather, many people want to become parents at some point in their lives and expect to do so in the context of a loving relationship. Some women report feeling surprised and dismayed to find themselves in their late 30s or early 40s without a partner or children. Many have been in relationships or marriages that ended, and they had remained childless because either the relationship or timing was not right. Some women have had relatively few or even no serious relationships. Some have been actively pursuing the goal of finding a life partner, while others have not. Some have been very involved in career development, therefore postponing marriage and childbearing. Some have delayed parenthood due to medical problems, mental illness, or family of origin commitments.

Given the variety of reasons why individuals may consider single parenthood by choice, it is not surprising that their attitudes about this decision also vary greatly. Some approach the idea of single parenthood with many fears and trepidations, while others feel optimistic and eager to proceed.

> *"I am an extremely self-sufficient, independent, strong-minded person and I was absolutely confident that this was what I wanted, and more importantly, this is how it was supposed to be. I felt in my bones it was the right choice for me! I still worry about whether my son will suffer one day because I decided to have him without a father in the picture; but – at the same time – I just can't say I'm sorry. If I had done it another way, I would not have the son I do now and he is entirely too precious for me to be anything other than thrilled to have him."*
>
> *"First off, I never wanted to do this by myself. I am heartbroken that I will never truly have the family I always wanted. I will never have a husband who is the father of my children. I am already heartbroken for my future child that they will never have a father."*

The reasons for single people to want parenthood are usually no different than for married people (e.g., "I have always wanted to be a mother") and do not require further justification. Most women report that the reason to start trying to become a parent when they did was that they were getting older, they felt the time was right and they felt financially ready [29]. Some women have not always wanted to become mothers, but find themselves seriously considering it later in life.

Often, the decision to become a single mother is difficult because it means relinquishing the traditional image of becoming a family, including falling in love, getting married and expecting a baby (in that order). For some, attachment to this traditional conceptualization of family is very strong. These women struggle with such issues as grief over the loss of the idea of a two-parent family and self-perception of failure at traditional family building. For example, the woman below remarked on her initial consideration of becoming a single mother.

> *"The closer I got to my 39th birthday, the more I lost hope that I would find a relationship lasting and meaningful enough for me to want to start a family. When all of my tests were completed I was stunned when the doctor told me I could start immediately. Up to that point, I was just researching. I think I was still mourning the loss of the dream of a traditional family with mother, father, and children."*

Many women fear that they might lose the chance to have a genetically related child due to their "biological clock" running out. Many think about becoming a single mother for a long time, having told themselves when they were younger something like, "If I don't find the right person by the time I am 35 or 40, I will use a donor."

For some women, finding a romantic partner is not important, but many single mothers by choice do hope to find a future partner. Some are afraid that if they have a baby as a single woman, it will further reduce their chances of finding a partner. Pursuing single motherhood most likely will postpone finding a new partner. During pregnancy, dating is unlikely due to the emotional and practical complications. After becoming a parent, women experience the time demands of new parenthood and may be concerned about bringing a new partner into their child's life. Most women feel that male role models are at least somewhat important for children, and many are at least a little concerned about their child growing up without a father. The positive side, however, may be that women no longer feel the same intense time pressure to find a partner in order to become a parent and may be willing to consider a wider range of potential partners (e.g., those who already have children of their own).

Raising children well takes emotional, social and economic resources. Consideration of these factors is part of the decision about whether to become a single parent. Women consider job stability, maternity leave, childcare and financial planning. They consider their living arrangements, community and distance from family and friends. They consider their work – life balance and how they would fit the time needed for children. They review their social network for sources of emotional and instrumental support, evaluating how family and friends will react to the idea of single parenthood. They consider who would be able to help them if they had financial problems, got sick, and even who could raise their child if they were to die prematurely. They consider the possibility of having a child with special needs or medical problems. Although all these concerns apply to couples considering parenthood, they are amplified in the case of being the sole parent.

> *"While there are certain benefits to raising a child in the way that I see fit, without having to run decisions by someone else, being the only decision maker will also be a huge responsibility. I worry that I will not have the energy needed to raise a child on my own. I am concerned about the finances, how I will juggle working with childcare, how I will get my kid into a good school…"*

Men probably face similar considerations, though it is likely that their decisions are less biologically driven. That is, because men can become genetic fathers later in life than women, the situation may not take on the urgency that many women feel (though this may be changing due to recent research suggesting paternal age is related to risk of disorders, such as autism in the offspring [30]). Conversely, men likely face greater concerns about how their social network would react if they chose single parenthood, and they may worry they won't receive as much in the way of assistance or support.

Complications associated with current or recent relationships

In practice, we find that current or recent intimate relationships can complicate the process of considering single parenthood. Some women are in a relationship that does not appear to be leading toward having children in the near future (e.g., the relationship is too new or the partner is uncertain about having children). In such cases, it would be difficult to remain in the relationship while also pursuing single parenthood. Emotionally, trying to get pregnant and being pregnant are times when women want support from intimate partners. If the partner isn't intending to become a co-parent, she may feel very alone, and the partner may feel neglected or rejected. Practically, for heterosexual couples, it is difficult because the woman may need to avoid sexual intercourse to avoid possible pregnancy, particularly if her treatment protocol involves ovarian stimulation. Thus women often find themselves considering whether to continue the relationship with the hope that it will eventually lead to having children (knowing that this might risk waiting too long given their reproductive potential), or to sacrifice the relationship to pursue single motherhood.

> *"I never had a burning desire to become a mom, but at age 37, I discovered that I was finally really content in life, and had so much good to share with a child. I was in a go-nowhere relationship, neither good nor bad, but I knew I didn't want to have any legal, lasting ties with him. I did some research, and discovered the two major single moms by choice groups. Seeing that there were processes and methods to choose motherhood made it easier to move ahead. I started my testing and researching donors and gained more confidence. My relationship finally ended when I realized I was ready to do this on my own."*

Some women are struggling with recent relationship dissolution. An upsetting break-up can sometimes lead women to jump to single parenthood too quickly, out of fear they have wasted too much time on a disappointing relationship. Sometimes a relationship broke up because the man wasn't ready for commitment or for children, and the woman is hoping that starting the DI process will convince him of the intensity of her desire for children and he will change his mind and decide to proceed in trying to build a family with her.

Deciding the route to parenthood

The options for women are usually having a baby with donor sperm or adoption. Using donor sperm appears to be the more common method and is usually the one considered first. This option allows the woman to be genetically connected to the child and to experience pregnancy, which is often highly valued. Sperm donors are most commonly from a sperm bank but can also be a known donor, usually a close friend or more rarely an acquaintance. Possible benefits of a sperm bank donor as compared to a known donor include easy availability, previously completed medical testing and evaluation and a wide range of donor choices. Further, use of a sperm bank donor is often less expensive and does not have the complications associated with negotiating the emotional, financial and legal involvement of the sperm provider. Possible benefits of a known donor as compared to a sperm bank donor include knowing the donor's background and qualities in a more significant way than from a donor profile, as well as having the potential for the child to know or even have a positive, ongoing relationship with the sperm donor. In some cases, single women may intend for a known donor to have a role in raising the child (often thought of as an "uncle-type" relationship) even though she will be the only legal and custodial parent.

Working with a known donor is typically more complex emotionally, because both parties (and the donor's partner, if he has one) must consider their intentions regarding the relationship between the donor and the offspring, disclosure to the child and others and any legal and financial issues. Working with a known donor is more complex practically as well, because arrangements must be made for medical screening, psychological screening, semen analysis, infectious disease testing and providing samples for cryopreservation. If the donor doesn't live nearby, there may also be travel time and costs. Cryopreservation of sperm is generally the most practical plan because of the complexities of infectious disease testing, and because it allows the woman to proceed with multiple treatment cycles without repeat involvement of the sperm donor. Known donors can donate as a "directed donor" at a sperm bank, thus using the sperm bank's services but offering the sperm only to the intended recipient, or they can donate directly at the fertility clinic the woman is using. Although many women consider known donor arrangements, most do not proceed with them because they don't have a candidate they feel comfortable with or feel the unknown aspects of the future relationship are too complicated.

"The idea of a known donor appealed to me for maybe two seconds and then I thought of all the possible legal and social ramifications. What if he wants to be involved? What if he sues for custody or visitation? Will my child be confused as to the role this person plays in his or her life? Will others be confused? I felt going with a sperm bank was the safer option."

Choosing a sperm bank donor is relatively simple logistically, yet can present psychological challenges. Some women approach donor selection with relative ease, narrowing down the most important characteristics of their choosing without difficulty (e.g., physical characteristics, education, ethnic background). Some women experience significant discomfort taking this step because it means fully accepting not having a partner, not really knowing the person, and the fear that they will make a poor choice. Some women also have difficulty making the transition from internet dating to internet donor selection, having had many disappointing experiences with the former. Some women believe choosing someone to be the genetic father of one's child online feels too impersonal.

As they have become more available, many women are choosing donors who agree to potential contact with the child when the child is 18 [31]. Donors with this status are termed "willing to be known," "identity release," or "open" donors.

"I wanted an open ID donor so my child would have the option of contacting them at some point in adulthood if that was their choice."

An identity release donor seems to be a benefit for the child and the parent–child relationship as parents will likely feel better knowing that if their child wants more information about the donor in the future, they have done what they can to provide that option. Some prospective mothers are concerned that the donor might later interfere with family life, or that the child will discover negative information about the donor that could be upsetting. However, research shows that parents who chose an open identity donor felt positive about the idea of their child being able to have contact if they desired it, and none regretted the decision to choose an open-identity donor [32]. It is important to note that choosing a willing to be known or identity release donor is not a guarantee that a child will be able to have contact with their donor in the future, as illustrated in the thoughts expressed below.

> *"While I used an open donor, the fact is, it's a crapshoot. I have heard that there is no guarantee that the sperm bank will really contact him on my child's behalf. There needs to be more transparency surrounding open donors and what that means."*

Adoption tends to be considered after failed fertility treatment, or if the woman is already past a viable age for pregnancy. Some single women prefer adoption because the idea of becoming a parent to a child in need appeals strongly to them and they do not have a strong desire for pregnancy. The adoption process, however, is complex (see Chapter 14). Many countries do not allow single women to adopt; those that do often involve long waits and rarely offer the adoption of infants. US domestic adoption is possible for single women, but this may also involve long waits. Further, there is a presumption that many birth mothers prefer to place their child in a two-parent family.

Some women do not use any of the above options and instead decide to try to become pregnant via fresh home inseminations or intercourse with a man whom they plan on not involving in raising the child, either by prior agreement or by not telling him. Women who pursue this path do not usually see fertility counselors unless they are experiencing fertility problems. The major appeal of this path is that it requires no medical treatment, no financial costs and may be readily available. A major issue is that it leaves the woman at higher risk for sexually transmitted diseases. Further, in most jurisdictions, the man would be considered the legal father of the child, meaning he would have rights and responsibilities to the child and could assert them unexpectedly. In addition, having a known sperm provider who did not consent is likely not a benefit to the child compared to a sperm bank donor; conflict between parents could have a negative impact on the child and the father is unlikely to play a positive role in the child's life.

The options for single men are adoption or having a baby with an egg donor and a gestational carrier. Adoption options for single men are perhaps even more limited than for single mothers, due in part to continued strong societal beliefs in the importance of having a mother [33]. Moreover, media reports suggest that the intentions of single men are still considered suspect [27,28]. The benefits of egg donation and surrogacy are that this allows the man to be genetically connected to the child, to have more control over the process, and to be involved in the pregnancy. The major barrier is that it is costly ($75 000–$100 000), which is likely prohibitive for most men.

In terms of the process for the latter option, egg donors may be recruited through an agency or may be someone known to the man (friend or acquaintance). The decision about known versus anonymous egg donors is similar to the decision about sperm bank donor versus a known donor for women. Gestational carriers can also be recruited by an agency or via websites, or they could be a friend, sister, or acquaintance. Because the surrogacy process requires the involvement of two women at the time of treatment, men experience significantly less control over the pregnancy process, thus making the barriers greater for single men to proceed (for more on surrogacy, see Chapter 9).

Facing infertility

Single women are often at high risk of facing age-related infertility as they often try to become parents in their late 30s or early 40s. As noted above, going through the fertility treatment process on one's own can be challenging as one copes with the emotional, financial and logistical challenges of treatment.

> *"Going through fertility treatments as a single person is incredibly difficult. I can do a lot of things myself and I am highly independent, but it would be so much easier to have a spouse to help bear it. I didn't have a husband who I could force to give me shots. I basically had to tell myself, if I was planning to be this kid's mother and father, I better 'man up' and get over my fear."*
>
> *"I think that for anyone going through fertility treatments it is hard emotionally – whether it's more of a challenge for single people is up for debate; because as nice as it would be to have someone going through the struggle beside you, even a coupled person isn't guaranteed comfort from that other person. It's all very isolating. The only difference between the single woman and the coupled woman is that the single woman has no choice but to face those feelings alone. If the coupled woman is lucky and has a supportive, sensitive partner, she'll have some measure of comfort that another person is sharing her exact pain. I don't think that necessarily makes it easier though."*

Further, if fertility treatment is unsuccessful or unaffordable, the experience of not being able to have a child from one's own eggs can be emotionally devastating.

> *"Overall, to characterize the experience, it is tough. It has been frustrating, exhausting, disheartening, draining, depressing, anxiety-filled, not to mention physically challenging. It is an awful feeling, as a woman, to not be able to manage what we are biologically intended to do. It makes you feel like a failure at a level you never anticipated. I realized at a very young age that my purpose in life was to raise children. So realizing that the possibility of this actually happening was now slim, is rough, to say the least."*

Trying to have a child with egg and sperm donation is an option some women pursue, depending on financial resources, but it is often difficult to accept and means that the child will not have a genetic connection to any parent. Single infertile women sometimes consider adoption after failed fertility treatment but often face difficulties associated with being single and their older age. Embryo donation is a promising option for single women who cannot use their own eggs, but in practice it is often not available, particularly to single women as some agencies and donors do not support single women as embryo recipients.

While facing infertility as a prospective single mother by choice can be daunting, there may be a positive side as well. Specifically, a single woman can make the treatment decisions she is most comfortable with without needing agreement from a partner. Some women feel there is relief in not having someone else to be disappointed and to have to negotiate decisions with. This may help in giving her a greater sense of control over the infertility treatment process.

Raising a child as a single parent by choice

Single parents by choice generally experience the same joys and challenges as any other parent. Below are some of the unique challenges. First, single parents of any type face the entire parenting load without someone to share in the day-to-day care of the child or navigate times of crisis.

> *"I struggle financially because even though I have a good job, it is still only one income. I struggle to save money for a rainy day and still afford preschool, retirement, savings for my son and future college. I also felt the need to get a will done quickly because I am my son's sole parent and if something happens to me, I wanted to make sure my estate went to him and set up the chain of guardianship ..."*

Again, however, the flip side is that single parents have the freedom to make the decisions they want for their child and they may experience more closeness with their child. In addition, their children may be less likely to experience interparental conflict, and they may become more independent and mature. When asked about experiences raising their child, many single mothers by choice did not feel that they were having more difficulties than other mothers.

> *"I suppose the challenge will always be managing alone, whether it's the financial constraint, running simple errands, or having another person to bounce ideas and child rearing strategies with. However, the benefit is that you won't have to negotiate at every turn either. The name gets to be 100% your choice as does the nature of discipline and even the sports/activities that they play."*

Single parents of any type are vulnerable to disapproval from family, friends and their community. Some experience criticism from others regarding their decision to become a single mother. While single parents by choice may feel their decision to raise a child alone is justified by their preparation and resources, others may challenge that idea and believe that the child is not getting the right upbringing.

> *"I have had mostly positive responses to what I have been doing, but I definitely have friends who think what I am doing is very selfish. I do not disagree. I am intentionally having a child who will not have a father. This is obviously about creating happiness and fulfillment in my life. But I also am not sure why, just because I am a single person, people seem to think I have less of a right to create that happiness."*

Men may face even more stigmatization and judgment from others, as well as disbelief in their ability to effectively parent alone, given societal beliefs about the primacy of the mother–child relationship. Because they are less common, single fathers may feel more isolation and have fewer opportunities for socializing with other parents. They also may be left out of single-parent support groups.

Knowing how to ask for or accept support can be a challenge. For example, some single parents by choice feel that since they decided to have a child willingly, they aren't entitled to complain or ask for support. In other cases, because some individuals have been single for significant part of their adult lives and are quite self-sufficient, they may not be accustomed to asking for help. They may need to strengthen their support network and learn to ask for support, both practical and emotional.

Talking to the child about biological origins

One of the major challenges single parents by choice face is how and when to talk to their children about their family constellation, why they don't have another parent, how they were conceived, and the role of any other individuals who were part of their story (e.g., donors, gestational carrier). Most single-parent families intend to tell their child their family building story. It appears that single mothers using DI disclose to their children at a younger age than heterosexual couples do, and parents and offspring report primarily neutral or positive experiences associated with disclosure [32,34–36]. The largest study to date of DI offspring (ages 9–40) found that most children of single mothers report no negative effects of being donor-conceived, with about 36% reporting they feel "different," 47% reporting that it "makes no difference," and only 7% reporting they feel "confused" [37]. These reactions were highly dependent on the age they were told about their origins, with those who had "always known" reporting very low levels of confusion and those who learned after age 18 reporting much higher levels of confusion.

Donor offspring may want information about their donors and about other offspring conceived via the same donor [35,38]. This strong interest is reflected by the fact that several networks have been organized to enable this type of contact (e.g., the Donor Sibling Registry), as well as from the growth in the number of sperm banks in the USA and Europe that offer open-identity donor programs. It appears that donor sperm offspring of single mothers may have the highest level of interest in making contact with their donors and with other offspring born from the same donor, as compared to donor sperm offspring of heterosexual couples or lesbian couples. This may be because they do not have another parent who might feel hurt by the child's interest in the donor [37–39]. The primary reasons offspring seek contact appear to be: (1) to see what the donor looks like; (2) to see what the donor is like as a person; and (3) curiosity about genetic ancestry and medical history. In some cases, offspring are also interested in establishing an ongoing relationship with their donor [35,37]. Thus far, existing evidence suggests that when donor offspring make contact with their sperm donor (or other offspring of that donor), the effects tend to positive or neutral rather than negative. Table 12.1 offers a spotlight on offspring for single parents by choice.

Table 12.1 Guidance for single parents by choice.

Spotlight on the offspring
• *Historical conceptualizations.* In the past, it was erroneously believed that children born to single mothers by choice would experience poor psychological development and might not develop normal gender identity.
• *Effects of family structure.* Current research shows that there is nothing inherently less optimal about being raised by a single parent by choice.
• *Child adjustment.* Families created by single mothers by choice are generally not different from other types of families; where differences exist, they are in the direction of more positive functioning in single mother by choice families.
• *Disclosure decisions.* Single parents by choice must decide how and when to talk to their children about their family constellation, why they don't have another parent, and how they were conceived.
• *Timing and effect of disclosure.* Early disclosure can help promote a feeling of security and strength within the family. Most children of single mothers report no negative effects of being donor-conceived.
• *Seeking contact with the donor.* Some offspring seek contact with their donor, with the primary reasons being to see what the donor looks like, what he is like as a person, and to learn more about genetic ancestry and medical history.
• *Preparing parents for talking with children.* The counselor should discuss when and how to talk with children about their donor origins and provide sample stories for clients.

Psychosocial consultation with prospective parents

Setting the goals

The counselor should begin by orienting the client to the purpose and goals of the session, indicating that they will be covering the primary concerns and decisions that single people considering parenthood face. Although fertility counselors may be asked to evaluate a single person's suitability for parenthood or appropriateness for treatment, we argue that this is not an appropriate role. Instead, counselors should be conducting psychoeducational sessions to review the clinical issues presented above as they relate to the individual, help the individual assess whether single parenthood is right for them, clarify decisions and future plans, share information and resources, and identify areas in which further support or exploration may be beneficial. Typically, the counselor helps the individual to review and assess his or her own readiness.

It is essential to share with the client that the session is not intended to determine his or her fitness for parenthood. Prospective single parents may be worried about being judged and can be resentful of any requirement that they see a counselor. The successful counselor needs to directly address these concerns at the beginning of the session. Even so, some individuals may be resentful of the counseling mandate or may be reluctant to share concerns out of fear that the counselor may recommend against proceeding with treatment. If the session is made optional, this may likely lead to few people opting to take advantage of it.

> *"I was forced to meet a counselor by my clinic. I felt that because I was single, I needed to justify wanting a baby. I thought it was horribly discriminatory and offensive. I had already done my research, and could have taught her a few things. It was a complete waste of $250. I feel counseling should be offered to those who desire it, but it should not be forced."*
>
> *"Counseling was a routine part of the pre-treatment protocol. I was surprised to find it interesting and stimulating, I thought I'd worked everything out already! Eighteen years later I'm still discovering aspects I'd not thought of…"*

Background

The next step is to review how the individual got to where they are today with regard to considering single parenthood. This usually involves a brief review of personal and relationship history as it pertains to the goal of parenthood. Understanding how the individual arrived at their current plan to pursue single parenthood by choice helps both the counselor and the client consider the context in which decisions are being made. For example, if there has been a recent relationship dissolution, it is important to consider whether sufficient grieving of the relationship loss has occurred and if the individual is ready to face the challenges of pregnancy and single parenthood. Note that this should *not* be a detailed review of all relationship history or of reasons why relationships have not been successful; this is not relevant to the goals of the session and can increase feelings of failure and fear of judgment. As discussed previously, there is no profile for the single parent by choice and thus attempts to fit individuals into one can break the therapeutic alliance.

Review of the decision to become a single parent

When individuals decide to move forward with becoming a single parent, it is typically a confluence of several factors working together: they perceive adequate financial security; there is at least some support in their social network for the idea; becoming a parent currently feels like a stronger goal in their lives than finding a partner; they feel reasonably positive about bringing a child into the world or their lives without another parent; and, for women, they feel the time for biological parenthood cannot wait any longer. Still, even for those who feel sure about moving forward, counselors should encourage clients to express fears or concerns about whether this is the right choice for them. This can help them work through potential current and future challenges and feel more confident in their decisions.

If a client is unsure, the fertility counselor can help the person judge his or her level of readiness and use interventions aimed at reduction of decisional conflict. This might involve using imagery. For example, the counselor could ask the client to imagine his or her life over the next five to ten years and consider whether it feels more important to become a parent or to find a partner. Sometimes at this point, it becomes clear that poor self-esteem, unresolved previous relationship issues, or mental health problems exist, and the counselor can recommend ongoing counseling aimed at further emotional processing.

Social support review

The fertility counselor should initiate a discussion of how the client has talked (or will talk) to family, friends, acquaintances and co-workers about their decision to become a single parent. If support from family and friends is not strong, it may be important to help support the individual in creating opportunities to build their social support network. Most prospective single parents are not yet aware of the support organizations available to them (see Addendum 12.1). Helping them connect with these resources is very important as it helps individuals to feel less alone, provides practical information about how other people have considered the decisions about donor choice, and can provide parenting support. Mikki Morrisette, author and originator of the organization Choice Moms states, "Our children tend to grow up feeling extremely loved, benefiting from dedicated and attentive parenting. We tend to be fiercely determined women, if we make this choice, and that comes out in our role as mothers. My biggest piece of advice tends to be that we need to build a social life, and a support network, from the beginning. Women who are feeling isolated, highly stressed about career or lack of partner, need to apply resiliency to their thinking process, to find solutions with the help of community" (personal communication, February 11, 2014).

Deciding how to proceed

If the client is considering a known gamete donor, counselors should discuss the nature and history of the relationship between them, and review issues such as plans for the relationship between the child and the donor and disclosure to the child and others. Individuals should further be asked to consider the donor's role in the case of illness, financial problems, or death of the single parent in order to clarify expectations. This discussion can be difficult because people will often feel they are unable to know in advance how they will feel later. It is important to help the client to consider that either party could change their feelings or views in the future. Known donors (and the donor's partner, if any) should be scheduled for a psychological consultation appointment in which all of the aforementioned issues are reviewed. Gestational carriers (and their partner, if any) require a psychological screening. In this case, psychological testing is often used to supplement the information obtained from the clinical interview with the carrier. (See Chapters 9 and 10 for more information.)

Our clinical experience suggests that known-donor arrangements can be very satisfactory for all involved, as they provide the possibility for the child to have first-hand knowledge about their donor and his genetic heritage. However, if the relationship between the donor and the child's parent is conflictual or strained, or if there are unmet expectations, this can be quite challenging for the donor, the recipient parent and the child to cope with. For example, the potential recipient and donor must discuss how they might feel if the child wanted more time with the donor than he was willing to give, or if the donor wanted more involvement in the child's life. Some clients may be considering gamete donation from prior or even current intimate partners. Such potential known donors should be considered only with extreme caution, as expectations about the future nature of the relationship are often murky and the question of parental rights and responsibilities are quite unclear.

For individuals in the process of choosing sperm bank donors or recruited egg donors, the fertility counselor should help the recipient consider what he or she feels are the most important characteristics. Initial considerations often center around ethnic background, physical characteristics, health history, educational background and personality. Recipients should be encouraged to consider the profile in light of what it would be like to share the information with offspring in the future. They can also be instructed to ask themselves if they would feel positive about the concept that some aspects of who the donor is are part of who their child is, and that the donor helped them become a family. Often this reframing helps the recipient view donor selection more positively.

For clients considering conceiving via intercourse or insemination at home with a known donor, the counselor should provide information about risks including sexually transmitted infections. They should also be educated that in most jurisdictions, the known-donor concept and its protections only applies when there is a licensed medical provider involved and legal consultation should be recommended. For clients considering adoption, referrals listed in Addendum 12.1, plus other local referrals should be given and support through the process should be offered.

Talking to children about how they were conceived

Many single men and women planning to become parents have not thought in much detail how they would approach this topic. The counselor should discuss when and how to talk with children about their donor origins. In our experience with prospective mothers, while this discussion is welcomed by some, others seem to feel it is premature, particularly if they are anticipating difficulty getting pregnant. Such women may feel frustrated by being asked to consider what they would do in the lucky circumstances in which they are successful, when they are mostly concerned that they won't have that opportunity. The counselor must acknowledge these fears before a useful discussion of future disclosure can be initiated. Specific issues to help clients consider include: what they will say to their child, how the child might feel about this information and how the child might feel about not having another parent. Some women are hoping not to have to disclose if they find a new partner when the child is young; the fertility counselor should then address why disclosure is still important in these circumstances. If the woman is not using her own eggs to conceive, she may feel less comfortable disclosing the need for egg donation than sperm donation, feeling this might be too confusing for a child. In these cases, the fertility counselor should address why disclosure about egg donation might seem more difficult due to feelings associated with infertility and why it is still important.

Based on research and clinical experience, we recommend that the disclosure process should start when the child is young. Early disclosure can help promote a feeling of security and strength within the family. Prospective parents are often concerned that if they start too young the child will be confused. The fertility counselor can help with this concern by describing how to talk to children in a developmentally appropriate manner. It is helpful to provide sample stories for clients. Even for those who feel talking to children about their origins sounds reasonable, they may be unsure about how to begin and often feel comfort from hearing a concrete example. The counselor can remind the person that the actual story would be in the parent's own words and would grow in a gradual, natural way from conversations with their child. Here is a very simple sample story for a young child:

> *"Let's talk about the story of how we became a family. A long time ago, I wanted so much to be a mommy and have a family of my own. I knew I had a lot of love to give a baby, but I also knew it takes a seed from a man and seed from a woman to have a baby, and I didn't have any seeds from a man. So, I went to a special place where men who had more seeds than they needed had given their seeds to share with someone else who didn't have any. A doctor helped me use those seeds and mix them together in mommy's tummy, so that I could have a baby. My tummy got bigger and bigger, and one day the baby came out. It was you! Then I was so happy because I finally had my baby to love and we were finally a family."*

A story like this provides a foundation for healthy family development. The parent can be encouraged to look for opportunities over time to bring up the story again and respond to questions. Parents-to-be often wonder how they would respond to questions such as, "Do I have a daddy?," "Where is my daddy?," or "Is the donor my daddy?" The counselor can discuss the client's feelings about the questions and encourage honest, straightforward responses like,

> *"All families are different. Sometimes people get married and have a family with that person and it makes a family of three. We are a family of two, and that is just the way I planned it. You don't have a daddy, you have a mommy who wanted you and loves you very much. And you also have lots of others special people who care a lot about you like your grandma and grandpa. They are part of our family too."*

Another question parents-to-be often struggle with is how to refer to the donor. Language such as "biological father" or "donor daddy" can be confusing for children, because these terms confuse the concept of genetic material and parenthood. Children understand fathers or daddies as someone actively involved in a child's life and may not understand why if the person is a father, they are not there. Instead the term "donor" or "special helper" is probably easiest, and can be explained as someone who gives a very important gift of a seed so that someone else can have a family. The parent can then express that he or she is thankful that there are people who help other people to have families by being donors.

As children grow older, their understanding of the idea of sperm donation and the donor's role in their own life story will develop and become more complex. Older children can determine for themselves the words they feel most comfortable using to refer to their donor.

Teens and young adults may have questions about the donor. They specifically may wonder what, if anything, they see in themselves that may come from the donor, and how being born with the help of donor sperm affects their identity. They may have a strong desire to receive more information about the donor, and possibly about other children born with the help of the same donor. The fertility counselor should reassure the parent that the child's curiosity about the donor, while often confusing for parents, is healthy. Prospective parents need to think about how they feel about the idea of contact between their donor-conceived offspring, the donor, and other offspring born from the same donor. There is no right answer to whether these types of contacts should be made or not, and each family will have to make sense of the meaning of such contact for themselves. Prospective parents need to know that their desires and intentions may not always match that of their child. Children may show little interest in contact even when parents made detailed plans for contact and, conversely, children may have a deep desire for more information about their genetic makeup when the parent thought it was of little importance. (See Chapter 18 for more discussion on disclosure.)

Reflection and summary

As recently as the 1970s, there was still significant controversy about whether donor insemination should be offered to single women in the USA. Now, in the USA and in many parts of the world, single parenting by choice is seen as another constellation in which healthy families grow. While single parenting by choice may be a more common and accessible an option than in the past, it is still inaccessible in many locations. Counselors should be aware of both public and private forms of stigma associated with single parenting, as well as feelings of loss that are sometimes associated with letting go of the idea of the "traditional" two-parent family.

As a fertility counselor, facing one's own biases is imperative: fertility counselors who personally believe children and families need both a mother and father in order to thrive should probably not work with prospective single parents or they risk compounding the existing stigma. A major challenge fertility counselors face is that our clients may view our role as judgmental or evaluative and, as a result, they may be reluctant to openly share their concerns. We want our clients to leave our offices feeling supported, strong and prepared. Counseling with prospective single parents by choice is often inspiring because it means sharing in the process of people taking active steps to forge a desired life path for themselves.

As a group, single mothers by choice tend to be demographically distinct from other categories of single parents (e.g., older, financially secure, well educated). Less is known about single fathers by choice. As we consider the ways in which single parents by choice are unique in their determined pursuit of parenthood, it is important not to set "choice" single-parent families as the model of good single-parent families, as doing so may serve to further emphasize negative connotations of other types of single-parent families (i.e., those created via divorce, death, or unplanned pregnancy). We hold that it is essential for counselors to believe in and support that *any* family arrangement can be a great way to raise healthy and happy children.

Acknowledgments

We thank all of the women who shared their fertility treatment experiences with us for this chapter. Their contributions provide a real-life portrait of the stories of single people pursuing parenthood.

References

1. Artificial insemination: Its socio-legal aspects. *Minn Law Rev* 1949; 145: 150–1.
2. Curie-Cohen M, Luttrell L, Shapiro S. Current practice of artificial insemination by donor in the United States. *N Engl J Med* 1979 Mar 15; 300(11): 585–90.
3. Kerr MG, Rogers C. Donor insemination. *J Med Ethics* 1975; 1: 30–3.
4. Strong C, Schinfeld JS. The single woman and artificial insemination by donor. *J Reprod Med* 1984 May; 29(5): 293–9.
5. Baetens P, Ponjaert-Kristoffersen I, Devroey P, Van Steirteghem AC. Artificial insemination by donor: an alternative for single women. *Hum Reprod* 1995 Jun; 10(6): 1537–42.
6. Englert Y. Artificial insemination of single women and lesbian women with donor semen. Artificial insemination with donor semen: particular requests. *Hum Reprod* 1994 Nov; 9(11): 1969–71.
7. Kritchevsky B. The unmarried woman's right to artificial insemination: a call for an expanded definition of family. *Harv Women's Law J* 1981 Spring; 4(1): 1–42.
8. Ethics Committee of the American Society for Reproductive Medicine. Access to fertility treatment by gays, lesbians, and unmarried persons. *Fertil Steril* 2006; 86: 1333–35.

9. Human Fertilisation and Embryology Act (c. 22), (2008).
10. International Federation of Fertility Societies. International Federation of Fertility Societies Surveillance 2010. Available from: http://c.ymcdn.com/sites/www.iffs-reproduction.org/resource/resmgr/newsletters/iffs_surveillance_2010.pdf. Accessed October 2014.
11. Hamilton BE, Martin JA, Ventura SJ. Births: Preliminary data for 2010. *National Vital Statistics Report* [Internet]. 2011. Available from: http://www.cdc.gov/nchs/data/nvsr/nvsr60_02.pdf. Accessed October 2014.
12. Mosher WD, Jones J, Abma JC. Intended and unintended births in the United States: 1982–2010. *National Health Statistics Reports* [Internet]. 2012; 55. Available from: http://www.cdc.gov/nchs/data/nvsr/nvsr60_02.pdf. Accessed October 2014.
13. French HW. Single mothers in China forge a difficult path. *The New York Times*. 6 April 2008.
14. United Kingdom Office of National Statistics. *Statistical Bulletin: Families and Households, 2013.* 2013.
15. Pakizegi B. Emerging family forms: single mothers by choice – demographic and psychosocial variables. *Matern Child Nurs J* 1990 Spring; 19(1): 1–19.
16. McCartney CF. Decision by single women to conceive by artificial donor insemination. *J Psychosom Obstet Gynaecol* 1985; 4(4): 321–8.
17. Mechaneck R, Klein E, Kuppersmith J. Single mothers by choice: A family alternative. *Women Ther* 1987; 6(1–2): 263–81.
18. Eiduson BT, Kornfein M, Zimmerman IL, Weisner TS. Comparative socialization practices in traditional and alternative families. In: Lamb M, editor. *Nontraditional Families*. Hillsdale, NJ: Erlbaum; 1982.
19. Jadva V, Badger S, Morrissette M, Golombok S. 'Mom by choice, single by life's circumstance…' Findings from a large scale survey of the experiences of single mothers by choice. *Human Fertil (Camb)* 2009 Dec; 12(4): 175–84.
20. Lamb ME. Mothers, fathers, families, and circumstances: Factors affecting children's adjustment. *Appl Dev Sci* 2012; 16(2): 98–111.
21. Patterson CJ. Children of lesbian and gay parents: Psychology, law, and policy. *Am Psychol* 2009; 64(8): 727–36.
22. Golombok S, Tasker F, Murray C. Children raised in fatherless families from infancy: family relationships and the socioemotional development of children of lesbian and single heterosexual mothers. *J Child Psychol Psychiatry* 1997 Oct; 38(7): 783–91.
23. Murray C, Golombok S. Solo mothers and their donor insemination infants: follow-up at age 2 years. *Hum Reprod* 2005 Jun; 20(6): 1655–60.
24. Maccallum F, Golombok S. Children raised in fatherless families from infancy: a follow-up of children of lesbian and single heterosexual mothers at early adolescence. *J Child Psychol Psychiatry* 2004 Nov; 45(8): 1407–19.
25. Golombok S, Spencer A, Rutter M. Children in lesbian and single-parent households: psychosexual and psychiatric appraisal. *J Child Psychol Psychiatry* 1983 Oct; 24(4): 551–72.
26. Shechner T, Slone M, Meir Y, Kalish Y. Relations between social support and psychological and parental distress for lesbian, single heterosexual by choice, and two-parent heterosexual mothers. *Am J Orthopsychiatry* 2010 Jul; 80(3): 283–92.
27. Navarro M. The bachelor life includes a family. *The New York Times*. 7 September 2008.
28. Tuttle I. Single fathers by choice: The newest trend. *National Review Online*. July 2, 2012.
29. Morrissette M. *Choosing Single Motherhood: The Thinking Woman's Guide*. New York: Houghton Mifflin Company; 2008.
30. Reichenberg A, Gross R, Weiser M, Bresnahan M, Silverman J, Harlap S, et al. Advancing paternal age and autism. *Arch Gen Psychiatry* 2006 Sep; 63(9): 1026–32.
31. Scheib JE, Cushing RA. Open-identity donor insemination in the United States: is it on the rise? *Fertil Steril* 2007 Jul; 88(1): 231–2.
32. Scheib JE, Riordan M, Rubin S. Choosing identity-release sperm donors: the parents' perspective 13–18 years later. *Hum Reprod* 2003 May; 18(5): 1115–27.
33. Pakizegi B. Single-parent adoptions and clinical implications. In: Javier RA, Baden AL, Biafora FA, Camacho-Gingerich A, editors. *Handbook of Adoption: Implications for Researchers, Practitioners, and Families*. Thousand Oaks, CA: Sage Publications, Inc; 2007. pp. 190–216.
34. Jadva V, Freeman T, Kramer W, Golombok S. The experiences of adolescents and adults conceived by sperm donation: comparisons by age of disclosure and family type. *Hum Reprod* 2009 Aug; 24(8): 1909–19.
35. Scheib JE, Riordan M, Rubin S. Adolescents with open-identity sperm donors: reports from 12–17 year olds. *Hum Reprod* 2005 Jan; 20(1): 239–52.

36. Murray C, Golombok S. Going it alone: solo mothers and their infants conceived by donor insemination. *Am J Orthopsychiatry* 2005 Apr; 75(2): 242–53.

37. Beeson DR, Jennings PK, Kramer W. Offspring searching for their sperm donors: how family type shapes the process. *Hum Reprod* 2011 Sep; 26(9): 2415–24.

38. Scheib JE, Ruby A. Contact among families who share the same sperm donor. *Fertil Steril* 2008 Jul; 90(1): 33–43.

39. Freeman T, Jadva V, Kramer W, Golombok S. Gamete donation: parents' experiences of searching for their child's donor siblings and donor. *Hum Reprod* 2009 Mar; 24(3): 505–16.

Chapter 13

Counseling lesbian, gay, bisexual and transgender patients

Sarah R. Holley and Lauri A. Pasch

Susan (businesswoman, age 40) and Evan (lawyer, age 31) are a married couple in a major metropolitan city in California. Susan is female and Evan is a female-to-male transgender individual. They married in 2008 when same-sex marriages were first allowed, so they had legal marital status in the state. They had their first child (a daughter) in 2011, followed by a son in 2013.

To obtain sperm, they initially pursued known-donor options and asked a few men they thought might be a good fit. When one said no, they were crushed. Another agreed to do it, but by then they had moved toward the idea of using an anonymous donor. While they would have preferred a close friend who would leave the parenting to them but who the children could know, they were also highly aware of "horror stories" that could be involved in such a scenario. In the end, they chose to use an anonymous donor from a sperm bank, selecting a "willing-to-be-known" donor. They selected a donor with features similar to those of Evan's "so that our first child would look like a mix of us."

They decided Susan would carry both children. Evan noted, "It just made sense in our family for my partner to carry our child because she liked being pregnant and as a gender non-conforming person, I had decided that being pregnant, and all the femininity that is inextricably attached to that experience, would not work for me." For their first child, they used Susan's eggs because she was the one who wanted to have a baby more, and due to her age, it felt like it was "now or never." For their second child, they used Evan's eggs as they felt the younger eggs offered a better chance to successfully conceive. This brought up very mixed feelings for Evan. He noted, "As a genderqueer/trans person ... it was a somewhat challenging and awkward experience to be at a fertility clinic and doing estrogen shots to retrieve the eggs. I also ... gained a whole new level of gratitude around what my body was able to create, even though sometimes I wished that my body couldn't create them."

They described the process of becoming parents as "a bit stressful and incredibly expensive." Susan was 36 at the time they started treatment. Like many women at that age, she was not sure whether she could successfully become pregnant, so each attempt was emotionally trying. Susan's insurance did cover infertility, but according to the policy, they had to go through three rounds of insemination attempts before they could get any aspect of treatment covered. For their first child, they used IUI and were successful on the seventh cycle. Evan had to go through the second-parent adoption process to ensure he would have legal rights to their daughter. For their second child, they had to go through in vitro fertilization (IVF) due to their decision to use Evan's eggs. They used the same sperm donor for both, stating, "We thought it would be cool to have two kids that shared genetics with the same sperm donor but be genetically linked to each of their parents that they were raised by." They were successful on the first IVF cycle.

Evan observed that one of the largest challenges of the whole process was dealing with the insurance. He noted, "They don't view you the same, and I believe it costs us more as LGBT people. With IVF, it was really challenging around how to label me as the egg donor? And my partner as the surrogate? This was confusing for insurance, for the doctors, the hospital and for us. It was confusing to do the birth certificate as we didn't know which name should go where." Though they noted feeling lucky to have

The addenda referred to in this chapter are available for download at www.cambridge.org/9781107643116. Password: AX164BKR7.

Fertility Counseling: Clinical Guide and Case Studies, ed. Sharon N. Covington. Published by Cambridge University Press.

doctors and hospital staff who were supportive, knowledgeable and accustomed to working with diverse types of families, they still felt that the paperwork was insensitive and did not reflect all the types of family configurations that can be involved in the LGBT childbearing process.

Now, having successfully conceived two children, Susan and Evan have found that they have become repositories of information for queer couples looking to start families of their own. While in some ways they enjoy being able to help others figure out this process, they observed they had not known anyone they could turn to with questions when they were going through it and had felt very much on their own. Evan noted, "I think this could be helpful for fertility counselors to know just how little is out there comparatively to the experience of non-LGBT people/families. There is a lot of education around how cognizant we need to be around language and experience for folks that don't fit into the heterosexual binary model."

Introduction

This chapter provides the background needed for counseling lesbian, gay, bisexual and transgender (LGBT) women and men as they undergo fertility treatment. The story of Susan and Evan illustrates many of the challenges that LGBT couples may face, including making complex childbearing decisions, navigating a treatment system designed for infertile heterosexual couples and confronting barriers such as insurance issues and uncertain legal rights. The goal of this chapter is to highlight the primary issues that many LGBT couples confront during treatment, and to provide guidance for fertility counselors on specific considerations to factor in when working with this group of prospective parents. Many aspects of treatment are no different for LGBT couples as for heterosexual couples and therefore are covered elsewhere in this book. As such, this chapter focuses on aspects of treatment particular to sexual minority patients. Further, while many of these issues pertain to LGBT individuals who seek treatment, this chapter will focus on couples since the experience of single parents by choice is covered in Chapter 12.

The experiences of LGBT families are highly diverse, so case examples (in the form of vignettes provided directly by real patients) are included to illustrate the range of issues that can arise. Lesbian couples comprise a dyad with two women, and gay couples are a dyad with two men. Given this chapter's focus on couples, the experiences of bisexual patients (i.e., those who identify as sexually attracted to both men and women) will depend highly on the context of their current relationship. For example, if a bisexual woman is pursuing pregnancy with a male partner, the experience will be similar to that of heterosexual couples. If the bisexual woman is pursing pregnancy with a female partner, the experience will be similar to that of lesbian couples. Since lesbians represent the greatest proportion of LGBT fertility treatment patients, and because most research in this area is on the experience of lesbians, we note that much of the literature and vignettes presented come from lesbian couples. Specific information associated with gay and bisexual patients and their partners is highlighted when available.

For transgender individuals, their experience with fertility treatment will depend highly on the biological sex of the two partners. In the case of Susan and Evan, they were both biologically female. For the purposes of fertility treatment, their experience was that of a lesbian couple, with certain considerations linked to Evan's transgender identification. Thus, couples with a transgender partner may have fertility treatment options more similar to that of heterosexual couples (i.e., a male-to-female transgender individual partnered with a female, or a female-to-male transgender individual partnered with a male), a lesbian couple (i.e., a female-to-male transgender individual partnered with a female), or a gay couple (i.e., a male-to-female transgender individual partnered with a male). What is different is that transgender patients may have to contend with extra levels of bias or discrimination during treatment, as well as consider the effects that steps required for gender transitioning (e.g., hormone therapy, surgery) may have had on their reproductive functioning.

Of note, guidelines for appropriate LGBT-related terminology are ever evolving, so part of the fertility counselor's task is to be aware of contemporary conventions. For example, in current practice in the USA, the words "lesbian," "gay," "bisexual," and "transgender" are used as adjectives, not nouns (e.g., "Sam is a gay individual," rather than "Sam is a gay.") The term "homosexual" has largely fallen out of favor and should generally be avoided. Conversely, the term "queer" is coming back into use as a self-affirming umbrella term encompassing all non-heterosexual identities; fertility counselors, however, should only use this term if there is a compelling reason for doing so (e.g., quoting someone who self-identifies as queer). The term "transgender" is now commonly used as the term for individuals whose gender identity does not match his or her physical sexual characteristics. More specifically, "transgender man" refers to a person who was considered female at birth but identifies as male (this is also represented by the term "female-to-male transgender person," the acronym "FTM," or the colloquial term "trans man"); vice versa for the term "transgender woman." The term "transsexual" is considered antiquated and should generally be avoided. Some transgender individuals will use the term "genderqueer" to characterize all gender identities other than the binary categories of "male" and "female." The process by which transgender individuals change their characteristics is termed "gender transition" (not "sex change") and may include a change of name and/or pronouns, clothing, legal documentation and medical treatments. In general, the best rule of thumb is to determine what terms and gender pronouns the patient prefers, and to honor those preferences. For example, Evan identified as a "genderqueer/trans person" and used male pronouns. Other transgender people may prefer using gender neutral pronouns (e.g., ze, zir, sie, hir). A full review of all current conventions in LGBT terminology is beyond the scope of this chapter, but helpful resources can be found online (suggested links are provided in Addendum 13.1).

Background

It is important to have a sense of the various social and political forces that may influence LGBT patients' feelings about pursing fertility treatment, their access to services, or the attitude of treatment providers. Historically, homosexuality and the family were viewed as incompatible categories [1]. LGBT parents typically had children within a heterosexual relationship and then came out after the relationship dissolved [2]. But in recent years, a growing number of couples are *choosing* to become parents in the context of a same-sex relationship. US Census data indicates that, in 1990, 1 in 20 male couples and 1 in 5 female couples were raising children; these number rose to 1 in 5 males couples and 1 in 3 female couples by 2000 [3]. The trend will likely continue as same-sex couples gain marriage rights and as social attitudes shift toward greater acceptance [4,5].

Fertility treatments, however, have not always been accessible to LGBT couples. In the past, discrimination against LGBT patients was overt, with providers citing legal, ethical, or moral arguments against same-sex parenting [6,7]. In certain countries, this still remains the case. For example, there is no access to fertility treatment for lesbian women in Austria, Czech Republic, France, Italy, Portugal and Slovenia [8]. These laws are not always relics of the past. In 2013, in Denmark, the law was amended to allow non-anonymous sperm donation for only heterosexual couples; in Croatia and Malta, new laws expressly ban women in same-sex relationships from access to fertility treatment [9]. But, fortunately, the situation in many places has improved. In the United States, in 2006, the Ethics Committee of the American Society for Reproductive Medicine (ASRM) published a statement declaring, "The ethical arguments supporting denial of access to fertility services on the basis of marital status or sexual orientation cannot be justified" [10, p. 1333]. ASRM went on to conclude that there is no basis for denying LGBT patients access to treatment, highlighting the absence of scientific evidence that parenting effectiveness is affected by parental sexual orientation [11,12]. In the USA, the ethical directive garnered some legal enforcement in 2008 when the California Supreme Court ruled that refusal to treat a lesbian based on the physician's religious views violated state law [13]. Other countries have even stronger protections in place.[1] For example, in the United Kingdom, the 2008 Human Fertilisation and Embryology Act protects patients from discrimination on the basis of sexual orientation, and both partners in a same-sex couple (provided they are in a civil partnership or conceived in a licensed clinic) have legal parenting rights to their child from birth [14,15]. In Canada, the law unequivocally states that those seeking reproductive services cannot be discriminated against on the basis of sexual orientation [16].

Even in countries that provide ethical and legal protections, however, potential barriers are still present. Fertility treatment services are still largely

[1] The European Society of Human Reproduction and Embryology (ESHRE) has not published an ethical position paper on LGBT reproductive treatment, and thus is not mentioned when discussing ASRM policies. They do, however, provide information on the legal policies in each of the European Union countries (see Addendum 13.1).

designed around a partnered, heteronormative paradigm [6,17]. As examples, clinic forms may not be designed appropriately for non-heterosexual clients, written materials may presume infertility and insurance coverage may be difficult to access or blocked altogether [17–19]. LGBT couples may also encounter overt homophobia or heterosexist practices. For example, while the ASRM issued a clear ethical directive, the guidelines are not legally binding, and different US clinics may have widely discrepant access policies [16]. In general, it is important to recognize that the policies and laws governing LGBT access to reproductive services vary dramatically from state to state and country to country, and all are subject to change. As a result, prospective LGBT parents may be still be subject to biased attitudes or denied service, and they cannot necessarily rely on policies to remain stable as they pursue parenthood. Taken together, these social, political and legal factors may significantly impact the experience of fertility treatment for LGBT couples.

Clinical issues: decisions, decisions, decisions

For same-sex partners on the path to parenthood, there are no "oops babies" or opportunities to just try "naturally" for a period of time. Rather, the process is an inherently intentional one that requires considerable planning and coordination. The start of this "child project" first involves making a choice: to become parents [20]. By the time LGBT couples sit down with a fertility counselor, they typically have made this first decision [2]. From that point, a series of choices must be evaluated and decisions made: What reproductive options to pursue? Whose egg will be used? Whose sperm will be used? Who will carry the child? Where can LGBT-friendly services be found? What are each partner's legal rights? Will any of this be covered by insurance? A primary function of the fertility counselor is to help couples understand their options and the implications of their choices, as well as to support them through the evolving process of treatment. The counselor must additionally take into account complex interrelationships between social, legal, political and economic factors that may uniquely impact treatment options for LGBT patients [7].

Routes to parenthood

One of the first major decisions is what route to take to parenthood. For lesbian couples, there may be many possible options, while for gay couples, options are typically limited to surrogacy with egg donation or adoption. As noted above, for couples in which one member is bisexual or transgender, options will stem from the biological composition of the couple and their fertility potential. Specific considerations for LGBT couples are highlighted below.

Home insemination

Lesbian couples may use home insemination. This route involves vaginal insemination performed at home, either with the help of a known donor or with sperm from a sperm bank. Couples can use what has been called "turkey-baster technology" (e.g., a needleless syringe, eye dropper, cervical cap). Home insemination does not involve any medical staff, and couples may therefore feel a greater sense of autonomy and intimacy [20]. Further, it often represents the least expensive route.

> *"We did a home insemination using 'fresh' sperm from a known donor (my partner's brother)... the alternative insemination program route was going to take quite a long time – there was a lengthy application and interview process for our donor, he was going to have to travel to our city to make the 'donations,' and then there would be the six-month quarantine on the sperm. The cost of collection, processing and storage was also going to be very high. We decided to try the 'low tech' method in the interim as we got the application process underway."*

There are important considerations to keep in mind with home insemination. Some couples carrying out self-insemination may not feel supported or safe, or have easy access to professional support or medical assistance should they need it [14]. If using fresh sperm from a known donor, the donor may not have been screened for sexually transmitted diseases (STDs), so there may be a higher level of health risk. Finally, and perhaps most crucially, in some jurisdictions, known-donor sperm must pass through the hands of a licensed medical professional, otherwise the donor can be granted legal rights and responsibilities for the resulting child.

Clinic-based treatments

Clinic-based treatments may involve an initial meeting with a gynecologist or reproductive endocrinologist, a fertility evaluation and genetic testing. Some clinics require a meeting with a fertility counselor. The most common treatment option used is intrauterine insemination (IUI), but couples can make use of the full range of fertility services depending on their needs, including IVF, egg donation, or embryo donation. Often multiple medical interventions (e.g., blood work, ultrasounds, medications) are also part of the treatment. Some LGBT couples may be uncomfortable with the degree of medicalization, while others will welcome the interventions as helpful tools for conception [7,21].

> *"We did our procedures at a clinic, mainly because we wanted to do whatever we could to increase our odds for success. We figured if something like an IUI can ensure the sperm gets right where it needs to go, then let's do it. It took us seven cycles. The doctor always offered to let me squeeze the syringe. I can see why some people would like that – like they were a part of the conception. I always declined. For me, the syringe (and what was in it) was not a part of me, just a means to an end."*

Clinic-based treatments offer LGBT couples benefits that home insemination do not. If working with a known donor, the donor will have infectious disease testing. Working with a clinic offers greater protections of parental rights as the treatment process requires legal documentation defining parental status [7]. If pregnancy doesn't occur, fertility interventions can be added to the treatment protocol as needed. However, some clinic policies may seem involved and cumbersome. Further, as reflected in one of the vignettes above, these procedures add a great deal of time and cost to the process.

Surrogacy

For gay couples, the options include surrogacy with egg donation and adoption. Surrogacy allows one of the partners to have a genetic link to the offspring, which is often valued by couples. Building a family with surrogacy means involving several outsiders in the process, including an egg donor and a gestational carrier, as well as a fertility doctor, legal counsel and an agency to help find the donor and carrier.

Surrogacy is expensive (typically between \$75 000 to \$120 000) and the legal issues can be complicated. In some states and countries (e.g., New York and Japan), surrogacy is prohibited (regardless of sexual orientation). In other states and countries, surrogacy may be permitted, but policies may prevent same-sex couples from accessing these services. For example, in Florida, Nevada and Texas, gestational services are restricted to married couples. Because same-sex couples can't marry in these areas, they are by extension unable to use surrogacy [22]. In general, LGBT couples need to be very clear about the laws in their home state/country, the laws of the gestational carrier's home state/country and the laws of the state/country in which the carrier delivers. Gay men are advised to use a gestational carrier who will deliver in a jurisdiction where the men can obtain a pre-birth order recognizing one or both of them as legal parents – otherwise the carrier will be a legal parent until her rights can be terminated. In some states/countries, if the gestational carrier is married, they will additionally need an order of non-parentage so that her husband's name is not placed on the birth certificate [23]. Regardless of location, gay couples must also be certain to have legal contracts in place to define the rights and responsibilities of all parties involved [23].

Adoption or foster care

While adoption or foster care is an option for prospective LGBT parents, they again may face certain barriers. LGBT couples must first determine the policies of the state or the country from which they are attempting to adopt or foster. For example, as of 2014, 21 states in the USA (and Washington, DC) allowed same-sex couples to petition for a joint adoption; seven states had explicit obstacles to equal treatment (e.g., in Mississippi, same-sex couples are expressly prohibited from adopting); and in the remainder of states the regulations were unclear and decisions made on a case-by-case basis [24]. Policies for international adoptions can also vary dramatically. Due to the extreme variability of the laws, prospective parents should find out about laws in their jurisdiction and seek consultation at the outset of the adoption or foster process from either a family lawyer, state equality organization, or a national organization like the Human Rights Coalition (HRC) or the International Lesbian and Gay Association (ILGA) if needed [25].

Adoption agencies themselves can either function as supports or barriers. While many agencies work with LGBT prospective parents and are very helpful, others may not accept LGBT clients, may be less likely to place a child with LGBT families, or may demonstrate negative views toward same-sex families. Some agencies may operate on a "don't ask, don't tell" policy, which can be upsetting and confusing for clients [2,26]. Prospective parents should ask the agency about its track record in placing children with LGBT families, as well as the number of LGBT families it has worked with [25].

Complex arrangements

Until recently, LGBT families were frozen out of the institution of marriage and more "traditional" family structures. As a result, some couples have chosen to fully redefine what the notion of family entails. For example, a lesbian couple and a gay couple may decide to conceive children together and rear them together [27]. Other researchers have found that some lesbians may seek out gay donors, in part to give the donor an opportunity to take part in a parenting role that they might not otherwise have had [2]. Given the diverse paths lesbian and gay parents may take to family formation [27], fertility counselors need to be open-minded in supporting patients who may be creating relatively unique family structures. In these cases, the primary role of the counselor may be to help all parties involved consider the roles, rights and responsibilities of all of the individuals involved in the family system.

Gamete selection

Another major decision stems from whose gametes (i.e., sperm or egg) will be used. For cross-sex couples (i.e., in some dyads with a bisexual or transgender partner), the options are straightforward. For same-sex couples, presuming intact fertility in both partners, decisions will be based on a number of factors such as age, health and genetic history, family relationships and intensity of the desire to be a genetic parent. Some couples know in advance that they want to try to have more than one child, so then it becomes a question of whose gametes to use first. In some cases, infertility actually is an issue. For same-sex couples, this might mean that the other partner then becomes the gamete provider. Many times, some combination of any or all of these factors will be weighed in deciding which partner will provide half of the needed genetic material.

Same-sex couples are typically accepting of the fact that the child will only have a genetic link to one of the partners [2], though one job of the fertility counselor will be to make sure that any perceived loss around this issue has been processed. In surrogacy arrangements, some gay men ask that two embryos, one fertilized by each partner, be transferred to give the opportunity for both partners to have a genetic offspring. This scenario must be considered very carefully, however, because of the high risk of twins, the associated medical complexities for the carrier and the fetuses, and because (in cases when only one child is born) one partner may be disappointed in the end when he learns he was not the genetic provider. Sometimes men report that they do not want to know who the genetic provider actually was, but experience suggests that this is not advisable because of the uncertainty and confusion that can result (e.g., with the child's pediatrician, and later for the child him or herself).

Sometimes one partner in a same-sex couple has a sibling (i.e., a brother or sister of the partner who will be the non-biological parent) who is willing to be the donor and provide the missing gamete. This arrangement can bring up complicated emotional and relational dynamics, so couples will often forgo this route [28]. For those who do use a sibling donor, the fertility counselor will play an important role in helping the individuals involved carefully think through their roles and consider the long-term implications of this decision.

Carrier selection

For same-sex female couples, the choice to use one partner's eggs and which partner will carry often go hand in hand, though that is not always the case, as with Susan and Evan. A study by Goldberg [29] highlighted what is probably the most significant determining factor for lesbian couples: who has the greatest desire to experience pregnancy and childbirth.

> *"The first decision was that we would plan for two kids – one to be carried by me, the other by my wife … The hardest decision was which of us would go first. We both wanted to. In the end, I went first because I was ready first. She just wasn't quite there yet, in terms of thinking of physically carrying a child, and I was."*

Other factors that can impact the decision of who carries the child include: age of each partner, medical history, insurance benefits, attitudes of extended family and the presence of existing children [30]. Some considerations stem from practical implications, such as who has the most job flexibility or can most easily take time off.

Donor selection

For same-sex couples, a third party donor will inevitably be a part of the picture, but the decisions around the donor can vary greatly. For some couples, having a known donor is a major part of the process of family formation [7]. Prospective parents may want the child to know the donor and have some contact with them. This does not mean the couple necessarily wants the donor to take a parenting role, but they may want to give the child the chance to know more about his or her biological origins [2].

"Anonymous donor sperm was never an option for us. This was especially true for my partner. She said, 'I would just look at the kid and think Who Are You?' Likewise, we did not consider adoption – it's just not for us. Finding the perfect donor took time, painful experience and dumb luck. We were really looking for intangible things – character, ability to love and be loved, resilience – not just because we wanted to see those traits in the child, but because we wanted the donor to be a positive, loving presence in our child's life."

Other people prefer a known donor because they feel it gives them more control over the insemination process, or because they want more direct access to the donor's health and genetic history. Regardless of the motivation, an important consideration for LGBT couples using known donors is to openly discuss, in advance, what role that individual will play in the family unit, as well as to have a legal agreement in place wherein the known donor relinquishes all legal rights and responsibilities to the child

Some couples have a strong preference for an unknown donor. Two major motivations stem from legal reasons (i.e., nobody else can lay claim to the child) and from the desire to raise the child without outside interference from a third party [2]. Non-biological parents may prefer unknown donors as it would pose less of a threat to his or her status as an equal co-parent [31]. Many sperm banks have increasingly popular "identity release" (or "willing-to-be-known") options, wherein the donors allow the sperm bank to pass along requests for contact information from the offspring after they turn 18 [30]. This may be an appealing option for many LGBT couples as it enables them to engage in family formation without the involvement of an outside party, but still provides the offspring the later possibility of obtaining information about their biological origins.

"We used anonymous donor sperm from a bank. We chose ID release so our child would have the option to contact him if desired... We started our search limiting it to ID release donors and using characteristics of my wife – eye color, hair color, skin tone. We don't expect our offspring to look like my wife but we wanted our child to look like she was born into this family, as she was. We then read profiles and likes and interest. My wife and I met working at summer camp and the donor we ended up choosing also indicated his love of working with kids at camp. We call him 'camp guy.'"

Specific challenges for LGBT patients and their partners

This chapter will now examine some of the specific challenges that LGBT couples face when receiving fertility treatment. While each area is addressed individually, it should be recognized that these social, legal, political and economic forces are often inextricably interwoven in ways that may significantly affect treatment for LGBT couples.

Navigating a heteronormative system

The majority of fertility treatment services are targeted toward heterosexual women, and partners are presumed to be husbands. This heteronormative approach is reflected in the very term "infertility counseling" or "infertility treatment" that is used by providers. That is, these services were designed for people who met the criteria for infertility (defined as 12 months of regular, unprotected heterosexual intercourse without a successful conception). This construct does not create space for the experiences of LGBT couples. Take the example of a perfectly healthy lesbian in the USA with no known risk factors for infertility using anonymous donor sperm, who goes to a fertility clinic for IUI treatment. Based on clinic policy (and in accordance with ASRM guidelines), this patient would receive a fertility work-up and psychological counseling. All of this adds time and money to the process, and it can medicalize or pathologize a relatively straightforward situation.

"If you are going into a fertility clinic for help getting pregnant, it is difficult for them to get out of problem-solving mode. Everyone they deal with suffers from infertility issues. They default to interventions. As we told our doctor, the only problem we are solving for is that neither one of us makes sperm."

This heteronormative framework has far-reaching implications for non-heterosexual persons attempting to access services. On a practical level, it may create a mismatch between service offerings and the patients' needs. Clinic forms may not be designed appropriately for LGBT patients (e.g., they may specify "husband" and "wife"), and seminars or literature may presume infertility and focus on coping with loss [17]. For lesbian couples, the non-birth mother may experience a sense of invisibility throughout the entire conception process and beyond [2,17]. As examples, treatment providers may fail to acknowledge the non-birthing partner in office visits, and that partner may be systematically denied markers of parental rights to the offspring.

"We weren't allowed to put one of us on the birth certificate. All of the paperwork stated 'husband' or 'father' and had no language to support us in such a wonderful time in our life. The paperwork at times made us feel not the norm and very excluded."

The heteronormative framework can also have large implications for insurance coverage. Even when insurance provides some coverage for assisted reproductive technology (ART), the policy may contain criteria related to marital status (i.e., defining infertility as a condition of married couples or requiring use of the spouse's gametes) or require a diagnosis of infertility (which, defined in medical terms, presumes heterosexual sex) [18,19]. As reflected in Susan and Evan's case, this may create an undue cost burden for same-sex couples as compared to their heterosexual counterparts.

Confronting heterosexist bias

With firm support from the ASRM and some degree of legal protection in various countries, overt discrimination against treating LGBT fertility patients appears to be waning. Unfortunately, that does not mean it has disappeared. At the most severe, biases against LGBT parents may prevent access to services altogether. This is certainly true in countries that prohibit LGBT couples from receiving treatment, but it may also be the case where services are theoretically available. For example, a survey of ART programs in the USA found that (of those with data on sexual orientation), 17% reported they were likely or very likely to turn away a lesbian couple wanting donor insemination, and 48% reported they would turn away a gay couple wanting to use surrogacy [32]. Another study found that 14% of practicing obstetrician–gynecologists would discourage a woman in a lesbian relationship from using ARTs, and 13% would not help the woman obtain services [33]. Bias may also be manifest in more subtle ways. That is, services may not be explicitly denied, but they may be made more difficult to access for LGBT couples. This is reflected in the following vignette, shared by a couple wherein both partners are obstetrician–gynecologists:

"Our first donor lived in another state. So we contacted a local sperm bank there and tried to arrange for him to donate, and have them ship the sperm to us. When my partner called them as 'Dr. Smith' making arrangements for a patient, they readily agreed. Then, after talking to our donor, they learned that he was donating to a lesbian couple. All of a sudden their 'policies' did not allow them to ship sperm out of state."

At its most insidious level, stigmatizing attitudes about same-sex parents may be internalized and contribute to feelings of defectiveness or shame, or they might foster a sense of anxious anticipation [34,35]. Yager and colleagues [36] found that lesbian and bisexual women who were trying to conceive described expectations of encountering biased attitudes when meeting with ART service providers. This anticipation of discrimination, even absent actual discrimination, may contribute significant psychological distress to LGBT patients [35,36].

"I suppose the one challenge is the constant coming out. At the clinic or hospital there is always that moment of explaining – 'no, this is not my sister or friend, she is the mom of these babies too.' And you never know what you are going to get in response. We had no real problems but I guess an added anxiety."

Legal issues

The legal considerations for LGBT prospective parents can be complicated and may vary dramatically based on geography. As noted above, different states within the USA and different countries have differing policies regarding LGBT adoption and surrogacy, and these policies are subject to change. While the discussion in this section highlights considerations within the USA, similar issues occur in other countries.

Beyond the 2008 statute prohibiting discrimination based on religious beliefs, there currently is no federal policy in the USA regulating access to ART. As such, the law has limited ability to respond to LGBT barriers, and the question of who legally qualifies as a child's parents may be up for significant debate [22,23]. For LGBT couples, then, consultation with attorneys who specialize in family law may have to be an integral part of family creation. These legal specialists, who ideally are consulted before conception or adoption efforts begin, are involved in defining the rights and responsibilities of all involved parties, as well as planning for things such as the disposition of embryos and making arrangements in the event of the partners' separation or death [23]. Such legal issues can add cost, time and stress to an already long and arduous process.

"We have put a lot of thought, time and money into protecting our family legally and financially – things that straight families rarely have to think about. We're lucky to have the resources to do that. There are some scary things out there – what if our donor's parents freaked out and tried to take custody of the baby? What if something happened to me before my partner's adoption is complete? What if...?"

A major issue for LGBT couples pertains to getting legal recognition in place for both parents. For example, when a lesbian couple conceives a child, typically only the birth parent is recognized[2]. Similarly, in states where same-sex joint adoption is not allowed, often one person is on record as the adopting party. In these cases, same-sex couples have to go through a "second-parent" (or step-parent) adoption. Second-parent adoption allows a same-sex parent to adopt her or his partner's biological or adoptive child without termination of the first parent's rights, thereby providing all parties with legally recognized relationships with one another [30]. Unfortunately, however, second-parent adoption is not allowed in all states. Further, this process entails a period of ambiguity after the birth of the child wherein the non-biological or non-adopting parent has to wait for her or his rights to be instated. Second-parent adoption is a time-intensive and expensive process. It can also feel discriminatory to LGBT couples, who are the only real *parents* the child will ever know.

"Because I am not the birth mother, I have to complete a second-parent adoption... I have to get references from four people, fill out a ton of paperwork, be interviewed by a social worker, and get my work to fill out an employment verification, among other things... It's a little insulting that I'm somehow the 'step-parent' by legal definition when I'll always be known as Mom to our child."

Because policies related to LGBT treatment access and patient rights show such geographic variability, a growing issue has arisen in the form of cross-border reproductive service (i.e., patients traveling outside their state or country of residence to seek services) [37,38]. While people may seek cross-border care for a number of reasons (e.g., higher quality, lower cost), this is highly relevant to LGBT couples who may face legal restrictions in their own jurisdiction but be able to procure treatment elsewhere. While the exact worldwide rates of cross-border service-seeking are unclear, the fact that LGBT couples do cross borders for legal reasons was supported by a 2010 study in Europe [39]. Results showed that in countries with more restrictive laws, the majority of patients who

2 An exception occurs in the case of a lesbian couple where one partner provides the egg and the other partner is the gestational carrier. This method, however, while conferring legal rights to both partners, is not typically the first choice for treatment due to elevated cost and health risks as compared to less invasive methods (i.e., IUI).

crossed borders did so for legal reasons, and that many of these individuals were sexual minority patients. For example, 39.2% of the sample of women who originated from France were lesbian (where lesbian treatment is illegal). In contrast, no lesbian women traveled from the UK (which has among the most progressive laws) for legal reasons. For gay men using surrogacy, another emerging trend is to pursue this service in India, where there is access to a large pool of potential carriers and costs are substantially lower. In general, cross-border reproductive service is seen as a major issue as it can add extra cost and stress to the reproductive process, as well as raise concerns for the safety of the patient [37,38].

Cost issues

Fertility treatments are expensive, and these costs can be prohibitive for any couple, regardless of sexual orientation. As such, many treatment options remain the exclusive province of those with access to resources or insurance coverage [6]. For LGBT couples, however, the cost burden may be even higher as compared to their heterosexual counterparts due to many of the issues highlighted above: limited access to insurance coverage, second-parent adoption costs, the need for legal counsel and so forth. Even when insurance will cover services, it will typically not cover sperm or egg donation. Thus, even for straightforward treatment plans (e.g., a lesbian couple who want to use IUI), the costs can add up quickly and become a limiting factor for prospective LGBT parents.

> *"We were lucky; we had resources. I can't imagine how other couples with a lower socioeconomic status could possibly afford this – we paid $650/vial of sperm and $450/IUI – that's $1100/cycle* ***before*** *shipping costs, time off from work for appointments, copays, etc. Insurance covered all tests and diagnostics, but still – it was so expensive."*

Social support issues

Social support from friends, family, or support groups is important for anyone going through the fertility treatment or adoptive process. Novel issues may arise, however, for LGBT prospective parents. Some individuals may not have disclosed their sexual orientation to family members – the transition to parenthood may end up "outing" them [17]. Families, in turn, may or may not be supportive. While friends can be a crucial source of support in general, research indicates that some LGBT couples may encounter a lack of support, or in some cases, overtly negative attitudes from the gay community when they become parents [36,40]. In such cases, it may be that their entry into parenthood goes against the norms that have been established within that group. Conversely, some LGBT prospective parents find that their desire to parent is more understood and accepted by heterosexual friends, for whom parenthood tends to be an expected stage of the lifecycle [2]. For many, they may not know how people will react until it happens.

> *"I've encountered a lot of unexpected reactions from family and friends. This ranged from people who were happier about it than we anticipated, to those who reacted with unexpected scrutiny and criticism. Our donor's brother, a very conservative southerner with some pretty homophobic attitudes, suddenly feels like he can 'relate' to his brother around fatherhood, and now calls regularly and sends us pictures of his kids. A few of my partner's friends (older lesbians) were baffled that she would want to become a parent relatively late in life, and were less than supportive of her decision."*

The LGBT transition to parenthood may be associated with significant social network shifts. These changes may stem both from the aforementioned issues with family/friend attitudes, as well as from a general realignment of priorities. For example, in a study examining gay men adopting children, Goldberg [41] found that many fathers reported a sense of alienation from gay non-parent friends and increasing closeness to heterosexual parent friends. The shift from non-parent to parent friends is common for new heterosexual parents as well, but as Goldberg notes, the shift for gay couples is qualified by the fact that their friendships with gay non-parents are not easily replaced by friendships with gay parents. This may be particularly true for couples living outside of major urban areas, where there are simply fewer LGBT parents in the vicinity [26]. As such, some LGBT parents may feel they lack a community of parent friends who really "get" their full experience.

Transgender patient considerations

Above and beyond the heteronormative or heterosexist systems already mentioned, transgender fertility treatment patients may be subject to additional biases and barriers to services [42]. Therefore, when working with transgender patients, fertility counselors should be aware that these individuals may be particularly wary of the attitudes and/or discriminatory practices of those in the healthcare system. In addition, a specific consideration for transgender patients pertains to those who are considering physical modifications that may impact their fertility potential (e.g., surgical removal of testes, penis, ovaries, and/or uterus that would render the individual sterile). Discussions regarding fertility preservation may be needed as research has demonstrated that there are cases of people who have received these treatments who later regretted their inability to produce genetically related children [43].

Gender modification may also involve use of hormone therapies. While not irreversible, these therapies may impact reproductive potential, and patients may need psychoeducation around this. Transgender individuals may elect to discontinue hormones in order to engage in reproductive measures. For example, as in the case of Evan, transgender men who keep their uterus and ovaries may stop hormones in order to provide eggs; others might even seek to become pregnant if this makes sense for the couple. In such cases, counseling may be important to help patients anticipate and cope with identity discordant changes that may occur in their body while off the hormones, or while going through the pregnancy process [44]. While some of the scenarios involving transgender patients may sound novel or difficult to counsel in theory (e.g., a transman pursuing pregnancy), in reality the fertility counselor is still fulfilling his or her typical role in helping the prospective parents build their family in the manner they feel is best, anticipating any consequences of their treatment decisions, and guiding the couple to the necessary social and legal supports.

Counseling approach

The work the fertility counselor will do with LGBT couples will depend on where they are in the decision-making process, as well as what the reproductive options are for the dyad. Counselors are most likely to get involved once the decision to pursue parenthood has been made but before formal treatments have begun. Couples may or may not have done independent research on the conception process, so the level of knowledge and preparation may vary greatly. Thus, the role of the counselor is to help the couple navigate whatever issues are relevant to their situation and provide psychoeducation and support as needed. Below is an overview of suggested areas to cover in a counseling session, as well as a list of recommended practices.

Components of the session

Set the stage

The fertility counselor should begin by providing an orientation to the purpose of their meeting, which is to discuss the major decisions and concerns that LGBT couples may have when pursuing parenthood. Specific stated goals may involve: (1) helping the couple think through their reproductive options; (2) considering the implications of their decisions; (3) answering questions they may have about the treatment process and (4) providing guidance to supportive and/or informational resources. Because LGBT clients may have already encountered (or be apprehensive of) biased attitudes or practices, the counselor should be aware of ambivalent or negative feelings that LGBT couples may bring to the meeting. In particular, for some couples, this meeting may have been a mandatory part of their treatment. As such, there may be resentment about having to attend the session or concerns that the meeting is a screening for parental fitness. In these cases, the fertility counselor should make it clear that this is not an evaluation, and state that the meeting is required for all patients using a donor. Empathy and validation of negative feelings about the mandated counseling requirement may be important to help foster a therapeutic alliance with the couple.

Collect background information

It may be helpful to start the dialogue with an open-ended question, such as, "Tell me about how you got to where you are today." This will help the counselor assess what issues need to be addressed during the session. Some couples may be at the very start of their treatment process, whereas others may have tried various methods (e.g., home insemination, surrogate search) that either failed or are in process. The counselor will want to gather as much information as possible about what decisions still need to be made, and how comfortable each of the partners are with the elements that have been decided already. This will also be a chance to see how well-oriented the couple is (or not) with any upcoming fertility treatment procedures. Counselors can work to fill in the gaps as needed with psychoeducation around any relevant medical, legal, financial and emotional demands of their treatment plan.

Address LGBT-specific challenges

The fertility counselor will want to be particularly attuned to LGBT-specific challenges that the couple may have encountered. Sensitivity to issues related to bias or discrimination will be important, both in terms of allowing LGBT patients to feel heard and supported, and to make space for corrective, positive interactions with members of the fertility treatment system. When possible, the counselor may be able to offer the couple suggestions or resources to help address the issue (see examples in "Best Practice" section). The fertility counselor can also listen for indications of internalized stigma that need to be addressed. It will help if the counselor is very familiar with the research literature on LGBT parenting and can point to evidence demonstrating that, for example, parental sexual orientation has no deleterious effects on the development, adjustment and well-being of children [12]. For couples in which one or both members are not yet "out" or are in the process of revealing their relationship to others, the counselor will want to be able to provide referrals to the appropriate therapeutic services so that the patients can get the support they need around the coming out process.

Regarding legal issues, the fertility counselor will want to make sure that LGBT couples have thought through any relevant legal considerations. While the counselor is not equipped to provide legal advice, he or she needs to make sure that the couple is at least aware of any legal implications of their fertility treatment plans. If indicated, fertility counselors should strongly encourage couples to consult with counsel and take whatever precautions needed (e.g., second-parent adoption, pre-birth orders) to protect the rights of the parents to the child.

For couples using a known donor, the considerations may not be unique to LGBT couples but may be amplified due to a lack of legal rights or recognition on the part of the non-biological parent. The fertility counselor should work with the couple (possibly in conjunction with the donor as well) to clarify each party's expectations for what their relationship will look like once the child is born. LGBT couples will need to get legal documentation in place relinquishing the donor's rights and responsibilities. Beyond that, the counselor can help the couple to consider the more emotional or relational aspects of having the donor in the child's life. Questions to consider might include what to call the donor, or how much time they want the child to spend with him or her. Making sure that all parties have thought through the long-term implications of their prospective arrangements will save everyone involved a lot of potential conflict down the road (see Chapter 10 for more on known donor use).

Same-sex parents are not likely to keep their use of third party assistance a secret, but they may have questions about when and how to talk to the child. The counselor can help the couple generate strategies for disclosure and discussion. Based on our experience and research, it is recommended that parents start the disclosure process early, explaining the situation to the child in a way that is appropriate for his or her developmental stage. Early disclosure helps promote a sense of security within the family, and the birth story becomes naturally integrated into the child's narrative of his or her life story. Parents might start the disclosure process with a simple "bedtime story" that introduces the idea that they received help from an outside source. Two examples are below – the stories can be adapted to fit the family's situation. Parents can then develop the story, filling in details as the child gets older and is prepared to understand more (see Chapter 18 for more on disclosing information on donor origins).

> Lesbian parents who used anonymous donor sperm: *"A long time ago, Mommy and Mama wanted to have a family of our own. We knew we had a lot of love to give a baby, but we also knew it takes a seed from a man and seed from a woman to have a baby and we didn't have any seeds from a man. So, we went to a special place where men who had more seeds than they needed had given their seeds to share with other families who didn't have any. A doctor helped us use those seeds and mix them together in my tummy, so that we could have a baby. My tummy got bigger and bigger, and one day the baby came out. It was you! Then we were so happy because we finally had a baby to love."*
>
> Gay parents who used donor eggs and a gestational carrier: *"A long time ago, Daddy and Papa wanted to have a family of our own. We knew we had a lot of love to give a baby, but we didn't have all the ingredients we needed to make a baby. We knew we needed seeds from a man, seeds from a woman, and a special place called a uterus to grow the baby. We had the seeds from a man, but we were*

missing the other pieces. Fortunately, there are really nice people in the world who were willing to help us build our family. One woman offered to give us the eggs we needed. Another woman offered to let us grow the baby in her uterus. Now we had what we needed. A doctor helped us mix the seeds together, and put them in the woman's uterus. A baby started to grow in there, and that baby was you! After nine months, you came out, and we were right there waiting for you. Then we were so happy because we finally had a baby to love."

Assess social support

The fertility counselor will want to assess the degree of social support the couple perceives from family, friends and coworkers. If, for example, family members have not demonstrated support (or were outright rejecting) of a LGBT individual due to his or her sexual orientation or transgender status, that family is likely not expected to be a reliable source of support during the conception or childrearing process. In this situation, helping the couple connect to sources of peer support will be particularly important. Conversely, if it is the LGBT peer community that is less than supportive, couples may seek tighter connections with family supports. Regardless, if family and friend support networks are not strong, a major role the counselor can play is to help direct the couple to sources of social support. This may take the form of web or community based LGBT-specific support groups, or simply helping them connect with other prospective or new parents, regardless of sexual orientation.

Assess mental health state

It is well-established that heterosexual couples receiving fertility treatment are at elevated risk for psychological distress [45]. But in this context, the distress may be linked to infertility and a history of failed reproductive attempts [46,47]. In contrast, LGBT couples are not necessarily facing fertility problems, and their entry into treatment may be associated with a greater degree of excitement or optimism as they begin the process of family formation [48]. Alternatively, because LGBT couples are confronted with their own stressors, high levels of distress may be present, but for different reasons. Further, for some couples, the initial enthusiasm of embarking on treatment may quickly start to mirror the distress of heterosexual couples as they confront the reality of failed attempts and waiting periods. Fertility counselors should conduct a careful assessment of each partner's mental health state at the beginning of treatment, and ideally will be available to reassess as treatment progresses to determine if changes have occurred. When needed, couples may benefit from ongoing psychological support services (either from the fertility counselor or another LGBT-friendly therapist) aimed at managing anxiety, depression and/or relationship distress.

"The process of insemination started out as just funny and awkward and sweet, but has become increasingly more stressful. At this point, the insemination itself is still very sweet and intimate, but the process of tracking, planning and waiting has been incredibly stressful and difficult on our relationship. I feel like my partner's entire world is wrapped up in tracking her cycles ... She has become very depressed, likely both from the progesterone and the process ... I feel pretty burnt out and I just miss having our partnership when it was just the two of us and not this hypothetical baby. I think that when there is a real baby on the way it will be a more than welcome intruder, but the process of making a baby has become an unwelcome third party."

General best practices

Fertility counselors are in an excellent position to identify areas where treatment services can become more supportive of LGBT couples. As a starting point, fertility counselors need to develop the necessary *cultural competency* for working with LGBT patients. In the context of fertility counseling, cultural competency involves recognition of the types of issues highlighted throughout this chapter that LGBT couples may confront during treatment [36]. In addition, based on our own experiences and a review of the literature [e.g., 16,17,22,26,36,49], here is a checklist that helps to establish a set of best practices in serving LGBT patients. This list is not comprehensive but at minimum provides a starting point for fertility counselors (and clinics) to provide the best possible support to the LGBT patient population (summarized in Table 13.1).

- Check printed materials for heteronormative assumptions or heterosexist biases. Forms should reflect possible variability in family structure. Either make forms gender neutral or have alternative versions available for different couple

Table 13.1 Summary of recommended practices with LGBT couples.

- *Create inclusive printed materials.* Forms should be gender neutral (i.e., Parent 1 and Parent 2) or available in alternative versions for LGBT families. Websites and clinic literature should include language and images that are inclusive of LGBT families.
- *Use inclusive verbal communications.* For example, refer to unions instead of marriage, partners instead of husband/wife. Frame treatment in terms of creating a family, not treating infertility.
- *Respect term and pronoun preferences.* Use the terms that the patient and her or his partner prefer regarding sexual orientation and/or gender identity.
- *Involve the partner.* The partner is an equal parent to any offspring resulting in treatment and should not be marginalized during the conception process.
- *Know relevant literature sources.* This includes resources that do not focus on infertility, and ideally includes resources that are written specifically for LGBT prospective parents.
- *Know relevant supportive services.* Be able to direct patients to local or internet-based services that address the social and emotional support needs of LGBT prospective parents.
- *Know relevant legal information.* Get familiar with the laws for marriage, adoption and surrogacy in your state or country, and have referral information available for LGBT-friendly adoption agencies and family planning lawyers in your area.
- *Troubleshoot for the patient.* Notice if other treatment providers are creating an uncomfortable environment, and make efforts to provide psychoeducation.
- *Adjust treatment protocol as needed.* Fertility treatment clinics may want to make certain service components (e.g., full pre-treatment fertility work up, fertility counseling) are recommended but optional, after discussing with the patient the type of information they may miss by opting out.
- *Transparency in services.* Provide clear, written, defensible treatment policies for all patients. Ideally, also provide a description of patient demographics to enable prospective patients to know the extent to which the clinic is welcoming of LGBT patients.

configurations. Websites and clinic literature should include language and images that are inclusive of LGBT families.

- Be aware of the messages that are communicated verbally. Use neutral terms – refer to unions instead of marriage, partners instead of spouses or husband/wife. Frame treatment in terms of creating a family, rather than solving the medical problem of infertility.
- Determine what terms the patient and her or his partner prefer regarding sexual orientation and/or gender identity, and respect those preferences.
- Be sure to involve the partner. The partner who is not providing gametes (and/or serving as the gestational carrier, in the case of lesbian couples) may be overlooked throughout treatment. They will be equal parents to any offspring that result in treatment and should therefore not be marginalized during the conception process.
- Be able to direct patients to appropriate literature sources. This minimally includes resources that do not just focus on infertility or refer to "husband and wife," and ideally includes resources that are written specifically for LGBT prospective parents. (For a list of books and resources, please refer to Addendum 13.1.)
- Be knowledgeable about supportive services that address the social and emotional support needs of LGBT prospective parents (e.g., local or internet-based LGBT-specific support groups like "Dykes Planning Tykes" or "Daddies & Papas 2B").
- Be aware of the laws for marriage, adoption and surrogacy in your state or country as they pertain to LGBT couples, or where to direct patients to look for finding out this information (e.g., the HRC website). Have referral information available to LGBT-friendly adoption agencies and family planning lawyers in your area.
- Be aware of treatment providers who may be creating an uncomfortable environment, and make efforts to provide psychoeducation. Or proactively provide education to all clinic staff, addressing any discomfort or concerns they have about treating LGBT patients.
- Fertility treatment clinics may want to consider adapting policies so that certain service components (such as a full pre-treatment fertility work up, or fertility counseling) are recommended but optional, after discussing with the patient the type of information they may miss by opting out.
- To provide the highest level of transparency, fertility treatment clinics should provide clear, written, defensible treatment policies for all patients. Clinics can additionally provide a detailed description of patient demographics, thus enabling prospective patients to know the extent to which the clinic is welcoming of LGBT patients.

Reflection and summary

It is remarkable to us how much has changed regarding fertility care for LGBT couples in a relatively short time. For example, a "debate" article published in 1994 in the journal *Human Reproduction* on the use of insemination services for lesbian women stated: "The sexual minorities now have an increased confidence which has led them to assert their rights for social recognition, encouraged by a new talk of tolerance towards minorities (even if it does not always fit in with reality)" [50, p. 1969]. The author's clinic had decided to welcome these "special requests" for donor insemination using a stringent psychological screening protocol involving approval by the doctor and psychologist, as well as the head of the fertility unit. He noted that this decision to treat lesbian women was not for everyone, and that "every practitioner must have the right of non-participation should their moral conscience tell them so." That this was the prevailing dialogue of the day (and one that appeared to represent an "inclusive" attitude at the time) reflects the extent to which the decision to deny fertility treatment services to LGBT patients was both socially and medically sanctioned.

While there is still progress to be made, we view a sea change underway with regard to LGBT rights and reproductive options. Twenty years ago, few would have predicted that same-sex couples would hold the right to marry in 17 US states and 16 countries worldwide (and counting). Or that research would resoundingly debunk questions about LGBT parental fitness, and that prominent medical and ethical governing bodies of the day would make clear statements supporting equal rights to fertility treatment services. As a result of these kinds of changes, the debate regarding fertility treatment has made a profoundly important shift from *if* LGBT patients should be treated to *how to best* deliver treatment to this steadily growing patient population.

We believe fertility counselors working with LGBT patients have the important task of remaining abreast of new developments regarding treatment options and the ever-changing legal and social barriers our patients encounter. They must also work to provide a supportive environment to facilitate family building within a societal framework that is often not fully supportive. A major challenge fertility counselors face is that patients may view our role through a lens colored by previous experiences of discrimination – as a result, developing a positive working alliance can be hard. Overcoming this challenge requires openness to diverse family building scenarios, staying up to date with new developments, seeking consultation from colleagues when faced with unfamiliar concerns, and requesting feedback from patients about their experiences in order to continue to improve counseling skills.

The goal for this chapter was to provide a summary of many of the major contemporary considerations to keep in mind when providing fertility counseling to LGBT patients. While LGBT couples do share many commonalities with heterosexual couples receiving fertility treatment, there are also many aspects of their experience that are unique. Even within the population of LGBT patients, there will be a great deal of variability in terms of the options couples have and the decisions they make on their path to family formation. The fertility counselor can play a critical role in providing LGBT couples guidance, psychoeducation and support as they navigate a treatment system that was not designed with their needs in mind. As reflected in this final vignette, the process may be trying for myriad reasons, and the fertility counselor can help couples learn and grow along their winding path to family formation.

> *"The experience, as a whole, was ... a growing one. I have never worked so hard at something and failed so many times. I have never been so physically and psychologically tested (and I did a four-year surgical residency, so that's saying something). I have scars that will never fade. I know it was deeply painful and stressful for my partner, and our relationship was profoundly tested more than once. But I came out stronger, more dedicated, more humbled, more honest, more real. We came through deeply in love and committed to each other. I'm a more compassionate physician, a more loving partner, and a real grown-up. I hope it will make me a better mother."*

Acknowledgments

We thank all of the people who were willing to share their fertility treatment experiences with us for this chapter. Their contributions provided vibrant illustrations of both the trials and successes of LGBT couples navigating the world of fertility treatment options.

References

1. Allen KR, Demo DH. The families of lesbians and gay men: A new frontier in family research. *Journal of Marriage and the Family* 1995; 57(1): 111–27.
2. Goldberg AE. *Lesbian and Gay Parents and Their Children: Research on the Family Life Cycle.* Washington, DC: American Psychological Association; 2010.

3. Gates GJ, Ost J. *The Gay and Lesbian Atlas.* Washington, DC: Urban Institute Press; 2004.

4. Baetens P, Camus M, Devroey P. Counselling lesbian couples: Requests for donor insemination on social grounds. *Reproductive Biomedicine Online* 2003 Jan–Feb; 6(1): 75–83.

5. Pratesi A. A respectable scandal: Same-sex parenthood, emotional dynamics, and social change. *Journal of GLBT Family Studies* 2012; 8: 305–33.

6. Agigain A. *Baby Steps: How Lesbian Alternative Insemination Is Changing the World.* Middletown, CT: Wesleyan University Press; 2004.

7. Mamo L. *Queering Reproduction.* Durham, NC: Duke University Press; 2007.

8. Embryology ESoHRa. *Comparative Analysis of Medically Assisted Reproduction in the EU: Regulation and Technologies.* Brussels, Belgium; 2013.

9. ILGA-Europe. *ILGA-Europe: Annual Review of the Human Rights Situation of Lesbian, Gay, Bisexual, Trans and Intersex People in Europe, 2013.* Brussels, Belgium: ILGA-Europe, 2013.

10. Ethics Committee of the American Society for Reproductive M. Access to fertility treatment by gays, lesbians, and unmarried persons. *Fertility and Sterility* 2006 Nov; 86(5): 1333–5.

11. Ethics Committee of the American Society for Reproductive Medicine. Access to fertility treatment by gays, lesbians, and unmarried persons. *Fertility and Sterility* 2009 Oct; 92(4): 1190–3.

12. Ethics Committee of the American Society for Reproductive Medicine. Access to fertility treatment by gays, lesbians, and unmarried persons: A committee opinion. *Fertility and Sterility* 2013 Dec; 100(6): 1524–7.

13. North Coast Women's Care Medical Group v. Benitez, 44 Cal. 4th 1145 (2008).

14. Wykes KA. Fertility services for same-sex couples: Policy and practice. *British Journal of Nursing* 2012 Jul 26–Aug 8; 21(14): 871–5.

15. Human Fertilisation and Embryology Act (c. 22), (2008).

16. Corbett SL, Frecker HM, Shapiro HM, Yudin MH. Access to fertility services for lesbian women in Canada. *Fertility and Sterility* 2013 Oct; 100(4): 1077–80.

17. Chabot JM, Ames BD. "It wasn't 'Let's get pregnant and go do it':" Decision making in lesbian couples planning motherhood via donor insemination. *Family Relations* 2004; 53(4): 348–56.

18. Rank N. Barriers for access to assisted reproductive technologies by lesbian women: The search for parity within the healthcare system. *Houston Journal of Health Law & Policy* 2010; 10: 115–46.

19. Johnson KM. Excluding lesbian and single women? An analysis of U.S. fertility clinic websites. *Women's Studies International Forum* 2012; 35: 394–402.

20. Baetens P, Brewaeys A. Lesbian couples requesting donor insemination: An update of the knowledge with regard to lesbian mother families. *Human Reproduction Update* 2001 Sep–Oct; 7(5): 512–19.

21. Ross LE, Steele LS, Epstein R. Service use and gaps in services for lesbian and bisexual women during donor insemination, pregnancy, and the postpartum period. *Journal of Obstetrics and Gynaecology Canada* 2006 Jun; 28(6): 505–11.

22. Kissil K, Davey M. Health dispartities in procreation: Unequal access to assisted reprodutive techologies. *Journal of Feminist Family Therapy* 2012; 24(3): 197–212.

23. Smith D. What are the reproductive options when a same-sex couple wants a family? *Sexuality, Reproduction & Menopause* 2011; 9(3): 30–6.

24. Human Rights Campaign. Parenting Laws: Joint Adoption. HRC [Internet]. June 4, 2013. Retrieved from: www.hrc.org.

25. Child Welfare Information Gateway. *Frequently Asked Questions from Lesbian, Gay, Bisexual, and Transgender (LGBT) Prospective Foster and Adoptive Parents.* Washington, DC: US Department of Health and Human Services, Children's Bureau; 2011.

26. Kinkler LA, Goldberg AE. Working with what we've got: Perceptions of barriers and supports among small-netropolitan same-sex adopting couples. *Family Relations* 2011 Oct 1; 60(4): 387–403.

27. Patterson CJ. Children of lesbian and gay parents: Psychology, law, and policy. *American Psychologist* 2009; 64(8): 727–36.

28. Kranz KC, Daniluk JC. Living outside the box: Lesbian families created through the use of anonymous donor insemination. *Journal of Feminist Family Therapy* 2006; 56: 1–33.

29. Goldberg AE. The transition to parenthood for lesbian couples. *Journal of GLBT Family Studies* 2006; 2: 13–42.

30. Amato PR, Jacob MC. Providing fertility services to lesbian couples: The lesbian baby boom. *Sexuality, Reproduction & Menopause* 2004; 2(2): 83–8.

31. Ben-Ari A, Livni T. Motherhood is not a given thing: Experiences and constructed meanings of biological and nonbiological lesbian mothers. *Sex Roles* 2006; 54(7–8): 521–31.

32. Gurmankin AD, Caplan AL, Braverman AM. Screening practices and beliefs of assisted reproductive

technology programs. *Fertility and Sterility* 2005 Jan; 83(1): 61–7.

33. Lawrence RE, Rasinski KA, Yoon JD, Curlin FA. Obstetrician-gynecologists' beliefs about assisted reproductive technologies. *Obstetrics & Gynecology* 2010 Jul; 116(1): 127–35.

34. Herek GM, Gillis JR, Cogan JC. Internalized stigma among sexual minority adults: Insights from a social psychological perspective. *Journal of Counseling Psychology* 2009; 56: 32–43.

35. Meyer IH. Prejudice, social stress, and mental health in lesbian, gay, and bisexual populations: Conceptual issues and research evidence. *Psychological Bulletin* 2003 Sep; 129(5): 674–97.

36. Yager C, Brennan D, Steele LS, Epstein R, Ross LE. Challenges and mental health experiences of lesbian and bisexual women who are trying to conceive. *Health & Social Work* 2010 Aug; 35(3): 191–200.

37. Ethics Committee of American Society for Reproductive M. Cross-border reproductive care: A committee opinion. *Fertil Sterility* 2013 Sep; 100(3): 645–50.

38. Ferraretti AP, Pennings G, Gianaroli L, Natali F, Magli MC. Cross-border reproductive care: a phenomenon expressing the controversial aspects of reproductive technologies. *Reproductive Biomedicine Online* 2010 Feb; 20(2): 261–6.

39. Shenfield F, de Mouzon J, Pennings G, Ferraretti AP, Andersen AN, de Wert G, et al. Cross border reproductive care in six European countries. *Human Reproduction* 2010 Jun; 25(6): 1361–8.

40. Ross LE, Steele L, Sapiro B. Perceptions of predisposing and protective factors for perinatal depression in same-sex parents. *Journal of Midwifery & Women's Health* 2005 Nov–Dec; 50(6): e65–70.

41. Goldberg AE. *Gay Dads: Transitions to Adoptive Fatherhood.* New York, NY: New York University Press; 2012.

42. Murphy TF. The ethics of helping transgender men and women have children. *Perspectives in Biology and Medicine* 2010 Winter; 53(1): 46–60.

43. De Sutter P, Kir K, Verschoor A, Hotimsky A. The desire to have children and the perservation of fertility in transsexual women. *The International Journal of Transgenderism* 2002; 6(3).

44. Murphy TF. The ethics of fertility preservation in transgender body modifications. *Journal of Bioethical Inquiry* 2012 Sep; 9(3): 311–6.

45. Cousineau TM, Domar AD. Psychological impact of infertility. *Best Practice & Research in Clinical Obstetrics & Gynaecology* 2007 Apr; 21(2): 293–308.

46. Petok WD. The psychology of gender-specific infertility diagnoses. In: Covington SN, Burns LH, editors. *Infertility Counseling: A Comprehensive Handbook for Clinicians (2nd edn.).* New York, NY: Cambridge University Press; 2006. pp. 37–60.

47. Burns LH, Covington SN. Psychology of infertility. In: Covington SN, Burns LH, editors. *Infertility Counseling: A Comprehensive Handbook for Clinicians (2nd edn.).* New York, NY: Cambridge University Press; 2006. pp. 1–19.

48. Ehrensaft D. Just Molly and me, and donor makes three: Lesbian motherhood in the age of assisted reproductive technology. *Journal of Lesbian Studies* 2008; 12(2–3): 161–78.

49. Ross LE, Steele LS, Epstein R. Lesbian and bisexual women's recommendations for improving the provision of assisted reproductive technology services. *Fertility and Sterility* 2006 Sep; 86(3): 735–8.

50. Englert Y. Artificial insemination of single women and lesbian women with donor semen. Artificial insemination with donor semen: Particular requests. *Human Reproduction* 1994 Nov; 9(11): 1969–71.

Chapter 14

Adoption

Anne. F. Malavé

"'Why don't you just adopt?' she said ... I was so upset ... I felt like saying 'If you think adoption is so great then why did you have your two biological sons?' I don't want to adopt ... I don't want someone else's child. I want my own child!"

Susan is a woman suffering from infertility describing an exchange with a close friend that captures a common interaction around infertility as well as the profound longing for a child "of my own": the biogenetically related child. Susan is now a proud and happy adoptive parent. How did this change happen?

This chapter presents information for Mental Health Professionals (MHPs) to help people with infertility problems explore adoption and, when relevant, prepare for adoptive parenting. For some people this means learning about adoption as a viable alternative family building option. For others it means embracing a child "as one's own" through social, legal and interpersonal connections instead of through a biogenetic link. For adoptive parents this means embarking on a personal and social life-long journey involving additional parenting tasks. Fertility counseling may be instrumental in preparing future adoptive parents like Susan by promoting an understanding of the lifelong experience of adoption, strengthening coping skills, facilitating personal growth and healing, and promoting resilience. In the best-case scenario, adoption exploration initiates a journey of adaptation and transformation concerning what it means to belong in a family. This journey may begin in the office of an MHP working in fertility counseling.

Susan's story

Susan is a professional woman, married in her mid 30s, who sought counseling because of her deep distress about her infertility and the constant failure of fertility treatments. At the beginning of counseling I urged Susan and her husband to explore all their family building options, including adoption, in order to learn about these alternatives and also to create continuity in the event that their original plan was unsuccessful. Reluctantly, Susan researched the third party reproduction and adoption options. With time, as Susan started to lose hope for a biogenetic pregnancy, she began to grieve the immense loss of a longed-for genetically related child. The middle part of the treatment involved processing her profound pain and losses while also finding hope for a way forwards. In working through her feelings, and with self-examination and reflection, Susan began to feel hope that a non-genetic path to parenthood would be successful. Her feelings of failure and self-blame gradually gave way to faith and hope that she would have a child to parent. Susan desperately wanted to be pregnant, but after more disappointments with egg donation, she and her husband decided to adopt. Susan described this as "climbing another mountain," but felt more confident that adoption would be successful. Susan's initial fears about adopting were about attachment. She worried that she would not be able to love the child. She feared rejection and imagined an angry teenager saying: "You're not my real mother!" These fears and other concerns gradually dissipated as she read about adoption, talked to adoptive families and attended adoptive parent meetings and conferences. She found herself surprised at one adoptive parents'

Fertility Counseling: Clinical Guide and Case Studies, ed. Sharon N. Covington. Published by Cambridge University Press.

meeting when she realized that she was feeling identified with adoptive parents. Initially interested in domestic adoption, she had a strong negative reaction to the idea that she had to be chosen by a birthmother, which made her feel out of control (replicating feelings of infertility). She was also worried that the birthmother would change her mind. She was initially angry about being evaluated in a "home-study" process by the adoption agency social worker. She felt threatened by the idea of an open adoption and imagined that this would interfere with her future family integrity. Time passed as Susan kept processing her losses and learning more about adoption. After disappointments with domestic adoption she and her husband eventually adopted a daughter in an intercountry and transracial adoption. By the end of the counseling Susan was a strong adoption advocate, questioning why she had waited so long to adopt (her grief crowded out by joy at this time) and, ironically, wondering out loud about her friends who were still undergoing fertility treatments: "Why don't they just adopt!"

Although finally a parent, Susan's story as part of an adoptive family has just begun. In the future she will experience the common joys and difficulties of being a parent, as well as the additional layers of adoptive family life.

Adoption today

Adoption is currently practiced around the world in a family, social and global system. Adoption has served both public and private needs as a social solution to the problem of finding safe and permanent families for children whose birthparents are unable or unwilling to raise them and a personal solution for people who seek children to parent. In adoption, traditionally, a child is born to one set of parents and raised by other parent/s in permanent social arrangements, after having been orphaned, abandoned, relinquished, or taken away from parents who were unable to look after them by the state. Adoption terminates the parental rights of the birthparents to children and provides those children with the same rights and responsibilities in their adoptive families as other children who join their families through birth. All adoptive families are created by laws, social contracts and attachment relationships, rather than by birth, blood or genetic ties.

Adoption today includes domestic, international, intercountry, transracial and familial (relative/kinship) adoptions; adoption by a step-parent; "stranger" adoption; adoption by single parents and Lesbian, Gay, Bisexual and Transgendered (LGBT) parents; through agencies, government child welfare systems, or directly from relinquishing parent(s). People adopt because they are unable to have children, to expand their family, for social, economic and legal reasons including access, and availability, protection of legal parenting rights in ART family building and for purposes of inheritance and political alliances. The focus of this chapter is on people who adopt after experiencing infertility through "stranger adoptions." With advances in ART, adoption is no longer a linear process: there is a bidirectional influence and overlap between adoption and ART and an increase in blended families with children from increasingly diverse origins.

All adoptive parents must fulfill their region-specific legal requirements in areas such as psychological and physical health, financial stability, home environment and motivation to adopt. There are barriers for some people wanting to adopt including age limitations, laws and discrimination, prohibitions against criminal backgrounds, and health and medical conditions. Other obstacles include the diminishing availability of desirable children (i.e., infants) who are eligible for adoption. Approval can be lengthy with many steps and much paperwork. Intercountry adoptions require additional steps, including fulfilling the legal requirements for sending and the receiving countries as well as the Hague International Treaty [1]. Increasingly mandatory formal pre-adoption training and post-adoption supervision is required.

Adoption is not a onetime event but a life-long process that affects all parties within the adoption triad/triangle, other members of their families and extended families for present and future generations, and the society and world in which they live. The focus of this chapter is on adoptive parents. The life-long journey of the adoptive family is heavily influenced by that family's particular individual, extended family, social, cultural and geographic environment as well as the socioeconomic and racial and ethnic diversity (heterogeneity vs. homogeneity) of the country in which they live. All families formed through adoption share characteristic similarities and differences with mainstream biogenetic families. The adjustment to family building through adoption as well as the life-long experience of being part of an adoptive family, for parents and their children alike, is fundamentally related to the navigation and integration of these similarities and differences.

As an experience, adoption contains the profound polar opposite experiences of tragedy and joy, fortune and misfortune, solution and problem, loss and gain, and risk and resilience. Therefore it draws forth highly emotional and polarized responses in individuals and in groups. Although in the Western developed world the guiding principle is "in the best interests of the child," the history and practice of adoption is filled with conflict and controversy, rhetoric and debate, competing interests, and diverse reactions to different parts of the adoption experience, including issues of social justice. In learning about adoption, it is important to hold its full complexity in mind rather than oversimplify in response to external or internal polarizations and pressures.

Adoption today is increasingly heterogeneous as social and political forces impact on individual, family, social and global systems. Adoptive families continue to become more diverse as a wider range of potential adoptive parents have access to adoption and as the range of available children changes. Despite this multiplicity there remain groups who lack access to children that they wish to adopt.

History of adoption

Adoption is the oldest and original family building choice after infertility, and historically it was the only alternative. Adoption has existed in all societies from ancient times onwards, across all periods of history and all cultures [2]. The earliest adoptions were informal, arranged mainly for economic purposes of inheritance, religion, peacekeeping, political alliances, providing for care in old age and labor needs. The first orphan asylums were created in the fifth century in the Byzantine Empire and in AD 787 in the West [3]. Foundling homes were first created in the thirteenth century [4]. During the nineteenth century, migrations from Europe to countries including the United States, Canada and Australia, combined with the industrial revolution and urbanization, resulted in disrupted families and increasing numbers of orphaned children. In the USA these children were first housed in almshouses, then in orphanages: by the mid nineteenth century, public concerns about poor conditions in these institutions led to adoption [5].

Table 14.1 Top sending countries in order of total number of children sent worldwide [7].

1980–1989	1998	2003	2006
Korea	China	China	China
India	Russia	Russia	Russia
Colombia	Vietnam	Guatemala	Guatemala
Brazil	Korea	Korea	Ethiopia

As adoptions became more common, laws were developed to protect these children. The earliest adoption law is found in the Code of Hammurabi in 2800 BC [6]. In much of Europe adoption laws were created in the 1700 and 1800s. England developed adoption laws in 1926 [6] and Canada and Australia also developed adoption laws in the 1920s. In the United States the first adoption law was passed in 1851 [6].

In recent history there have been changes in the origins of children who have been adopted. Intercountry adoption developed mainly due to wars (World War II, Korean and Vietnam wars), internal conflicts in Latin American countries, the fall of communism in Romania and Russia and the one-child policy of China. Almost always poverty has played a fundamental role, with an exception being Korea, which has one of the strongest economies in the world [7]. Politics has also played a role in governmental policies in adoption: for example, after embarrassing publicity during the 1988 Korean Olympic Games about South Korea's status as a "leading exporter" of children, these adoptions slowed down considerably; this was repeated during the 2009 Chinese Olympic Games. And recently Russia placed a ban on US adoption of Russian children, partly in response to a US law that targeted alleged Russian human-rights violators and also in protest about Russian children adopted by Americans who have died from abuse, neglect or other causes while in the care of their adoptive parents [8].

According to Selman's 2009 estimate, nearly one million children were adopted internationally between just after the end of World War II (1948) and 2010 [7]. By 2004 there was a peak of a minimum of 45 000 international adoptions worldwide [9]. On a global level, some countries are mainly "sending countries" and some mainly "receiving countries." Some countries are both a sending country and receiving country: for example, the USA sent 99 children to be adopted in other countries in 2012 [10]. Tables 14.1–14.3 summarize changes in intercountry adoption and the shifts of the top sending and receiving countries [7,9].

Table 14.2 Sending countries: total number of children sent worldwide [9].

Country	2003	2004	2007
China	11 228	13 404	8753
Russia	7745	9425	4873
Korea	2287	2258	1265
Ethiopia	854	1527	3031

Table 14.4 Intercountry adoptions to 23 receiving states: 2003–2012 [12].

Year	Total Number of Adoptions
2003	41 535
2004	45 229
2008	34 785
2012	19 540

Table 14.3 Total adoptions in receiving countries per 100 000 [7].

Country	Total Adoptions per 100 000 in 1980	Total Adoptions per 100 000 in 2004
Sweden	20.5	12.3
Denmark	15.0	9.8
The Netherlands	11.0	8.1
USA	2.2	7.8
UK	unknown	0.6

Table 14.5 Top ten states of origin: 2003–2011 [12].

Rank	2003	2007	2009	2011
1	China	China	China	China
2	Russia	Russia	Ethiopia	Ethiopia
3	Guatemala	Guatemala	Russia	Russia
4	South Korea	Ethiopia	Vietnam	Colombia
5	Ukraine	Vietnam	Ukraine	Ukraine

The USA is the largest receiving country with approximately a half million children adopted since 1971: two-thirds from Asian countries, and the rest from Latin America, Eastern Europe and (recently) Africa. However the USA has by no means the highest concentration per 100 000 population, as seen in Table 14.3 [7]. The fluctuation has been extreme in some countries: for example, the growth of intercountry adoption in Spain has been dramatic, with numbers almost tripling between 1998 and 2004 when it was one of the countries receiving the highest number of children in relation to its population [11]. In some countries, particularly in Western Europe, adoption predominantly consists of intercountry adoptions, most of which are also transracial adoptions.

Concerns about the international abuses and corruption in adoption, including trafficking in children, have led to the development of an international treaty called The Hague Adoption Convention on Protection of Children and Co-operation in Respect of Inter-Country Adoption, established in 1993 to safeguard and protect the best interests of the child and promote best intercountry adoption practices [1]. According to this agreement, intercountry adoption should only be pursued after proper effort has been made to find a domestic adoption placement within the child's country of origin. Although many proponents of this treaty applaud its efforts, opponents are concerned that it has resulted in fewer children finding permanent homes.

These worldwide policy changes in adoption have resulted in a significant drop in intercountry adoptions from 45 299 in 2004 to 19 540 in 2012 [12]. Tables 14.4–14.5 summarize intercountry adoptions to 23 receiving states and top 5 states of origin ("sending countries") between 2003 and 2011 reported on October 7, 2013 [12]. As an example of this decreasing trend, figures from the US State Department for 2013 showed 7094 adoptions into the USA, a decrease of 18% from 8668 in 2012, and 69% from the high of 22 884 in 2004 [13,14]. This decrease is partly due to Russia's ban on adoptions by Americans [8]; adoptions from South Korea and Ethiopia also dropped significantly.

Adoption continues to evolve over time as it seeks solutions to problems for the three parties involved: the child who needs a family, the birthparents who are unable to raise their child, and the adoptive parents who seek a child to parent. The balance between the needs of members of the adoption triad as well as reactions to adoption corruption has led to adoption reforms and international laws including greater attempts at placing children domestically within their countries of origin. These changes mean that sources for children available for adoption have become limited for some people. Therefore it is expected that in the future prospective adoptive parents will expand the range of children they seek to adopt, and increasingly cross boundaries of race (in transracial adoption), age (adopting older children and sibling groups), type of adoption (adopting from the public/foster care system) and health (adopting children with special needs).

Adoption theories

The first adoption theory, developed by H. David Kirk, a Canadian sociologist, was based on research in the 1950s at a time when most adoptive parents (and professionals) expected adoptive parenthood to replicate birth parenthood [15]. Kirk suggested that all members of the adoption triad experience role handicaps that impact adoptive family adjustment. Kirk determined that parents who acknowledged difference (AD) were more likely to be empathic with their children, and better able to communicate about adoption and establish a healthy family life than parents who rejected or denied difference (RD). Others have built on Kirk's work, in particular Brodzinsky, who amended this model by adding an "insistence on difference" (ID) category and argued that there is a curvilinear relationship between RD and AD, with problems at both extremes [16].

Attachment theory, based on the work of Bowlby, has direct relevance for adoption, with its focus on attachment, loss and separation [17,18]. Here, every child develops an internal working model of attachment through a reciprocal process of responsive interactions with a parenting figure, which then informs how that child will interact with other people thereafter. Changes in care-givers put a child at risk for attachment difficulties, although the experience of making one attachment makes it more likely that a child will be able to attach again. Due to pre-adoption risks, there are attachment difficulties in some adopted children. Adoptive parents may also have their own attachment difficulties.

While most adoption theories have focused on the children, some have focused on adoptive parents. Daniluk and Hurtig-Mitchell presented a "Hope and Healing" model of adjustment to adoptive parenthood based on their research [19]. Their subjects went through a process of needing to know they had done all they could do to have "their own child," of acknowledging their losses, of separating the desire to reproduce from the desire to parent, of evaluating the options of childlessness and adoption, and a process which Daniluk and Hurtig-Mitchell called "resocialization" during which they changed their personal identity from biological to adoptive parents. Other aspects were the suddenness of becoming parents, the fears the child would be taken away from them, and negotiating open relationships with birthfamilies. These parents were able to attach to the children they adopted and transform into adoptive parents comfortably. Hendry and Netherwood address the emergence of infertility issues over the lifespan and the accompanying additional challenges [20]. They suggest that infertility feelings can be triggered throughout the lifespan for parents (into grandparenting) and adopted individuals alike; and that infertility feelings also re-emerge when individuals search for birthparents, which is often triggered when they become parents themselves. Shapiro, Shapiro, and Paret and Palacios have developed theoretical approaches that emphasize the influence of context [21,22]. From this perspective, past adoption research that emphasized psychopathology has negatively affected perceptions about adoptive families in the general public, while current adoption research emphasizes "normality" and resilience within the complexity that adoption requires and deserves [22].

Theories of adoption have come full circle from the sociological approach of H. David Kirk, through an emphasis on the losses and identity formation of individuals who have been adopted and communication within adoptive families, to the increasingly complex process of recognizing the context and environmental influences and healing and resilience within adoptive families [15,16,23–25].

Adoption research

Adoption as a field of inquiry began around the middle of the last century as mental health and other professionals became interested in adoption as a unique experience. Prior to that time, adoption was viewed under the domain of child welfare and social services, when society-emphasized sameness and attention primarily addressed practical concerns. Early adoption research was largely atheoretical and primarily focused on clinical populations and the topics of the psychological and behavioral adjustment and outcomes of children who had been adopted. Research has demonstrated that most children who have been adopted function within the normal range. However, these children are overrepresented in the mental health field. Some children experience increased psychosocial, emotional and behavioral struggles in the middle childhood and adolescent years, which remit by early adulthood. Adoptive parents seek the help of MHPs more frequently and more readily than other parents. Pre-adoption risk factors include prenatal intrauterine difficulties, malnutrition, poor medical care, deprivation in nurturance and deficits in sensory stimulation, abuse experiences, a history of multiple placements, older age and institutionalization. Adoption is a protective and buffering experience that reduces risk and promotes resilience. "Catch-up" (e.g., developments in cognition and behavior) after adoption is significant but within limits. Curiosity about origins and searching behaviors are normal. Adoption discrimination exists, and being different from family and peers is difficult for some people who have been adopted. For reviews of adoption research, see Palacios and Brodzinsky and Van Ijzendoorn and Juffer [26,27].

Over the last 30 years adoption research has changed dramatically, leading to an increased complexity in investigating and interpreting research findings, increased consideration of known and unknown pre-adoption risk factors, the use of qualitative and meta-analytic as well as quantitative studies, and changes in methodology such as using more appropriate control groups. There is a growing interest in international collaboration and a multidisciplinary approach, including social scientists and professionals in fields as varied as Immigration, Law, Ethics, Social Anthropology and Sociology. It has been largely assumed by MHPs that the experience of infertility remains alive in the adoptive family system over the course of that family's lifetime; however, there has been very little research on the experience of adoption after infertility. Instead research has focused more on motivation for adoption after infertility and the adjustments involved in adoptive parenthood after infertility.

Adjustment to adoption after infertility

In the first nationally representative survey of adoptive parents in the United States, 72% listed infertility as a primary motivation for adoption [28]. Other motivations included wanting to expand their family (92%) and wanting to provide a permanent home for a child (90%). According to health statistics in the USA from 2002, approximately one-quarter (26%) of infertile women who had used fertility treatments unsuccessfully and not given birth adopted a child by the ages of 40–44 [29].

In a prospective longitudinal study of 1338 couples initiating infertility treatment in Denmark (a country that offers socialized healthcare and free infertility treatments) Pinborg and colleagues found that only 5.9% of the women adopted [30]. In a US study, Zhang and Lee investigated the motivations behind the high demand for intercountry/international adoption [31]. Beyond the common motivation of infertility, the researchers reported that race played a part in the decision due to "… a perception that American children available for adoption (i.e. mainly Black children) presented difficult problems whereas foreign children presented interesting challenges." White adoptive parents had a "hierarchy of race," and some parents adopting transracially showed a preference for adopting non-Black children. Other motivating factors for intercountry adoptions reported by the researchers were fears of potential problems with birthparents, wanting a young child, shorter waiting periods and possible health issues of older children.

In a Swedish study, Hogström and colleagues compared the quality of life among couples who had adopted a child 4–5.5 years previously, couples who had undergone successful or unsuccessful IVF treatment, and couples who had conceived spontaneously (control group) [32]. The researchers found that adoptive couples had the highest quality of life scores, while the couples who had undergone unsuccessful IVF living without children had lowest quality of life scores. The researchers concluded that quality of life was independent of the IVF outcome as long as there were children in the family.

In a study from the United Kingdom, Triseliotis and colleagues explored the experiences and perspectives of 93 birthmothers and 93 adoptive parents [33]. Of the adoptive parents, 79% reported that feelings of loss and sadness about infertility did not persist over time and described adoption as a healing factor. The 21% of adoptive parents for whom feelings of loss persisted rated the closeness of their relationship to their adopted adolescents lower than the other parents. Of the adoptive parents who later gave birth, over 87% found their relationships with their adopted and biological children similar.

Adoptive family formation

In a qualitative study of 43 infertile American couples, Weir examined the transition to adoptive parenting [34]. She identified what she called a "leap-frogging pattern" in the rapid transition to adoptive parenthood. Within 10 years of child placement, the couples had caught up with other parents in their adjustment to parental roles, the developmental tasks of parenting their children, and engagement in social activities with other parents and their children. In Canada, McKay and colleagues conducted a study that reviewed the literature on adaptation to parenthood during the three years post-placement [35]. The researchers found only 11 studies that examined parental mental health, physical health and intimate partner relationship satisfaction. They found that the adoptive parents reported lower levels of distress than biological parents, although post-adoption depression was relatively common. In addition, the researchers noted that almost all of the support services for early parenting (e.g., breastfeeding) were aimed at biological parents, suggesting the need for more research into the needs of adoptive parents in order to improve services to adoptive parents that better match their needs.

Atkinson and Gonet interviewed 500 adoptive families in the United States to investigate adoptive family formation and adjustment [36]. The majority of the adoptive families (more than 60%) included children from foster care, while 20% of the families were from private adoptions and 15% from international adoptions. The forms of assistance families identified most frequently as helpful were support groups with other adoptive parents, followed by adoption-competent counseling and respite care. The parents reported the most progress in strengthening of their parenting abilities primarily through increasing their capacity to understand and cope with their children's behavior. Atkinson and Gonet concluded that adoptive families needed continuing education on the developmental aspects of adoptive parenting by adoption-competent counseling.

In a recent qualitative study in the United States, Klevian found that in examining decisions about the race of their child, some adoptive parents experienced personal growth through "transformational processing" and "racial renegotiation of self" based on race-based choices in adoption [37]. For some parents this meant an additional layer of self-analysis beyond the acceptance of not having a biogenetically related child, to giving up the dream of having a child who shares racial resemblance.

In summary, the field of adoption research has primarily focused on individuals who have been adopted, demonstrating that adoption remains a protective solution for children in need of families, within limits associated with various risk factors. Research on adoptive parents has focused mainly on motivation for adoption after infertility and the adjustments involved in adoptive parenthood after infertility. Adoption remains a solution for people with infertility who seek children to parent. Adjustments to adopting after infertility include changes in personal identity and expectations regarding the kind of children that are adopted, which may result in additional processing which leads to choosing a child of a different cultural or racial background.

The fertility counselor as an adoption guide

People who are beginning to learn about adoption feel overwhelmed and want a roadmap, and it may be useful to approach adoption as a journey into new territory with the counselor as a guide. This journey into the unknown can be described as "making the strange familiar." The journey of change is not linear, and the idea of being at a crossroads and journeying down different pathways and back to the crossing in the road can be a safe way to start the exploration.

Beginning the journey

Julie and David decided to start the adoption process while they were approaching their third and (possibly final) IVF treatment. They initially called adoption their "insurance plan." After years of failed treatments and disappointment they were shocked to learn that in today's private, domestic adoption in the USA they had to be chosen by a birthmother (they had fully expected that they would be the ones doing the choosing). They had difficulty adjusting from being the clients in the fertility clinic to adoption's focus on the "best interests of the child." Julie found the home-study (evaluation) process to be especially painful and invasive: "... first I have been poked and prodded physically ... and now I am being poked and prodded psychologically." They resented the social worker's questions about their ability to become adoptive parents. It took them some time to recognize that they had approached adoption as an altruistic act and had expected to be rewarded and compensated for their past suffering and losses.

At the beginning of adoption exploration people are approaching adoption through the lens of their fertility failures and by fitting the idea of adoption into their existing framework of what it means to be a family. Typically, adoption begins as a second or third choice, or even "last resort," and may therefore appear to be inferior to mainstream parenting and be devalued. It is very important that the counselor allow for the open expression of all thoughts and feelings, which lays the groundwork for the open acknowledgment of mixed feelings. Familiar principles of psychotherapy hold true here: feelings that are resisted get stronger, and awareness and ambivalence are achieved only through the open receptivity to all states of mind.

Because the subject of adoption is emotionally laden for most people and has typically been on theirs and other people's minds throughout their infertility experience ("Just adopt!"), the counselor may encounter the least resistance if adoption exploration is introduced early on in the infertility journey along with all other possible family building options. Furthermore, when people do not feel forced to choose then they are better able to explore challenging topics.

If the counselor has been able to facilitate an early introduction to adoption then the transition to exploring adoption is less disruptive. As adoption is investigated more seriously, the counselor needs to help people grieve and process their feelings of the losses in adoption, which include an absence of a genetic connection and pregnancy. The counselor can help people understand that it is not just that the child who will be adopted who is different from the child they thought they would parent, but it is also they themselves who will become different. The counselor needs to reinforce the relational, systemic experience and the reality that in adopting people become *adoptive parents* and part of an *adoptive family*.

The exploration of similarities and differences is the backbone of adoptive parenting and also fundamental to all learning and change. If the counselor can help people become aware of how connecting through sameness feels safe, and that differences may initially feel more distant and even threatening, then this understanding can become a foundation for the life-long journey of adoptive family life.

Couples' dynamics: taking different routes

Clare wanted to move on to adoption but Justin believed they would get pregnant if only Clare would "... stop being so stressed out." Clare was angry: "... it's ok for you, you are not the one in the stirrups! I can't take it anymore!" Justin complained: "... in adoption you don't know what you are going to get!" Their deadlock was finally broken after Justin (reluctantly) attended an adoption conference. This experience, in addition to counseling, enabled Justin to become open to exploring adoption. As Justin gradually became enthusiastic, Clare suddenly felt a new reluctance. Learning about familiar couples' systemic dynamics during counseling helped this couple learn how to collaborate. Clare developed a new appreciation for Justin's cautiousness while Justin took charge of the new adoption checklist, thereby helping Clare to finally feel supported.

Many couples feel painfully distant from each other when approaching adoption. The fertility counselor can help couples learn about common couples' dynamics such as polarizations and the couple as a system. This idea of polarization helps promote the development of a vitally important skill for adoptive parenting, namely to understand that when one party emphasizes the differences in adoption then the other party feels pressure to respond with similarities, and vice versa. The idea of the couple as a system prepares the couple for the idea of the adoptive family as a system, the adoption triadic system of adoptive parenting and parenting within a particular social context. The counselor can also encourage the couple to work together as a team, which can be profoundly healing after the past unevenness in fertility treatments.

The counselor can promote personal growth and resilience by encouraging people to take risks in exploring adoption and to reflect on progress that has been accomplished. This tracking of progress promotes hope and perseverance: looking backwards at distance traveled can create encouragement to keep moving forwards. Reminders of previous developments, such as the gradual acceptance of IVF (typically also initially encountered as both daunting and overwhelming), are helpful. If the counselor can help people learn that even when powerful feelings are present this is only part of their psychic landscape, they will be contributing greatly to a solid foundation for future adoptive parenting challenges.

Once there is openness to exploring adoption then people are more likely to focus on the advantages of adoption, such as the opportunity to parent, love and nurture a child. This understanding leads into the formation of entitlement and claiming of future children who will be adopted. The counselor can help people gradually identify and critically evaluate existing beliefs, expectations, fears and myths about adoption. By encouraging people to "try adoption on for size" and making adoption more real, the counselor is providing important steps towards parenting. In helping people understand, for example, how the common idea that adoptive parents are altruistic by "saving" or "rescuing" a child leads to the consequence that their child may feel intensely indebted to those parents, the counselor is helping those people learn how to take the perspective of the child and to become adoptive parents.

Gravitational pulls along the journey

James and Stefan sought counseling because they felt stuck: While James was enthusiastic and wanted to learn about adoption, Stefan did not appear to be at all interested. A discussion about the birthparents resulted in Stefan becoming annoyed: "… the person who raises you is your parent, what is the big deal here?" Initially angry, further investigation moved him to tears, as he finally came in contact with feelings of sadness that he had not been raised by his "own" father, but rather by his (beloved) stepfather. Counseling helped Stefan recognize how his feelings of loyalty towards his stepfather had interfered with his capability to approach adoption. This couple were able to be helped to see how Stefan's particular step-family formation could be an advantage as a resource for the triangularity and potential "loyalty conflicts" inherent in adoptive family life.

Counseling can do much to promote the psychosocial health of adoptive families by recognizing predictable forces and pressures. One of the main challenges in adoptive parenting is acknowledging the reality of the birthparents. Counselors can normalize how people initially fit adoption into a mainstream perspective where there is no room for two sets of parents, and help them find room in their minds for this more complex family structure. This leads to a more direct consideration of the birthparents, often conceptualized as a birthmother who may return to take back the child, or to whom the child will return after rejecting adoptive parents with the much dreaded and commonly imagined "you're not my real mother." Counselors can help people accept the reality that birthparents are in fact psychologically present in the adoptive family system even when it is a closed or confidential adoption. If the counselor can explain that the feeling of being threatened by birthparents is partially connected to a heightened fear of future loss, and partly to fitting adoption into the mainstream "either/or" perspective where it is imagined that a child will have to choose one set of parents over another, then this can create a counterpoint for people to start to challenge their fears and anxieties.

Acceptance of birthparents is a crucial element of adoptive parenting, which takes time to mature and as such requires patient and careful ongoing exploration. If the counselor can give voice to the perspective and needs of the future child and humanize birthparents, this normalizes the adjustment and reduces anxiety. Counseling can raise people's awareness of how adoption decisions are often motivated by future loss prevention, for example by choosing an adoption plan in which it is anticipated that the birth connection will be disconnected.

The counselor can help people understand how the existence of birthparents adds additional layers of triadic experience to everyday family life. One way to introduce this concept is to reference the common experience of how families attribute aspects of biogenetic children to "one side" of the family or the other. Typically talents are claimed while problematic behaviors are disavowed, as in, for example: "… this (problem) must come from your side of the family!" The counselor can then build on this experience by explaining how in adoption the existence of the birthparents provides more opportunities for triadic processes for both positive and negative traits and behaviors to be attributed to this additional "other side of the family" along nature/nurture lines.

Choosing the "right" path

Vanessa and Paul, a Caucasian couple, wanted a child who would "fit in" with their extended family. Neither was initially conscious of their own fears of being visibly different if the child did not resemble them. Moreover, their past experience in the fertility field had emphasized the need to "match" them with potential gamete donors. However, as they became comfortable with adoption, their feelings changed. After counseling and attending adoptive parents meetings and conferences they learnt more about the challenges of transracial adoption and decided to adopt from Ethiopia. While they became aware that their child became simply that, "their child" rather than someone who looked different from them, actual encounters in parks and in their home towns later brought stares and comments which were harder for them than they had initially anticipated.

The counselor can help people face the challenges of deciding which kind of child they would feel comfortable parenting, with the associated issues of race and ethnicity. Counselors can help people explore their fantasies of parenting children from different backgrounds, including in transracial adoptions where the child and the whole family becomes visibly different: a transracial adoption creates a *transracial adoptive family*. Counseling can help people recognize the additional challenges of helping a child develop a dual identity and, where relevant, a different racial identity, as well as the additional parenting responsibilities of helping a child learn how to navigate in a world which includes racism. Other areas where counseling can be profoundly helpful include helping people think through being motivated by feelings of urgency when choosing which child and when to adopt instead of taking time to evaluate and become comfortable with choices and the consequences of those choices. Counseling needs to help people create a space in their minds to imagine and recognize the needs of each child.

Once a decision has been made to adopt then there will be a focus on both similarities and differences. The counselor can point out the natural rewriting of the personal and family narrative, often accompanied by references to fate and destiny and the common reflection of: "I've always wanted to adopt!" For those people who choose to adopt transracially, the counselor can help them learn the necessary racial socialization skills to support the positive identity formation of their children and prepare them for issues associated with racism. Likewise, for those parents who pursue intercountry adoptions (many of which are also transracial adoptions), the counselor can be helpful in encouraging adoptive parents to learn how to promote cultural continuity and integration for their children.

Social support is extremely important for adoptive families. People who have experienced infertility typically withdraw from family and friends, and the counselor can help people find ways to reconnect with family and friends and to expand their social network to accommodate membership in a new group of adoptive families while maintaining connection with biogenetic families. The transition to actually becoming adoptive parents can be a vulnerable time, and the counselor can play an important role by raising awareness and looking out for a possible post-adoption depression.

Communicating in a new language

"Who are her real parents?," Joseph and Anna reported how scrutiny and curiosity about their transracial family evoked this typical question from the general public. A parallel also occurred in the playground and at school where their daughter is often asked "Where are your real parents?" "I tell them I'm her real mother and I tell her she should do the same" said Anna, sounding outraged. "I tell them you are looking at them right now!" said Joseph angrily. In counseling they learnt a wider range of responses and also to be aware of how their responses shaped their future interactions with others. They learnt how to discriminate between people whom they wanted to educate and when (e.g., on the line/queue at the supermarket) they wanted to cut short the interaction. They also learnt how to help their daughter choose when and how to handle unwelcome comments. This process brought up old familiar painful feelings about being different, as well as the profound fear and reality common to all parents of not being able to protect their child from pain.

A main focus of adoptive parenting has to do with communication with the child and others about adoption [38,39]. It is well established that the best to way to create an integrated sense of self for individuals who have been adopted is for parents to talk to their children about adoption from the very beginning as part of an *ongoing process*. Counseling can help parents understand the need for a calm and receptive state of mind in parents in order to promote an open atmosphere which will make it more likely that their child can establish an ongoing dialogue about adoption over the course of their lifetime together. The counselor can help people understand that children are acutely aware of their parents' discomfort and that

Table 14.6 Examples of positive adoption language.

Negative	Positive
Real parent or natural parent	Birthparent, birthmother, birthfather
My own child	My child by birth
Given up, put up for adoption, given away	Made an adoption plan or relinquished
Foreign adoption	Intercountry adoption
Child taken away from	Termination of rights
Is adopted	Was adopted
Decided to keep	Chose to parent

if children sense that talking about adoption makes their parents feel anxious they will avoid bringing it up. The counselor may need to reinforce the importance of parents refraining from making negative comments about the child's birthparents and background and also from trying to compensate through idealization. More psychoeducation is helpful to explain that children learn gradually according to their developmental level and to accept that curiosity is a normal part of being human.

Counseling can do much to help future parents develop fluency in positive adoption language by providing modeling and increasing awareness. (Table 14.6 provides examples of positive adoption language.) The counselor can, for example, help people examine and alter their use of the common phrase "my own child," typically reserved to describe a biogenetically related child. Talking about adoption also means talking to friends, families, and the general public, where scrutiny and curiosity may lead to unsolicited and intrusive comments in the presence of children. This is particularly likely in the case of adoptive families where adoption is noticeable, as with transracially adoptive families. There are important social skills that the counselor can teach adoptive parents about how to respond from a place of empowerment and strength rather than from being reactive or defensive [40]. The counselor can help parents understand the power of their emotional tone and suggest useful strategies for decreasing anxiety and increasing self-authorization, such as encouraging practice and role-play.

Adoptive parents can be trained by the counselor to clarify and reframe difficult and unwelcome comments, and take charge of the conversation by steering, reframing and setting positive limits, rather

Table 14.7 Examples of reframing reponses.

Comment/Question	Response
Where are his real parents?	I think you mean his *birthparents*...
She is so lucky you adopted her...	We are the lucky ones here.
I'm sorry you had to adopt.	This was our choice and we are very happy about it.
How much did he cost?	Nothing. Children must not be sold.
What do you know about her background?	We have information we shall share with our child as she gets older.
Aren't you worried the mother will take him back?	No. Adoption is forever.
Where is she from?	This country ... I can see you are curious ... let me suggest a website where you can learn more about adoption.
Aren't you worried she will grow up and find her real mother?	You mean his birthmother ... There are many common fears about adoption. Fear of future loss is one of them.
It is different from having your own child ...	S/he *is* our own child ... Adoption is one of many ways to form a family, and for the most part we are just like any other family.
I want to adopt ... tell me how you got her ...	Let me refer you to a website which will give you more information.

than responding from a defensive position that only alienates and leads to isolation. Adoptive parents can be reminded of their own prior lack of understanding about adoption as an equally viable and legitimate parenting choice. Adoptive parents can learn from the counselor how to develop flexibility in their responses to others. It is important to emphasize how modeling and their parents' capability to respond to others with limits and low defensiveness and reactivity will be internalized by and empower their child/ren. Table 14.7 provides examples of reframing responses.

Dealing with uncertainty in a new land

Cheryl sought counseling to find out whether her son's difficulties in school were "adoption issues." Initially defensive, once she expressed some difficult

feelings and fears and felt understood, she was able to consider various possibilities. Initially fearing she would blame herself (or be blamed by others) for not being a good enough mother (many adoptive parents are very hard on themselves) and also wondering if the problem could be attributed to the birthmother's pregnancy and lack of prenatal care, she gradually became less frantic. With encouragement she was able to join an adoptive parents' support group. "I came to you for answers," she said, "I hoped you would tell me exactly what was happening...and now I know that it is more complicated...I may never know exactly whether it is or it isn't an adoption issue. But at least I'm not so worried anymore. At least I don't feel so alone."

The counselor can do much to help adoptive parents with the higher level of uncertainty that accompanies adoptive parenting. Because adoptive parents nurture their children but have no biogenetic contribution they may overemphasize nurture and minimize the impact of nature and genetics. The counselor can encourage a more integrated approach that allows for nature and nurture, and interactional processes between both. There is increased uncertainty in adoption, from the time frame of waiting for a child, to unknown genetic inheritance, to the central question of whether any one particular issue is or is not "adoption-related." The counselor can normalize this uncertainty and help parents create continuums, openness and curiosity instead of certainties based on oversimplification and anxiety. The same nature/nurture split occurs socially, with other people responding to one pole or the other. Counselors can help people withstand the projections of others and respond from an integrated framework, weaving in both nature and nurture, rather than becoming polarized. Additionally counselors can help parents understand that curiosity about and searching for birthparents are both normal and not a sign of adoptive parents' inadequacy or pathology within their child [41,42].

The split between nature and nurture also occurs in some countries and cultures, with one set of roots (usually nature) being privileged over the other. Adopted people have two sets of roots to identify with, and therefore there are variations between and within families and between and within individuals over time. Adopted people can identify with either or with both sets of roots, and identifications may shift over time. This may be more striking when the differences between the two sets of roots appear to be further apart, such as in transracial and intercountry adoptions. As adopted people grow older they develop their own ideas about adoption, which may contrast with those of their parents. For example, while adoptive parents may emphasize the power of fate and destiny, their children may instead resonate with the randomness of being placed in one family when they might easily have been placed in another. When parents find themselves and their children lacking congruence in how they understand adoption this can produce conflict. The counselor can help adoptive parents process their feelings and remain open to allowing for the individuation of their children and also to developmental processes associated with separation. Ultimately adoptive parents, like all parents, have to come to terms with the fact that the children they have adopted are free to come to their own understanding about adoption as in all other matters. The goal of parenting, after all, is to have children grow up and separate, leave home and go out into the world. Children do not remain children and children who have been adopted grow up to be adults. Adoptive parents may also become grandparents. Adoption continues to be present in family life over time.

Besides the processing of loss and other challenges, the counselor needs to allow room for the recognition of potential advantages in adoption. For example, many adoptive parents appreciate the personal growth of adopting which can be healing as well as providing a powerfully different model of connection, identity and belonging. Adoptive parents also commonly report feeling freed to allow for the discovery of who their child is rather than feeling burdened by expectations. Some parents feel less guilty if their children have health or learning issues, which may partially explain why adoptive parents are able to seek help more readily than other parents. Some adoptive parents feel relief in not passing on their own genetic susceptibilities to various illnesses. Counselors can help parents consider that the additional complexity of adoptive family life can in the best-case scenario buffer their adopted children not only against their past but also against future adversity as the world becomes increasingly complex. The fertility counselor may help strengthen adoptive families by modeling an attitude of elasticity, flexibility and resilience. People who adopt after infertility learn firsthand many powerful lessons about the limitations and the immensity of being human.

For people who choose to adopt after experiencing infertility, this choice involves an adaptation, which may not only include choosing to parent a child who is initially a stranger, but also crossing economic, geographic and racial boundaries. Adoptive parents need ongoing support. Adoption presents expectable challenges to adoptive families at predictable developmental junctures across the lifespan. Adoption also presents advantages that include feeling freed from expectations. For people approaching adoption, this process may be likened to a journey into the unknown.

Reflection and summary

Adoption is a complex subject that is constantly evolving within a family, socio-political and global system. As a fertility counselor in the USA working in adoption, I find that the increasingly diverse array of ART options have had a significant and somewhat paradoxical effect on the way people with infertility problems approach adoption. On the one hand adopting a child is increasingly seen as more conventional, thereby undermining existing remnants of past associations having to do with the pathologization, marginalization and stigmatization of adoption. On the other hand, ART, with its potential for genetic connections and control over chosen gametes and pregnancy, has reinforced the idea that adoption is "not quite as good as having your own" [43]. Combined with the decrease in "desirable" children (i.e., infants) available for adoption, it "...seems to be a good idea...for someone else to do" [22]. I find that, for those people who have access to ART, adoption tends to be pursued only after all other reproductive possibilities have been exhausted. This means that some people approach adoption when they are more depleted, more overwhelmed and more desperate than in the past. This creates a greater need for counseling and also a more significant opportunity for the counselor to be profoundly helpful. I consider myself to be privileged to do this most important work. I feel a deep responsibility to help, protect and promote the integrity of future adoptive families. In the best-case scenario adoption becomes an adaptation that involves an expansion of human connection beyond existing limits. At its worst adoption can become human exploitation. I witness people at their best and at their most egregious; at their most vulnerable; and in their most flawed and their most valiant moments. Change is enormously hard. There is great resistance and a vast potential for growth. Adoption counseling is challenging, full of creative destructions and reconstructions. It fills my life with passion and meaning, as well as a deep admiration for the lengths (both external and internal) that people traverse in order to find their children. What could be a more important goal for a counselor than to be part of this primitive and essential task?

References

1. *Hague Adoption Convention on Protection of Children and Co-operation in Respect of Inter-Country Adoption.* Available from: http://www.hcch.net. Accessed February 8, 2014.
2. Volkman TA (ed). *Cultures of Transnational Adoption.* Durham, NC: Duke University Press, 2005.
3. Babb LA. Ethics in contemporary adoption practice. In: V Groza and K Rosenberg, eds. *Clinical Practice Issues in Adoption: Bridging the gap between Adoptees Placed as Infants and as Older Children*, revised and expanded. Westport, CT: Bergen and Garvey, 2001: 105–55.
4. Van IJzendoorn MH, Juffer F. The Emanuel Miller Memorial Lecture 2006: Adoption as intervention. Meta-analytic evidence of massive catch-up and plasticity in physical, socio-emotional, and cognitive development. *Journal of Child Psychology and Psychiatry* 2006; 47: 1228–45.
5. Freundlich M, Lieberthal JK. *Adoption and Ethics: The Impact of Adoption on Members of the Triad.* Washington, DC: Child Welfare League of America, 2001.
6. Cole ES, Donley KS. History, values, and placement policy issues in adoption. In: D. Brodzinsky and M. Schechter, eds. *The Psychology of Adoption.* New York: Oxford University Press, 1990: 273–94.
7. Selman P. From Bucharest to Beijing: Changes in countries sending children for international adoption 1990 to 2006. In: G Wrobel and E Neil, eds. *International Advances in Adoption Research for Practice.* New York: Wiley, 2009a: 41–69.
8. Herszenhorn DM, Eckholm E. Putin signs bill that bars US adoptions, upending families *New York Times* December 27, 2012; Available from: http://www.nytimes.com/2012/12/28/world/europe/putin-to-sign-ban-on-us-adoptions-of-russian-children.html?pa. Accessed April 6, 2014.
9. Selman P. The rise and fall of intercountry adoption in the 21st century. *International Social Work* 2009b; 52 (5): 1–20.

10. *U.S. Department of State: FY 2012 Annual Report on Intercountry Adoption*, January 2013; Available from: http://travel.state.gov/content/dam/aa/pdfs/fy2012_annual_report.pdf. Accessed October 24, 2014.
11. Selman P. The movement of children for international adoption: Developments and trends in receiving states and states of origin, 1998–2004. In: D Marre and L Briggs, eds. *International Adoption: Global Inequalities and the Circulation of Children*. New York: New York University Press, 2009: 32–51.
12. Selman P. *Key Tables for Intercountry Adoption: Receiving States 2003–2012; States of Origin 2003–2011*; Available from: http://www.hcch.net/upload/2013selmanstats33.pdf. Accessed February 8, 2014.
13. *U.S. Department of State: FY 2013 Annual Report on Intercountry Adoption*, March 2014 Available from: http://travel.state.gov/content/dam/aa/pdfs/fy2013_annual_report.pdf Accessed October 24, 2014.
14. *Wall Street Journal for the Associated Press*, March 22, 2014 Available from: http://online.wsj.com/news/articles/SB20001424052702303802104579453521021718870. Accessed March 23, 2014.
15. Kirk, HD. *Shared Fate*. New York: Free Press, 1984.
16. Brodzinsky DA. Stress and coping model of adoption adjustment. In: D Brodzinsky, M. Schechter, eds. *The Psychology of Adoption*. New York: Oxford University Press, 1990: 3–24.
17. Bowlby J. *Attachment and Loss: Vol. 1: Attachment*. New York: Basic Books, 2000.
18. Bowlby J. *Attachment and Loss: Vol. 2: Separation*. New York: Basic Books, 1973.
19. Daniluk JC, Hurtig-Mitchell J. Themes of hope and healing: Infertile couples' experiences of adoption. *Journal of Counseling and Development* 2003; 81, Fall: 389–99.
20. Hendry A, Netherwood PA. Child at last: Adoption and infertility. In: M Crawshaw and R Balen, eds., *Adopting after Infertility: Messages from Practice, Research, and Personal Experience*. London and Philadelphia: Jessica Kingsley, 2010: 151–63.
21. Shapiro V, Shapiro J, Paret I. *Complex Adoption and Assisted Reproductive Technologies*. New York: Guilford Press, 2001.
22. Palacios J. The ecology of adoption. In: GM Wrobel and E Neil, eds. *International Advances in Adoption Research for Practice*. London: Wiley-Blackwell, 2009: 71–94.
23. Grotevant HD, Dunbar N, Kohler JK, Esau AL. Adoptive identity: How contexts within and beyond the family shape developmental pathways. *Family Relations*, 2000; 49: 379–87.
24. Lee RM. The transracial adoption paradox: History, research, and counseling implications of cultural socialization. *The Counseling Psychologist*, 2003; 31 (6): 711–44.
25. Wrobel GM, Kohler J, Grotevant HD, McRoy R. The Family Adoption Communication (FAC) Model: Identifying pathways of adoption-related communication. *Adoption Quarterly* 2003, 7 (2): 53–84.
26. Palacios J, Brodzinsky DM. Review: Adoption research: Trends, topics, outcomes. *International Journal of Behavioral Development*, 2010; 34 (3), 270–84.
27. Van IJzendoorn MH, Juffer F. The Emanuel Miller Memorial Lecture 2006: Adoption as intervention. Meta-analytic evidence of massive catch-up and plasticity in physical, socio-emotional, and cognitive development. *Journal of Child Psychology and Psychiatry* 2006; 47, 1228–45.
28. Vandivere S, Malm K, Radel LF. *Adoption USA: A Chartbook Based on the 2007 National Survey of Adoptive Parents*. Washington, DC: U.S. Department of Health and Human Services, Office of the Assistant Secretary for Planning and Evaluation, 2009.
29. Jones J. Adoption experiences of women and men and demand for children to adopt by women 18–44 years of age in the United States, 2002. *U.S. Department of Health and Human Services, Center for Disease Control and Prevention, National Center for Health Statistics.*August 2008, Series 23, Number 27, pages 1–18. Available from: http://www.cdc.gov/nchs/data/series/sr_23/sr23_027.pdf Accessed October 24, 2014.
30. Pinborg A, Hougaard CO, Andersen AN, Molbo D, Schmidt L. Prospective longitudinal cohort study on cumulative 5-year delivery and adoption rates among 1338 couples initiating infertility treatment. *Human Reproduction* 2009; 24 (4): 991–99.
31. Zhang Y, Lee GR. Intercountry versus transracial adoption: Analysis of adoptive parents' motivations and preferences in adoption. *Journal of Family Issues* 2011; 32 (1): 75–98.
32. Hogström L, Johansson M, Janson PO, Berg M, Francis J, Sogn J, Hellström AL, Adolfsson A. Quality of life after adopting compared with childbirth with or without assisted reproduction. *Acta Obstetricia Gynecologica Scandinavia* 2012 Sep; 91 (9):1077–85. Available from: http://www.ncbi.nlm.nih.gov/pubmed/22708621. Accessed October 27, 2012.
33. Triseliotis J, Feast J, Kyle F. *The Adoption Triangle Revisited: A Study of Adoption, Search and Reunion Experiences*. London: British Association for Adoption and Fostering, 2005.

34. Weir KN. Adoptive family "leap frogging" patterns. *Adoption Quarterly* 2003; 7: 1: 27–41.

35. McKay K, Ross LE, Goldberg AE. Adaptation to parenthood during the post-adoption period: A review of the literature. *Adoption Quarterly* 2010; 13: 125–44. Available from: http://dx.doi.org/10.1080/10926755.2010.481040. Accessed October 2014.

36. Atkinson A, Gonet P. Strengthening adoption practice, listening to adoptive families. *Child Welfare* 2007; 86: 87–104.

37. Klevian M. Resolving race: How adoptive parents discuss choosing the race of their child. *Adoption Quarterly* 2012; 15: 2: 88–115.

38. Brodzinsky D. Children's understanding of adoption: Developmental and clinical implications. *Professional Psychology: Research and Practice* 2011; 42 : 2: 200–7.

39. Brodzinsky D. Family structural openness and communication openness as predictors in the adjustment of adopted children. *Adoption Quarterly* 2006; 9: 4: 1–18.

40. Smith B, Surrey JL, Watkins M. "Real" mothers": Adoptive mothers resisting marginalization and recreating motherhood. In: K Wegar, ed. *Adoptive Families in a Diverse Society*. New Brunswick, NJ: Rutgers University Press, 2006: 146–61.

41. Wrobel GM, Dillon K. Adopted adolescents: who and what are they curious about? In: GM Wrobel and E Neil, eds. *International Advances in Adoption Research for Practice*. London: Wiley-Blackwell, 2009: 217–44.

42. Howe D, Feast J. *Adoption, Search and Reunion: The Long-Term Experience of Adopted Adults*. London: BAAF, 2000.

43. Fisher AP. "Not quite as good as having your own"? Towards a sociology of adoption. *Annual Reviews of Sociology* 2003; 29: 335–61.

Chapter 15

Fertility preservation counseling

Allison B. Rosen

Maria, an elementary school teacher of Italian heritage, was 32 years old when she began psychotherapy. Three years earlier, she had cryopreserved embryos she created with her fiancé, Paul, after being diagnosed with Stage 2 breast cancer. When Maria called, she had just found out that her cancer had returned and that she had metastatic breast disease. She wanted therapy to clarify her thinking about the issues surrounding her death, her relationship with Paul, and whether or not to have children using a gestational carrier. Paul, age 29, from a large, Caucasian upper-class New England family, wanted to marry Maria. Maria's close, but controlling family, added stress to her life. As their only child, they wanted to be involved in all aspects of her decision-making and treatment.

First and foremost in Maria's mind was her desire for children. She looked surprisingly fit and healthy, and married Paul about a year after starting therapy. Maria reasoned that she might live several years and believed that her hope of giving life to her embryos/children and experiencing the role of loving mother was essential to her well-being. She knew that Paul would emotionally support her during her illness and wanted him to **want** to care for their children after her death. Maria felt that raising their children would be proof of his enduring love. However, Paul felt that caring for children during Maria's treatment for cancer would be more than he could handle. Her parents wanted to proceed immediately with gestational surrogacy, since they wanted to give Maria everything that she desired; in so doing they could also "replace" their only child with a grandchild, softening the blow of losing her. Paul resisted pressure from Maria and her family to create a family as soon as possible.

Maria's future death was a constant painful background note in her otherwise active life. She made videotapes for her future children. Messages were created for her children's important future events (e.g., entering school, birthdays and graduation). She hoped that even if Paul could not be a parent during their time together, he would use the embryos in the future.

During therapy, Maria mourned the loss of everything she valued. She mourned the loss of a chance to experience life, be a mother, and grow old. She mourned the loss of her physical vitality and beauty. She mourned not having a future to look forward to. The thought of children was her main hope and gave her the strength to continue treatment for her cancer. "Caring" for her future children (through fantasies, messages and videotapes) gave her a sense of motherhood in the present and "immortality" in the future. Intermittently, Paul came to treatment with Maria when her sadness at his not using the embryos interfered with their relationship.

After Maria died (fours years after the reoccurrence of her cancer), Paul briefly entered therapy. He felt guilty for not wanting to use the embryos during her life and after her death; therapy helped him work through these feelings. Maria's parents wanted custody of the embryos creating constant conflict with Paul. Three years later, Paul re-entered therapy. He wanted to destroy the embryos, a right that he had obtained from the consents he and Maria signed prior to cryopreservation. He felt angry, wishing the embryos had never been created; to him, they held his future hostage.

Introduction

The term fertility preservation refers to medical procedures that allow men and women to postpone

Fertility Counseling: Clinical Guide and Case Studies, ed. Sharon N. Covington. Published by Cambridge University Press.

childbearing. Fertility preservation may be used for both medical and social reasons and is performed throughout the world. There are many reasons for fertility preservation: cancer patients wishing to bear children after gonadotoxic chemotherapy regimens [1]; oocyte cryopreservation during IVF when sperm is unavailable [2]; patients at risk of losing their fertility potential due to genetic abnormalities [3]; patients with genetic disorders affecting fertility, such as Turner syndrome mosaicism [4,5]. Now, individuals undergoing gender reassignment surgery or men deploying to war may chose to preserve their fertility [6]. Importantly, oocyte cryopreservation has become a reality for women hoping to delay childbearing because of age-related fertility loss [7–9].

Fertility preservation is a rapidly changing field because of the developing nature of the underlying medical procedures necessary for successful preservation. Many of the procedures were initially considered experimental, then quickly evolved to be part of the reproductive specialists' standard armamentarium. For instance, while commercial sperm banks have existed since the early 1970s, the technology for oocyte cryopreservation is a relatively recent development. The first birth of a child after oocyte cryopreservation was reported in 1986, but because of the very low success rate of the procedure, there were only five live births for over a decade [10,11]. Thus, mature oocyte cryopreservation was considered experimental, to be performed only at specialized centers for patients needing fertility sparing procedures because of medical necessity. In 2012, the American Society of Reproductive Medicine (ASRM) changed its policy about the experimental status of oocyte cryopreservation since vitrification (fast freeze) of oocytes yielded fertilization rates comparable to fresh oocytes when combined with intracytoplasmic sperm injection (ICSI) [12]. In the largest random controlled trial, 600 recipients using fresh versus vitrified donor oocytes were compared. Investigators found that 92.5% of the vitrified oocytes survived warming and there were no significant differences in fertilization rates, implantation rates or pregnancy rates per transfer between groups [13]. Currently, young women using vitrified ooctyes have the same probability of live birth per embryo transfer as women undergoing IVF or ICSI with fresh oocytes [13].

Thus, the practice of cryopreservation of vitrified oocytes for social reasons has been increasingly accepted in a variety of countries. In the USA, more than 50% of IVF programs offer fertility preservation for social reasons.

This chapter will focus on the counseling issues of women seeking fertility preservation. While there are several effective methods to preserve fertility in men (e.g., cryopreservation of sperm), most men do not receive counseling prior to their fertility sparing procedures when undergoing fertility preservation for medical reasons. In general, they do not need to preserve fertility for social reasons because they do not suffer the same age-related decline in fecundity as women. While sperm quality deteriorates somewhat as men get older, the reduced quality does not usually create problems until after the age of 60 [14]. On the other hand, ASRM and ESHRE recommend that women receive counseling for both medical and social fertility preservation [15]. While it may be interesting to speculate the reasons for this difference in policy, more is known about the emotional experiences and counseling needs of women undergoing fertility preservation.

In one sense, the motivations for fertility sparing procedures for medical and social reasons are similar. In both cases, women who wish to postpone childbearing for the future are trying to prevent a problem that has not yet occurred, and may face similar benefits and potential negative consequences. Cryopreservation empowers both groups of women in that they are trying to maintain control over their lives and protect themselves. Both groups, however, face devastating loss if the procedures fail to work and the women are unable to have genetically related children. Both groups must be knowledgeable about the fact that fertility preservation involves some (small) medical risk to themselves and to their future offspring.

However, fertility preservation for women with medical illness differs from fertility preservation for social reasons (see Table 15.1). Medical fertility preservation occurs during an emotional crisis and the counseling may need to be rapidly scheduled between other medical appointments (e.g., oncologist, surgeon, etc.) because of medical necessity. Conversely, fertility preservation for personal reasons may be planned long in advance. Women in a medical crisis may have concerns that are unique to their diagnosis (e.g., passing the cancer to the children; exacerbating cancer growth because of the IVF stimulation protocol). Having time with a knowledgeable fertility counselor during a medical crisis may be more welcome than counseling for social fertility preservation. During a medical crisis, counseling is part of other appointments with medical

Table 15.1 Comparison of oocyte cryopreservation for medical and social reasons [46, adapted].

Freezing for Medical Conditions		Freezing for Social Reasons	
Pro	**Con**	**Pro**	**Con**
Physical Risk to Woman			
*Low risk for most patients	*Entails some risk to ER+ & PR+ breast cancer	*Low risk	*Medical procedures performed on healthy women *Risks exist *Pregnancy complications in older woman
Physical Risk to Child			
*Same low risk as IVF	*Congenital problems same as any pregnancy (3%) *May have increaed genetic problems due to ICSI	*Same low risk as IVF	*Congenital problems same as any pregnancy (3%) *May have increased genetic problems due to ICSI *Disadvantage of having an older parent (child taking care of the parent; early death of parent)
Money			
*Expenses may be covered by insurance as side effect of chemotherapy	*Occurs during other medical expenses for cancer; may not be covered by insurance; may not be able to afford GC	*May be worthwhile for peace of mind	*Elective procedure uncovered by insurance *$20K–40K to accrue enough oocytes
Societal			
*Allows woman to build family using her own genes *Avoids use of donor who must undergo medical procedures *Research may benefit other medical and social situations	*May involve a GS *No guarantee of successful pregnancy and childbirth	*Gives woman control over family building *Woman can complete education, find life partner and develop financial stability *Avoids rush into "bad" relationship *Avoids need for egg donation *Women can delay if partner unwilling to have children in present *Can donate unused oocytes to others or for research	*No guarantee of viable pregnancy and childbirth *False assumptions leading to decisions that limit the ability to have children *May encourage delay of marriage *Older parents may have to take care of children and parents at the same time *May never use oocytes *Discriminates against the poor *May allow society to ignore social support for working moms
Psychological Risks & Benefits			
*Provides hope during life-threatening illness *Avoids the need for a woman to choose between cancer treatments & biological children *May reduce overall stress due to active coping *Avoids pain of "double whammy" of cancer and loss of ability to have children	*May be false hope *Procedures may add stress *Worry that procedures may hurt cancer treatment and survival *Fear of passing on cancer genetically	*Women can control their reproduction *Women can assess benefits and risks in a reasonable manner	*False security and/or worry about the uncertainty of success *Psychological loss in accepting the reality of biology and life *Disappointment that procedure is not guaranteed to work *May have waited until too late for procedure to work and must confront loss
Oocyte Disposition			
*Same as IVF	*Must confront reality of cancer and possible death *Must ensure proper counseling about who receives oocytes in event of divorce or death	*Less of a moral problem for some because oocytes are used and not embryos	*Must confront what to do with her genetic material and its disposition if unused *May not be able to use eggs because of problems in creating or storing

personnel. On the other hand, counseling for women who want to delay starting their families for social reasons may cause some women to fear judgment about their reasons for delaying having children, or feel shame that they have not achieved their goals of marriage and family. Some fear the counseling, mistakenly believing that counseling is performed primarily to determine parental fitness.

The basic elements of fertility preservation counseling involve a counselor assuming several roles: psychoeducational, exploratory and supportive. The counseling is not unlike donor gamete recipient counseling. The fertility counselor may need to assess several factors in a relatively brief time frame and quickly prioritize the issues to address and the issues to ignore. However, a significant difference between fertility preservation counseling and recipient counseling is the lack of clarity about the use of the oocytes in the future. The fertility counselor does not know when (or if) the oocytes will be used and does not know the familial situation or context of their use.

Nevertheless, counseling for both groups is essential! Women with medical illness may be in crisis with attendant anxiety, panic, helplessness or feelings of loss of control. They may feel outside the norm and wonder "Why me?" They may want to talk about these issues or prefer to "remain strong," disinclined to let their feelings show. Women freezing for social reasons may feel that they did not achieve their dreams of finding the right mate and feel a sense of failure or blame themselves. It may be the first time they are really confronting the fact that they waited too long to have children. Counseling for both groups involves a rapid assessment of the individual's psychological strengths, weaknesses and coping styles. The counselor helps clarify and validate the complex emotions that may need to be sorted out. The emotional effects of important treatment decisions can be discussed at greater length than with other medical personnel. The counselor can serve as a present and future resource for the patient and most women are grateful that their medical team cares about their emotional well-being.

There is little or no research on the long-term psychosocial aspects of fertility preservation. Most research has focused on whether or not women actually *want* to preserve fertility. We know that they do, and that fertility preservation for cancer patients enhances the quality of life for women and men who want children [16–18]. Among young cancer survivors who are childless at diagnosis, approximately 75% desire children after treatment [19]. In one study of survivors of gynecological cancer, one-third of the patients identified with the statement that "part of one's self had died along with the idea of giving birth" [20]. Cancer survivors are at significant risk for emotional distress if they become infertile due to treatment for their cancer and may suffer unresolved grief, depression, increased anxiety and reduced life satisfaction [18]. Given the recent development of fertility preservation for social reasons, psychosocial research on the long-term impact of oocyte cryopreservation is understandably rare. Most research has focused on the motivations of women freezing for social reasons, their demographic characteristics and speculations about the societal impact of social freezing [21–23].

The fertility preservation interview

Counseling for fertility preservation occurs in different contexts: in hospitals and medical centers as part of an interdisciplinary team approach; in independent reproductive programs unaffiliated with major university centers; and in the private office of the mental health professional (MHP). The fertility counselor may be embedded in a particular program or serve as a consultant to different programs. The counseling may be one session for psychological evaluation "for medical clearance" or be several sessions to work through therapeutic issues. Counseling may be initiated by the patient or through referral by a reproductive program.

The consenting process will be different in the different contexts. It is important to be clear with the patient who (if anyone) will have access to the information obtained during counseling and the purpose of the interview. Is the interview a psychological evaluation for another party or a counseling session for the patient alone? When the purpose of the interview is psychological evaluation, consent forms need to indicate the purpose and nature of the evaluation; to whom the information obtained during the evaluation will be released; psychological risks (if any) of the counseling; and any conflicts of interest inherent in the counseling. Patients who are evaluated in a medical context need to be informed whether or not their physicians or other personnel will have access to information obtained during counseling or evaluation, where (and how) the records are kept, and how long the information will be retained.

Table 15.2 The fertility preservation interview.

The Fertility Preservation Interview
Reasons for preservation
Type of fertility preservation options
Individual's support systems (family, partner, friends)
Abuse history (physical, emotional, rape)
Alcohol or other pharmacological abuse
Mental health history
Psychotherapy/counseling (past and present)
Prior and present psychotropic medication use
Prior psychological traumas
Activities that are stress relieving
Probability of success of the FP procedures
Patient's perception of probability of success
Do FP procedures provide hope (realistic or not)?
Is it too late for FP to work?
Provision of legal and educational resources
What is individual's experience of the interview?

Suggested topics to cover during the clinical interview for fertility preservation are included in Table 15.2. The fertility counselor must use good judgment when deciding the issues to emphasize and the topics to ignore. S/he must try to balance different roles (psychoeducational, exploratory and educational), while being sensitive to the client's needs.

This chapter will illustrate the complex nature of fertility preservation counseling by presenting cases that bring up challenging questions. The case studies are not included to say that most of those preserving fertility have psychological problems. Rather, the fertility counselor or therapist needs to have knowledge of the questions and pitfalls in the fertility preservation process. For clarity in this discussion, "fertility counselor" or "counselor" will be used when referring to a MHP doing the consultative interview and "therapist" to an ongoing psychotherapeutic relationship.

In this chapter, countertransference refers to the thoughts, feelings and reactions that the care provider feels in the relationship with the patient that differ from the counselor's usual thoughts and behavior. Counseling involves balancing the supportive, psychoeducational and exploratory roles. If the fertility counselor places unusual and undue importance on one of these aspects, it may be helpful for the counselor to look at his or her own emotions. The feelings and emotional reactions may be conscious or unconscious and the reactions can be helpful or hurtful to either patient or counselor/therapist. The more self-aware the therapist, the more the therapist can learn about the experience of the patient and ameliorate hurtful reactions to the patient or self. Since life and death issues are involved in fertility preservation counseling, strong emotions can be elicited in the counselor. In addition, many counselors are trained to do counseling and psychotherapy over many sessions; the limitations of brief contact during standard fertility preservation counseling can be especially challenging. Each case discussion will include the fertility counselor or therapist's countertransference, as noted in the following discussion of the opening case of Maria.

Maria

Fertility preservation was undoubtedly a positive option for Maria. It provided hope during her darkest days before her death. Imagination, fantasy and dreams of her future children inspired her and gave her a sense of legacy beyond her life. Nevertheless, her grief at not being able to use the embryos during her lifetime was, at times, unbearable; in addition, the same fantasies and dreams were a potent source of pain and guilt for her husband, Paul. The videotapes for the children made "real" the fact that he would never have children with Maria and thus was losing both his wife and his children. Their intermittent marital discord over this issue was painful for both.

In general, patients are relieved that they have done what they could do to retain their ability to create a future family. However, Maria brings up the question of whether or not to use embryos when a parent will die before the child's age of majority. The customary answer to the question of preserving fertility in patients with advanced disease is that it depends on the support systems in place for the well-being of the child and for the people involved in the child's life. For Maria, fertility preservation was a positive experience. The thought of children was the one bright spot she had in a sea of pain and loss. Initially, her parents benefited from the preservation. The existence of embryos softened the loss of their daughter. Later, they experienced unbearable grief that they could not use the embryos. The loss of grandchildren compounded their pain. First they lost their only child and then they lost their grandchildren. The years following her death were filled with mourning, grief, anger and conflict.

It is easy to forget the multiple players in the patient's life. An individual who is going through cancer treatment or other serious illness may focus on themselves to the exclusion of others. For example, it may be hard for the patient to face the fact that a child will lose their parent or only know a mother who is very ill, if embryos are used during metastatic disease; the therapist may also find it difficult to hold in mind the multiple points of view. Once embryos are created, the family situation may evolve over time in directions not envisioned during cryopreservation. While treatment was going on, the therapist found it hard to "contain" the complexity of the different perspectives of Maria and her family. In addition, the therapist wanted to believe that Maria would live for a long time and denied the immediacy of her death. The therapist had fantasies about Maria's future children and she felt grief for Paul's loss and the loss of grandchildren for Maria's parents. The therapist understood the power of their desire for a grandchild but also knew that they wanted a "replacement child." This case illustrates the value of fertility preservation as well as its potential for creating pain. The therapist wanted to maintain a "happily ever after view" about the value of fertility preservation and its positive role in patients' lives.

Fertility preservation for medical reasons

As stated previously, before any information is obtained from the patient, the patient needs to understand the purpose of the interview and the individuals who will receive the information. The most important part of the interview is the opportunity to talk in a safe "holding environment." What this means is compassionately validating the patient's concerns without lecturing or judging [24–27]. Some patients are very emotional and find it to be a relief to express their feelings [28,29]. Others prefer to hold themselves together by not discussing their painful emotions. The patient may be in shock and denial. If so, the patient's defenses must be respected. Ignoring the warning signs of a patient's disinclination to talk about her feelings may flood her with unbearable anxiety and pain. The "elephant in the room" may be the patient's fear of death and her fear of the loss of the ability to have biological children [30–33]. The patient may not be able to talk to members of her family and/or support system about her concerns. Many individuals in the patient's environment are so distraught that the patient needs to "buck up" to reassure them. Some women are embarrassed to be emotional or discuss intimate matters with their physicians.

Danielle

Danielle, age 34, sobbed during her required interview for embryo cryopreservation prior to chemotherapy for breast cancer, Stage 1. She was planning to be married in three months. The large and expensive wedding had been planned for over a year. She was "petrified" and angry that she needed a mastectomy and would lose her hair just before her wedding. She did not want sex and could not envision a honeymoon. In the past, she had been treated for panic attacks, anxiety, depression and alcoholism. She was proud of her years sober but feared her current situation would cause a relapse in drinking. Her Prozac did not seem to be working. She felt embarrassed discussing her past psychological history but was relieved that her physicians would not know. (Records of the clinical interviews for fertility preservation were not included in the patient's medical record.) The interview with the fertility counselor helped her retain control of her emotions during her consultations with her oncology and reproductive specialists. She had a place to "let down" with the fertility counselor. Fertility preservation gave her hope that she would be able to have a family and lessened her fears that her fiancé would leave her because of the cancer and her perceived disfigurement. However, finances were an issue because of the wedding. Her parents spent most of their savings on the wedding. Should she change her wedding plans or ask for help from his parents?

Because of her cancer treatment, Danielle experienced a loss of self-esteem, shame and disfigurement. She feared judgment about past actions and feared she would be rejected by important individuals in her life. Danielle appreciated talking to the fertility counselor about fertility preservation because everyone she knew was telling her "everything would be alright." When with her physicians, she was in a "problem-solving mode," paying close attention to what she had to do for fertility preservation. The counseling session provided an opportunity to talk rather than reassure others. The positive and painful experience with the fertility counselor reminded her of the importance of "talking" and she contacted her former therapist.

It is important to determine who will be present during the counseling interview. Danielle's parents and fiancé wanted to be involved. In this case, the fertility counselor let her parents and fiancé be present during general discussion of the fertility preservation treatment. The counselor validated their concerns and discussed some of their fears (would the time frame of the wedding be "too much" for Danielle; would she lose her hair; would the fertility preservation cause the cancer to spread?). Then the fertility counselor asked her parents and fiancé to leave.

Danielle expressed concerns about whether or not her fiancé would be able to "stand it" before or after their marriage. While this fear could be addressed with her therapist, her concerns impacted fertility preservation. She wanted to cryopreserve both oocytes and embryos as an "insurance plan" to preserve her future ability to have children in the event her fiancé/husband left her. She felt guilty because she did not want to tell him about this fact. The fertility counselor discussed her ideas about privacy, keeping secrets from one's spouse and her fear of abandonment. Danielle decided to cryopreserve both oocytes and embryos and remain private about this fact. She felt she could "come clean" if they remained together and planned to say that she was not sure what to do at the time of cryopreservation.

The fertility counselor identified several problems during her one-hour fertility preservation counseling session with Danielle. Danielle was overwhelmed with the coincidence of a long planned-for wedding and her need for immediate medical treatment, as were her fiancé and parents. Danielle also suffered from depression and alcoholism. In response, the counselor wanted to lecture and advise rather than sustain an exploratory thoughtfulness. She feared exploration would strip off the Band-Aid and Danielle would relapse drinking. Swamped with her own opinions and feelings, the fertility counselor found it difficult to support and listen to Danielle and, more importantly, let Danielle's solutions to her problems emerge.

Although not overtly discussed, implicit in this session were issues of life and death, the nature of love, the symbolic hope of weddings, the importance of joy and pleasure obtained during ceremonies, the role of physical beauty, and Danielle's hope for a future. Because the counselor was flooded and she had trouble staying focused, her internal questions and thoughts silently dominated her thinking: Should one get married during a medical crisis? Would exploration of Danielle's life-long fear of abandonment open too many old wounds? Should Danielle wait to get married until she was sure her fiancé could remain a life partner? Should she wait until she could tell her partner about cryopreserving oocytes because of her fear that he would leave her? Are secrets damaging to a loving relationship? What is intimacy anyway? Would marriage during a medical crisis hurt Danielle's fiancé? What impact would Danielle's current physical disfigurement have on their present/future sex life?

The fertility counselor wanted more time and she wanted to tell her what to do to shut down her empathic stance and internal questions. She wanted to say, "It's not about the wedding, it's about your life. Focus on your treatment first." "Slow down, no need to rush!" However, for Danielle it WAS about the wedding. It gave her hope, it stamped a "happily ever after" signpost on her future and distracted her from the losses she experienced due to cancer. The fertility counselor was relieved that Danielle decided to contact her former therapist who knew her history of low self-esteem and fear of abandonment. The counseling session, though not psychotherapy, identified pertinent issues to discuss in therapy. Although Danielle was no longer the counselor's responsibility, she thought about the case for hours after the session. Several years later, the fertility counselor still wonders what happened to Danielle.

Fertility preservation for social reasons

The purpose of fertility preservation for social reasons is the ability to achieve parenthood in the future. When counseling for fertility preservation for social reasons, the fertility preservation is the center of the medical treatment. However, these women usually do not see themselves as an "infertility patient" but rather needing to "just freeze eggs." The woman enters counseling having thought about fertility preservation and considered whether or not it will benefit her. She may be optimistic, empowered and is not typically in the same kind of emotional crisis as occurs during counseling for fertility preservation for cancer or other medical illnesses. On the other hand, many who want to preserve fertility for future childbearing wait until the last possible moment to freeze. They may have achieved many goals and successes, but fear they will not be able to have the family of their dreams in the future. They may have given up on finding "Mr. Right," and must face the fact that if they wait to find him, they reduce their chances of childbearing. They may feel entitled; they have achieved financial stability or taken care of other responsibilities, now is "their time." They may have pride and empowerment; they know what they are doing and wonder why they need to "talk" to someone about their decision-making. In this context, counseling prior to social cryopreservation may be perceived as judging parental fitness or emotional stability, required on the program's "check list" for medical clearance. Sometimes, women feel shame at not achieving their dreams or feel resentment that life has not turned out as they wish. The counseling may elicit narcissistic issues and the women may be particularly sensitive to perceived criticism of their lives or decision-making process. Fertility preservation may be the last option to have biological children, and it may be difficult to set realistic expectations for the process.

It is a well-known fact that fertility declines with age. At about 32 years of age, fecundity gradually declines; it declines more rapidly after 37 years of age, primarily due to a decrease in egg quality. There are multiple factors involved in this decline that are just beginning to be understood [34]. At age 40, women have a 40% chance of miscarriage if they can get pregnant with their own eggs; by the age of 45, the risk of miscarriage is 75% [34]. Thus, women need to cryopreserve oocytes when young (when a woman is in her 20s or early 30s) to have a reasonable chance of success. In one large investigation of oocyte vitrification, age-stratified pregnancy rates per embryo transfer were 48.6% in women under 34 years of age but half that percentage in 41 to 43-year-olds (22.2%) [35].

In general, maternal age is inversely correlated with delivery rates regardless of the type of cryopreservation used (fast vs. slow freeze) [36–38]. Despite the age induced decline, live births have occurred as late as 44 years of age with vitrified oocytes [38]. Currently, calculators exist that show women their probability of success for live birth given their age and number of oocytes frozen [38]. Recent studies show that programs accept older women for social egg freezing. An investigation reporting on the status of elective egg freezing in the United States through 2009 found that half the programs accepted women between the ages of 38–40 years; one-third of the programs accepted women over 40 years of age [7]. Similarly, an investigation of 491 women showed that the reported mean age of the women cryopreserving their oocytes for social purposes was 38 years [39]. Similarly, other investigations report that 80% of women undergoing fertility preservations for social reasons are over 35 years old (range: 36–41) [40,23,6].

A large barrier to fertility preservation for social reasons is the lack of knowledge of the reduced fecundity associated with advanced maternal age. Many women think that they can postpone families, often until it is too late to have children through cryopreservation. In a large survey study of female university students, Drukenmiller et al. found that 72% of the women lacked fertility knowledge [41]. Since the mean age for fertility preservation is presumably 35 years old and 80% of programs accept women over 36 years old, two important issues must be addressed during the clinical interview for fertility preservation for social reasons: false expectations and plans for using oocytes [40,23].

The counselor should be attentive to any false expectation of the success of cryopreservation. Individuals respond to statistics in different ways. If quoted a 1% chance of working, some individuals will believe that they have a 99% chance of failure; others see themselves on the "success" side of statistics and believe they are the 1% for whom the procedure will work. If one-third of programs accept women over 40 years of age and half accept women between the ages of 38 and 40, these women must be counseled that there is a strong possibility that they will not have a child utilizing the procedures (22.2% success; 77.8% failure) [42]. Some women realistically undergo many procedures for fertility preservation. How many is too many? Should there be a limit?

The second important counseling issue is the woman's plan to use the oocytes. How old will she be? What are the health consequences of her decision? Will it be safe to be pregnant? What are the health consequences for her future children of pregnancy during advancing age and are there any health consequences for her offspring? Sometimes women feel younger than their actual age, and may not have considered the psychological consequences for their children of their advancing years. It may be a challenge to bring up such topics without offending the patient. (Please see Chapter 11 for more discussion on older parenting.)

With these issues in mind, the Fertility Preservation Interview (Table 15.2) may serve as a template or menu from which to choose necessary and relevant topics for social fertility preservation counseling. Women utilizing fertility preservation procedures are often grateful for the opportunity to discuss their concerns with a knowledgeable and supportive fertility counselor.

Carole

Carole, age 53, a native New Englander, was referred for required counseling prior to cryopreservation for social reasons. As Carole described, she had spoken to two reproductive endocrinologists who informed her that she had very low odds of conceiving after cryopreservation using her own oocytes. One physician suggested that she might consider waiting for future technological breakthroughs rather than vitrification of her oocytes.

Carole had never been married or been in a long-term relationship. As a devout Christian, she lived her life according to Biblical tenets. As a virgin, she wanted a man who was also a virgin; together they could share in the sanctity of marriage and children. Oocyte donation was not to be considered since it would violate the holiness of their marital bond.

Carole was a care-taker of several members of her family. She was actively involved in youth programs for her church. These activities fulfilled her, but now was her time to have the joys others experienced. She did not want to believe that time had run out. She knew that having a child after cryopreservation "would be a miracle." But, as she said, "I believe in miracles."

When asked how long she might wait for future stem cell technology (because of her age), Carole became angry. She was also angry at the idea that due to her age, fertility preservation and pregnancy involved some medical risk. She was aware of the potential for miscarriage. As she said to the counselor, "You are a very negative person; why talk about problems?" She indicated that she was aware of the problems of raising a child at her age and the chance of death or ill health before her child was an adult. She was angry that the counselor brought up such issues, though she had not made plans for such occurrences. "Do others need to justify their desire for parenthood?" She did not want to discuss any other option than oocyte cryopreservation.

The fertility counselor wondered if this case was a "kick the bucket down the road" situation. She wondered why the program where Carole wanted to freeze oocytes didn't just say "no." Leaving this question aside, the counselor felt Carole was being very unrealistic. It was hard not to judge Carole's assumptions, especially about miracles and the low probability of finding a partner with her requirements, a 50-year-old male virgin. The counselor wanted to argue with the patient and try to convince her not to proceed. She felt judgmental. Although not said, she thought, "You waited this long and you want to wait longer?" On the other hand, the fertility counselor internally debated, "Would effort and the cost of cyropreservation give Carole piece of mind?" Not wanting to serve as a gatekeeper, the counselor provided the reproductive program with a note describing the situation and Carole's understanding of the implications of proceeding (i.e., low probability of success). Ultimately, Carole did not cryopreserve at this program. Maybe counseling made a difference or maybe Carole decided to take her business elsewhere.

Carole's case illustrates the difficulty in bringing up "reality" to an individual in denial. Carole did not know the negative consequences of delay of childbearing when she could have cryopreserved oocytes (i.e., when she was younger). Her wish to have her life meet her expectations caused her to wait until it was too late. Carole felt optimistic about her option to have children through fertility preservation, believing that God would give her a miracle, though she also knew "the facts." Carole did what many patients do. She had many responsibilities that delayed her from having children. She was unrealistic about her reproductive options as are many women. She dreamed of finding Mr. Right, a not unusual hope. Yet her sanctimonious air elicited a corresponding self-righteous, incredulity in her counselor. Although the fertility counselor tried not to let her internal dialogue and judgments affect her actual behavior ("You've got to be kidding?" "Is this a joke?" "Are you a reporter?"), Carole probably sensed her reactions.

Post-cryopreservation counseling

Whether a woman cryopreserves her oocytes for medical or social reasons, there will come a time in the future when she will need to decide whether or not she will use them, and may be advised or seek counseling. In addition, reproductive programs may refer women due to advanced maternal age, as suggested by ASRM guidelines for women older than 50 years of age [43]. Common fears of women cryopreserving for medical reasons are a concern about safety for themselves and their children; that is, when (and if) is it safe to proceed with a pregnancy? Women cryopreserving for social reasons must be informed about the risk that the cryopreservation will not work and the potential risks of pregnancy when postponed until after 45 years of age.

If the woman has hoped to have a child through fertility preservation methods and is unable to achieve a pregnancy, the sense of failure is profound. Prior maladaptive coping methods may resurface and the patient may again feel rage at the injustice of having a medical illness that denies one the ability to have a child. In addition to grieving this loss, patients may become clinically depressed and need psychiatric assessment. Marital discord may occur. The survivor may fear partner rejection. It has been noted that cancer survivors may feel a dual loss, the loss of a full life as well as the loss of the wished-for child. Glazer and Huber have observed that infertile cancer survivors often report a sense of exclusion from the infertile community [44]. In fact, the cancer patient may be discriminated against in the adoption process and suffer a sense of failure and reduced self-esteem [45]. Parenting options are available, but the survivor must mourn their reproductive loss before feeling ready to use third party options such as donor gametes, gestational surrogacy, or adoption.

Gina

Gina was 42 years old when she first began cryopreservation of embryos for social reasons. As a very busy professional and successful single woman, Gina cryopreserved embryos in order to protect her ability to have a family in the future. Oocyte freezing was still experimental at the time she began cyropreservation. As a single woman, she used sperm donation to create the embryos. She reported having over 12 back-to-back IVF cycles in one year alone and happily reported having "hundreds" of frozen embryos. She did not have any romantic relationships during the ensuing ten years and focused on her career and caring for her elderly and sick parents. When oocyte cryopreservation for social reasons was no longer considered experimental, she cryopreserved oocytes as well. She felt very close to the physicians in her reproductive program and socialized with them. At 52 years of age, she retired from her profession and planned to become a mother. Her parents had died and she had ample financial resources and could retire. Now, she could start her new career – motherhood. She planned to move to a small community in rural Maine to create her family. She had no social support in her proposed new home but felt she would make friends now that she had time for them. In the event of her death prior to her children's age of majority, she planned to have her older single sister raise her children. She had not discussed this fact with her but felt sure her sister would want to have a family.

The denial of one's age is a common reaction of infertility patients. "I feel young, I won't have trouble conceiving." It may come as a shock to learn that looking and feeling young doesn't make a difference in childbearing capacity if one is actually much older. Now, however, a woman can preserve fertility until she is ready to become a parent. The irony in Gina's case is that she resented caring for her own elderly parents. When asked if she felt that she might be creating the same situation for her own future children, she became annoyed. "Of course it's not the same." "I'm not like my mother; she was crazy." The fertility counselor felt that Gina did not understand the reality of parenthood as a single person in a new community without social support. Gina did not plan to have help. Gina reasoned that she had waited this long to have a baby and she wasn't going to have another person deprive her of enjoying the experience. The fertility counselor felt Gina had substituted the reproductive program for "family" during the ten years she cyropreserved oocytes and embryos. Freezing oocytes and embryos was Gina's light at the end of the tunnel. Her life during cryopreservation consisted of two things: work and caring for her "disturbed" and sick parents. Visiting the welcoming reproductive program and her fantasies about her family in a small town with friendly neighbors carried her through days of hard work, career development and a life without many relationships. Gina said that she was glad that the fertility counselor brought up the possibility of predeceasing her child. She had never thought of it.

The fertility counselor found it hard not to react to Gina's "know it all" demeanor. Was Gina's sense of superiority in discussing her future parenthood plans ("I won't have any problems, I'm a successful career woman!") eliciting a similar reaction in her counselor ("I know what it is to be a single mother, you don't!") or were the counselor's concerns about Gina's ideas about her rosy future irrelevant? After all, many individuals are surprised about the joys and difficulties of actual parenthood vs. their fantasies of it. The fertility counselor found it hard to contain her wish to "lecture" (i.e., educate her about child development; common difficulties in parenting; the stresses on single, older parents) and felt she lacked the skill to delve tactfully into potentially legitimate concerns. She worried that Gina's cryopreservation of oocytes and embryos was potentially "false hope," and that for a woman used to success and control of her environment, failure to conceive would have significant impact on her emotional well-being.

Alice

> Alice sought psychotherapy to deal with her feelings about her recent diagnosis of breast cancer. She had just been diagnosed and was "freaked" out. After a year of trying unsuccessfully to have a child, Alice, age 35, and her husband of 15 years did two cycles of IVF. The first IVF was unsuccessful; however, two embryos were cryopreserved. During the second IVF cycle, Alice was diagnosed with breast cancer, Stage 2. All 13 embryos were cryopreserved before transfer. Her cancer was aggressive, hormonally sensitive, and had different kinds of cancer cells necessitating different types of chemotherapy regimens. She required radiation to shrink the tumor, a lumpectomy and two years of chemotherapy. After completing chemotherapy, she was put on five years of tamoxifen. She was advised not to get pregnant at any time in the future. If she wished to use her embryos, she would need a gestational surrogate. Although insured, medical expenses were large. During the years of chemotherapy, she became increasingly fatigued and depressed. She did not like her job, and wanted to quit, but she needed the medical benefits. She could not even think of parenthood during this time. She feared a reoccurrence of cancer and wondered if she would even have a future. She felt dead inside. After chemotherapy, Alice was menopausal and felt fat and "stupid." She felt older than her peers and outside her social group. Her friends wanted to help, but Alice was too tired to go out and activities that interested her prior to cancer did not interest her after diagnosis. She wondered if she should even think of having children given her emotional state. However, her husband wanted to use the embryos and have children. When she was initially diagnosed, her best friend offered to serve as a gestational surrogate. Alice was grateful but also felt that such a "gift" was too much to ask of anyone.

Alice entered therapy when she was initially diagnosed with cancer. She wanted someone to help her work through her depression, anxiety, ambivalent feelings toward her husband and career. In addition, she wanted help thinking through treatment decisions such as whether or not to have a mastectomy or lumpectomy. During the ensuing years, psychotherapy was supportive. Alice was firm about her decision not to take psychotropic medication. After she started to heal, she felt cancer had given her the "gift" of not needing anyone else's opinion to feel good about herself. She felt "centered." Though she feared that the cancer would return, and that she would have no future to offer a child, she decided to approach her friend to see if she would still be willing to serve as a surrogate. Circumstances in her friend's life had changed, so she declined. Alice said she understood her friend's decision but was disappointed. She approached two other distant relatives. No one could help her. Surrogacy in the United States was out of the question because of the expense. She is exploring surrogacy in other countries but fears she will never be able to use her embryos.

When Alice found out her friend could not be a surrogate, her therapist became so involved in finding an alternative surrogacy arrangement that surrogacy became a center of therapy. The therapist felt rage at the injustice of the situation. Alice could not have children through surrogacy and would find adoption difficult due to her cancer diagnosis. While Alice had legitimate concerns about her ability and desire to mother, her therapist was angry Alice was denied a choice. The therapist became aware of her role in making motherhood the central issue in Alice's therapy. Alice may decide to pursue the possibility in the future, but is enjoying the fact that she is less depressed and is regaining pleasure in life before assuming the responsibilities of motherhood.

Summary

Cryopreservation for medical or social reasons is at the heart of ethical debates about the role of childbearing in society. The capacity to postpone parenthood has political, ethical and religious implications. If society values children, it will educate men and women about the dangers of delaying parenthood and remove obstacles to childbearing when young. Until then, fertility preservation may provide hope and a sense of comfort for individuals and families able to utilize fertility sparing procedures. Problems with fertility preservation and unintended consequences are to be expected as we enter the new age of increased reproductive possibilities. The complexity involved in the development of the technology has caused an understandable focus on the medical aspects of fertility preservation. There is scant evidence about the real lives of those utilizing the technology. This chapter discussed the actual experiences, both good and bad, of those who hope to have children in their future and why counseling for fertility preservation is important. The complex emotional interplay between the fertility counselors and women utilizing fertility preservation techniques is presented to illustrate the difficulties and rewards of working in this new and evolving field.

Reflections

I never envisioned the course my career took when I began. However, I was at the right time and place in history to understand the importance of fertility preservation. I had been working with infertility patients for several years when I was diagnosed with breast cancer. The value of family, the pain of infertility and the possibility of death caused me to throw myself into fertility preservation for cancer patients, and to widen my role serving the emotional needs of men and women experiencing infertility through serving as the Executive Director of Resolve of New York City. I knew that cancer patients needed the technology to preserve their fertility and I also knew that the technology was available to safely stimulate women with cancer. At that point, oncology was wary of reproductive medicine, worried that stimulation and pregnancy might be dangerous. In my role as Executive Director, I was able to hold the first conference (I believe) in the United States about fertility preservation for medical reasons. Thus, a new dialogue began between the various professions. I approached ASRM to develop the Fertility Preservation Special Interest Group to stimulate research and dialogue among fertility specialists, oncology and allied professionals. Now, several years later, I'm proud of the developments in the field and that I had some part in highlighting the importance of attention to the emotional needs of women preserving fertility.

When young, I thought fertility preservation for social reasons might allow women to take charge of reproduction and level the playing field with men in that women could postpone parenting until they were ready. However, now I see the limits of my initial vision. With hindsight, I can see the pros and cons of employing the technology. Typically, women wait too long or can't afford to cryopreserve when young. I have found that fertility preservation for medical and social reasons brings me up close to life and death, dashed dreams, unrealistic hope and human folly. At times, I fear the reoccurrence of my own breast cancer and I can "taste" the pain (as I recently discovered with yet another scare). However, the work has enabled me to see the best of people in their darkest times, the power of courage and hope and it has given me a passionate purpose for my life. For these reasons I am immensely grateful to the women I have treated.

References

1. Cobo A, Domingo J, Perez S, et al. Vitrification: an effective new approach to oocyte banking and preserving fertility in cancer patients. *Clin Transl Oncol.* 2008;10:268–73.
2. Song W, Sun Y, Jin H, et al. Clinical outcome of emergency egg vitrification for women when sperm extraction from the testicular tissues of the male partner is not successful. *Syst Biol Reprod Med.* 2011;57:210–13.
3. Rodriguez-Wallberg KA, Oktay K. Fertility preservation and pregnancy in women with and without BRCA mutation-positive breast cancer. *Oncol.* 2012;17:1409–17.
4. Oktay K, Rodriguez-Wallberg KA, Sahin G. Fertility preservation by ovarian stimulation and oocyte cryopreservation in a 14-year-old adolescent with Turner syndrome mosaicism and impending premature ovarian failure. *Fertil Steril.* 2010;94:753, e15–753e19.
5. Cil A, Seli E. Current trends and progress in clinical applications of oocyte cryopreservation. *Curr Opin Obstet Gynecol.* 2013 June; 25(3):0.1097/GCO.0b013e32836091f4.
6. Wierckx K, Van Caenegem E, Pennings G, et al. Reproductive wish in transsexual men. *Hum Reprod.* 2012;27(2):483–7.
7. Rudick B, Opper N, Paulson R, et al. The status of oocyte cryopreservation in the United States. *Fertil Steril.* 2010;94:2642–46.
8. Dondorp W, de Wert G, Pennings G, et al. ESHRE Task Force on Ethics and Law. Oocyte cryopreservation for age-related fertility loss. *Hum Reprod.* 2012;27(5):1231–7.
9. Stoop D, Nekkebroeck J, Devroey P. A survey on the intentions and attitudes towards oocyte cryopreservation for non-medical reasons among

women of reproductive age. *Hum Reprod.* 2011; 26(3):655–61.

10. Chen C. Pregnancy after human oocyte cryopreservation. *Lancet* 1986 Apr 19;1(8486):884–6.
11. Oktay K, Cil A, Bang H. Efficiency of oocyte cryopreservation: a meta-analysis. *Fertil Steril.* 2006; 86:70–80.
12. The Practice Committees of the American Society for Reproductive Medicine and the Society for Assisted Reproductive Technology. Mature oocyte ccryopreservation: a guideline. *Fertil Steril.* 2013; 99:37–43.
13. Cobo A, Meseguer M, Remohi, M. Use of cryo-banked oocytes in an ovum donation programme: a prospective, randomized, controlled, clinical trial. *Hum Reprod.* 2010;25(9):2239–46.
14. Paulson R, Milligan R, Sokol R. The lack of influence of age on male fertility. *Am J Obstet Gynecol.* 2001; 184:818–22.
15. Peterson B, Boivin J, Norre J, et al. An introduction to infertility counseling: a guide for mental health and medical professionals. *J Assist Reprod Genet.* Mar 2012; 29(3):243–48.
16. Tschudin S, Bitzer J. Psychological aspects of fertility preservation in men and women affected by cancer and other life-threatening diseases. *Human Reprod Update* 2009;1(1):1–11.
17. Rosen A, Rodriguez-Wallberg K, Oktay K. Psychological issues of cancer survivors. In: Donnez J, Kim S, eds. *Principles and Practice of Fertility Preservation.* Cambridge: Cambridge University Press. 2011; pp. 473–84.
18. Partridge A, Gelber S, Peppercorn J, et al. Web-based survey of fertility issues in young women with breast cancer. *J Clin Oncol.* 2004;22:4174–83.
19. Schover L. Patient attitudes toward fertility preservation. *Pediatr Blood Cancer.* 2009;53:281–84.
20. Carter J, et al. Gynecologic cancer treatment and the impact of cancer-related infertility. *Gynecol Oncol.* 2005;97:90–5.
21. Cobo A, Garcia-Velasco J, Domingo J, Remohi J, Pellicer A. Is vitrification of oocytes useful for fertility preservation for age-related fertility decline and in cancer patients. *Fertil and Steril.* May 2013;99(No 6):1485–95.
22. Lockwood G. Social egg freezing: the prospect of reproductive "immortality" or a dangerous delusion? *Reprod Biomed Online.* 2011;23:334–40.
23. Vallejo V, Lee J, Schuman L, Witkin G, et al. Social and psychological assessment of women undergoing elective oocyte cryopreservation: a 7-year analysis. *Open J Obstetric Gynecol.* 2013;3:1–7.
24. Kerr J, Engel J, Schlesinger-Raab A, Sauer H, Hölzel D. Communication, quality of life and age: Results of a 5-year prospective study in breast cancer patients. *Ann Oncol.* 2003;14:421–7.
25. Baile W, Aaron J. Patient-physician communication in oncology: Past, present, and future. *Curr Opin Oncol.* 2005;17(4):331–5.
26. Hack T, Degner L, Parker P. The communication goals and needs of cancer patients: A review. *Psychooncol.* 2005;14(10):831–45.
27. Fagerlind H, Lindblad A, Bergström I, et al. Patient-physician communication during oncology consultations. *Psychooncol.* 2008;17(10):975–85.
28. Stanton AL, Danoff-Burg S, Cameron CL, et al. Emotionally expressive coping predicts psychological physical adjustment to breast cancer. *J Consult Clin Psychol.* 2000;68(5):875–82.
29. Byrne A, Ellershaw J, Holcombe C, et al. Patients' experience of cancer: evidence of the role of "fighting" in collusive clinical communication. *Patient Educ Couns.* 2002;48:15–21.
30. Cimprich B, Ronis D, Martinez-Ramos G. Age at diagnosis and quality of life in breast cancer survivors. *Cancer Pract.* 2002;10:85–93.
31. Ganz P, Greendale G, Petersen L, Kahn B, Bower J. Breast cancer in younger women: Reproductive and late health effects of treatment. *J Clin Oncol.* 2003; 21:4184–93.
32. Avis N, Crawford S, Manuel J. Psychosocial problems among younger women with breast cancer. *Psychooncol.* 2004;13:295–308.
33. Goodwin P, Ennis M, Pritchard K, et al. Association of young age and chemotherapy with psychosocial distress and health-related quality of life (HRQOL) during the first year after breast cancer (BC). *Proc Am Soc Clin Oncol.* 2004;22(14s):732s.
34. American Society for Reproductive Medicine, Birmingham, Alabama. Age-related fertility decline; a committee opinion. *Fertil Steril.* 2008;90:S154–5.
35. Ubaldi F, Anniballo, R, Romano, S, Baroni, L, et al. Cumulative ongoing pregnancy rate achieved with oocyte vitrification and cleavage stage transfer without embryo selection in a standard infertility program. *Hum Reprod.* 2010;25(5): 1199–1205.
36. Rienzi L, Cobo A, Paffoni A, Scarduelli C, Capalbo A, Vajta G, et al. Consistent and predictable delivery rates after oocyte vitrification: an observational longitudinal cohort multicentric study. *Hum Reprod.* 2012;27: 1606–12. Level II-2.
37. Cil A, Oktay K. Age-based success rates after elective oocyte cryopreservation (EOC): a pooled analysis of 2281 thaw cycles. *Fertil Steril.* 2011;96(Suppl):S211. (P-354).

38. Cil A, Bang H, Oktay K. Probability of live birth with oocyte cryopreservation: an individual patient data meta-analysis. *Fertil Steril.* 2013 Aug;100(2):492–9.e3.

39. Hodes-Wertz B, Druckenmiller S, Smith M, et al. Tick Tock: can the clock be stopped? The use of elective oocyte cryopreservation (EOC) as a means to preserve fertility. *Fertil Steril.* 2012;98(Suppl):S235. (P417)

40. Mertes H, Pennings G. Social egg freezing: for better, not for worse. *Reprod BioMed Online.* 2011;23:824–9.

41. Druckenmiller S., Knopman, J, DeVore, S., Noyes, N. Psychology behavior and ethics of fertility preservation. *J Assist Reprod Genet.* 2011 November;28(11):1031–6.

42. Ubaldi F, Anniballo R, Romano S, Baroni, A, et al. Cumulative ongoing pregnancy rate achieved with oocyte vitrification and cleavage stage transfer without embryo selection in a standard infertility program. *Hum Reprod.* 2010;25(5):1199–1205.

43. Ethics Committee of the American Society for Reproductive Medicine. Childrearing ability and the provision of fertility services. *Fertil Steril.* 2009; 92:864–7.

44. Glazer E, Hubner M. Coping with the double blow: Facing cancer and infertility. Resolve Fact Sheet, Boston, MA: Resolve Inc., 1992.

45. Rosen A. Third-party reproduction and adoption in cancer patients. *J Natl Cancer Inst Monogr.* 2005;34: 91–93.

46. Galst J. What's a young woman to do? The pros and cons of social egg freezing. Fact Sheet. American Fertility Association. http://www.theafa.org/article/whats-a-young-woman-to-do-the-pros-and-cons-of-social-egg-freezing/. Accessed October 21, 2013.

Chapter 16

Pregnancy and loss counseling

Irving G. Leon

Alice, a tall woman in her early 40s, began the session almost cheerfully, recalling how happy she was when she learned almost a year ago that she was pregnant with twins. She described in much detail the long journey of trying to become pregnant over the prior ten years. This included many unsuccessful attempts, tensions with her husband over her unwillingness to consider adoption yet, and finally becoming pregnant with a donor egg. She beamed with pleasure, proudly announcing how she won the jackpot. It was two for the price of one. Wistfully, she momentarily recalled her high school days as a star athlete. She gave birth abruptly at 30 weeks. Her daughter, thankfully, was fine. Pushing back tears, she said how her son, Jim, had a rampaging sepsis which he succumbed to within a day. While this occurred over three months ago, she still can't believe it happened, starting to cry more openly. She pulled back again from crying, voicing her fear that her daughter, Jill, would pick up on her sadness, preventing her daughter from having a happy life. She was also afraid this would blot out how thrilled she felt over being a Mom. She paused long enough for me to comment. I told her I could see (more accurately feel) how painful it was to so unexpectedly lose Jim. "What a shock it must have been. Perhaps you are just coming out of it now. The emotional gestation was much longer than 30 weeks. It was more like ten years. I could also see how great it was not only to be pregnant, but pregnant with twins. It brought back those great high school athletic days when you felt your body was strong and capable of doing anything." She smiled appreciatively. "You bet," she said, "no more losing and failing for me."

Perhaps that was why, I went on, it was so important that she made these babies rather than their being adopted. She looked dismayed, saying that making the babies seemed less important than her being able to nurture them during pregnancy. After all, it was not her eggs and that felt OK to her. I told her I could see the distinction she was making and appreciated her correcting my misunderstanding. Over the course of the session, she reported a happy childhood, no prior history of depression or other emotional problems, and a very supportive husband, many friends, and a caring family.

No matter how deeply she grieved, I told her I was very impressed with how well she could control its expression, showing us over the course of the session when to allow the tears to flow for Jim and when to nurture Jill. She said, "Yep. It's hard to read books about parenting during the day and reading about grieving at night." I completely agreed with how difficult that can be. But I strongly believed she would not be in this position a year from now and would not have to be doing nightly or even necessarily weekly readings on grief.

The next session a week later, she said our first meeting helped a lot. Being able to talk about the whole experience lifted a load off her shoulders. But she was very upset, hurt, and angry with the doctor on that night who told her that her son died without giving his condolences. She did talk to him later about it and she was relieved that he had tears in his eyes when he apologized. "Those tears let you know he cared which meant a lot. It also helped you to be forgiving." Despite the difficult tasks of concurrent parenting and grieving, Alice was quite resilient. We met for about a month weekly, reducing at her request to every other week for another month and then once a month for the final three months.

We will frequently return to this case summary because it illustrates many of the key ingredients in working with pregnancy loss. Alice tells us how her

Fertility Counseling: Clinical Guide and Case Studies, ed. Sharon N. Covington. Published by Cambridge University Press.

loss is embedded not only in her pregnancy but in her reproductive past and life before. The therapist's empathy enables her to process this traumatic loss, facilitate grieving and repair self-esteem. When there is a benign psychological history with effective coping, a supportive social network and a solid marriage – predictors of adaptive recovery from pregnancy loss [1,2] – it is usually possible to anticipate major resolution of the loss within six to twelve months.

This chapter will guide therapists in dealing with the range of the most frequent reproductive losses, including miscarriage, ectopic pregnancy, stillbirth, infant death and pregnancy termination for fetal anomaly. Working with infertility will be considered only in the context of having additional reproductive losses. We will explore many of the common themes in dealing with these losses, while never losing sight of how individualized a loss is for each woman or man, each couple and each family. The reader is directed elsewhere for a more general description of the nature of and differentiation among the range of reproductive losses. (See references [4,37].)

Cultural differences can have a profound effect on how these losses are experienced and grieved. Space constraints limit the thorough discussion that ethnic, religious and national differences deserve. These differences influence when a loss is defined as a baby or something else; how publicly or privately grieving is allowed expression; the stigmatizing or normalizing function of mental health intervention; feminine versus masculine models of grieving and so forth, which significantly contribute to the emotional impact of these losses around the world. Practitioners who work with particular cultures are advised to become familiar with their different orientations to these losses. However, one should never assume an individual simply represents (i.e., caricatures) the norms of a larger group. It never hurts, and usually helps, when a clinician asks questions in an open, curious and respectful manner in order to better understand the impact of those cultural factors on those particular parents.

Before examining therapeutic interventions for reproductive loss, reviewing the unique features of this kind of loss is necessary [3,4]. These losses feel less real than the death of a person one has known in the "outside world." Grieving is more elusive without the rich store of memories upon which grief is based. Thus, while reproductive loss involves "prospective" grieving for the life and relationship projected into the future, other grieving is retrospective, based on painfully remembering the interactions with and images of the lost loved one. Accustomed to only understanding retrospective grieving, well-intentioned family and friends frequently minimize these losses, telling the bereaved couple to "forget," "move on" and "just have another child." They do not realize that encouraging remembering these losses helps the bereaved to gradually return to embracing the living and future, and not remain "stuck" in the past. Because the unborn baby often represents the best parts of oneself, defying mortality by projecting oneself into a new future life, a pregnancy loss is a tremendous assault on one's self-worth. If there are no other children, it may also block the normal transition into a crucial stage of adult development, that of parenthood. Finally, as cherished as the unborn baby is, his/her identity is nebulous, making it quite common for past, unresolved grief to merge with the baby, making this loss even more profound. All of these unique aspects of reproductive loss will be discussed and illustrated in this chapter. Too often paternal grief is overlooked and will occasionally be examined here. However, space constraints lead me to focus on the impact these losses have on mothers.

Models of counseling and psychotherapy

A variety of therapeutic approaches are available to treat reproductive loss. While psychodynamic versions are oriented to an examination of the client's emotional and cognitive experience, they tend to be eclectic and not traditionally psychoanalytic. They focus on resolving current repercussions from the loss, not seeking broader characterological change via transference interpretation, and build on the power of the therapeutic alliance with a highly interactive give and take. Each has its own particular emphasis. Jaffe and Diamond [5] follow a developmental perspective, contrasting one's "reproductive story" (anticipated life, especially family-to-be, narrative) with the unexpected subsequent losses in order to resolve traumatic grief. Covington [6] often employs cognitive behavioral techniques of creating mementoes, planning memorial activities, and advocating self-care activities in providing a place to safely grieve these losses. Leon [7] considers the therapist's empathy as the critical healing agent in fostering a secure attachment enabling the client to concurrently grieve and move forward.

Table 16.1 Guidelines for working with pregnancy loss.

- First session is usually telling the story. Listening fosters understanding.
- Take several sessions to acquire history and establish rapport.
- Give and get feedback to promote collaboration.
- Acknowledge longer-term issues even if not the focus of the work.
- Do not medicate grief. Reserve medications for major depression and other disorders.
- Be flexible. Individualize therapy.
- Include the partner whenever feasible.
- Be aware of maternal versus paternal differences in grieving.
- Empathy is more critical than insight.
- Work with past dynamics as they influence current issues.
- Respect, highlight, and support strengths.
- Making meaning of this loss – "why did it happen?" and "what good can come from it?" – may subdue trauma.
- Tune into cultural differences in grieving.
- Acknowledge and appropriately challenge stigmatization.

Cognitive-behavioral therapies (CBT) are oriented towards exposure to (and extinction of) stimuli provoking anxious and/or grief-related reactions, and cognitive re-appraisal which shifts negative, more depressive ideas towards more positive affirmative responses. One preliminary study by Bennett and her colleagues [8] had a sample size of only five, severely limiting the validity of its positive outcomes. However, with a sample size of 78, Kersting et al. [9] reported very impressive, significant reductions in grief, depression and PTSD following a pregnancy loss when CBT was administered over the Internet with individualized therapist responses to client writing assignments.

Differential diagnosis appears to be especially important in deciding upon psychopharmacologic treatment. Antidepressant medications are unneeded or ineffective in dealing with, respectively, normal or complicated (prolonged) grief. However, antidepressants were found to be very helpful in treating grief-related major depression – with symptoms no different from non-bereavement major depression – especially when combined with a supportive and individually tailored psychotherapy [10]. Guidelines for working with pregnancy loss are summarized in Table 16.1 and will be discussed at length throughout this chapter.

Key components in treating pregnancy loss

Flexibility

A cornerstone in working with pregnancy loss is flexibility. As Covington [6, p. 204] describes her practice, "I advise, analyze, educate, advocate, console, and support while employing a variety of treatment modalities." Ideological purity should take a far back seat to therapeutic efficacy. How directive and structured one is should be determined by the need for crisis intervention (if the loss is very recent) and not a pre-set, one-size-fits-all treatment plan. Similarly, the length of therapy should be customized. Three or four sessions may be sufficient for a more normative counseling: A mother with a young child was initially shocked and dismayed by her miscarriage at nine weeks. Given a license to grieve by her therapist that had been derailed by family and friends, she readily obtained closure once she decided to honor her loss by constructing a life lesson session on pregnancy loss for her middle school health students. Grief counseling (not specifically applied to reproductive loss here) may do more harm than good when universally administered to those with normal bereavement [11].

However, when earlier, especially depressive, problems associated with emotional neglect and insecure attachment intervene, a longer therapy is usually necessary to more painstakingly establish a safer tie. A chronically depressed 35-year-old woman entered therapy in the midst of losing her preterm twins. Intertwined with the deep grief and despair of losing them and a subsequent pregnancy, she mourned the absence of emotionally available parents, frequently moving from country to country during her childhood to support her father's successful business career. Now, as in the past, her relentlessly upbeat and grief-avoiding parents would hear none of her sadness. Over the course of five years of weekly therapy, she was able to grieve the loss of her three children, forge on to give birth to a healthy child whose pregnancy she was understandably convinced would never successfully conclude, and with much less anxiety and despair have a relatively calm fourth healthy pregnancy. The therapist's consistently empathic and emotionally available stance provided a solid chamber to contain her at times seemingly bottomless despair. Very fulfilled over having the relationship with her sons that she never had with her parents, her depression has subsided considerably.

Many such extended treatments involve incipient prolonged or complicated grief, which while having elements of depression and PTSD can be clearly distinguished from those conditions [12], even if that diagnosis is only provisionally accepted in DSM-5 [13]. As many as 25% of bereaved women go on to have more chronic difficulties [2] with the majority not in fact following the "normal" model of a steady decline in grief, but instead some variant [14]. Because in the midst of such a recent loss, it often is not possible, clinically, to know how quickly emotional problems are likely to be resolved, it can be critical to be flexibly attuned to new issues as they arise and not be rigidly harnessed to a standardized treatment manual for all clients. An initial consultation of three to five sessions enables getting to know the woman as a whole person, including her childhood, adolescence and young adulthood, not simply as a victim of a traumatic loss. Discussing extended feedback and recommendations at that point may provide a clearer sense of direction as well as establishing a collaborative relationship, which is indispensable for change.

Boundary and confidentiality concerns often mitigate against concurrent individual and conjoint work by the same therapist in general psychotherapy. However, with reproductive loss absent earlier significant individual and marital problems, such multimodal work is often effective. Typically (though not inevitably) the mother's more enduring, deeper and self-blaming grief than her partner's is given additional time individually, while tensions created by those differences may be worked through in conjoint sessions. It is neither necessary nor natural to expect men and women to grieve equivalently for these losses, particularly because the loss is so much more personal and immediate for the woman, it being within her body. It is crucial, however, that those differences be acknowledged and respected. Men especially need to be able to support, not reject, and join in – when honestly felt – their partner's grief. He may need to be told by his partner that sharing his grief will not burden her, but bring them closer, as often happens following this loss. A bereaved father will rarely come to therapy for pregnancy loss of his own accord, but is quite willing to participate to help his partner. Usually that motivation is sufficient for him to meaningfully engage in the therapy. Conjoint sessions are usually not as critical for pregnancy loss as they are for infertility because the course of treatments, multiple stressors and marital decisions that need to be made are so much greater for the latter.

Rarely do I feel it is helpful to directly include children in the therapeutic work. That may inadvertently reinforce a parent's sense of failure after such a loss by usurping a parenting function. It is better to empower parents by coaching them on addressing a child's concerns based on their own intimate knowledge of their children. (For a more thorough discussion of dealing with sibling issues see reference [37].)

Strengths

In her very first session, Alice highlighted her ability to focus on the positives in her life – her being pregnant with twins, her high school days as an athlete and the survival of her daughter – even before she describes the loss of her son. Her resilience in being able to transcend adversity with an active sense of personal control is a critical asset in effectively coping with pregnancy loss [15]. A dual-process model of coping with bereavement [16] depicts how effective grief resolution balances the painful reckoning of grieving with an orientation to distraction and avoidance of grief in the service of establishing new identities and a changed reality without the deceased. Compartmentalizing grieving can be adaptive so long as grief is not wholly denied. Alice's ability to parent by day, while grieving by night (as do many bereaved parents with another live child to parent), similarly demonstrates such a dual track in which self-regulation enables grieving which is modulated, oscillating with unimpaired functioning. Clinically, the therapist needs to echo her strengths, respect and sometimes encourage the legitimate need to have breaks from grieving and "come up for air." Using humor during therapy – when it is not being used by the therapist to avoid his own discomfort with grieving – can offer needed relief, sense of normalcy and some occasional distancing from grief.

Empathy

Empathizing with the client's experience in general and grief in particular engenders healing. In a meta-study of all psychotherapy, empathy is a moderately strong predictor of therapeutic success [17]. The utter sense of feeling abandoned among all kinds of bereavement may make empathy critical in facilitating grief. Grieving pregnancy loss may make therapeutic empathy even more indispensable due to the usual minimization, avoidance, and pat solutions others often apply to this loss if not personally familiar with it. Empathy is a key ingredient appreciated in medical care after miscarriage [18] and perinatal loss [19]. If we understand one form of empathy as being intuitively attuned to what kinds of statements or emotional expressions would be hurtful (i.e., how would

I feel if that was said to me, taking the "I" to include what one knows about the client), empathy can occupy a helpful self-censoring function.

Empathy embodies three arenas [17]. By taking the other's perspective, it fosters a cognitive sense of what the client is experiencing, promoting feeling understood. There is an emotional resonance felt within the therapist for the client, enabling the client to feel less alone. Finally, authentic caring actions including tears and providing realistic reassurance help the client to be genuinely cared for, aiding in the regulation of distress. The load lifted off of Alice's shoulders could be traced to feeling understood by the therapist's words, not feeling so alone and burdened due to his emotionally sharing her loss and providing a realistic basis for a happier future once her grief had subsided.

Ironically, while empathy is often belittled for its soft, soggy, unscientific connotations, its neurological credentials are quite impressive. Empathy is a mammalian trait rooted in the brain's mirror neurons, which are activated by another's actions and emotions [17]. The three different empathic processes described above have been associated with different areas of brain function, including, respectively, temporal cortex, limbic system and orbitofrontal cortex [17]. Different areas of brain activation can similarly distinguish between empathy, which preserves a *distinction* between self and other, versus a *merging* of self and other [20] (termed *identification* in psychoanalytic nomenclature). The client's affective experience of feeling understood, appreciated and cared for takes precedence over the cognitive aspects of insight and interpretation, whether defined as an "implicit relational knowing" [21] or a neurological re-coding of more secure attachment paradigms via emotional engagement [22].

Empathy is at the crossroads of several overlapping clinical models: the client-centered approach of Carl Rogers [17], Kohut's self-psychology using empathy as the crucial tool to accessing the client's experience [23], and an attachment model of psychotherapy which, in part, through empathic attunement can provide a form of a secure attachment [24] from which many of the therapeutic tasks of integrating trauma, grieving the loss and repairing self-esteem may be resolved. This work proceeds at a much quicker and direct pace with the majority of clients who can readily draw upon the prevalence of earlier secure attachments. More characterologically disturbed clients often require longer treatments due to their heightened sensitivity to narcissistic slights, resulting in more therapist empathic failures re-enacting earlier hurts [23,25].

Even without re-enactments of earlier paradigms, our empathic failures are inevitable and potentially therapeutic. It enables the therapy to be truly collaborative with the therapist's willingness to acknowledge mistaken understandings (without being willy-nilly or pleading mea culpa about it) and the client to feel more empowered in defining her own experience. It may promote resilience by fostering adaptation to an empathically imperfect world, perhaps akin to Kohut's reference to therapeutic progress occurring following the reparation of empathic errors [23]. Alice was able to confront and readily forgive her doctor's empathic failure of not expressing condolences over her son's death once he more openly demonstrated by tears how much the loss meant to him. It was a powerful lesson to both, demonstrating to her that she could help effect the support she needed in her medical environment and it made clear to him that completely avoiding his own sadness and grief does no good for his patients.

In our initial session, Alice corrected my empathic misunderstanding of her deferring adoption due to preferring genetic parenthood (which she reminds me, she did not have) when she longed for the nurturance experienced in gestational parenthood. At the outset, clients may be encouraged to share when inevitable misunderstandings occur. We may be more susceptible to empathic errors when we expect clients to follow our prior clinical experience and/or what "the literature" suggests, rather than their own path. Our own personal (especially pregnancy) losses may facilitate empathy while ironically encourage empathic mistakes when we expectantly project our personal loss experience onto our clients. As wisely noted, "Empathy should always be offered with humility and held lightly, ready to be corrected" [18, p. 48]. It is an ongoing, evolving inter-subjective feedback loop, not a static, one-way expression of therapeutic sensitivity.

Therapeutic tasks in working with reproductive losses

Most clients dealing with these losses will need to address most of the following issues, but each client will have her particular emphasis, combination and texture of issues. These tasks are also very inter-related, distinguished here for didactic purposes while naturally occurring together.

Processing trauma

After briefly reviewing the consultation process, I typically begin the first session by asking, "Where would you like to begin?" This is an invitation to tell the story of usually traumatic losses. For many (as with Alice) it began years back with the diagnosis and treatment of infertility, telling you the other crucial issues and events leading up to the specific loss. Typically, the details become more painstakingly specific, indicating the tell-tale imprinting of trauma on the mind, leading up to the shock and tears at the moment of loss. More traumatized and less trusting clients may not initially be able to tell their story with full intensity. Constructing a narrative, done over time with many repetitions, becomes an important, active way of processing a traumatic loss, that in one's utter helplessness and initial shock felt beyond assimilation. Re-living the loss makes it more real. As Alice noted, even three months later, she still can't believe it happened.

Therapeutic empathy and responsiveness leads to the client feeling less isolated and more supported, allowing the traumatic emotions and memories to be processed. It offers a "holding" environment in which the client feels safe with the therapist, solidifying the bond felt between them. This explains why the psychologically healthy client (as was Alice) almost always reports feeling much better after the first session. The emotionally overwhelming residues of the traumatic experience may be primed in later sessions by asking what continues to be the most difficult, painful or unforgettable aspects. Inquiring into what has helped the most may reveal what sources of strength and resilience can be mobilized, whether internal (e.g., fortitude, sense of humor), interpersonal (e.g., connection with others, emotional intelligence) or spiritual (e.g., faith in God, hope).

Cognitive-behavioral therapy similarly emphasizes the importance of exposure to the most traumatizing stimuli in order to extinguish the anxiety response [8,26]. However, if the CB therapist is not empathically attuned to what might re-traumatize the client, certain exposure practices (e.g., going to the baby section at Target) [8] may be exactly what is recommended to be *avoided* in the early work because it is just too painful. Interestingly, qualitative results from a CBT study indicated that one of the most helpful aspects of the intervention was "having an empathic, nonjudgmental person to talk to about their emotions and experiences around the loss" [8, p. 172].

These losses may be traumatizing not only due to anxiety producing, affective overstimulation, but because of "shattered assumptions" [27] of the world being viewed as safe, just and predictable. Schemas defining our security in the world undergo massive cognitive disruption, sometimes uprooting the foundations of religious beliefs. Reassuring cornerstones, often of one's religious faith (e.g.,"If I am good and work hard, my just rewards will follow"), are now replaced by disorganizing, confusing questions of "What did I do to deserve this?" A crucial task of resolving these traumatic losses is making meaning and sense of what happened, assimilating what one can to one's existing beliefs, and gradually modifying those schemas accommodating to the new harsh reality [11,28]. Multiple schemas are often simultaneously violated. Not only is one's basic safety in the world eradicated by this loss, but the prior confidence in modern medicine and dependability of friends being sources of support and understanding may be casualties as well.

It is not the therapist's job to prophetically resurrect the client's infrastructure of meaning. But by articulating the areas of disrepair, encouraging a process of making sense of this loss and, crucially, offering an emotional climate of respect, patience, understanding and confidence in her finding, not alone, her way through this, usually allows the client to adaptively integrate past and current good in her life with the current tragedy. A new, more realistic and sober view of the world can co-exist with a renewed, though wary, confidence.

Both forms of trauma may besiege the bereaved, singly or in combination, and sometimes reviving earlier traumatic events. A 32-year-old woman expressed muted grief at her son's premature birth and death, avoiding his name and thinking about him. It soon became evident that she was emotionally repeating the secrecy of a rape at 14 about which she never told her neglectful parents. Once this earlier trauma could be processed in re-telling what happened, reducing her shame and self-blame, she was better able to more emotionally grieve her son's death, with less dissociative-like detachment. An understandable, lingering sense of vulnerability from the earlier rape could be challenged and modified by appreciating her capacity for assertiveness as an attorney.

The decision to end a pregnancy due to fetal anomaly may be especially traumatizing. One never imagined oneself getting such news or making such a decision. With the window of having a choice ever narrowing, a woman needed to decide within a week whether to terminate her Down's pregnancy. What initially appeared to be a pathologic self-punitive paralysis of spending weeks obsessively reviewing her choice after the termination, later became understood as a necessary process of validating a decision that had to be made too soon for her psyche to absorb.

Traumatic residues are normal and to be expected in the pregnancy following a prior loss. Anticipating another shocking death, re-living cues of the last pregnancy, and detaching oneself from the much wanted child as one lives in a state of low-level hypervigilant anxiety, keeps her "one step in and one step out" of that difficult pregnancy [29]. One woman who endured multiple pregnancy losses was so convinced she would lose another one that she guiltily acknowledged wishing it would happen already, finding it intolerable to endure the wracking helplessness defining how traumatic those losses were. Her husband was troubled by her seeming indifference to the pregnancy, defined as "it." Yet, once she gave birth to a healthy girl, her attachment quickly blossomed. In this situation, support figures – medical, mental health, family and friends – need to empathically and patiently accept her anxiety and responses as understandable based on her earlier loss(es), not trying to minimize or "talk her out of it," encouraging additional ultrasounds if that relieves anxiety and maintaining an air of quiet hopefulness.

Husbands are very susceptible to these traumatic repercussions, often feeling as helpless bystanders to their wives' bodily injuries. One man was always able to comfort and reassure his anxious wife, until his firm guarantee that their baby would be OK was shattered by a stillbirth. No longer could he maintain the aura of being her protector, requiring a slow process of accepting the limitations of his sense of power. Too often the man is left out of the grieving process, asked by family and friends how his wife is doing, with no acknowledgment of his own sadness and hurt. Cultural prohibitions against men expressing grief (i.e., viewed as weakness) may make it more acceptable for him to show anger rather than loss. Often he may show more grief by vicariously sharing with his wife's tears.

Defining the loss

A crucial therapeutic task is helping the couple appreciate what or who has exactly been lost. My own clinical work indicates that there is a typical sequence of experiencing an ongoing pregnancy, first as a fetus, then as a baby, culminating as a son or daughter, usually in the last trimester. Couples vary considerably on how rapidly they progress through that sequence in any particular pregnancy. Both the nature of the loss and the degree of maternal–fetal attachment will determine the intensity and nature of the grief reaction. Typically, the termination of an unwanted pregnancy (i.e., elective abortion) experienced as a fetus with very limited maternal–fetal attachment will not evoke significant grief [30], in contrast to a later termination for fetal anomaly of a much-wanted pregnancy, akin to grieving a spontaneous perinatal loss [31]. A miscarriage may be experienced as a devastating, shocking blow to a woman's feminine potential and/or the loss of a baby as well, depending upon whether personhood has been conferred in viewing it as the loss of a baby. Because the pregnancy is within the woman, she is more likely to experience a deeper attachment with an earlier sense of it being a baby than her male partner, generally resulting in deeper and more prolonged grief [32].

Listening carefully to whether the bereaved parent refers to the child by name, as a baby or something else usually indicates where the loss is on the trajectory of personhood. One may ask more specifically if it was felt as the loss of a baby or something else if the clinician is unclear.

Clinical experience along with anthropological and research data suggest three factors impact maternal–fetal attachment and development of personhood. Societal expectation of a healthy pregnancy and baby in the developed world accelerates the establishment of babyhood and promotes maternal–fetal attachment. Conversely in the developing world, such as in Tanzania, with a very high perinatal mortality rate, babies born with visible defects are often not considered humans and miscarriages and stillbirths not worthy of mourning [33]. Similarly, the normative frequency of pregnancy loss among Irish Catholic women at the turn of the twentieth century resulted in such losses being usually not deeply grieved, being instead, "just one of those things" [34, p. 189].

Motivation to parent is another important factor influencing maternal–fetal attachment and development of personhood. When there is no desire to parent a child, whether in elective abortion [30] or relinquishing a child by a third party surrogate [35], there is little maternal–fetal attachment or resulting grief.

Analogously, psychosocial factors that mitigate focusing one's energies and hopes on the pregnancy, such as lack of family support, emotional disturbance including depression, anxiety and substance usage, are significantly associated with less maternal–fetal attachment [36].

Finally, increased interaction with the fetus/baby accelerates both the experience of personhood and maternal–fetal attachment. Perinatal loss often results in a deeper and more prolonged grief than earlier losses, with quickening usually marking a more profound sense of the baby being separate from the mother [37]. Similarly the magnified, increasingly refined image of the fetus in ultrasound often accelerates the experience of personhood and maternal–fetal attachment [36]. Over the past 30 years with the improved technology and greater usage of ultrasound, women are much more likely, in my clinical experience, to view a miscarriage after the first eight-week ultrasound as the more personal death of her baby, not the loss of a pregnancy.

Of course, these models are intended as guidelines to understanding the variability of response to different pregnancy losses. Clinical acumen best determines what such a loss will mean to a particular woman and time in her life. A 38-year-old woman experienced her terminating her Down's pregnancy as the deeply disappointing loss of a potential, not actual, child, a "pre-human creature." Reporting neither guilt nor regret about her decision she was readily able to share her sadness, feeling minimal grief and soon ready to attempt another pregnancy, concerned about her advancing age. A 42-year-old woman expressed a deep and lonely grief for the entirely unexpected ectopic pregnancy following a history of successful infertility treatments and birth of twins six years earlier. Her prior history of reproductive frustration heightened this loss, felt as that of a baby, much to the chagrin of her relieved family who did not believe having more children made sense.

Pregnancy termination for fetal anomaly is perhaps the most variably experienced loss. Clinically, the sense of what has been lost is fluid, not statically determined once and for all. Frequently it is perceived as the loss of a potential child, clearly not a baby, especially if not seen. Others who choose to view the body sometimes uncomfortably consider the loss as "it," somewhat less than a baby, but more than a potential. Over the course of our work, many choose (their decision, not my agenda) to transform that loss into the more personal death of a named son or daughter. Only the couple can decide whether to endure the potentially greater guilt in feeling they ended their child's life while allowing them to acquire the rudiments of that child's existence (i.e., mementoes, memories, rituals, and so forth) which can catalyze mourning.

Facilitating grieving

Grieving the loss of the baby is generally what is most equated with counseling for perinatal loss. This unique form of grieving entails transforming the loss of a baby into the death of a specific, named son or daughter. There is a two-step process of establishing the identity of the baby and then constructing the memories of interaction which is the raw material of grieving. Much of this may be accomplished in the hospital with seeing and holding the baby, making a memory box with mementoes, and so forth. Psychotherapy can continue that process as well (see reference [4] for a useful table of interventions to facilitate grieving), especially since a brief hospital stay laden with traumatic shock usually deters much overt grieving. Imparting a child an identity also enables the rituals around memorials and remembering which help to make sense and meaning of such a loss, increasingly understood as an important ingredient in adaptation to loss [11,28]. Alice recognized in grieving the loss of her baby son, Jim, she would review and remember the precious hours she had with him and the tokens he left behind. It is quite striking and poignant to observe in the midst of the sadness of grieving parents, the momentary pleasure they may take in a therapy hour of the love they felt in the time together with their child. One father especially appreciated taking a video of his very premature son's movements soon after birth, documenting his brief life.

Because so much of grieving perinatal loss is projected prospectively into the future, anniversaries and birthdays often take on great importance in missing what might have been. "Weaving babies lost in pregnancy into the fabric of the family" [38] through rituals, symbols, a visible presence and other means enables a continuing bond with one's child that is now recognized as a normative adaptation to this loss [39] rather than a defense against resolving grief. Some parents need to briefly take their baby home to create memories of his/her place concretely in the family. One mother planned a family picnic by the grave of her deceased son on his birthday as a way of celebrating his brief life. A special song, memory, or dream may conjure up the spiritual presence of and connection to the baby. While we need to encourage and validate parents' own actions that sustain their unique everlasting, ongoing parental relationship with their child, it can sometimes be useful to offer memorializing activities that have helped other parents. Remembering such a young loss is so important due to others not knowing him and the constant fear of that child being forgotten.

For some parents an earlier, unresolved loss or trauma becomes fused with a current perinatal death, extending and complicating the therapy. The earlier loss must be identified and often grieved to some degree in its own right, before reconciliation with the perinatal loss can be achieved. A 35-year-old woman relentlessly grieved the intra-uterine fetal demise of her 16-week pregnancy month after month with no relief. It was only when she was able to discuss in considerable detail the suicide of her psychotic, bipolar father (which was a family secret) and openly grieve the loss of him that she was able to more effectively relinquish the loss of her daughter. A 32-year-old father reported increasing anxiety about the safety of his 2-year-old son and distancing from the family following several miscarriages. Being able to explore in greater depth traumatizing sexual abuse when he was 4 years old significantly alleviated his anxious reactions.

Sometimes grieving is more diffuse, not of a son or daughter but of a sense of failed parenthood or reproductive capacity, especially with an earlier miscarriage or pregnancy terminated for fetal anomaly. While this will be discussed in greater detail in the following section, it is worth recognizing that not following the parental path one expected [5] entails prospective grieving a loss of one's future and identity, analogous to not parenting the deceased child one loves. There may also be significant losses associated with pregnancy demise. A 40-year-old woman did not grieve the loss of a baby due to an elective abortion at 16, but sorrowfully missed the relationship with her boyfriend, the only figure at that time who genuinely cared for her, and who faded from her life soon after.

Grieving does not occur in an interpersonal vacuum. The empathic support, sharing of sadness and crying at a funeral powerfully facilitates grieving. Similarly and more deeply, a secure attachment with a therapist enables an open expression of multifaceted parental grief embodying sadness, rage, despair, loneliness and so forth. Such emotional support for grieving perinatal loss may be painfully missing due to the tendency of family and friends to quickly minimize or avoid discussing the death. The heightened yearning of the recently pregnant woman for maternal nurturance is a normal regression in preparing to empathically care for the vulnerable infant [40,41]. This also makes the need of the newly bereaved mother for empathic understanding so critical.

Repairing the self

Pregnancy loss is almost inevitably a major if not devastating blow to the self. As we will examine, the multiple strands of the "bio-psychosocial" foundations of the self are challenged. One's helplessness in the face of identity being shaken can be traumatizing.

Pregnancy loss shatters a basic bodily function, that of reproduction. A young woman in her mid 20s called her miscarriage not so much the death of a baby but a "loss of invincibility." The sense of omnipotence and immortality through projecting one's genes into the next generation is dismantled, sometimes permanently. Shame, commonly felt after any bodily malfunction, can be intense, along with feeling defective.

Psychologically, pregnancy loss assaults a woman's self-worth in general, and gender identity in particular. Even when a woman rationally understands she did nothing wrong and everything right to ensure the health of her baby, there is a virtually ubiquitous tendency to emotionally blame herself and feel the resulting guilt. A very successful Latina businesswoman in her mid 30s relentlessly attacked herself for not going to the hospital sooner when she felt unusual pains at 20 weeks, even though she was told by the hospital to wait and see if it got better by morning. Her baby was prematurely born that dreadful night. Her motto in life, that she could fix anything she set her mind to, was left shattered.

There are multiple interventions to keep in mind in addressing these biological and psychological assaults on the self. For many, simply identifying these multiple injuries is therapeutic, broadening the understanding that more has been taken away than solely the loss of a baby. Amid the self-blaming and bashing, having someone take the time to understand her pain conveys the sense that she matters. Different strategies will work for different women. Understanding what caused the loss will go a significant way for some in subduing irrational self-blame and guilt [42]. For others, blaming oneself – if specifically designed to be able to avoid another such traumatic loss – may in fact improve mood and sense of competence by increasing one's sense of efficacy [43]. This seemed to work effectively for the businesswoman, serving to preserve a sense of control over the future rather than being left with her shredded self-confidence. Reinforcing other areas of self-esteem in one's life – that of career, parent (if one has surviving children of course), marriage and so forth – can significantly ameliorate, over time, one's wounded self-worth. When prior infertility has taken its toll, as occurred with Alice, simply becoming pregnant can be validated as a legitimate boost to one's self-esteem.

CBT techniques may be useful in addressing unrealistic self-blame. Cognitive re-appraisal [8,26] directly challenges the irrational underpinnings of these beliefs as well as recognizes what has been gained in adapting to these losses. This may be done, respectively, by having the client "put her thoughts on trial, and weigh the evidence" [28, p. 528] or considering "The Gifts" [6, p. 209] given by the lost baby, such as greater marital closeness, gratitude for the good in life and such like. When applying these techniques, one needs to be very careful in timing them not too soon, when in the midst of intense sorrow, or in any way justifying this loss as something positive. Once again, accurate empathy will guide when, how and ultimately if those interventions are made, directed by the client and not a manual.

Interactions in one's social world can be a critical determinant of the depletion or sustenance of self-worth. A 42-year-old woman became intolerably infuriated by the lack of acknowledgment and minimization of the loss of her 16-week-old twins by her extended family. When attempts to encourage more empathic responses failed, recommending avoidance of them – typically not the best alternative – in this case seemed warranted. The impact of the social world becomes even more malignant when one encounters the stigma against certain pregnancy losses, such as pregnancy termination for fetal anomaly [44]. A therapist's identifying and allying oneself against such stigmatization can be appropriate. At the same time, one must be careful to consider whether the anticipation of social criticism for this decision may be a projection of the woman's own guilt, especially if one senses a supportive social network. In order to reduce the tremendous shame this loss can elicit, it is usually very helpful to encourage the couple to share the nature of this loss with at least one figure (and optimally more) in their support system with whom they feel completely safe.

Finally, when pregnancy loss occurs before parenting a live child, there can be tremendous disruption in one's psychosocial adult development, interfering with attaining "generativity" [45]. One not only experiences estrangement from family forming peers, but feels out of synch with one's own life plan and vision of the future. Men can profoundly feel such frustration when these losses prevent entering fatherhood. Empathically identifying the source of this social and personal isolation as well as supporting steps to realize other important developmental goals (e.g., career aspirations) and for now finding alternatives to parental wishes (e.g., mentoring) can be important therapeutic tasks.

Preserving social connections

Due to the vulnerability of social isolation and the increased probability of feeling one's loss has been misunderstood and minimized by others, maintaining supportive social ties is significantly related to a quicker adaptation to this loss [1,2]. Just as was the case in defining optimal therapist and health provider support, empathy in its multiple ingredients (i.e., comforting, listening, being nonjudgmental, etc.) registered as the most helpful form of support that could be provided by family and friends [46]. Support groups have emerged as a particularly valuable resource offering a safe place to share one's loss and feel validated, whether meeting face-to-face [47] or over the Internet [48].

While a therapist's empathy with the inevitably painful and tactless comments the bereaved will receive is necessary, when clinically feasible it can be helpful to underscore family and friends' desire to be helpful, even when they fail. Modeling ways to non-aggressively but assertively confront repeatedly hurtful remarks ("I know you mean well but when you say that, it doesn't help me") is often necessary, along with educating family and friends as to what actions will be helpful. If the offending family member or friend persists, limiting contact for now may be the best solution. Finally, in recommending support groups as a useful adjunct to therapy, it is important that it be conveyed as supplementing, not replacing, the work (and support) in therapy, lest the bereaved feel rejected.

Weathering termination

While termination varies among clients in this kind of work, it trends towards brevity. In brief therapy it may be announced that session, though in longer work I encourage at least several sessions to allow for a usual expression of some loss over ending, especially meaningful as it is loss which brought them in. Because traumatizing helplessness is usually such a critical ingredient in the loss, I am reluctant to challenge what may feel like a rushed exit. Even if you may wish for a more planned departure (in part, perhaps, to deal with one's own sense of loss in ending), it may be most important for the client to feel in control of *this* loss compared to the last traumatizing one. Sometimes ending soon becomes an understandable desire to put this loss behind them, especially if a ticking biological clock has them thinking of a subsequent pregnancy before it is too late.

A more maladaptive, shockingly sudden termination may be unconsciously designed to provoke the abandonment the parents have felt by their loss, which may be re-activated by interruptions in the therapy. Parents of a stillbirth many years prior suddenly announced their decision to end therapy in the final minutes of their first appointment following my three-week summer vacation, after having worked productively for over a year. The better approach, I believe, is not to metaphorically slam the door on their way out, but to express one's disappointment in not having more time to say goodbye, while letting them know the door is open should they choose to return (a message I convey in all terminations).

Reflections

The more experience I gain in working with pregnancy loss, the less of a sense I have that I have the answers. Despite commonalities in reactions, profound individual differences persist. A couple who I saw but hours earlier today shared a common deep Christian faith in grappling with the neonatal loss of their son due to an extremely rare metabolic disorder. While the father was furious with God for not hearing his prayers, the mother was at peace with Him, knowing her son was whole, resting in heaven.

More research is needed to more accurately direct clinical practice. Despite the almost universal recommendation to encourage parents' viewing and holding their baby after perinatal loss, one of the few studies which examined the impact of that contact reported significantly greater PTSD, depressive and anxious reactions in a subsequent pregnancy among those who chose such contact [49]. The increasing belief in the value of sustaining bonds with one's deceased child is qualified by considering those situations where relinquishing one's attachment may be optimal [50].

One is likely to stay on the right track by listening to what the bereaved has to say, feeling what they are going through, asking questions about what may be omitted in their account, empowering them to be as much as possible the authors of their experience and providing guidance when they feel lost.

References

1. Lasker JN, Toedter LJ. Predicting outcomes after pregnancy loss: results from studies using the Perinatal Grief Scale. *Illness, Crisis & Loss* 2000; 8: 350–72.
2. Bennett SM, Litz BT, Maguen S, et al. An exploratory study of the psychological impact and clinical care of perinatal loss. *J Loss Trauma* 2008; 13: 485–510.
3. Leon, IG. Understanding pregnancy loss: helping families cope. *Postgrad OB & GYN* 1999; 19: 1–7.
4. Covington, SN. Pregnancy loss. In Covington S, Burns L, eds. *Infertility Counseling: A Comprehensive Handbook for Clinicians* (2nd edn.). Cambridge: Cambridge University Press. 2006; 290–304.
5. Jaffe J, Diamond MO. *Reproductive Trauma: Psychotherapy with Infertility and Pregnancy Loss Cients*. Washington, DC: American Psychological Association. 2011.
6. Covington, SN. Miscarriage and stillbirth. In Rosen A, Rosen J, eds. *Frozen Dreams: Psychodynamic Dimensions of Infertility and Assisted Reproduction*. Hillsdale, NJ: Analytic Press. 2005; 197–218.
7. Leon IG. Understanding and treating infertility: psychoanalytic considerations. *J Am Acad Psa Dyn Psychiatr* 2010; 38: 47–76.
8. Bennett SM, Ehrenreich-May J, Litz BT, et al. Development and preliminary evaluation of a cognitive-behavioral intervention for perinatal grief. *Cog Beh Pract* 2012; 19: 161–73.
9. Kersting A, Kroker K, Schlicht, S, et al. Efficacy of cognitive behavioral internet-based therapy in parents after the loss of a child during pregnancy: pilot data from a randomized controlled trial. *Arch Wom Ment Health* 2011; 14: 465–77.
10. Zisook S, Shear K. Grief and bereavement: what psychiatrists need to know. *World Psychiatr* 2009; 8: 67–74.
11. Neimeyer RA. Searching for the meaning of meaning: grief therapy and the process of reconstruction. *Death Studies* 2000; 24: 541–58.

12. Boelen PA, van de Schoot R, van den Hout MA, et al. Prolonged grief disorder, depression and posttraumatic stress disorder are distinguishable syndromes. *J Affect Disord* 2010; 125: 374–78.
13. American Psychiatric Association. *Diagnostic and Statistical Manual of Mental Disorders, DSM-5 (5th edn.)*. Washington DC: American Psychiatric Association. 2013.
14. Lin SX, Lasker JN. Patterns of grief reaction after pregnancy loss. *Amer J Orthopsychiatr* 1996; 66: 262–71.
15. Lang A, Goulet C, Aita M, et al. Weathering the storm of perinatal bereavement via hardiness. *Death Studies* 2001; 25: 497–512.
16. Stroebe M, Schut H. The dual process model of coping with bereavement: rationale and description. *Death Studies* 1999; 23: 197–224.
17. Elliott R, Bohart AC, Watson J, et al. Empathy. *Psychotherapy* 2011; 48: 43–9.
18. Swanson-Kauffman K. Caring in the instance of unexpected early pregnancy loss. *Top Clin Nurs* 1986; 8: 37–46.
19. Gold KJ. Navigating care after a baby dies: a systematic review of parent experiences with health providers. *J Perinatol* 2007; 27: 230–7.
20. Jackson PL, Brunet E, Meltzoff AN, et al. Empathy examined through the neural mechanisms involved in imagining how I feel versus how you feel pain. *Neuropsychologia* 2006; 44: 752–61.
21. Lyons-Ruth K, Change Process Study Group. Implicit relational knowing: its role in development and psychoanalytic treatment. *Inf Ment Health J* 1998; 19: 282–9.
22. Amini F, Lewis T, Lannon R, et al. Affect, attachment, memory: contributions towards psychobiologic integration. *Psychiatry* 1996; 59: 213–39.
23. Kohut H. *How Does Analysis Cure?* Chicago: University of Chicago Press. 1984.
24. Sable P. *Attachment and Adult Psychotherapy*. Northvale NJ: Jason Aronson. 2000.
25. Wallin DJ. *Attachment in Psychotherapy*. New York: Guilford. 2007.
26. Kersting A, Kroker K, Schlicht S, et al. Internet-based treatment after pregnancy loss: concept and case study. *J Psychosom OB GYN* 2011; 32: 72–8.
27. Janoff-Bulman R. *Shattered Assumptions: Towards a New Psychology of Trauma*. New York: Macmillan. 1992.
28. Davis CG, Wortman CB, Lehman DR, et al. Searching for meaning in loss: are clinical assumptions correct? *Death Studies* 2000; 24: 497–540.
29. Cote-Arsenault D, Marshall R. One foot in – one foot out: weathering the storm of pregnancy after perinatal loss. *Res Nurs Health* 2000; 23: 473–85.
30. Cameron S. Induced abortion and psychological sequelae. *Best Prac Res Clin Ob Gyn* 2010; 24: 657–65.
31. Zeanah C, Dailey J, Rosenblatt M, et al. Do women grieve after terminating pregnancies because of fetal anomalies? A controlled investigation. *Ob Gyn* 1993; 82: 270–5.
32. Peppers L, Knapp R. *Motherhood and Mourning: Perinatal Death*. New York: Praeger. 1980.
33. Wembah-Rashid JAR. Explaining pregnancy loss in matrilineal southeast Tanzania. In Cecil R, ed. *The Anthropology of Pregnancy Loss*. Oxford: Berg. 1996; 75–93.
34. Cecil R. Memories of pregnancy loss: recollections of elderly women in Northern Ireland. In Cecil R, ed. *The Anthropology of Pregnancy Loss*. Oxford: Berg. 1996; 179–96.
35. Hanafin H. Surrogacy and gestational carrier participants. In Covington S, Burns L, eds. *Infertility Counseling: A Comprehensive Handbook for Clinicians* (2nd edn.). Cambridge: Cambridge University Press. 2006; 370–86.
36. Alhusen JL. A literature update on maternal-fetal attachment. *J Ob Gyn Neonat Nurs* 2008; 37: 315–28.
37. Leon, I. Helping families cope with perinatal loss. Nov, 2008. http://www.glowm.com/section_view/item/417. Accessed November 4, 2013.
38. Cote-Arsenault D. Weaving babies lost in pregnancy into the fabric of the family. *J Fam Nurs* 2003; 9: 23–37.
39. Klass D. *The Spiritual Lives of Bereaved Parents*. Philadelphia: Brunner Mazel. 1999.
40. Brazelton TB, Cramer BG. *The Earliest Relationship: Parents, Infants and the Drama :of Early Attachment*. Reading, MA: Addison-Wesley. 1990.
41. Leon IG. *When a Baby Dies: Psychotherapy for Pregnancy and Newborn Loss*. New Haven, CT: Yale University Press. 1990.
42. Nikcevic AV, Tunkel SA, Kuczmierczyk AR, et al. Investigation of the cause of miscarriage and its influence on women's psychological distress. *Br J Ob Gyn* 1999; 106: 808–13.
43. Affleck G, McGrade B, Allen D, et al. Mothers' beliefs about behavioral causes for their developmentally disabled infant's condition: what do they signify? *J Ped Psychol* 1985; 10: 293–303.

44. McCoyd J. Pregnancy interrupted: loss of a desired pregnancy after diagnosis of fetal anomaly. *J Psychosom Ob Gyn* 2007; 28: 37–48.

45. Erikson E. *Childhood and Society* (2nd edn.). New York: Norton. 1963.

46. Kavanaugh K, Trier D, Korzec M. Social support following pregnancy loss. *J Fam Nurs* 2004; 10: 70–92.

47. Cacciatore J. Effects of support groups on posttraumatic stress responses in women experiencing stillbirth. *Omega* 2008; 55: 71–90.

48. Gold KJ, Boggs ME, Mugisha E, et al. Internet message boards for pregnancy loss: who's on – line and why? *Wom Health Issues* 2012; 22: 67–72.

49. Hughes P, Turton P, Hooper E, et al. Assessment of guidelines for good practice in psychosocial care of mothers after stillbirth: a cohort study. *Lancet* 2002; 360: 114–8.

50. Neimeyer RA, Baldwin SA, Gillies J. Continuing bonds and reconstructing meaning: mitigating complications in bereavement. *Death Studies* 2006; 30: 715–38.

Chapter 17

The view from the fertility counselor's chair

Janet Jaffe

> *A deep understanding of one's own pain makes it possible to convert weakness into strength and to offer one's own experience as a source of healing to those who are often lost in the darkness of their own misunderstood sufferings* [1, p. 87].

Fertility clients come to us in crisis: they have been traumatized and have experienced multiple losses – perhaps of a child, a pregnancy, or yet another failed cycle, perhaps how they feel about themselves, their intimate relationships with family and friends, and of their hopes and dreams for the future. Whether they are seeking ongoing psychotherapy or a consultation, their *reproductive story* – their conscious, but often unconscious, ideas about becoming parents – clearly has not gone as they had hoped [2]. What is often not addressed is that you, as a mental health professional and a human being, also have a reproductive story. The nature and course of your own personal story, whether you have children or not, are in the midst of a crisis now or have long resolved it, has an impact on the clinical work you do. You even may have been motivated to enter this field because of your personal story. Calling upon your inner psychological narrative can have a powerful effect on your therapeutic relationships; this chapter discusses how to use your own history to avoid pitfalls and foster healing in your patients.

The purpose of this chapter is to explore the complexities of our relationships with our clients: the impact their fertility struggles have on us, and how our life's challenges and crises can affect them. Being aware of our own conflicts and wounds allows us to use them constructively in the service of our clients. How we use these emotions to enhance the psychotherapy of fertility clients – by the controversial use of self-disclosure and awareness of countertransference feelings – is addressed. Additionally, as we are exposed to a great deal of grief and loss by our clients' stories, we may experience vicarious trauma and/or compassion fatigue. Thus the need for therapist self-care also is discussed.

Along with theoretical constructs and ethical considerations, clinical vignettes illustrate these concepts. These examples, however, are not meant to provide a recipe for the right or wrong way to approach clients: each client and each therapeutic relationship needs to be assessed for its own unique set of circumstances. As such, this chapter hopefully will make you, the fertility counselor, more acutely aware of the ramifications of the relationship between you and your clients.

Anna: a case of self-disclosure

A woman, Anna, calls to set up an initial appointment. She found you through your website which describes your work with infertility and pregnancy loss clients. When you ask her what is going on, she breaks down and reveals that she has just experienced her second IVF failure: another chemical pregnancy. Without knowing anything else about her, her relationships or history, your genuine response, "I am so sorry to hear that," reveals much about you and your capacity to empathize, and can set the tone for the therapeutic relationship.

When she comes in for her first session with you, Anna asks if you have any children. A seemingly innocuous question, one that is asked all the time in social situations, undoubtedly is loaded for Anna. Thus how you answer Anna's question, or if you do, is not to be taken lightly. What does it mean to her if you have children or if you don't? How is your answer going to

Fertility Counseling: Clinical Guide and Case Studies, ed. Sharon N. Covington. Published by Cambridge University Press.

make her feel? How much is too much to tell, and is saying nothing too little? What is the potential impact on the therapy?

Anna's question pushes the conventional boundary of therapist privacy and anonymity [3]. She has delved into territory that may be loaded with profound feelings for you. What if you have had your own series of losses, perhaps similar or completely different from hers? What if your reproductive issues are in the past and have been resolved? On the other hand, what if you are in the midst of trying to have a child yourself? What if you or your partner is pregnant? With new clients, do you address this on the phone? With ongoing patients, do you wait until they notice? How do you answer if having children was easy for you? These are essential questions to consider because not only does Anna have a reproductive story, so do you. The question is: Do you answer her question, and if so, how?

Therapist self-disclosure is a provocative topic: some practitioners believe that revealing personal information will contaminate the therapeutic treatment, while others strongly support it [4]. Although a highly controversial and rarely used clinical strategy (only about 3.5% of all therapeutic interventions) [5], a review of empirical research indicates that more than 90% of therapists have used self-disclosure in their work [6]. This section explores therapist disclosure and addresses if, how, why, and when you answer a question such as Anna's. Included in this discussion are:

- A definition of self-disclosure.
- The different types of therapist disclosure.
- The risks/benefits of therapist disclosure for the client.
- Theoretical viewpoints.
- The ethics of self-disclosure.
- The implications of answering direct, or not-so-direct inquiries (i.e., how did you get into the field of reproductive psychology?).
- The timing of disclosures.
- The impact of your reproductive story on the client and the therapy: case example.

These issues are important, regardless of theoretical orientation, as the dynamic between the client and the counselor accounts for so much in the therapeutic process. Indeed the strength of the therapeutic relationship has been found to be the best predictor of both positive and negative clinical outcomes [7]. Additionally, when a client asks a direct question, or if personal information about the therapist is inadvertently exposed, the therapist must be prepared. In the moment when a clinician's private life is revealed, whether intentionally or not, s/he may not have time to ponder all the pros and cons of the most therapeutic response, and may feel a loss of composure and professional control. Thus, thinking about these matters ahead of time can help when clinical decisions need to be made quickly [8–10].

What is self-disclosure?

Broadly speaking, everything a counselor does or does not say is a self-disclosure [11]. Disclosures can be deliberate or accidental, verbal or non-verbal, avoidable or unavoidable. From the way one dresses to one's office décor, one's physical attributes, ethnicity, gender and age – these are self-revealing unavoidable, non-verbal disclosures [9,12]. One's body language – a smile, a look of concern, a change of position – are also non-verbal disclosures revealing instinctual expressions of the therapist's feelings. If the counselor has a home office or resides in a small community, his/her personal life becomes more transparent as inevitable boundaries may cross. Unexpectedly running into a client in a grocery store with one's kids in the shopping cart is an unavoidable, unintentional, and perhaps very awkward disclosure. Additionally, with information readily available on the Internet and Facebook, it is common today for clients to search for reviews or other information about the therapist. A click of a mouse can reveal intentional postings (articles, websites), but also may make known information that was posted by others – without the therapist's knowledge. Anonymity has become virtually impossible with personal information readily available, and may include a home phone number and/or home address, information about family members or other people the therapist knows, reviews, photos, lawsuits, political affiliations and donations [13]. The access to information can feel like a boundary violation with the client potentially knowing more about the counselor at the onset of treatment than the counselor is aware of. Depending on the client's issues and diagnosis, this kind of information about the therapist can affect the course of treatment.

When therapists think about self-disclosure, they usually refer to deliberate, verbal disclosure of personal information, perhaps prompted by a client's question, sometimes by the clinical material they are presenting. Seven different types of therapist disclosures have been proposed:

- Facts: sharing your professional experience and credentials.
- Feelings: validating the client's feelings by comparing your own feelings in a similar situation.
- Insight: revealing perceptions of your own life in a comparable situation.
- Strategy: advising the client in ways you have handled like circumstances.
- Reassurance/support: normalizing the patient's experience by acknowledging your own experience.
- Challenge: divulging information about your own similar life trials.
- Immediacy: providing feedback to the client as to how their behavior with others is occurring in the therapy with you [14].

Whether intentional or unwitting, disclosures affect the therapeutic alliance. They may create "a real moment of human sharing of vulnerability and helplessness that has the potential to bring the patient to a new level of feeling and enrich the treatment" [10, p. 15]. On the other hand, a therapist disclosure can have the opposite effect, interfering with transference feelings and/or burdening the patient with concern about the counselor. (See Table 17.1 for the benefits and risks of therapist disclosure.) Decisions about disclosure are influenced by one's theoretical perspective; the patient's diagnosis; the strength of the therapeutic alliance; whether it is at the beginning, middle or end of treatment; and, ultimately, by ethical concerns of what is in the best interest of the client. Additionally the therapist's personal history of loss and trauma plays a factor in these choices.

Table 17.1 Benefits and risks of therapist self-disclosure.

Benefits of Therapist Disclosure	Risks of Therapist Disclosure
Model behavior & expression of feelings	Focus on therapist rather than client
Offer alternate ways of thinking	Burden client with information
Reduce shame; increase trust	Violate boundaries
Decrease sense of feeling alone	Contaminate transference
Enhance therapeutic alliance	Overshadow client's needs
Normalize & validate	Create role reversal
Decrease power differential	May create desire to take care of therapist
Allow view of therapist as human/imperfect	May not promote a therapeutic goal
Expand client's self-awareness	
Increase client's self-disclosure	
Demystify therapeutic process	
Repair therapeutic ruptures/misunderstandings	
Promote insight	

To disclose or not: theoretical orientation

When Freud first discussed self-disclosure, he suggested that the therapist should be "like a mirror," reflecting back only what the patient reveals [15, p. 18]. Traditional psychoanalytic therapists were trained to be neutral and not to self-disclose. The theory purports that the key to successful treatment is the working through of transference: the feelings that clients have from earlier significant relationships that are displaced onto the therapist [16]. Self-disclosure is seen as a detriment to therapy because it shifts the focus away from the patient and onto the therapist; by introducing "real" elements of the clinician, the client's fantasies and transference may be disrupted and contaminated.

Much has changed since Freud's early work. Some of the more recent psychoanalytic/psychodynamic thinking views therapy as a two-person model, with both patient and therapist contributing to the relationship, and recognizes that strict neutrality is not only impossible, but also may be harmful to the therapeutic experience [17,18]. A therapist who comes across as distant and withholding may in fact do damage to a patient whose self-esteem is already battered and who is feeling depressed and isolated, as many infertility patients feel. In a treatment outcome study at a university counseling center, it was found that an increase in therapist disclosure lowered clients' symptoms [19]. Thus infrequent and judicial use of self-disclosure may actually facilitate healing: the therapist can serve as a role model, reassure clients that they are not alone, and help normalize their struggle [14].

Other theoretical approaches consider self-disclosure to be an essential component of therapy. Fundamentally different from the psychoanalytic perspective, humanists advocate therapist self-disclosure as a means to foster change. By being authentic and real, counselors help minimize the power differential in the therapeutic relationship, thus aiding their clients' openness and willingness to share their own struggles. The genuine dialogue between therapist and client is used to address problems that may arise in the therapist–client relationship. Similarly, feminist theories espouse the use of self-disclosure in fostering an egalitarian relationship. Appropriate disclosures are seen as a way to transmit feminist values, and are used to validate and normalize struggles, decrease feelings of shame and promote empowerment of the client. Therapist self-disclosure in the Lesbian Gay Bisexual Transgender (LBGT) community has been used to create a safe space to process feelings of marginality [20]. Cognitive-behavioral therapists (CBT) use self-disclosure to challenge clients' distortions about themselves or others by providing feedback and modeling more effective behavior [14]. Dialectical behavior therapists (DBT) also judiciously use disclosure to support the emotional experience of the client. As many of the client's issues are interpersonal in nature, it can be validating, for example, to hear that a therapist also would react in a similar way, given the situation the client described [21].

Disclosure and ethical considerations

Regardless of theoretical orientation, it is important to understand the consequences of disclosing or not. Under what circumstances should a counselor disclose when working with reproductive patients? What types of disclosures are necessary? What is it that the client needs? How will a particular disclosure affect the client and the therapy? Will it be helpful or harmful?

The most salient question to consider is: *Is this disclosure in the client's best interest?* The motive for disclosure should be to promote a therapeutic goal and be in the service of the patient [12]. Professional organizations for psychologists, social workers and counselors in the United States as well as in other countries provide guidelines for addressing the issue of therapist disclosure. For example, the American Psychological Association (APA) Ethical Principle A states, "Psychologists strive to benefit those with whom they work and take care to do no harm" [22, p. 3]. Regardless of training, mental health professionals should strive to practice *beneficence* (do what is helpful for the patient) and *nonmaleficence* (avoid doing harm) [8,9,23]. Similarly, APA Ethical Standards 3.04 (Avoiding Harm) and 3.08 (Exploitative Relationships) raise the issue of the potential power differential in the therapist–client relationship. If a boundary is broken with a therapist disclosure, is it for the therapist's need, or is it in service of the client? Clearly, taking advantage of a patient is an ethical breach. A counselor who unburdens him/herself with no clear benefit to the client is in violation of the professional ethical guidelines.

Equally important to consider is therapist nondisclosure. It has been suggested that a refusal to disclose, especially when asked a specific question by a client, is a kind of disclosure in and of itself [8]. In an empirical study with current therapy clients, nondisclosures were twice as likely to be experienced as unhelpful [24]. Non-disclosures can be read as rejections, felt as withholding and increase a sense of alienation and inferiority [13,14]. As many reproductive clients already have low self-esteem from the trauma of infertility treatments and/or pregnancy loss, a counselor who comes across as cold or aloof would not be in the client's best interest. Non-disclosures have the potential to compromise the therapeutic relationship, but too much disclosure also can be perceived as a burden to the client. Too much information about the counselor's life circumstances or emotional state can make the client feel as if they are in a role-reversal, having to take care of the counselor. This can feel overwhelming, frightening, unsafe and intimidating – creating a non-therapeutic climate for the client. The questions then arise: If, when, and how much? And should infertility and pregnancy loss clients be treated differently than the general therapeutic population?

Back to Anna's question: Do you have children?

All of us, clinicians and clients alike, experience illness, death and loss throughout life. As mental health professionals, we are in the unique position of dealing with our own distressing life situations while helping our clients through theirs. The intersection of these events can create feelings of emotional chaos in the patient and a loss of feeling safe and cared for [10]. Likewise, shared experiences with clients can generate uncertainty in therapists, and throw them off their normal professional footing and objectivity [14]. In other words, when the counselor is personally challenged by life events, there may be a disruption in the connection/relationship with clients. Thus, where you are in your own reproductive journey and how that intersects with your client's will affect the therapy.

As Anna's new counselor, her question provides you with an array of opportunities and dilemmas. Because you know that Anna may be particularly sensitive to your answer, it is essential to give it some thought and be mindful of what it means to her. Some issues to consider in your response to Anna's question:

- **Therapeutic Alliance**: Research has shown that the effectiveness of therapist disclosure is highly dependent on the strength of the therapeutic alliance [24,25]. This is bi-directional: not only is it important for the patient to trust the counselor, but for therapists to reveal personally sensitive material they, too, must trust the patient deeply [3].
- **Client Traits**: There may be traits in the client that would make disclosure harmful to them. For instance, those with poor boundaries or reality testing, those who might try to take care of the therapist, or clients who are self-absorbed may actually be harmed by a counselor disclosure [9].
- **Stage of Treatment**: Early in treatment, therapist disclosures (your office decor, how you dress, etc.) are inevitable. In the middle phase of treatment, disclosures are likely to be used when therapeutically necessary [23], whereas disclosures at the end of treatment serve a different function. During termination with a client, it can be empowering to demystify the therapeutic process, discuss what was effective in treatment and what was not, and see the counselor as a genuine human being [14,16].
- **Your Reproductive Story**: Are you in the midst of a reproductive crisis yourself or is this something that has been worked through? Disclosure has been found to be much more risky if the therapist's issues have not been resolved [14].

As this is your first meeting with Anna, and you are just getting to know each other, it may not be possible to explore her fantasies about you at this juncture of the treatment. You may not yet have a sense of her needs, her personality traits, or her history. You may not want to expose private information with concerns of how she will receive it, nor do you want to be dismissive. A question like Anna's, about whether you have children or not, can elicit a variety of reactions in you depending on your own personal story.

Some possible scenarios for the mental health professional:

A. *Yes*, you do have children and you struggled to have them (this includes biological, third party, or adopted child(ren), and this is in the past.
B. *Yes*, you do have children, and you did not struggle with infertility or pregnancy loss.
C. *Yes*, you have a child or children, and are still in the family building phase, actively trying to conceive.
D. You (or your partner) are *currently pregnant.*
E. *No*, at this point you do not have children, and know you want them someday.
F. *No*, you do not have children and are in the midst of trying.
G. *No*, you are child free, not by choice.
H. *No*, you are child free by choice.

Let's say, for example, that you have recently found out that you are pregnant with your first child. Because the changes of pregnancy are gradual, you can decide, case by case, when it is appropriate to discuss it with your clients. You may decide it is important to let certain clients know as soon as possible, while with other clients, you may decide to wait. Processing clients' emotional reactions to the pregnancy can be challenging depending on their background, history and the strength of the therapeutic alliance. What are some of the issues that may arise in therapy when the counselor becomes pregnant? Clients may feel abandoned, as the fantasy of the therapist's care shifts from them to a baby. They may feel angry and jealous, especially if they are trying to conceive as well, but may feel too inhibited to express their negative feelings. Issues of mistrust may surface and patients may leave treatment prematurely. Therapists, on the other hand, may feel more vulnerable because of their pregnancy, and may not want to invite patients' hostile feelings about them or the pregnancy [10].

In Anna's case, because you know she is struggling to have a child, you may decide to let her know about your pregnancy when she asks if you have children. To wait may create feelings of tension and anxiety for you; likewise, she may trust you less if she knows you were not forthcoming. Saying something like, "I imagine this will be difficult to hear: I have recently learned that I am pregnant. It has not been an easy journey for me either. I realize this may be hard for you to tolerate, and I would understand if you would like to see another therapist, but perhaps we can work through your feelings about this together." It may feel like a relief for Anna to be able to process her emotions with you. If she can work through her anger, envy, resentment and grief with you, it is possible that she will cope better with the pregnancies of friends or family members.

A risky and challenging situation is if the fertility counselor and the client are both trying to conceive at the same time. Should the therapist become pregnant, self-disclosure will eventually become a necessity and, as above, a sensitive and honest discussion is called for. If the situation is reversed, that is, if the client should become pregnant, the counselor may feel jealous, angry and competitive. It may be difficult to celebrate the client's hard-won battle and hard to maintain therapeutic neutrality. If the client is aware that the therapist is "trying" to conceive, she may feel guilty about her own success and may feel the need to take care of the therapist. The client should be reassured that the therapist has her own support and, indeed, it is recommended that the therapist seek consultation.

The wounded healer

Many of us become involved in the mental health professions because of our own history of pain or loss [26]. Studies have found a link between a therapist's history of trauma, his/her desire to specialize in trauma care, and the effects on the clinical work [27]. For example, in the area of substance abuse and eating disorders, it is not uncommon, and often preferred, for the clinician to have "been there" [28,29]. Specific to reproductive medicine, a survey of nurses and mental health professionals revealed that more than half had a history of infertility, and almost three-quarters of those surveyed began working in the field after their diagnosis [30]. In a small sample of psychologists working in reproductive medicine, it was found that about 42% specialized in the field because of their own infertility [31]. Thus it is not uncommon, but not necessary, to choose to work with reproductive clients because of our personal life events.

A "wounded healer" is a formidable image suggesting that the healer's wounds carry curative power. Having a similar "wound" as the client may increase greater empathy and understanding of what they are experiencing. It is important to emphasize, however, that *simply being wounded does not make one an expert.* It is the process of understanding one's own wounds and recovering from them that facilitates healing in others [32]. If the counselor's wounds are not mended, processed and understood enough, his or her own healing may interfere with his or her work with clients [33]. Indeed, therapist disclosure has been found to be much riskier if the therapist is in the midst of unresolved problems [14]. If the wound is fresh, therapist objectivity may be lost; the focus may shift from the patient's needs to the therapist's. The challenge is to use our wounds in the service of the client.

The wounded healer: personal stories of therapists' crises

There are times when counselors are able to prepare, strategize and discuss personal life changes (as in a pregnancy). However, when a therapist has a miscarriage, stillbirth or other perinatal demise, there is no time to prepare herself or her clients, and it may not be possible to keep the loss private. A sudden absence from clinical work can evoke a multitude of feelings in clients, from anxiety and concern about the counselor's well-being, to antagonistic and aggressive feelings. Some patients may express relief regarding a pregnancy loss (i.e., the therapist will not abandon them or be in competition with them), while others may struggle with guilt over destructive fantasies [34]. Clients also may worry that their reproductive story may overwhelm their counselor; they may feel the need to minimize their own grief and loss in order to protect and take care of the therapist. Several mental health professionals have courageously written about their own reproductive traumas, and how these struggles affected their clinical work. Through the personal accounts of these clinicians, we learn how they managed the impact their loss had on their clients.

Dana Comstock was teaching at a university as well as doing clinical work when, about halfway through her pregnancy, her daughter was stillborn. Her medical emergency, followed by a three-month absence from work, made it necessary to disclose to her students and clients. When she did return to work, feeling raw and vulnerable, she was able to discuss her loss with clients as it affected them. "[T]hose explorations felt really different in the context of my now being a 'touchable' therapist, versus being perceived as 'untouchable' prior to my loss" [35, p. 262]. As a wounded healer, she was able to shift to a deeper level with her clients.

Additionally, she noted that details of her personal life did not need to be discussed in depth. In a case that shared some similarities to her own loss, and with the hope that sharing would validate the pain her client was experiencing, Comstock simply stated that she, too, had lost a baby. No details were discussed, but that self-disclosure let the client know that her therapist "got it."

When analyst Barbara Gerson was put on bed rest because of problems following an amniocentesis, she continued to see some of her patients at home, thus unavoidably disclosing a great deal about her personal life. Sadly, she had to terminate the pregnancy, and this "real" experience brought core issues to the foreground for her patients. Her own grief brought up feelings of loss for some clients; others became overwhelmed with fear and anger as boundaries loosened. A genuine person replaced the fantasy of the omnipotent therapist; a shift occurred in the authenticity of the therapist/patient relationship. Because she was in the midst of acute grief, her therapeutic "armor" was weaker and it was, at times, difficult to tolerate her patient's negative reactions. Her personal crisis, however, elicited some of the most intense work for her patients as they confronted, together, difficult and deep-seated issues [18].

What happens if the therapist and client face experiences that are psychologically similar? Jo Ellen Patterson discussed her active pursuit of fertility treatments while working with a couple that had a disabled child. "We were similar ages and all struggling with a major developmental milestone – the transition to parenthood – that had gone awry" [36, p. 24]. Patterson chose not to disclose any information about her personal life, but was able to use her own experience of grief and loss to empathize with the couple. Other counselors found that disclosing traumatic life events to their clients enhanced the therapeutic alliance; it allowed patients to have a genuine give and take with their therapist, and deepened the sense of collaboration [37]. The important point is that each counselor/client dyad needs to be assessed for its unique dynamics. What is right for one patient may not be right for others. The amount of disclosure, if any at all, will depend on the strength of the therapeutic relationship, the trust that has been established, whether or not the client has asked a direct question, the psychological needs of the client, and on the therapist's clinical judgment regarding the client's needs [3,36,38].

Lessons learned: my own story

My own reproductive trauma consisted of four miscarriages and five years of fertility interventions and procedures. This was before IVF was readily available, using a donor was not even on the horizon, and it seemed as if our reality was that we would not have children. I was in graduate school when I had my third miscarriage. None of my fellow students/colleagues knew my secret; the shame I felt was overwhelming as if I were defective (a theme I since have heard repeatedly from clients). I can remember a lecture in one of my classes about grief and loss – it was all very theoretical to me until the professor said, "Even miscarriages need to be grieved." My heart began to race, I glanced around to see if anyone was staring at me (of course not!), I felt sick to my stomach, and couldn't wait to bolt from the room. That's how humiliated I felt. It was also at that point that I realized I could probably help others through this kind of trauma, but I had to get through it first myself.

My son was born a year later. His birth was one of those miraculous events – after all the interventions, it just happened. It was only after he was about 4 years old that I felt ready to take on my first reproductive clients. I realized that as much as I wanted to help others through their reproductive traumas, it would have been too painful had I not resolved my own grief [14,33]. And so, when the question arose – "do you have kids?" – I found myself facing an interesting internal dilemma. Like so many clinical psychologists, I had been trained that disclosure is taboo. I did my best to understand the reasons why the question was being posed and to focus on what my answer might mean to that particular client. Sometimes I would explore the fantasies before I responded, at other times I would respond directly and then get deeper into the client's feelings about my personal admission. I let them know that I was willing to answer their questions, but that we had to talk about it. It was important for our work together to know how my answers made them feel. To be clear, I did not go into details about my reproductive journey; I simply said that I had been able to have a child. For the most part, clients felt comforted by this; it seemed to give them hope. Additionally I tried to reassure patients that their life crisis could have any number of resolutions, with or without children; being open to new endings to their reproductive story was key to working through the grief.

I have been fascinated about the assumptions my clients have made about me over the years: some thought that I had gone through IVF, others concluded that I had adopted, others said, "Oh you are one and done!" as if that was by choice. Interestingly, their conjectures often ran parallel to their own decisions, almost as if they were projecting their choices onto me (if I did it, it must be okay). While I was (and am) willing to answer the "do you have kids question" I try to maintain my neutrality; I do not want to influence clients one way or another, nor do I want to presume to know how they feel. While this is a good rule of thumb, it is also valuable to be a realistic sounding board as clients rethink their story. The following case, a woman who I call Kathy, illustrates a valuable lesson learned: the use of self-disclosure to assist in working toward treatment goals [23].

Kathy: taking a risk with disclosure

Kathy began once-a-week individual psychotherapy to cope with infertility and its impact on her relationship, and to sort through decisions about her life. Her lifelong dream had been to become a mother; infertility caused her self-esteem to plummet. This came out in multiple ways: she had difficulty making decisions, would acquiesce to the needs of others, and even felt insecure calling people on the phone. It was often difficult for her to get started in our sessions; she felt awkward and clumsy talking about herself. Her transference feelings toward me were positive. I was aware of her deference to me and was concerned that she was in constant need of my approval.

She had been getting a great deal of pressure from friends and family to seek out alternate ways to have children. Part of our work together was to process the plusses and minuses of third party reproduction, as well as adoption. Over the course of several months, we explored her wavering feelings, especially regarding adoption. Part of me was secretly hoping she would embrace it; I wanted to see her fulfill her dreams, and I was feeling as stuck as she was. I did not, however, want her to make any decision in order to please me, and so I was acutely aware of not offering an opinion and maintaining my neutrality. She vacillated back and forth; she clearly was tormented by social pressure, with the belief that if she truly were a "good" person she would open herself up to adoption.

In one of our sessions, after she had gotten another dose of, "Why don't you just adopt?" from a close relative, it occurred to me that she assumed I felt the same way. Her distorted belief that I thought negatively of her because she did not want to adopt was: (1) not at all what I was feeling, and (2) keeping her from choosing her own path. My intuition propelled me to take a risk. I said, "You know, adoption isn't for everyone. It wasn't for me." This disclosure turned out to be a turning point in her therapy. Her relief was palpable: Here was someone whom she respected (clearly I was not a "bad" person in her mind), giving her permission not to adopt. Although it felt risky to share something that I had struggled with as well, I believe it was my ability to truly feel her anxiety that allowed me to call upon my own.

Soon after that, Kathy began talking about the positives of a child-free life. She was able to be more forthright with her husband, began taking writing classes (something she had always wanted to do), started a small business, and put more energy into her nieces and nephews. The result of loosening my boundaries gave her the authority to let go of societal pressures and turn the page to a new chapter in her life.

What is countertransference? It's not just Freudian any more

Akin to therapist self-disclosure is the concept of countertransference. Our personal history, intrapsychic struggles and interpersonal relationships make us who we are. Even the most neutral clinician brings his or her personality and life experiences into the therapy arena, which when used correctly can have a positive impact on the patient.

When Freud first described countertransference – therapists' unconscious, defensive response to their clients – it was not thought of as something beneficial to the therapy, but rather something to be avoided [39]. As psychological theory has evolved, however, so has the understanding of countertransference. It has now been defined as the "internal and overt reactions to clients that are rooted in therapists' unresolved intrapsychic conflicts" [25, p. 173]. It is not merely the definition that has broadened, but countertransference is seen now as a valuable self-reflective tool that therapists can use to gain insight into the therapy. While many believe that countertransference is strictly a Freudian concept, others view it as a universal phenomenon, regardless of theoretical orientation.

As noted by Hayes, Yeh and Eisenberg, humanistic, existential, feminist and cognitive-behavioral theorists all have emphasized the importance of the therapist's personal history and mental health on the quality of therapy [40].

How does countertransference apply to the fertility counselor? If a client's struggle with infertility or pregnancy loss triggers unresolved personal conflicts in the therapist, it may adversely affect interactions with the client. Research suggests that therapists may become anxious, have distorted perceptions of clients and exhibit avoidance behavior when unresolved issues have been aggravated [41]. If a client is coping with reproductive issues that provoke a reaction in the counselor, it is important for the counselor to examine his/her personal issues. Not only can this introspection lead to greater understanding of one's own wounds, but also it can help to better understand the patient.

An interesting study on countertransference in bereavement therapy found that the more the therapist missed a deceased loved one, the less empathy clients perceived their therapist to have. The researchers speculated that if therapists had unresolved grief, their focus would be on themselves and they would have fewer emotional resources available to empathize with their patients. Conversely, if the grief had been sufficiently worked through, therapists would have more capacity to empathize, especially with a client's loss. Using their own losses as a guide, therapists who had resolved their grief were able to "reflect on their own experiences to inform treatment decisions, make judicious self-disclosures, and offer genuine hope born of their own pain" [40, p. 347].

In another study, subjects rated therapists by watching one of two videos in which the therapist either disclosed relatively resolved or relatively unresolved personal issues. Results indicated that when therapist's issues were resolved, they were found to be more attractive, trustworthy and instilled more hope [42]. Applying these results to fertility counseling, *the therapist's own reproductive history can either impede or facilitate the client's therapy.* As previously discussed, if the therapist's issues have not been adequately resolved, disclosure may be more for the therapist than the client [14,33]; likewise, where the therapist is in his/her own reproductive story will have an impact on countertransference reactions and affect his/her ability to be able to remain objective.

The following case illustrates how countertransference initially interfered with the therapy; it then describes how awareness of these feelings was used to gain a better understanding of the client and help her through her grief and loss.

Melissa: Countertransference in action

When Melissa, 41 years old, began weekly psychotherapy with me, she was distraught over secondary infertility. She had struggled with primary infertility as well, and through IUI had a daughter, age 4. All her attention, however, was on the son she hoped to have one day. She spent endless hours on internet forums obsessed with increasing her chances of having a boy; she went so far as stockpiling little boy outfits and toys that she found on sale. As Melissa had been trying for a second child for a couple of years to no avail, she met with her reproductive endocrinologist; her goal was to do IVF and test for gender selection. Unfortunately, her IVF cycle failed, leaving her devastated and hopeless.

Melissa was challenging to work with in therapy. She arrived late to nearly every session by at least 15 minutes. Her tardiness extended to other situations as well; she had been reprimanded at work, not only for being late, but also for surfing the web. Invariably her searches were pregnancy related. When confronted about her ongoing late arrivals to our sessions, she became defensive: because this was "her time" she felt at liberty to do with it whatever she wished.

Melissa brought up a multitude of feelings in me. Her lateness was irksome as was her sense of entitlement. I understood her behavior as a way of acting out feelings of depression and anger. I also saw it as a way to defensively avoid the reality of her situation, that is, she would most likely not be able to conceive a son and have her dream come true. If I represented realism and common sense, she was doing her best to evade it, and that included dodging me.

It is very likely that Melissa's behavior would evoke irritation in most counselors; it felt like we were in an ongoing standoff with little to no progress being made. If I confronted her, she became defensive; if I empathized with her disappointment, she sobbed uncontrollably, which also had the effect of keeping me at a distance. I began to realize that my frustration with Melissa went deeper; I was forced to address my negative countertransference towards her. I realized that we had several things in common: although my son was considerably older than her daughter (the fact that I had a son was never discussed in therapy), we both had one child after primary infertility, we both wanted another child, and we both were "older" mothers who grappled with secondary infertility. This internal understanding helped me identify my anger: she tugged at my own loss. While I had long since resolved pursuing another pregnancy, this was still a "sore-spot" in my personal history that got called to light because of Melissa's issues.

It should be noted that I did not disclose any of my self-revelations to Melissa. However, by reflecting on my own experience, I felt that I understood her better and could use it to better serve her. As my anger abated, so did her defensiveness. It was at this point in the treatment that she began to process her grief. Interestingly, she became more connected with her daughter and gained insight into her relationship with her own frustrating and distancing mother. We were able to dig deeper into what it meant to have a son (in her view, boys could not disappoint a mother the way she felt she had let down her own; boys were powerful and could compensate for her own sense of weakness). Although she continued to come late to her therapy appointments (it became a running joke between us), she had a much better understanding of her issues with her own mother and was determined to parent her daughter differently.

This case made me appreciate the importance of reflecting on my own defensive countertransference reactions. Although my losses felt resolved to me, this case brought to the forefront that reproductive losses change us in profound ways. As noted previously, when therapists' internal conflicts are triggered, they may react to their clients with anxious, angry, avoidant behaviors [41]. How fertility counselors manage their countertransference reactions may be central to building and maintaining a good therapeutic alliance, thereby affecting clinical outcome. If countertransference acting out is harmful to the working alliance, it stands to reason that managing one's countertransference constructively promotes positive therapeutic effects. Fertility counselors can use self-insight and mindfulness, through personal therapy or supervision, to promote their own psychological health and, in turn, allow themselves to understand how their clients' issues personally affect them [39].

Fertility counselors and self-care

Working in the field of reproductive psychology can be incredibly satisfying and meaningful. We help people in crisis move through the process of grieving; we help them go from the depths of despair to feeling positive about themselves and about their life, whether they are successful at having children or not. But working with this population is not without risk to the fertility counselor as we are confronted with trauma and loss, sadness and anguish, on a daily basis. This section focuses on the need for self-care; the concepts of vicarious trauma and compassion fatigue are explored, as are ways to prevent these from interfering with our work and our lives.

A trauma, by definition, is exposure to an "actual or threatened death, serious injury, or sexual violence" that one witnesses or experiences, or learns has occurred to a close family member or friend [43, p. 271]. Trauma, whether physical or psychological, overwhelms people's ability to cope, and unlike other traumas that are one-time incidents, it is the chronic nature of infertility and other reproductive events that overpowers clients' coping resources [2]. Traumatized people often try to avoid triggers of the traumatic experience [43], but it is virtually impossible for reproductive clients to do so. They may try to steer clear of pregnant women and baby showers, but the inescapable reminder of a women's monthly menstrual cycle, as well as the trauma from repeated intrusive treatments which must be endured (and repeated) in order to conceive, is a painful and unavoidable trigger of yet another loss.

By the nature of our work with clients struggling with infertility, miscarriage, or other perinatal demise, we are exposed to a great deal of trauma and loss. These stories are difficult to hear; fertility counselors repeatedly listen to accounts of sadness, defeat and death in our practices. When these stories include unsuccessful cycles or failed pregnancies, the pain can be overwhelming not just for our clients, but for us as well, especially poignant if we have experienced some aspect of the trauma ourselves. The need for therapist self-care is important no matter what issues clients bring to therapy, but for fertility counselors, awareness of countertransference, vicarious trauma and compassion fatigue are of particular importance. Understanding the differences among these phenomena is important; although there may be overlap, each requires different forms of self-care. (See Table 17.2.)

Table 17.2 Comparison of compassion fatigue, vicarious trauma and countertransference.

Compassion	Vicarious	Counter-Fatigue Trauma Transference
Based on caring for those who are suffering	Based on developing trauma secondary to client's traumatic experience	Based on interaction between client's world and clinician's unconscious
Cumulative experience of care-giving	Working with victims of trauma	Pervasive to all clients
Feeling generally exhausted, burnt-out	Reaction specific to trauma	May be difficult but not exhausting
Can interfere with clinical work	Can interfere with clinical work	Can be used as a tool to enhance clinical work
Self-care: A need to replenish: yoga, meditation, relaxation, connecting with nature, exercise, creativity, social support, individual or peer supervision	Self-care: In addition to the compassion fatigue self-care, limit number of trauma clients	Self-care: Self-reflection to understand intrapsychic roots of reactions to clients, supervision, psychotherapy

As discussed, countertransference refers to a therapist's unresolved personal issues that are evoked by a client. Rather than serve as a detriment to the treatment, our own inner conflicts can help inform us of the intrapsychic world of our clients. Vicarious trauma, on the other hand, describes a counselor's negative transformation after being exposed to a client's trauma [44,45]. Listening to the details of a client's traumatic experience can affect us deeply; in essence their trauma can "rub off" on us. Hearing the specifics of a premature birth, viewing photographs of a baby who has died, witnessing the anguish of an IVF that has failed – these are all client traumas that have an impact on us. Vicarious trauma is different than countertransference in that vicarious trauma "is a direct reaction to traumatic client material and is not a reaction to past personal life experiences" [45, p. 32]. Vicarious trauma, however, can evoke countertransference issues: when the traumatic experiences are shared or similar, for example, if the therapist has had his/her own reproductive losses, the therapist is even more vulnerable.

Compassion fatigue occurs when a therapist is overexposed to client suffering and becomes exhausted by the cumulative effects of this exposure. This can happen to any counselor (as well as any medical caregiver) at any time; essentially, it is defined as a therapist who becomes tired of caring. When counselors experience compassion fatigue, they may feel worn out, depleted and drained, may become impatient and irritable, may feel depressed, and may be less available to process their clients' issues [46]. Although this can occur with all kinds of therapeutic issues, the concerns that reproductive clients raise, with multiple losses, medical traumas and psychological pain, can feel particularly emotionally draining.

While countertransference is a part of every clinical encounter and can be used constructively in our work, vicarious trauma and compassion fatigue have a negative impact. Saakvitne suggests that we ask ourselves, "How am I doing?" on a regular basis [44]. Making an assessment of our own well-being is imperative if we are to be present and available to our clients. Essential for every fertility counselor is to find a balance among work, play and rest. Finding time for enjoyable activities outside of work (physical activity, meditation, vacations, spiritual and/or creative endeavors) is key. Making time to socialize with friends and family can re-energize and re-invigorate one's sense of self. Being able to talk with colleagues, as in a peer supervision group, helps to eliminate isolation and can validate the demands of working with this population. It is also helpful to find a balance within the workday itself. This may mean not scheduling back-to-back clients who are emotionally draining, building in breaks, and as obvious as this may seem, making sure to eat and hydrate. In order to be present for our clients, fertility counselors must figuratively put their oxygen mask on first in order to help others. Additionally, it is important to know when to refer a client to another clinician. If the client's issues are too close to one's own, or if the clinician is in the midst of a life-crisis, it may better serve the client to see another therapist.

Summary and reflection

While working with infertility and reproductive loss clients can be meaningful and rewarding, it is not for the faint of heart. There are times when fertility counselors are left with their own feelings of helplessness and sadness as they bear witness to the upsetting details of clients' lives. These feelings may be intensified if the therapist has had his/her own difficulties in having children. Regardless of the counselor's personal reproductive story, the events of one's life have an impact on interactions with clients. Whether the clinician chooses to disclose or not, drawing on one's internal narrative and emotions will bring increased understanding and depth to the therapy. Just as important as it is to attend to the client's needs, it is equally important to attend to our own. Seeking consultation, especially if a case touches on the therapist's own losses, is highly recommended.

Writing this chapter has enabled me to reflect on my own life experiences, my own reproductive story and my clinical work; as such, I have learned a great deal. My hope is that reading this will do the same for you.

References

1. Nouwen H. *The Wounded Healer*. Garden City, NY: Image. 1972.
2. Jaffe J, Diamond MO. *Reproductive Trauma: Psychotherapy with Infertility and Pregnancy Loss Clients*. Washington, DC: American Psychological Association. 2011.
3. Leibowitz L. Reflections of a childless analyst. In: Gerson B, ed. *The Therapist as a Person: Life Crises, Life Choices, Life Experiences, and Their Effects on Treatment*. New York: Routledge. 2009; 71–87 (Original work published 1996).
4. Hill CE, Knox S. Self-disclosure. *Psychotherapy* 2001; 38: 413–17.
5. Hill CE, Knox S. Self-disclosure. In: Norcross JC, ed. *Psychotherapy Relationships That Work: Therapist Contributions and Responsiveness to Patients*. New York: Oxford University Press. 2002; 255–65.
6. Henretty JR, Levitt HM. The role of therapist self-disclosure in psychotherapy: A qualitative review. *Clin Psychol Rev* 2010; 30: 63–77.
7. Hill CE, Knox S. Processing the therapeutic relationship. *Psychol Res* 2009; 19: 13–29.
8. Gutheil TG. Ethical aspects of self-disclosure in psychotherapy: Knowing what to disclose and what not to disclose. *Psychiatr Times* 2010; 27: 39–41.
9. Peterson ZD. More than a mirror: The ethics of therapist self-disclosure. *Psychother* 2002; 39: 21–31.
10. Ulman KH. Unwitting exposure of the therapist: Transferential and countertransferential dilemmas. *J Psychother Pract Res* 2001; 10: 14–22.
11. Gutheil TG, Brodsky A. *Preventing Boundary Violations in Clinical Practice*. New York: Guilford Press, 2008.
12. Stricker G. The many faces of self-disclosure. *J Clin Psychol* 2003; 59: 623–30.
13. Zur O. Therapist self-disclosure. In: Bloomgarden A, Mennuti RB, eds. *Psychotherapist Revealed*. New York: Routledge. 2009; 31–51.
14. Knox S, Hill CE. Therapist self-disclosure: Research-based suggestions for practitioners. *JCLP* 2003; 59: 529–39.
15. Freud S. Recommendations to physicians practicing psycho-analysis. In: *The Standard Edition of the Psychological Works of Sigmund Freud*. London: Hogarth Press. 2000; 1–120 (Original work published 1912).
16. Gelso CJ. *The Real Relationship in Psychotherapy*. Washington, DC: American Psychological Association. 2011.
17. Bloomgarden A, Mennuti RB. Therapist self-disclosure: Beyond the taboo. In: Bloomgarden A, Mennuti RB, eds. *Psychotherapist Revealed*. New York: Routledge. 2009; 3–15.
18. Gerson B. An analyst's pregnancy loss and its effects on treatment. In: Gerson B, ed. *The Therapist as a Person: Life Crises, Life Choices, Life Experiences, and Their Effects on Treatment*. New York: Routledge. 2009; 55–69 (Original work published 1996).
19. Barrett MS, Berman JS. Is psychotherapy more effective when therapists disclose information about themselves? *J Consult Clin Psych* 2001; 69: 597–603.
20. Patton J. Engendering a new paradigm: Self-disclosure with queer clients. In: Bloomgarden A, Mennuti RB, eds. *Psychotherapist Revealed*. New York: Routledge. 2009; 181–92.
21. Filetti L, Mattei S. To share or not to share: Self-disclosure in the treatment of borderline personality disorder. In: Bloomgarden A, Mennuti RB, eds. *Psychotherapist Revealed*. New York: Routledge. 2009; 71–83.
22. American Psychological Association. Ethical principles of psychologists and code of conduct. *APA*; 57: 1060–73. Retrieved from http://www.apa.org/ethics/code2002.html. Accessed October 2014.
23. Barnett JE. Psychotherapist self-disclosure: Ethical and clinical considerations. *Psychother* 2011; 48: 315–21.
24. Hanson J. Should your lips be sealed? How therapist self-disclosure and non-disclosure affects clients. *Couns Psychother Res* 2005; 5: 96–104.
25. Myers D, Hayes JA. Effects of therapist general self-disclosure and countertransference disclosure on

ratings of the therapist and session. *Psychother: Theory, Res, Pract, Train* 2006; 43: 173–85.

26. Barnett M. What brings you here? An exploration of the unconscious motivations of those who choose to train and work as psychotherapists and counselors. *Psychodynamic Practice* 2007; 13: 257–74.
27. Weingarten K. Intersecting losses: Working with the inevitable vicissitudes in therapist and client lives. *Psychother: Theory, Res, Pract, Train* 2010; 47: 371–84.
28. Jackson SW. The wounded healer. *B Hist Med* 2001; 75: 1–36.
29. Bloomgarden A, Mennuti RB. Lessons learned from adolescent girls. In: Bloomgarden A, Mennuti RB, eds. *Psychotherapist Revealed.* New York: Routledge. 2009; 101–14.
30. Covington SN, Marosek KR. Personal infertility experience among nurses working in reproductive medicine and mental health professionals. *Fertil Steril* 1999; 72:S129.
31. Marrero SJ. *The role of the psychologist in reproductive medicine. Unpublished doctoral dissertation.* Rutgers University, New Jersey. 2013.
32. Zerubavel N, Wright MO. The dilemma of the wounded healer. *Psychother* 2012; 49: 482–91.
33. Gelso CJ, Hayes JA. *Countertransference and the Therapist's Inner Experience: Perils and Possibilities.* Mahwah, NJ: Erlbaum. 2007.
34. Lazar S. Patients' responses to pregnancy and miscarriage in the analyst. In: Schwartz HJ, Silver AL, eds. *Illness in the Analyst.* Madison, CT: International Universities Press. 1990; 199–226.
35. Comstock DL. Confronting life's adversities: Self-disclosure in print and in session. In: Bloomgarden A, Mennuti RB, eds. *Psychotherapist Revealed.* New York: Routledge. 2009; 257–73.
36. Patterson JE. A birth gone awry. In: McDaniel SH, Hepworth J, Doherty WJ, eds. *The Shared Experience of Illness.* New York: Basic Books. 2003; 23–9.
37. Mendelsohn EM. More human than otherwise: working through a time of preoccupation and mourning. In: Gerson B, ed. *The Therapist as a Person: Life Crises, Life Choices, Life Experiences, and Their Effects on Treatment.* New York: Routledge. 2009; 21–40 (Original work published 1996).
38. Chasen B. Death of a psychoanalyst's child. In: Gerson B, ed. *The Therapist as a Person: Life Crises, Life Choices, Life Experiences, and Their Effects on Treatment.* New York: Routledge. 2009; 3–20 (Original work published 1996).
39. Hayes JA, Gelso CJ, Hummel AM. Managing countertransference. *Psychotherapy* 2011; 48: 88–97.
40. Hayes JA, Yeh Y, Eisenberg A. Good grief and not-so-good grief: countertransference in bereavement therapy. *J Clin Psychol* 2007; 63: 345–55.
41. Rosenberger EW, Hayes JA. Therapist as subject: A review of the empirical countertransference literature. *J Couns Dev* 2002; 80: 264–70.
42. Yeh YJ, Hayes JA. How does disclosing countertransference affect perceptions of the therapist and the session? *Psychother* 2011; 48: 322–29.
43. American Psychiatric Association: *Diagnostic and Statistical Manual of Mental Disorders, Fifth Edition.* Arlington, VA: American Psychiatric Association. 2013.
44. Saakvitne KW. Shared trauma: The therapist's increased vulnerability. *Psychoanal Dialogues* 2002; 12: 443–49.
45. Trippany RL, Kress VEW, Wilcoxon SA. Preventing vicarious trauma: What counselors should know when working with trauma survivors. *J Couns Dev* 2004; 82: 31–7.
46. Berzoff J, Kita E. Compassion fatigue and countertransference: Two different concepts. *Clin Soc Work J* 2010; 38: 341–49.

Chapter 18

Disclosure

Helping families talk about assisted reproduction

Jean M. Benward

George and Lilly Thomas were seen for a counseling session before their scheduled treatment with donor sperm. Mrs. Thomas had always felt they should disclose the donor conception but because her husband was uncomfortable with disclosure, she had deferred to him in this decision. After a more detailed discussion with the fertility counselor about his concerns, Mr. Thomas concluded that he understood his wife's reasons for wanting to disclose but he thought it best to wait until the child was "old enough to understand," perhaps at age 16 or older.

Introduction

The use of donor gametes in the medical treatment of infertility has a long history, beginning with the first recorded case of sperm donation in 1898. Historically advised to keep the sperm donation a secret, parents were isolated from social support and the opportunity to talk with others about the impact of using gamete donation to build a family. Professionals and parents alike believed donor insemination would become unimportant as the children grew up in what appeared to be conventional families. In the last 25 years, social science research, personal accounts by the adult donor-conceived and parents, openness associated with the expanded use of oocyte donation, along with professional discourse have led to the understanding that gamete donation is highly complex with long-term psychosocial implications for the donor-conceived family.

The addenda referred to in this chapter are available for download at www.cambridge.org/9781107643116. Password: AX164BKR7.

In recent years, we have seen a change in legal policy and clinical practice with increased openness in the United States (US) and throughout the developed world. A more open approach has occurred on two fronts: professional recommendations in support of disclosure of donor conception and the legislated removal of donor anonymity. The first country to remove donor anonymity was Sweden in 1985. Over the next 20 years, more countries enacted legislation allowing the donor-conceived access to the donor's identity, including Switzerland (1992), Austria (2002), Norway (2003), New Zealand (2004) the Netherlands (2004), the UK (2005), Finland (2007) and several states in Australia [1]. The United Kingdom's Human Embryology and Fertility Authority (HFEA), the British Infertility Counselling Association, the Swedish National Health and Medical Research Council, and the Australian National Health and Medical Research Council have explicitly recommended that disclosure is in the best interests of the donor-conceived. While donor anonymity is still the norm in the USA, there has been an increase in the number of sperm banks and egg donor agencies offering open-identity donors.

While debate continues about the relative importance of disclosure, the two largest assisted reproductive technology (ART) professional bodies, the European Society of Human Reproduction and Embryology (ESHRE) and the American Society for Reproductive Medicine (ASRM), agree that counseling is an essential component of parent preparation prior to donor procedures. Likewise, several key associations of fertility counselors in the USA, UK, Canada, Australia, New Zealand, and Germany recommend counseling about disclosure [2]. In 2004, The ASRM Ethics Committee issued a document,

Fertility Counseling: Clinical Guide and Case Studies, ed. Sharon N. Covington. Published by Cambridge University Press.

stating, "*while ultimately the choice of recipient parents, disclosure to donor conceived persons of the use of donor gametes in their conception is encouraged*" [3]. This statement reflects an emerging consensus among American professionals that openness in gamete donation is an important value and consideration, especially for the donor-conceived.

In this changing legal, social and professional context, research suggests that an increasing number of parents plan to disclose donor conception to their children and will seek counseling help with their decision [4]. In light of the increased need for counseling, this chapter will explore parents' concerns about disclosure, counselor preparation of parents for disclosure, and recommendations for helping parents create the family disclosure story. In addition, the chapter will explore how children and young adults understand the role of the donor, the ongoing process of disclosure and its long-term implications. (Table 18.1 summarizes recommended practices in disclosure counseling.) The chapter will conclude with an examination of several complex cases of disclosure.

Table 18.1 Recommended practices in counseling parents about disclosure.

- **Importance of Parent Preparation.** 1) Disclosure is anxiety producing 2) Parents need support and help creating a "telling story."
- **Components of Preparation.** 1) Family is based on relationships not genetics 2) Education about appropriate language 3) Education about bonding in donor-conceived families.
- **Exploring the Meaning of the Donor.** 1) Children's curiosity about the donor is normal 2) Importance of preserving donor information 3) Interest in the donor does not represent looking for the "real parent."
- **Basic Components of Telling the Story.** 1) Parents couldn't have child on their own 2) They needed help from a doctor and/or a donor 3) This is the story of how we became a family.
- **Refer Parents to Children's Books, Parent Resource Books and Material, and Support groups.** See Addendum 19.1
- **Advantages of Early Telling.** 1) Associated with better outcomes 2) Is not about "getting the facts right" 3) Is known from the beginning.
- **Telling in the School Age Years** 1) Developmental changes observed between ages 7 and 10 can prompt disclosure 2) Children's reactions vary 3) Research indicates children may not discuss their thoughts with parents, unless parents pro-actively seek opportunities.
- **Parents who Wait "Until They Are Old Enough to Understand" are at Risk to Postpone Disclosure If They Do Not Receive Support.** 1) They don't think of disclosure as a process 2) They associate "understanding" with the facts of reproduction.
- **Disclosure Involves Sharing Information about the Donor.** 1) During childhood children endeavor to understand the meaning of having a donor and the connection between their donor conception and genetics (what they get from the donor) 2) Information about the donor can be important in identity formation.
- **Concerns about Gamete Donation Can Re-surface Throughout the Donor-conceived and the Family's Life Cycle.**

Parent preparation

Parents choose to disclose for a number of reasons, including prevention of inadvertent disclosure, personal beliefs about openness and honesty, key events in their personal history, and the belief their children have the right to know about their genetic heritage. Parents interested in disclosure seek information about "telling scripts," the best age for disclosure and available resources. Helping parents discuss donor conception with their children requires preparation prior to the actual "story telling." Information sharing, both the decision and process, is a significantly emotional experience in which parents feel a variety of uncertainties and anxieties. The fertility counselor can play an instrumental role in helping parents' explore their fears, decrease their anxieties, articulate a plan and increase their confidence in disclosure.

Before discussing the "when and how" of disclosure, the counselor first needs to explore what disclosure means to the parents; how they see themselves as parents in light of donor gamete use; how they expect others, including their child, to react; and what they expect the outcome of disclosure will be [5]. Counseling parents about disclosure occurs within a cultural context where parenthood and family are defined by biogenetic relationships. This "blood tie" is seen in the larger culture, and often among the parents themselves, as a powerful and exclusive connection, in which there is room for only one "real parent." Thus, cultural beliefs can create a primary fear in the non-genetic parent that they will not be a "real parent," and ultimately that they will be rejected by their child.

The first critical counseling intervention is to help the parents explore and reframe the meaning of family. If "real families" and "real parents" are created by genetic relationships, then our job is to help disclosing families create a new family narrative. It is important then to think about the language they will use. The language used in all family narratives plays a significant role in defining relationships. Hence, we have a father, stepfather, mother, mother-in-law and so forth, each describing a unique relationship. Parents want to tell their child about donor conception without conveying that the non-genetic parent is not the "real father" or "real mother." It is therefore important in the disclosure narratives that the person who provided the gametes be referred to as the donor, and not the other *parent,* the real parent, another Daddy, or the "Donor Dad or Donor Mom." Other approaches can be problematic for children. One mother in her first telling of the story talked to her child about having "two daddies". Realizing this had been distressing and confusing to her child, she used the word "donor" in her subsequent conversations [6, p. 1395]. Beyond the importance of language, the other key piece of the disclosure story is defining family as based on loving relationships, and parental intent, not genetics. Accordingly, the husband in a couple using DI becomes a father because he plays an active role in bringing his child into the world and committing himself to parenthood.

The second counseling intervention is to educate parents about the nature of bonding, family development and findings from current research. Some parents fear that using a donor will generate distance in their relationship with their child. Bonding is a complex two-way process that begins in utero with both mothers and fathers primed hormonally before birth to attach to infants. Because bonding, attachment and comfort with a new infant take time, some parents may fear that because they do not "instantly love" the infant, they are poor parents or that the "disconnect" derives from the lack of genetic connection. Despite these fears, research has consistently revealed long-lasting bonds in donor-conceived families, and that over time, parents are less worried about their relationship with their child, feel greater confidence in their parental roles and place less significance on the genetic difference [7,8]. Further, parents view their choice of donor conception as a positive one, the quality of parenting among those who have used donor gametes is as good as, if not higher, than those in natural conception families and the children in donor-conceived families thrive [9].

The third intervention is to explore the psychological meaning of the donor for the family. The fertility counselor will prepare parents to understand that as children grow they may ask questions about the donor. Parents often fear their child's interest in the donor, believing that the curiosity represents a failure on their part or the child's rejection. It is important to emphasize that the child's curiosity about the donor suggests just the opposite. In fact, the questions are an indication of attachment, security and trust in the relationship with the parents, all of which allow them to raise the questions in the first place. While patients may not be interested in saving donor information in the pre-treatment phase, they or their children might find the information important in the future. Accordingly, fertility counselors should advise parents to save all the donor information they have, especially pictures, for a time when their child may want to know more about the donor.

Beginning the story

Starting with young children

Parents who plan to disclose have varying views about when to do this, including from "when it's the right time," when they believe their children can "understand," or from an early age, before the school years. Some view disclosure to a young child as meaningless, since children in this stage of cognitive development do not understand the cultural or biological meaning of genetic heritage, or how reproduction occurs. However, the emphasis on the importance of cognitive understanding, offered as support for later disclosure, overlooks the significance of the affective and relational components of the story for both the child and the parents.

Fundamental to any family's identity are stories of conception, birth, family history and stories of "how our family came to be." It is through stories that family members understand themselves and their place in the family [7]. Thus, many parents in donor-conceived families begin sharing their family story when their children are between 2 and 5 years old and find that early telling has several advantages. First, the parents establish the foundation for ongoing discussion of their family's creation, by introducing a vocabulary, and providing a reference point that the child and parent can return to as the child's development continues [6]. Early telling allows parents to practice their "telling" skills and, for some, get over the first emotional hurdle, leaving them freer to engage in future conversations. The donor-conceived family story, like other family stories, becomes a normal part of life, one that the children have always known.

Effective "telling stories" used by parents share several features, which are noted in Table 18.2. Woven

Table 18.2 Components of the telling story.

Effective "telling stories" used by parents share several features. The most common components of the story include:

1. the parents' inability to have a child on their own;
2. the need for help, from a donor and/or from a doctor;
3. the specialness of their child;
4. the parents' joy when their child was born; and
5. this is how we became a family.

together, the parent's explanation may sound like this: [6,10].

"Mommy and Daddy wanted a baby for a long time. We found out we could not make one on our own. We went to a special doctor who helped us."

"Babies are made from an egg from a Mommy and seed/cell/sperm from a Daddy. Mommy's eggs couldn't make a baby. We got help from this nice lady who gave us some of her eggs." Or, *"A kind man gave some of his sperm to help men like Daddy. This kind lady/man is called a donor."*

"The eggs and the sperm grew together inside Mommy, and now we have you, which made us the happiest parents in the world. This is how our special baby was born."

Parents' stories can differ in the language used to describe the building blocks of reproduction. Sperm are referred to as "sperm", "seeds", "tadpoles" or a "special ingredient". Oocytes are most often referred to as "eggs" or sometimes "a special cell." A baby grows in "a nest," a "baby sac," "mommy's tummy" or "a uterus". Analyzing the themes of parents' disclosure stories, researchers have concluded that the stories serve several functions including normalizing donor conception, decreasing stigma, differentiating the donor from the parents, reinforcing the role of the parents, separating genetics from relationships in families and introducing a vocabulary [7,11].

There are many children's books depicting different kinds of families, written to assist parents in sharing their family's story. (See Addendum 18.1.) The books range from those for preschool age children with appealing colorful illustrations, to books for older children that can be read together or separately by the child. Parents often view children's books as helpful tools, because the narrative is ready made, the stories can be easily shared and the narratives can encourage children to talk about their own story. Some parents make their own books for their children in which they add more detail to their story such as pictures of an embryo, sonogram images, history about the parents "falling in love," photos of the pregnant parents and description of the parents' feelings. However the story is shared with a young child, it becomes an anchor and a source of pleasure for parent and child. Many parents also read books about "different kinds of families," in which the overarching message is "a family is people caring about each other." Ideally, parents will leave these books where the child has easy access, allowing the child autonomy when s/he wants to read or look at the book.

And how do young children respond to the early stories and books? In general, young children will react with curiosity and ongoing interest in the story, *"Tell me the story again about how I was born."* If parents do not bring up the topic or read books to their children, the children are more likely to seem disinterested. Although Mr. Thomas thought disclosure was about getting the facts right, it is more importantly about an evolving shared family experience. The best-assembled script will not lead to "getting the facts right" when the child is young. In the end, as s/he hears the family narrative, the child will first experience the closeness of the relationship with his/her parents and secondly process the facts according to his/her stage of development. This anecdote below, shared by a parent, illustrates how facts can become interwoven with both the child's developmental (oedipal) stage and her attachment to and identification with her mother.

"I have shared our story with my 3-year-old daughter as a bedtime story … we were reading and she began to tell me that when she grew up, she would find a nice lady to give her some eggs, and that they would be mixed with daddy's sperm, and then would be put in her belly to grow into a baby. She said that she wanted to have babies the same way that I had her."

Parents report different reactions after their first conversations with their children. Some report they wished they had been able to talk to other parents first, some parents feel uncomfortable, others report that telling brought up emotional issues such as memories of their own infertility [6]. In light of these reports, fertility counselors are encouraged to direct patients to written accounts of other parents, and to refer them to online and face-to-face support groups where they can interact or just listen to other parents. (Refer to Addendum 18.1.) Despite the range of initial feelings, few parents express regret. Most report feeling good about sharing the information, reporting no negative effect on their child or the relationship with the child [6,12]. Some research found more positive parent–child relationships within disclosing families and that disclosing couples view themselves as more competent than their non-disclosing counterparts [13].

The school age years

Some parents choose to wait until latency age, when their children are between ages 7 and 11, to bring up their children's donor conception. Beginning around age 7, children make significant advances in their cognitive and emotional capacities including an increased ability to connect old and new information and greater curiosity about the world around them. This noticeable change in their child's developmental abilities can trigger parents to begin disclosure. As one parent noted, "And I look at [him] now, and I think he is a person in his own right. He has rational thought, and all of those things, and he has an absolute right to know" [14, p. 424]. Prior research has characterized some parents as "right timers" who believe there is a "right time" to tell and feel they will be able to identify when this is [6,7,11,14]. Parents who prefer the "right time" approach often anticipate disclosing when their children are between ages 10 and 12. Research has indicated that some "right timers" end up disclosing when their children are between the ages of 6 and 7 years [11,15]. Other "right time" parents perceive the disclosure story as one shared when the children "are old enough to understand." If these parents don't receive assistance, they are at risk to postpone telling because they have no active plan, need help working out an age appropriate telling script, and perceive the telling as something more like an announcement than an ongoing process [6,7,14].

Disclosure during the school years typically means that the parents will tell the story in one piece, not gradually. The reactions of children in this age group can vary tremendously, but parents often report a first response of disinterest. Importantly, there is no one "correct way" that children respond to disclosure in this age group and the same child can show changing levels of interest over time. Both research and parents' reports suggest that children may be thinking about their donor conception but not discussing it with their parents. In Vanfraussen's 2001 study, nearly half of the 41 children were interested in having more information about the donor, but only one-third of those reported discussing this with their parents [16]. Similarly, Blake et al. found that by age 10, most of the donor-conceived children did not talk to their family about the subject, perhaps reflecting their parents discomfort in discussing it [17]. It is important that counselors recommend parents find opportunities periodically to raise the subject, update the story and explore any questions.

The ongoing story

Interest in the donor

Disclosure is a multilayered process. First, parents must decide when and how to share with children the basic information about their donor conception; and second, determine when and how they will share information about the donor. In early conversations, with young children, parents tend to depict the donor as a generic "nice person" who contributed "missing parts" and downplay any significance attached to the donor as a person. However, as young children make sense of their social world, creating a mental image of their social network and placing people in it, they will think about where to "put" the donor and how to integrate the donor into their understanding of their family story.

One mother's story describes how her 5-year-old son drew a picture of his family and included the donor: "Adam was ... making a Mother's Day Card. He had drawn people on the front, inside and on the back of the card. Inside he drew a picture of himself, his mother, his father and two sisters. I asked who the man on the front is: 'He's the guy who gave you sperm'" [18, p. 173].

The process of understanding the meaning of the donor to the individual child and the family continues throughout childhood. Young donor-conceived children are often expressive in their thoughts and feelings, sometimes in surprising ways. Many comments affirm the child's positive feelings about donor conception. "I would not have been born without help from the donor"; "I don't care how you made me, as long as you made me" [7, p. 2239]. Some comments reflect distinct feelings about the donor, "I think of him as a friend since he helped us" [18, p. 175], and about the parent's infertility, "Why doesn't Daddy have any sperm?"

[6, p. 1396] or as a father reported, "Did it make daddy feel sad that he didn't have any sperm." Some ask questions about the donor that are insightful or make the parents uncomfortable such as "Does he have a family?" or "Why can't I know his name" [6, p. 1396]. During the school years, the early story may now be understood with a shock, as with the 8-year-old boy who asked, "Is it right what that book says, that I don't come from daddy's seeds? It was somebody else?" [18, p. 142] or as reported by her mother, a girl the same age who asked, "You are still my mom, right?"

In late childhood, the interest in their own story can shift to an interest in the actual person who gave the eggs or sperm. Children typically will ask questions about the donor or ask for more information, such as whether the parents have a picture of the donor, if they can meet the donor, or if the parents have the donor's name. Parents are often ambivalent about their child's interest in the donor, who while grateful to the donor, may prefer not to think about him/her. One mother put it this way, "I had trouble with my daughter's looks at first because it drove home the fact that we had used a donor." While one parent, in response to her child's questions, reported, "I don't think she [child] would be normal if she wasn't curious." Another more reluctant parent reported, "I'm just hoping that [my children] won't have that huge curiosity to go out and try to find the donor" [14].

It is common for children in middle to late childhood, 8–11, to explore how genetics play a part in their story, seeking to connect the donor's genetic contribution to their own traits. Only one children's book for older children addresses this directly, depicting a girl who does not look like her mother, and who is told she gets her red hair from the donor [19]. While they have a greater understanding about conception, children of this age are often still uncertain about how it exactly works. Consider as 9-year-old Lisa tries to puzzle out the connection between genetics, her donor conception, and her relationship with her parents.

> *"...I was born in my mom's uterus, but I was born from another lady's egg. My mom's hair is brown, my dad's hair is black and...mine is blond. The...reason is that the lady that made the egg that I was born from...her hair was blond, like mine. So, I have my dad's 'chubby' cheeks, my mom's curly hair and the lady's blond hair."*

The process of putting together the puzzle of how are they related and to whom, continues as children ponder what it means to have parents and a donor. For some, the answer is straightforward, "No, the donor isn't my parent. A parent is someone who raises you, feeds you and takes care of you" [20, p. 2239]. Lacking a concept that can explain a genetic connection that is not parenthood, children qualify the donor's genetic connection as "not parenthood," in their own idiosyncratic fashion. Parents have shared their children's musings: "I am half adopted"; "Mom, technically speaking, you aren't my mother"; or "Yes, it's almost like [the donor] is our ex-mother."

Resemblance talk and disclosure

> Mr. and Mrs. Thomas, whom we first met in the opening of the chapter, have returned for counseling 12 years later. They now have two school-aged sons, ages 9 and 11, conceived with donor sperm. The parents' decision to postpone disclosure had become increasingly uncomfortable for them. As the children had gotten older, they frequently asked their parents questions about whom they looked like and where they got this trait or that.

The importance of genetic inheritance in families is evident in what anthropologist Becker called "resemblance talk" [21]. Resemblance talk in families is a way of reaffirming relationships by talking about the genetic similarities between children, their parents and grandparents. Children's questions about resemblance and inherited characteristics can be difficult for parents, like the Thomases, because they remind them of the donor's significance and his/her contribution to their children's genetic makeup. As one patient explained, "our son looks just like our egg donor; just knowing her features, her personality.... It gives me a wave of insecurity." Some parents try to manage resemblance talk by avoiding the topic, answering vaguely or "making up" believable resemblances. It is quite likely that the children in the Thomas family, who had repeatedly asked the same questions about similarities, noticed hidden cues from the parents' facial expressions, avoidance of questions, or avoidance of any "resemblance talk" conversation. After counseling the couple through the preparation stage, with information about scripts and expected responses from their children, I recommended that they address their sons' earlier questions by emphasizing, "Genetics contribute some of your features and those genetics came from the donors. You can talk about how the curly hair, blue eyes and dimples come from the donor, but that their love of animals, playing soccer, and camping is just like Daddy, Mommy, Grandma and Grandpa." Parents, like Mr. and Mrs. Thomas, face the task of acknowledging that genetics from the donor contribute important aspects to their children's identities, while at the same time preserving a sense of security for themselves and their children.

This family, like others that have been observed, is one that had not previously disclosed, subsequently regretted the decision, and changed their mind in favor of disclosure [22]. Mr. Thomas reported that the early years were difficult because of the shame he felt about his infertility, the difficulty talking about it compounded by the fear that he would not be able to parent because he did not have a genetic connection to the children. As the children grew, he saw himself in a new light as a good father, close to his children and became increasingly aware of their needs separate from his.

Adolescence

Adolescence is a time of intensified identity development. The donor-conceived adolescent, when asking "Who am I?" wonders not only who he is in a general sense, but also who he is in relation to his genetic origins, an identity task not faced by those raised in their genetic families. Thus, the donor-conceived person's pathway to identity might be more complex, but it is neither inherently pathological nor detrimental to the outcome. Adolescents' interest in their donor conception at this point can range from uninterested and unengaged, to highly interested and invested, even among children in the same family.

In general, identity formation is a life-long developmental process. It is likely then that the donor-conceived adolescent's construction of the meaning of donor conception and its place in their identity will be an ongoing life-long process [23]. Some donor-conceived might think little about it when younger, only to think more about it later in life, for example, when they have their own children. While early disclosure has been widely associated with better outcomes, some have concluded that, despite the benefits, there is no guarantee that early disclosure will mitigate the distress that some donor-conceived offspring feel about the loss of genetic identity [19]. This belief has formed the basis for the legislated removal of donor anonymity in many jurisdictions. Those who achieve a workable identity are likely to be those who learned the truth at an earlier age, whose families have facilitated conversations about donor conception, and who have access to the information about the donor that they wish to have [23].

Complex disclosure situations

Some parents face disclosure decisions that appear especially complex or more daunting for them. What follows is examination of four such clinical cases.

Single mother using embryo donation

Ms. Jenny Bravo is a 41-year-old single woman who, after several failed inter-uterine inseminations (IUI) and in vitro fertilization (IVF) cycles using her eggs and donor sperm, was advised that she was unlikely to become pregnant unless she used donor eggs. Foregoing another IVF cycle, she investigated using donated embryos and chose to work with an embryo donation program that facilitated donor/recipient information sharing. She requested non-identifying information to share with her child, donors who were willing to meet her child at age 18 and introduce any genetic siblings.

While still relatively uncommon compared to egg or sperm donation (i.e., created embryos using both donated gametes), there is evidence of a growing interest among patients in receiving donated embryos (i.e., created during treatment and no longer needed by patients), both in the US and internationally. While forbidden by law in 14 countries, it is permitted by law or performed without legislative framework in approximately 27 [24]. Nonetheless, embryo donation is comparatively uncharted territory for professionals and families. The fact that children born from donated embryos will most likely have full genetic siblings in another family makes the disclosure decision even more complex.

Ms. Bravo wanted to explain embryo donation in a way that her child would not feel abandoned by his "first parents" or "genetic family." I recommended that Ms. Bravo start by telling her child "All babies are made when sperm from a man joins an egg from a woman and this special cell, called an embryo, grows inside a mommy's tummy (uterus/special baby place). Mommy found a kind man and woman who had sperms and eggs they had used to create an embryo. They gave that special cell, the embryo, to Mommy and the doctor put it inside mommy's tummy. That special cell grew into you. These mommies and daddies who help other people have babies are called donors."

There are children's books about embryo donation that allude to the fact that the donors had had their own children before sharing their embryos. For example, "One mommy and daddy...already had babies of their own...so they gave us some of their own embryos" [25, p. 30] or "The...doctor found some very nice people who had an extra [embryo]" [26, p. 12]. There is a recent children's book created for families that have an "open" embryo donation, in which the donors and recipients have contact. This book describes 5-year-old Miles, who gets a gift from his "special friend," Mike. Mike's parents are the donors who gave their embryos to Miles's parents. This book explores the question of whether the two "genetic siblings" are brothers. Mile's parents, the recipients, explain that Mike and Miles "have a special relationship, more like cousins" [27, p. 15].

We discussed Ms. Bravo's concerns about how to explain the absence of a father in their family. Because others would notice that their family had no father present, her child could encounter questions from his/her friends as early as preschool. Typically, these questions, asked more out of curiosity than meanness, would be direct: "Why is there no dad in your family?" "How could you be born without a dad, since everyone has a dad?" I recommended language Ms. Bravo could use to help her child answer friends' questions such as, "We don't have a dad in our family"; "We have a 'mommy and me' family"; or, "We have a donor who helped make me; the dad/male part that made me was from a donor."

Ms. Bravo wanted her child to have the option to meet the donors and genetic siblings when s/he was older, but did not know how to manage this or discuss it with her child. Some families will not bring up the existence of the genetic siblings unless their child asks questions. Some will not use the word sibling because the term, for them, refers to children who grow up in the same family and they do not want to create or impose a sibling relationship where one might not develop. Other parents are proactive and disclose the existence of the donors and their family early, so the topic is out in the open. A few families initiate contact with each other when the children are young, even though the genetic connection might not be revealed to the children at the time.

In discussion, Ms. Bravo concluded that it was feasible for her to have periodic contact with the donors, facilitated anonymously by her agency, to maintain a basic communication link. Having then established a foundation for the initial contact, Ms. Bravo could choose to tell her child that she has information about the donors and contact information when s/he indicates an interest or asks specific questions about making contact. Parents vary in opinion about the appropriate age for their child to meet genetic relatives. Some will wait until their child is 18, believing that their child will be mature enough then to manage contact. Others think that 18 is an arbitrary age, since children can have an interest in their donors well before then and may be ready, in the parents' opinion, to meet the donor or donor siblings. There is no evidence that supports one approach over the other.

For some parents, especially single mothers by choice, these potential donor sibling relationships hold significant meaning [28]. Beyond presenting the chance to learn more about their child's genetic origins, genetic siblings can be seen as opportunities for the formation of extended family bonds, kinship networks and lasting sibling relationships [29]. These possible sibling relationships can be described as close family friends, genetic siblings, donor siblings, or sisters and brothers. Some families might make up expressions such as "diblings" for donor siblings or a "sibling who grew inside another mother."

Ms. Bravo's situation raises three additional points about contact with the donor family. First, because not all donor-conceived are interested in meeting the donor family, any contact with the siblings and the donors should be driven by the expressed needs of the child, and not the parent. Second, positive feelings about contact between recipient and donor families depend on successful matching of expectations and finding a good "fit" between the families. Third, the frequency of contact can vary widely from infrequent to regular and the amount of contact between the adults can differ from the amount between the donor-conceived [28,29].

Research across cultures in the USA, UK and Finland indicates significant differences in embryo donation recipients' beliefs about disclosure, views about openness and the availability of donor information [30,31]. Some parents compare embryo donation more to adoption, in which disclosure and contact occur, while others see it as being more similar to egg and sperm donation and are less likely to disclose. (See Chapter 12 for more information on single parents.)

Disclosure to young adults

> Allen and Joan Smith sought help in telling their 18-year-old twins they had been conceived with donor oocytes. Mrs. Smith explained her feelings about disclosure. "It had become the elephant in the room. It was always there and I was so uncomfortable whenever one of the twins asked questions about how they got this trait or that. I would freeze up whenever I thought of telling them."

Mr. and Mrs. Smith had always thought they would tell their children, Beth and Sam, about their donor conception. After years of postponing it, they now felt at a crossroads, since the twins were leaving for college in a few months. The mother's anxiety about disclosure had intensified over the years and she remained fearful of her children's reactions. Because joint parental disclosure is perceived more positively by the donor-conceived and is associated with better family relationships [35], I suggested that Mr. and Mrs. Smith approach this delayed disclosure together. We then prepared for how they might respond to their children's initial reactions, which could include a mixture of shock, silence, anger, pain and feeling lied to [32]. While initial disclosure conversations with young adults are likely to trigger issues of trust and betrayal, they are unlikely to sever the parent–child relationship. In fact, many donor-conceived young adults feel sympathy for their infertile parent, appreciate their parents' honesty in disclosing, and continue to love the parent [33].

I recommended the parents choose a time when the family would naturally be home together. I advised them to "Talk about your own process, as well as why you waited to tell them." I encouraged them to practice how they would share the information, what they might say to their children after the disclosure conversation, and how they might respond to any negative reactions. I encouraged them to respond, "We know this might be hard for you to hear for the first time." "We can understand if you are upset that we didn't tell you before." "We know that you might have all sorts of confusing feelings right now" [34, p .6]. I encouraged the parents to listen actively to their children, accepting their feelings and answering their questions, so that a healing process could move forward [32]. Some young adults and adults may feel relieved, as previously unanswered questions fall into place.

The parents contacted me a few weeks later, reporting that they had initiated the first conversation. Mr. and Mrs. Smith reported the conversation was awkward, there were tears, and the twins wanted to know if their parents were hiding anything else from them. Apart from asking a few questions, Beth and Sam did not say much. The parents reported, "We think it hit them strongly; they were quiet and, when we tried to raise questions and talk more about it, we got little response." In the days that followed, tears and more questions emerged. Beth mentioned that she had always wondered why she was the only one in their extended family who was tall, slender and blonde. Over much of her life, friends and others had asked, "How did you get so tall?" Now it made sense, she told them. Overall, the parents felt that the twins had received the information well.

What might we conclude from this case? First, while later disclosure has been associated with negative feelings of confusion, anger, betrayal and distrust, it does not necessarily negate a child's positive feelings about their parents [32,33]. Further, the association between age of disclosure and the acceptance of donor conception is complex. Mahlstedt's study of adults born through sperm donation, most of who learned of this after age 18, found no association between age of disclosure and attitude towards their means of conception. She also found that positive reactions strongly correlated with positive family relationships [35]. Along similar lines, Paul and Berg [36] reported that the positive impact of a mother's long-standing openness in communication was more relevant to family functioning than avoidance of communication about donor conception. Moreover, their study failed to find an association between age at time of disclosure and family functioning, which raises questions about what factors, other than age, contribute to positive disclosure outcomes.

Second, sensing their mother's vulnerability and the difficulty she had discussing their donor conception, the twins may have protected her from any of their more negative feelings. When young adults do not talk much about their feelings after disclosure, it may lead parents to believe that their children no longer think about it or to underestimate the time it will take their children to process this information [33]. Capturing this dynamic are the words of one 20-year-old young woman, "I love my mother. We are close, and I do not want to hurt her feelings. My mom will always be my mom. I have a lot of questions about the egg donor but it seems like a betrayal to ask them." Third, given the daughter's comments about her appearance, it would not be surprising if she had some inkling of a different family origin story. Some have argued that the donor-conceived subliminally sense or know of their donor conception.

Current research indicates that parents who state they intend to disclose may not actually do so until their child is an adolescent or young adult. Disclosure to young adults is a complex phenomenon influenced by multiple variables, including family relationships and communication patterns prior to the disclosure, and current levels of psychosocial adjustment. While late disclosure carries risks, parents can be counseled that in the long run, later may be better than never, which continues the burden of secrecy.

Using donated gametes for a second child

> Tom and Colleen Ward were preparing to do an IVF cycle with egg donation. They had one son, Josh, almost 3 years old, conceived with their own gametes. They had always wanted more children and wanted Josh to have a sibling. They were concerned about how this would affect their older child and the sibling relationship.

Tom's concerns centered on whether his family might treat their second child differently or whether the second child might feel less important. Colleen was concerned about whether she would feel differently about their second child than she did about their 3-year-old. Counseling focused first on the general experience of parents who have a second child, with a particular emphasis on the fact that the second child is never the same as the first, even when using one's own gametes. In many families, siblings are often dramatically different in personality, looks and interests. In addition, because parents often have a unique bond with their first born, it is typically hard for them to imagine having a second child who would seem as special. Mothers in particular can feel sadness or even guilt about no longer having the same exclusive relationship with the first child. Colleen reflected a sense of loss that she might not see herself in the second child in the same way she did with Josh. However, she went on to say that her bond with Josh started in pregnancy, had grown from the daily involvement since birth, and that her attachment was not based on genetics. In my clinical experience, mothers who already have a child reported an easier transition to using donor oocytes than first time mothers, because they felt established in their identity as a mother and had greater confidence in caring for a child.

Colleen and Tom went on to express concerns about how to handle disclosure with their children. They were not sure whether to tell the children together or if they should tell their donor-conceived child first before Josh. They worried that Josh might feel differently toward his younger sibling or tell the second child before they did. On the one hand, they did not want disclosure with Josh to come as a shock, but on the other, they did not want the younger child to worry that everyone else had known before he was told.

We focused on their reasons for wanting a second child. "If we shift the focus away from the genetic differences between your children, what stands out is your desire to build a family in which everyone cares for and looks out for each other. When parents discuss gamete donation as a chance to have a sibling and a larger family, their first child will see it that way as well." I added that "While Josh might want to 'send the baby back' because it cries too much, takes his toys, and takes too much of your attention, the means of conception is rarely a factor for kids in their sibling relationships." With regard to disclosure, some parents do, in fact, want the donor-conceived child to know before the older child. In this scenario, conversations with the younger donor-conceived child would take place between the ages of 4 and 8, postponing the conversation with Josh until he was between 8 and 12. From there, they could begin to include Josh in discussions.

Other parents prefer that both children know from the outset to avoid the older child being shocked when he learns about it. By waiting years before bringing up the topic, parents may inadvertently be placing too much emphasis on it. Tom and Colleen could start talking with Josh early, explaining "Mommy and Daddy want him to have a baby sister or brother and need to go to the doctor for help." As he got older, they could also tell him, "A nice lady had given them an egg so they could make the new baby that would grow inside Mommy."

A growing number of families turn to egg donation after experiencing secondary infertility. The disclosure questions they face are both similar to and different from the questions of couples having their first child. Like many couples, Tom and Colleen struggled with concerns that gamete donation would negatively impact their family and had critical questions about the sibling relationship. Questions about how the siblings will feel toward each other can sometimes be a veiled expression of concern about the second child's "belonging" as well as anxiety that "genetics" may create a hierarchy in the siblings' relationship. Parents can be educated about increasing their family through donor gametes with reassurance that they will bond with this second child, and that they can frame the sibling relationship in positive terms.

Lesbian couples using a known sperm donor

Kim and Stacey Lane are a married lesbian couple who will be using a known sperm donor to have a family. Kim will be pregnant and give birth. Kim's long-time gay friend Greg will be the donor. While they agreed that they would disclose the use of a sperm donor, they sought counseling because they disagreed about if or when to reveal the donor's identity.

Over the last 30 years, the number of planned lesbian-couple families has increased significantly with lesbian and single women now constituting the majority of sperm bank clients. More than heterosexual couples, lesbian couples doing donor insemination (DI) are interested in using a known sperm donor. For these women, the motivations for using a known donor include the existence of a prior relationship with the donor, and the value of providing the child with access to their genetic origins.

My conversation with Kim and Stacey focused on the disclosure implications of using a known donor. To start, Stacey did not share Kim's enthusiasm for using a known donor. She felt, "Our child will have two moms. That will be our family, and I do not think there is a need to bring a third person into it. I do not want our child thinking that the sperm donor is a parent. If the donor is just a nice man who gave us his sperm, why would our child need to know his identity when s/he is young?" Further exploration revealed that she feared if their child knew Greg was the donor at a young age, the child would view Kim and Greg as the parents, and she would be on the periphery of the family.

Children who have a known sperm donor grow up in families with varying arrangements, from minimal contact to ongoing significant involvement with the donor. Recent data from a longitudinal study of lesbian families found no differences in well-being between those conceived with a known donor and those with an unknown donor [37]. While many mothers who use a known donor will disclose the identity to their child at a young age, some mothers are less transparent and may withhold this information until pushed by their children for more honesty [38].

In defining their family, lesbian mothers make a distinction between the biological father/donor and the parent. Children in a lesbian family then typically do not view genetic relatedness as central to their definition of their family. Differentiating the donor's role from that of parent, they view their non-biological mothers as parents. When young children in lesbian families comment that they "don't have a daddy," parents respond in different ways, for example, "You don't have a daddy, you're right; you have a donor." Other parents reframe the family itself: "You have a family with two moms, instead of a mom and dad." Some families make up an entirely new word for the donor. A known donor who plays the role of a special uncle, for instance, might be called "Duncle Greg." For children and adults with known donors, "father" is a more ambiguous term and the donor's role can be described in a variety of ways, changing over time, as donor, donor dad, biological father, family member, or family friend. Sharing this information reassured Stacey that her child would easily distinguish between moms and donor, whether their donor was identified to their child or not.

I suggested that they disclose Greg's identity as the donor when their child is young (4 or 5), by including a picture of Greg in their child's "special storybook" and say, "This is the man who helped us make you, so we could be a family; he is the donor." The risk of waiting to disclose Greg's identity was that their child might figure out Greg was his donor on his own without his parents' support, since many in their social network knew Greg was going to be their donor. I recommended that if they did not disclose Greg's identity when their child was young, they do so by age 10, before middle school, so that it was less likely to be a shock and he would still be more stable developmentally.

It is common for spouses, whether heterosexual or lesbian, to disagree about different aspects of disclosure. In this case, the non-biological parent, Stacey, saw the donor as a potential threat to the family and, like many non-genetic parents, she wanted to diminish the donor's importance. She worried about how others, including their child, would view the legitimacy of her motherhood. This fear is intensified for lesbian mothers, because historically lesbians have lost custody to fathers and because non-biological parents may be in a less secure legal position. It is possible that Stacey will become more comfortable with disclosure of the donor's identity as she grows in confidence in her role as a legitimate and equal co-mother. Having a known donor adds another layer of complexity to Stacey and Kim's decision-making about disclosure, as they grapple with how to include the donor in the family narrative and when to share the donor's identity with the child. (See Chapter 13 for more information on LGBT counseling.)

Conclusion

Disclosure of donor conception is a significant issue for parents using donor gametes for family building. Despite the professional encouragement of disclosure and an increase in the number of recipients who intend to disclose, many remain unsure about how to do it and desire more information and guidance. It takes confidence and support for parents to tackle the complex layers and meanings attributed to genes and relationships in their family. Even as parents' confidence grows with the support of counseling, books, educational materials and support groups, concerns about discussion of donor conception resurface throughout the family's life cycle. Individual/couple counseling appears to be helpful and appreciated by patients, although peer support, often in the form of professionally led groups, may be more effective. Peer support reduces the sense of isolation and stigma and facilitates the sharing of feelings and experiences that increase parents' confidence in disclosing [39]. While the logistics and circumstances of providing ongoing support will vary by country, by the healthcare system, and by treatment program, information from fertility counselors, families' reports and research make clear that ongoing support is essential.

Reflection

As an adopted person growing up in the era of closed records, secrecy held personal and painful meanings for me. In the first part of my career, I did much of my clinical work with adult adoptees and adopted children. Fast forward, now an infertility patient, I had a new appreciation of the pain of infertile parents. It is easy, with my background, to be self-righteous about disclosure. So, how could I help the parents struggling with disclosure when secrecy held such painful associations? Then it hit me, what is now so obvious, that secrets are rooted in fear. So, I am less focused now on whether an intended parent will disclose, but more concerned about what they fear. We still have a great deal of work to do to help patients struggling with disclosure and we need to be honest with them. It is not necessarily an easy road to travel. I feel grateful that patients have been willing to share their fears with me and that in some small way I have been able to help them.

References

1. Blyth E, Frith L. Donor-conceived people's access to genetic and biographical history: an analysis of provision in different jurisdictions permitting disclosure of donor identity. *Int JLPF* 2009; 23: 174–91
2. Blyth E. Guidelines for infertility counseling in different countries: Is there an emerging trend? *Hum Reprod* 2012; 7: 2046–57.
3. Ethics Committee of the American Society for Reproductive Medicine. Informing offspring of their conception by gamete donation. *Fertil Steril* 2004; 81: 527–31.
4. Indekeu A, Dierickx K, Schotsmans P, Daniels KR, Rober P, D'Hooghe T. Factors contributing to parental decision-making in disclosing donor conception: a systematic review. *Hum Reprod* 2013; 19: 714–33.
5. Thorn P. The shift from biological to social fatherhood – counseling men and their partners considering donor insemination. *Hum Fertil* 2013; 16: 40–3.
6. Rumball A, Adair V. Telling the story: parents' scripts for donor offspring. *Hum Reprod* 1999; 14: 1392–99.
7. Kirkman M. Genetic connection and relationships in narratives of donor assisted conception. *AJETS* 2004; 2: 1–20.
8. Indekeu A, D'Hooghe T, Daniels KR, Dierickx K, Rober P. 'Of course he's our child': transitions in social parenthood in donor sperm recipient families. *Reprod Biomed Online* 2014; 28: 106–15.
9. Golombok S, Brewaeys A, Giavazzi M, Guerra D, MacCallum F, Rust J. The European study of assisted reproduction families: the transition to adolescence. *Hum Reprod* 2002; 17: 830–40.
10. Baxter N. *Our Story*. Nottingham, Donor Conception Network, 2002.
11. MacDougall K, Becker G, Scheib J, Nachtigall RD. Strategies for disclosure: how parents approach telling their children that they were conceived with donor gametes. *Fertil Steril* 2007; 87: 524–33

12. Blake L, Casey J, Readings V, Jadva V, Golombok S. 'Daddy ran out of tadpoles': how parents tell their children that they are donor conceived, and what their 7-year-olds understand. *Hum Reprod* 2010; 25: 2527–34.

13. Lycett E, Daniels K, Curson R, Golombok S. School-aged children of donor insemination: a study of parents' disclosure patterns. *Hum Reprod* 2005; 20: 810–19.

14. Hargreaves K, Daniels K. Parents dilemmas in sharing donor insemination conception stories with their children. *Child Soc* 2007; 21: 420–31.

15. Durna EM, Bebe J, Steigrad SJ, Leader LR, Garrett DG. Donor insemination: attitudes of parents towards disclosure. *Med J Aust* 1997; 16:256–9.

16. Vanfraussen K, Ponjaert-Kristoffersen I, Brewaeys A. An attempt to reconstruct children's donor concept: a comparison between children's and lesbian parents' attitudes toward donor anonymity. *Hum Reprod* 2001; 16: 2019–2025.

17. Blake L, Casey P, Jadva V, Golombok S. 'I was quite amazed': donor conception and parent-child relationships form the child's perspective. *Child Soc* 2013; DOI: 10.1111/chso.12014.

18. Daniels K. *Building a Family with the Assistance of Donor Insemination.* Wellington, Dunmore Press, 2004.

19. Stamm L. *Phoebe's Family: A Story About Egg Donation.* New York, Graphite Press, 2010.

20. Kirkman M. Parents' contributions to the narrative identity of offspring of donor-assisted conception. *Soc Sci Med* 2003; 57: 2229–42.

21. Becker G, Butler A, Nachtigall R. Resemblance talk: a challenge for parents whose children were conceived with donor gametes in the U.S. *Soc Sci Med* 2005; 61: 1300–09.

22. Golombok S, MacCallum F, Goodman E, Rutter M. Families with children conceived by donor insemination: a follow-up at age 12. *Child Dev* 2002; 73: 952–68.

23. Benward J. Identity development in donor offspring. In: Guichon J, Mitchell I, Giroux M, eds. *The Right to Know One's Origins.* Brussels, ASPnv. 2012; 166–91.

24. Ory SJ, editor. IFFS Surveillance. 2013. http://c.ymcdn.com/sites/www.iffs-reproduction.org/resource/resmgr/iffs_surveillance_09-19-13.pdf. Accessed May 5, 2014.

25. McKee A. *Our Story.* Nottingham, Donor Conception Network, 2008.

26. Kluger-Bell K. *The Pea That Was Me: An Embryo Donation Story.* CreateSpace Independent Publishing Platform, 2013.

27. Barrett CE. *Training Wheels: How Did I Get Here?* Knoxville, National Embryo Donation Center, 2011.

28. Scheib JE, Ruby A. Contact among families who share the same sperm donor. *Fertil Steril* 2008; 90: 33–43.

29. Freeman T, Jadva V, Kramer W, and Golombok S. Gamete donation: parents' experiences of searching for their child's donor siblings and donor. *Hum Reprod* 2009; 24: 505–16.

30. Soderstrom-Anttila V, Foudila T, Ripatti UR, Siegberg R. Embryo donation: outcome and attitudes among embryo donors and recipients. *Hum Reprod* 2001; 16: 1120–28.

31. MacCallum F, Keeley S. Disclosure patterns of embryo donation mothers compared with adoption and IVF. *Reprod Biomed Online* 2012; 24: 745–48.

32. Daniels K, Meadows L. Sharing information with adults conceived as a result of donor insemination. *Hum Fertil* 2006; 9: 93–99

33. Jadva V, Freeman T, Kramer W, Golombok S. The experiences of adolescents and adults conceived by sperm donation: comparisons by age of disclosure and family type. *Hum Reprod* 2009; 24: 1909–19.

34. Montuschi O. *Telling and Talking about Donor Conception with People Age 17 and Older.* Nottingham, Donor Conception Network, 2006.

35. Mahlstedt PP, LaBounty K, Kennedy WT. The views of adult offspring of sperm donation: essential feedback for the development of ethical guidelines within the practice of assisted reproductive technology in the United States. *Fertil Steril* 2010; 93: 2236–46.

36. Berger R, Paul M. Family secrets and family functioning: the case of donor assistance. *Fam Proc* 2008; 47:553–66.

37. Bos HMW, Gartrell NK. Adolescents of the US National Longitudinal Lesbian Family Study: the impact of having a known or unknown donor on the stability of psychological adjustment. *Hum Reprod* 2011; 26: 630–37.

38. Goldberg A, Allan K. Donor, Dad or…? Young adults with lesbian parents' experiences with known donors. *Fam Proc* 2013; 52: 338–50.

39. Crawshaw M, Montuschi O. Participants' views of attending parenthood preparation workshops for those contemplating donor conception parenthood. *J Infant Reprod Psychol* 2012; 31: 58–71.

Chapter 19

An evidence-based approach to counseling for fertility treatment compliance

Sofia Gameiro and Jacky Boivin

Case 1

Faatima is a 27-year-old South Asian woman who presented after two years of trying to conceive with her husband Balaji. She was diagnosed with polycystic ovary syndrome (PCOS) with pronounced hirsutism and an overweight status. The medical team advised Faatima to lose 5% (13 kg/28 lb) of her body weight to help minimize the PCOS-related risks of cardiovascular disease [1] and to improve her treatment success chances. However, Faatima was experiencing high anxiety due to her fertility problem and believed stress was the cause of her failure to conceive. This belief made her unwilling to spend additional time on weight loss. As a consequence, Faatima and her husband decided to end treatment because they perceived that treatment was unlikely to work and as they, and Faatima especially, thought they could not cope with the additional stress of another treatment, especially waiting for treatment results. The medical team referred Faatima to the fertility counselor to discuss her psychological concerns and effective weight-loss opportunities in the hope that Faatima would be more willing to lose weight and do treatment as recommended, as it was judged she would have a good chance of conception.

Case 2

Amy (29) and Petroc (32) attended a first consultation and underwent a full diagnostic workup. They were diagnosed with infertility due to tubal blockage and recommended for IVF. Amy and Petroc discussed the recommendation but could not reach agreement about whether to undergo treatment or not. Petroc was concerned with the idea that children conceived with IVF were more likely to have malformations and resisted the idea of doing treatment, whereas Amy felt the technique was safe and they should at least try one cycle. The couple had been discussing this issue for one month without reaching agreement and requested fertility counseling because they felt the counselor could help them reach a joint decision.

Introduction

Medical care models assume that patients will act in a way that optimizes their chance of good health. This usually implies complying with treatment recommendations. The World Health Organization [2, p. 3] defined treatment compliance as "the extent to which a person's behavior follows medical advice or corresponds with recommendations from the health care provider." In the case of fertility treatment, this means assuming that patients will be willing to undergo the treatment cycles recommended by their doctor until pregnancy is achieved or until there is a recommendation to end treatment. In treatment with assisted reproductive techniques (ART, e.g., in vitro fertilization, IVF, intracytoplasmic sperm injection, ICSI) the typically funded treatment regimen is three ART cycles, based on cumulative pregnancy rates [3]. Therefore, non-compliance can occur in the form of *premature discontinuation* from ART, when patients decide to opt out of (further) recommended treatment despite a favorable prognosis and ability to cover the costs of treatment [4]. Non-compliance can also take the form of persisting with treatment beyond the number of cycles the doctor recommends, which will not be discussed in the present chapter.

Fertility Counseling: Clinical Guide and Case Studies, ed. Sharon N. Covington. Published by Cambridge University Press.

Compliance is important to clinics and patients because patients who comply have a 15% higher pregnancy rate [5]. Given that non-compliance means fewer patients achieve their parenthood goal, it is important to understand decision-making in fertility treatment and how different factors impact on willingness to comply. In this chapter, we will review this research and identify why fertility counselors can play an important role in treatment compliance. We discuss ways mental health professionals (MHPs) can use Evidence-Based Medicine (EBM) principles to help support patients facing compliance decisions using the two illustrative cases we began with.

Current state of knowledge about treatment compliance

A systematic review and meta-analysis of treatment discontinuation data from ten studies on the treatment trajectory of 14 810 patients across three consecutive cycles of ART was performed [5]. The results showed that overall compliance was 78% but differed as a function of number of treatment failures: 82% after the first failed cycle and 75% after the second. These results mean two of every ten patients are likely to discontinue treatment before achieving pregnancy. Based on current available data on ART cycles performed in Europe [14], it was estimated that with full compliance each European clinic would carry out an additional 110 cycles per year.

A systematic review was also conducted to investigate patients' stated reasons for discontinuation at any stage of fertility treatment. This review also included treatment predictors of discontinuation. Twenty-two studies were included, referring to 21 453 patients from eight different countries. The main reasons for treatment discontinuation (in order of decreasing frequency) were postponement of treatment (for at least one year), physical and psychological burden of treatment, relational and personal problems, clinic/organizational issues, rejection of treatment and logistical and practical reasons. Some reasons were common across all stages (e.g., psychological burden, postponement of treatment, doctor recommendation) but others were dominant at a particular stage of treatment. For example, rejection of treatment, financial issues and relational problems were common at initiation of the first or subsequent new types of treatments but, of these, only finance and relational issues were relevant after a failed ART cycle. The reader is directed to the systematic review for a more in-depth analysis of the issues captured by these categories of reasons [6]. Brandes and colleagues [7] provided the only prospective empirical evidence indicating that patients discontinued for different reasons, at different treatment stages, based on data from their study which followed-up patients through the duration of their treatment pathway in the fertility clinic. Figure 19.1 summarizes the main reasons for discontinuation at different treatment stages reported in their study.

Finally, the review revealed a lack of consistent association between any socio-demographic (e.g., age, education), infertility (e.g., years infertile, prior live birth) or clinical (e.g., number and quality of oocytes and embryos) predictors recorded in medical charts at the start of treatment and discontinuation 12 months later.

More recently, a substantial body of research on Patient-Centered Care (PCC) has been focusing on how clinic and organizational factors related to the delivery of treatment may affect compliance behavior. This body of research is based on the assumption that care provided should be tailored to patient's individual needs, preferences and values. The dimensions of PCC are accessibility, information, communication, patient involvement, respect, continuity and transition in stages of treatment, competence and organization [8]. Cross-sectional research has shown that almost all aspects of PCC are associated with patients' intentions to comply with treatment [9] and the results of a preference study asking patient to choose between hypothetical scenarios (e.g., slightly lower pregnancy rate but more caring doctor attitude) showed that PCC was an important criteria for choosing and/or changing fertility clinics [10]. However, a prospective study implemented in the Netherlands with 693 infertile women undergoing fertility treatment at 32 different clinics showed that women's evaluations of PCC did not predict their compliance behavior one year later [21]. Conversely, the patients were not differentiated according to stage of treatment (e.g., diagnostic versus first, second, third cycle) and, as noted, stage determines which reason (including elements of PCC) will be relevant. On going research is examining whether other factors (emotional distress, relational issues) predict compliance.

In conclusion, there are many reasons why patients do not undergo treatment as recommended. A main reason is indefinite postponement and procrastination; patients intend to do it, but do not ultimately

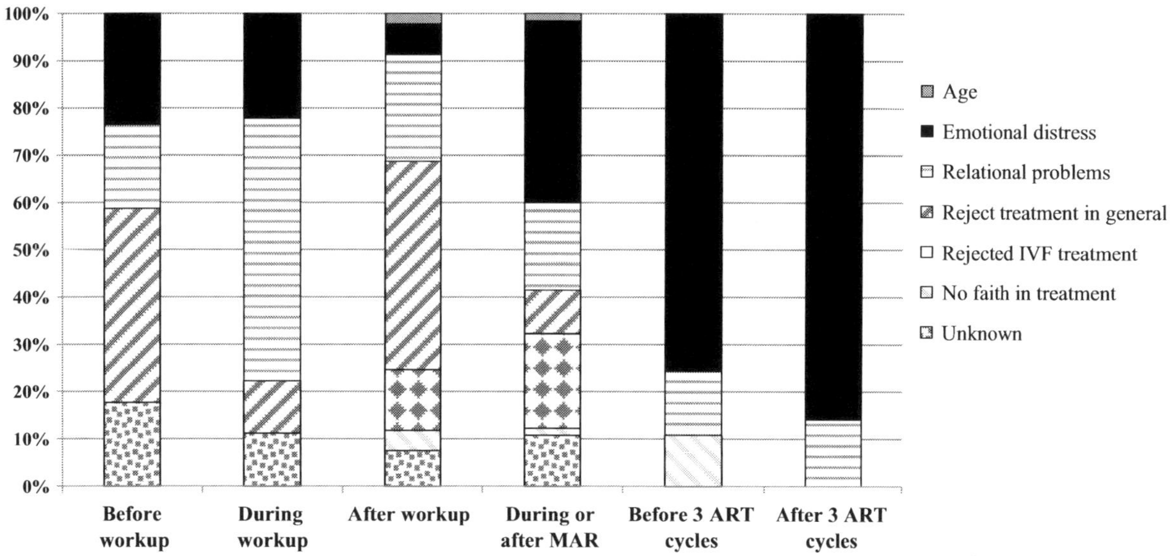

Figure 19.1 Reasons for discontinuation from fertility treatment across different treatment stages. Data concerning reasons that cannot be considered discontinuation because they refer to external constraints to treatment uptake (e.g., doctor censuring, financial issues) are not represented in the figure. Adapted from [7]. MAR = medically assisted reproduction, ART = assisted reproduction technology, IVF = in vitro fertilization.

do it. The physical and psychological burden of treatment is another common reason, as are relational and personal problems, which may or may not be related to the infertility. Research on the psychology of compliance with ART is not yet mature with many remaining questions concerning the specifics of the broad issues outlined; for example, which relational issues link to non-compliance, when and why. Given the lack of precision on the psychology of compliance in infertility there is also a dearth of studies on patient decision-making in this context. Currently it is known that patients find it stressful to decide about uptake of further treatment [11], especially when they have a very strong wish for children [12]. How this decisional process actually unfolds and who contributes to it (patient, partner [when present], physicians, nurses, etc.) is still not known. Patients themselves express the wish to receive counseling to help them with this decision [13] and 49% think that it should come from their physicians or nurses [14]. Nonetheless, fertility counselors also can play an important role in patient support and understanding during the decision-making process. Ultimately, knowledge from these two different strands (reasons/predictors and decision-making) need to come together if patients are to be better supported in their decision-making process about treatment. The latter is especially important considering the high rates of treatment postponement observed which most likely reflects decisional avoidance.

Enabling compliance from an evidence-based perspective

In the age of EBM, MHPs need to provide psychological care that has demonstrated efficacy, feasibility, cost-efficiency and generalizability [15] in regard to supporting decision-making or addressing the causes of non-compliance in the ART context. In short, practitioners are expected to follow a scientific approach to clinical decision-making and practice [16]. Boivin [15] has discussed extensively the increasing need for fertility counselors to integrate research findings into their everyday practice and has provided MHPs with a framework to meet this challenge using EBM principles. The five steps involved in this process are summarized in Table 19.1. Readers are referred to Sackett et al. [16] for detailed instructions on each step and to Boivin [15] for application in the context of infertility psychological care.

In the following sections, we apply EBM principles to the compliance issues described in the two case studies presented at the start of the chapter.

Table 19.1 The five steps of evidence-based clinical practice. Adapted from Sackett et al. [16].

Step	Description
1	Convert the need for information into an answerable question.
2	Track down the best evidence with which to answer that question.
3	Critically appraise the evidence for its validity (closeness to the true), impact (size of the effect), and applicability (usefulness in our clinical practice).
4	Integrate the critical appraisal with your clinical expertise and the patient's unique biology, values and circumstances.
5	Evaluate your effectiveness and efficiency in executing the previous steps and seek ways to improve them for the next time.

Case 1 – Faatina and Balaji: Discontinuation due to poor prognosis

An important reason for ending fertility treatment is anticipated prognosis of the recommended treatment being undertaken. Prognosis is a prediction about the likelihood of a pregnancy (live birth) with continued treatment. Perceived poor prognosis is an important reason why doctors advise patients to end treatment and why patients discontinue treatment. The systematic review presented showed that 15% of patients cited poor prognosis as a reason for discontinuation during first-line fertility treatments (e.g., insemination, ovulation induction) and 30–42% while undergoing ART [6]. In the review, patients perceived that doctors based their prognosis on issues such as a poor response (poor ovarian response, fertilization or embryo quality), absence or inaccessibility of a treatment that could help, and/or medical futility (defined as less than 1% chance of pregnancy [17]). Patients also referred to causes of a poor response (i.e., body mass index $> 30\ kg/m^2$, signs of ovarian aging) and inability to correct causes (i.e., failure to lose or gain weight), as per recommendation of the clinic. If patients end treatment because of a genuine poor prognosis, then patients are complying with recommendations.

However, there is evidence that patients perceive a poor prognosis, even when the doctors see a positive outcome. One study observed that 30% of patients who cited poor prognosis as a reason for discontinuation actually had a favorable prognosis according to their doctors, suggesting that patients may lose hope for success before the medical staff do [18] and/or that they define a "poor prognosis" differently. Indeed patients' stated reasons for discontinuation often refer to aspects such as lack of faith in treatment itself or in the possibility that it would be successful, feeling that success was not meant to be, giving up or simply feeling that all that could be done had already been done [6]. Such statements could corroborate an actual poor prognosis or could reflect patient hopelessness about efficacy of treatment. The fact that clinical indicators of poor prognosis are not significant determinants of compliance (as noted previously [6]) does lend weight to patient perception being a critical aspect for decision-making.

It seems clear that ending treatment due to a poor prognosis can hide different causes, and these need to be identified to select the best psychological support for the patient [4,19]. In particular is the need to counsel patients about the ways they can maximize their chance of success (i.e., adopt healthier lifestyles), how they can maintain hope during treatment, and how they can make the decision to end treatment following a definitive diagnosis of poor prognosis. The first case study presented in this chapter exemplifies the issues fertility counselors may encounter regarding discontinuation due to poor prognosis using EBM principles to identify the best option for support.

Step 1: The need for information is converted into an answerable question

The fertility counselor needs to consider the multifaceted case and select intervention targets consistent with the referral.

The most pressing issue for the medical team is for the patient to receive the necessary psychological support for the problems interfering with compliance. The problematic issues refer to worry about stress, a lack of motivation to achieve weight loss, perceived inability to cope with the stress of the waiting period, which altogether lead to the desire to end treatment despite recommendation to continue. To address these issues, the problems could be translated into the questions that would help the fertility counselor better understand the case and help the patient make an informed decision about pursuing further treatment, which is the subject of referral. The case raises multiple questions:

"In South Asian married women undergoing first-line fertility treatment...

a. ...is polycystic ovary syndrome associated with anxiety?
b. ...does anxiety decrease the chance of pregnancy?
c. ...what are the most effective interventions to reduce anxiety during the waiting period?
d. ...are lifestyle interventions effective for weight loss?

The answer to all questions is to some extent necessary to comprehensively understand and address the referral. The first three questions address the beliefs Faatima has about stress, which are reducing her motivation to comply with treatment. The fourth question concerns the issue of effective weight loss interventions, which is a priority area for the healthcare team, but not for Faatima. The fertility counselor can address some or all of these questions depending on resources, relevance to the problem solution, referral and, of course, can only do so if the couple attend for counseling.

Step 2: The best evidence with which to answer that question is identified

The MHP would need to use electronic databases to search for the best evidence for each question.

Some databases require a subscription (e.g., PsychInfo, Web of Science), while others are free (e.g., PubMed, Google Scholar). Free databases can yield relevant information because many authors can be contacted via email to obtain free text reprints of articles identified through the search. In addition, researchers are increasingly choosing to publish via open access, and some scientific journals also choose to make their papers open access after a period of time (e.g., one year for *Human Reproduction*, the journal of the European Society for Human Reproduction and Embryology). This reduces the disparity in access to information between academic and non-academic professionals. Recent studies comparing the effectiveness of searching via different databases show that Google Scholar out performs PubMed in retrieving twice as many relevant articles and in providing greater access to free-text articles when used by medical doctors [20]. However, skilled indexers may show improved search yields with PubMed [21].

The search terms to be used for the case of Faatima should refer to the problem context (i.e., polycystic ovary syndrome, anxiety, weight loss) but should be combined (in successive order) with terms indicating better quality research designs (e.g., meta-analysis, systematic review) to make the search as effective as possible. See Table 19.2 for quality ratings according to types of designs. The combination of the case and methodology search terms would have identified the following studies of relevance to the case of Faatima and Balaji. First, is a series of meta-analyses examining the prevalence of emotional distress in women with polycystic ovary syndrome [22–25]. Second, are two meta-analyses on the relationship between emotional distress and the outcome of fertility treatments [26,27]. Third, are a systematic review on lifestyle management in polycystic ovary syndrome [28] and a meta-analysis and meta-regression on factors predictive of the effectiveness of weight loss programs [29]. Finally there are a series of randomized controlled trials of coping interventions for the waiting period based on distraction [30,31], positive reappraisal coping intervention [32,33] and telephone support [34]. Overall, 13 studies were identified that could increase case understanding. It should be noted that the process of searching for evidence can be much more complex but is kept to a minimum here for the purposes of illustration. The interested reader is referred to The Cochrane Handbook for Systematic Reviews of Interventions (www.cochrane-handbook.org) [35] for more details of searching for best evidence.

Step 3: The evidence is critically appraised for its validity, impact and applicability

Critical appraisal is the process by which one judges the trustworthiness of the research being examined.

Critical appraisal varies according to study design (e.g., randomized trial, systematic review, cohort study). The fertility counselor needs to become familiar with the criteria that differentiate good and bad research designs. Although critical appraisal may seem a daunting task at first, many good-quality websites

Table 19.2 Evidence quality according to type of study design.

Quality of evidence	Study design	Definition
High	Systematic reviews and meta-analysis	The application of strategies that limit bias in the assembly, critical appraisal, and synthesis of all relevant studies on a specific topic. Systematic reviews focus on peer-reviewed publications about a specific health problem and use rigorous, standardized methods for selecting and assessing articles. A systematic review may or may not include a meta-analysis, which is a quantitative summary of the results.
	Multiple randomized control trials Single randomized control trial	An epidemiological experiment in which subjects in a population are randomly allocated into groups, usually called study and control groups, to receive or not receive an experimental preventive or therapeutic procedure or intervention. The results are assessed by rigorous comparison of rates of disease, death, recovery, or other appropriate outcome in the study and control groups.
	Large non-randomized trial	A trial in which subjects in a population are non-randomly allocated into groups.
	Case control/cohort studies	Cohort-study: The analytic method of epidemiologic study in which sub-sets of a defined population can be identified who are, have been, or in the future may be exposed or not exposed, or exposed in different degrees, to a factor or factors hypothesized to influence the probability of occurrence of a given disease or other outcome. The main feature of cohort study is observation of large numbers over a long period (commonly years) with comparison of incidence rates in groups that differ in exposure levels. Case control: The observational epidemiologic study of persons with the disease (or other outcome variable) of interest and a suitable control (comparison, reference) group of persons without the disease. The relationship of an attribute to the disease is examined by comparing the diseased and non-diseased with regard to how frequently the attribute is present or, if quantitative, the levels of the attribute, in each of the groups.
	Case reports/case series	A group or series of case reports involving patients who were given similar treatment. Reports of case series usually contain detailed information about the individual patients. This includes demographic information (for example, age, gender, ethnic origin) and information on diagnosis, treatment, response to treatment, and follow-up after treatment.
Low	Non-analytic studies: Cross-sectional surveys/qualitative	Cross-sectional survey: A study that examines the relationship between diseases (or other health-related characteristics) and other variables of interest as they exist in a defined population at one particular moment (i.e., exposure and outcomes are both measured at the same time). Best for quantifying the prevalence of a disease or risk factor, and for quantifying the accuracy of a diagnostic test. Qualitative study: Data-gathering techniques that are focused on the significance of observations made in a study rather than the raw numbers themselves.

Definitions adapted from [49]

exist to help practitioners do it and once learned the same design quality standards are applied in future appraisals.[1] Critical appraisal is a learning experience that will ultimately strengthen the counselor's confidence in being able to discuss and integrate the very best evidence into clinical practice. A further

[1] Useful websites with compilations of critical appraisal forms for different types of studies are http://www.cebm.net//o=1040, http://www.caspinternational.org/?o=1012, http://www.cardiff.ac.uk/insrv/libraries/sure/sysnet/criticalappraisalchecklist.html.

point to note about appraisal is that it should always include a consideration of fit between evidence and case characteristics.

a. . . . is polycystic ovary syndrome associated with anxiety?

Four meta-analyses were identified, but the one by Veltman-Verhulst et al. [25] included the earlier reviews, and was therefore the only one examined in greater detail. The review was a comprehensive meta-analysis of comparative studies reporting measures of depression, anxiety or emotional quality of life in women experiencing PCOS. It reviewed 28 studies (2384 patients and 2705 control women) and showed that women with PCOS reported significantly higher emotional distress (anxiety, depression, lower emotional quality of life) than did the comparison control group (other patients, other infertile women, other women with gynecological problems). As Faatima is from South Asia and is married, the review should be examined for information that might be relevant to these specific case characteristics. Marital status was not shown to impact results but studies carried out with American and European participants yielded lower emotional distress scores than did studies with Asian and Australian women. The meta-analysis was conducted according to a very good standard, as per its critical appraisal, and the data were relevant. The conclusions of the review should be examined to identify relevance to the present case. The authors concluded that women with PCOS are at risk for emotional distress and multiple factors could contribute to this distress (e.g., hirsutism, obesity, infertility).

b. . . . does anxiety decrease the chance of pregnancy?

Two meta-analyses were identified that examined the association between anxiety and outcome of fertility treatment. Boivin et al. [26] reviewed 14 prospective studies including 3583 women undergoing a cycle of in vitro fertilization and concluded no association between pre-treatment anxiety and depression (measured prior to day 5 of stimulation) and the success of a single cycle of IVF (i.e., biochemical or clinical pregnancy rate or live birth rate). In contrast, Matthiesen et al. [27] investigated 31 prospective studies including 4902 women undergoing treatment with assisted reproductive techniques (ART) over single or multiple cycles. The results showed an association between higher emotional distress (perceived stress, life events, occupational or other stress, anxiety and/or depression) and lower pregnancy rates in ART treatment. The reviews are relevant to the case of Faatima, but it should be noted that the samples were infertile women and not specifically women with PCOS. Further, the reviews sampled from many countries, yet none examined country of origin (i.e., South Asia) specifically. Similarly, none of the reviews provided information about marital status and its effect on the association between stress and fertility.

A critical assessment of the two meta-analyses suggests that one should be more cautious about the outcome of the Matthiesen et al. review [27]. The main difference and reason why is because the timing of the psychological and reproductive assessments in the Boivin review were better controlled, avoiding the possible confounding of factors such as poor prognosis and age. Given these confounds, the results of the Boivin review should be prioritized. Boivin et al. [26] concluded that emotional distress levels at the start of one IVF/ICSI cycle are unlikely to affect the outcome of that cycle. Additionally, the authors concluded that anxiety and depression should nevertheless be addressed to improve quality of life during treatment.

c. . . . what are the most effective interventions to reduce anxiety during the waiting period?

There were no meta-analyses or systematic reviews on coping interventions for the waiting period. Three randomized controlled trials (RCTs) were reported for waiting periods in infertility and cancer patients. Two RCTs considered the impact of active distraction in patients waiting for the outcome of a risk assessment for familial cancer [30,31]. These RCTs showed that an active distraction coping intervention (ADCI), teaching on the benefits of distraction, could reduce intrusive thoughts about risk assessment during the waiting period, but only in people who already had intrusive thoughts to begin with. There was no effect on general emotional distress, avoidant ideation (trying not to think of assessment) or emotions specific to risk assessment (e.g., fear, hope). Although this technique shows promise, a generalizability study in infertile patients facing the ART waiting period has not yet been performed.

The two other RCTs concerned a positive reappraisal coping intervention [32]. The Positive Reappraisal Coping Intervention (PRCI) was conceptualized using the cognitive model of stress and coping [36] and was designed specifically for the waiting period in fertility medical treatment [32,33,37]. The PRCI is a small laminated card that contains ten positive reappraisal statements and a leaflet with a detailed explanation about this coping approach. The ten statements were designed to stimulate the use of positive reappraisal coping techniques (e.g., "Focus on the positive aspects of the situation," "Focus on the benefits and not just the difficulties," "Make the best of the situation"). The leaflet describes the challenges of the waiting period and the expected benefits of using positive reappraisal techniques and provides instruction on using the PRCI card. The acceptability, feasibility [32] and effectiveness [32,33] of the PRCI in the waiting period of fertility treatment has been established in several randomized trials [32,33]. These studies also show that the main impact of PRCI is to help women sustain a more positive outlook during treatment (positive emotions, challenge appraisals, more positive reappraisal coping) which makes the stress of the waiting period seem more tolerable even when negative emotions such as tension and worry remain (i.e., helps them carry on). The critical appraisal of these RCTs shows some caution is required due to small sample size [32] or lack of double-blinding [33]. The authors concluded that PRCI could be a low cost way of providing additional support to women by making the two-week waiting period more tolerable. A final RCT of another intervention specific to the waiting period examined the effectiveness of two support telephone calls from a social worker after embryo transfer compared to routine care [34]. Although it was rated as helpful by 66% of those receiving the calls, there was no impact on perceived stress scores. Although there was no analysis of marital status or ethnicity in these trials, the randomization ensured that the groups were equivalent on these factors.

These RCTs are relevant insofar as they provide evidence of the effectiveness of interventions during the waiting period in helping to reduce intrusive thoughts (in cancer context only) or sustain a positive outlook. However, their fit to the specific case of Faatima will depend on whether the counselor believes Faatima needs a reduction in anticipatory anxiety or help to manage an unavoidable emotional state (i.e., waiting *is* stressful).

d. ... are lifestyle interventions effective for weight loss?

Fertility counselors are often asked to assist with behavior change interventions in clinics. A Cochrane systematic review of RCTs comparing lifestyle treatment to minimal or no treatment in women with PCOS was identified [28]. The review was performed on 6 studies (including 164 women). A meta-analysis could not be performed because the lifestyle interventions differed between studies (diet, exercise, behavior management techniques, or combined interventions). The lifestyle interventions were associated with reductions in weight (about 3.5 kg/7.7 lb. weight loss for programs of about six months) and waist circumference (about 1.95 cm/ .8 in. loss). However, there was insufficient data to conclude whether these had an impact on reproductive outcomes (i.e., pregnancy, live birth, miscarriage, ovulation or menstrual regularity) because too few or no studies examined these outcomes. Moreover, it was not possible to examine variations in these effects according to characteristics of the interventions (e.g., duration, content, motivational interviews) because too few studies used the same intervention. The systematic review is relevant to the case but some caution needs to be exercised because the interventions were heterogeneous and it was not possible to identify the cause of heterogeneity. There was no detailed analysis of country of origin or marital status. Moran et al. [28] concluded that interventions were effective to improve body composition (weight, waist circumference) in women with PCOS without evidence to conclude on reproductive outcomes.

A second meta-analysis was identified in the search, though this meta-analysis was not specifically with patients that had PCOS [29]. A primary question of that review was about the factors that predicted the most effective weight-loss interventions. The systematic review and meta-analysis was of RCTs of multicomponent behavioral weight management programs in overweight and obese adults with at least one follow-up at 12 months. The review included 37 studies (> 16 000 participants). The overall weight loss was lower than that reported in Moran et al. [28] and was 2.8 kg/6.2 lb at the minimum 12-month assessment. The meta-regression controlling for all factors simultaneously showed that the intervention components that remained significantly associated with weight loss were calorie counting, contact with a dietitian and the use of behavior change techniques that allowed participants to compare their behavior to that of others (e.g., information about others' approval, information about normative behavior, modeling or behavior demonstrations, and/or facilitating social comparisons) [29]. There was no evidence that supervised physical activity or more frequent in-person contact had an impact on the effectiveness of the program [29].

The meta-analysis [29] is relevant to the case of Faatima because it shows the effect of weight loss programs and because knowledge of predictors of effectiveness could help Faatima choose the most effective program. The critical appraisal suggests some caution because some of the comparisons reported were based on a small number of studies and some results (e.g., usefulness of calorie counting) could be confounded by other uncontrolled intervention differences (e.g., use of a self-monitoring device). Further the generalizability to patients with PCOS is not known. The authors concluded that most behavioral interventions were effective in reducing weight, but that some interventions were better than others (as described).

Step 4: The critical appraisal is integrated with the clinician's clinical expertise and with their patients' unique psyche, values and circumstances

Obesity and emotional distress should be a central focus of the psychological intervention because they are contributing to perceptions of poor prognosis for both the medical team and Faatima.

From a clinical perspective, the fertility counselor could feel confident in normalizing beliefs about the association between PCOS and emotional distress, and discuss with Faatima its possible causes, like the stigmatizing aspects of this disorder (e.g., obesity, hirsutism, infertility). This discussion could help contextualize the discussion of obesity and distress, and help Faatima take action on reducing weight and dealing with emotional distress as health problems in their own right and not just as a remedy for fertility problems. In the case of Faatima, erroneous beliefs about how her anxiety/stress influences the chances of treatment success are interfering with her motivation and therefore these misconceptions need to be addressed using psychological techniques. Although stress is not significantly associated with the outcome of a treatment cycle, this case provides an example of how it can indirectly affect patients' chances of pregnancy across multiple cycles via decreasing motivation to comply with treatment recommendations.

Faatima was also particularly concerned about further treatment because of her inability to manage the strain of the two-week waiting period. PRCI could be recommended to Faatima as a way of helping to sustain a positive outlook that could make the stress of this period seem more tolerable. Faatima would need other forms of support during the waiting period to produce an actual reduction in stress levels. The fertility counselor could then decide to apply psychological interventions known to generally be effective for stress reduction in infertile populations by executing another broad search. However, there would be no way of knowing whether the effectiveness of the identified intervention would generalize to the waiting context. The fertility counselor could see this gap in knowledge as an opportunity to collaborate with researchers on testing the generalizability of the identified intervention.

Faatima's healthcare team would like Faatima to take up a weight-loss intervention but she is not motivated to do so. The evidence identified poses a dilemma for the fertility counselor. Although it is known that obesity and a higher body mass index are associated with a lower cumulative pregnancy rate in ART [38], the review showed that the effect of losing weight on prognosis was unknown due to insufficient research. Given the state of current evidence, Faatima should not be misled. Weight loss should be promoted as an overall health benefit to minimize risks for cardiovascular problems associated with PCOS, as well as quality of life issues, but not for improved reproductive prognosis. Meta-analysis shows that generic advice from healthcare practitioners to lose weight is positively associated with weight loss [39]. The fertility counselor could encourage Faatima to look specifically for programs that have the characteristics known to be associated with more effective weight loss in adults (e.g., calorie counting).

A final point of reflection is that Faatima may have made an informed decision about ending treatment and, while the referral was to address issues of treatment compliance, the fertility counselor could focus on end-of-treatment issues with Faatima and Balaji.

This consultation would explore making the transition from active pursuit of the (biological) parenthood goal to other life pursuits [40].

Step 5: Practitioners evaluate their effectiveness and efficiency in executing the EBM process, and try to find ways to improve them

All aspects of the evidence-based process should be considered from formulation of questions to integration in the problem formulation.

The search process and examination of relevant literature was straightforward, and relevant literature was identified. One problem was that weight loss is a vast topic and many possible papers were identified. As a result, a *satisficing decision approach* was adopted which involved choosing the best evidence (most recent, better research designs, better critical appraisal) as the basis for decision-making. Satisficing (combination of satisfy and suffice) refers to a decision made on the basis of choosing the evidence that addresses *most needs*, rather than on choosing a potential optimal solution that could have addressed *all needs*, but which might have required considerably more investment to identify. A more thorough analysis that aimed to examine all possible best evidence could have generated other helpful advice. The reading of evidence was straightforward but a gap in knowledge with regards to meta-regression was identified. A third issue was that the reviews mainly concerned work published in scientific journals, but it is known that mobile applications and internet health interventions are increasingly available and used in infertility [41], but are not necessarily identified because they are in the gray literature (e.g., informally published technical reports and white papers from government, working papers from research) and may not have been detected. Finally, the fertility counselor could have detected that their expertise lay mainly in counseling approaches (emotional expression and support) with comparatively less knowledge in using educational interventions and/or supporting self-help psychological tools. In light of all these reflections, the fertility counselor could identify the following topics as targets for further continued professional development: understanding the impact of satisficing decision rules in evidence gathering, meta-regression statistical techniques, searching the gray literature, and self-help psychological tools.

Case 2 – Amy and Petroc: Supporting informed decision-making in compliance

Relational problems and rejection of treatment have been shown to be important reasons for discontinuation from fertility treatment [6]. Rejection of fertility treatment due to ethical objections, attitudes to the medicalization of fertility, fear of complications and possible adverse health effects on self and child or other factors are one of the most commonly cited reasons (42%) for not undergoing any type of fertility treatment [6]. Because often treatment is pursued with a partner, different views in relation to these personal beliefs and values, or the need to undergo any (further) treatment, may make it difficult for couples to reach agreement about which course of action to undertake. These differences may be one reason why patients frequently cite relational problems as a discontinuation reason at the stages of beginning treatment or transition to a new treatment type (20% before the start of any treatment, 19% before the start of ART [6]). It may also be that problematic relationships make reaching agreement on these or any issues difficult due to, for example, poor communication and negotiation skills. However, to date the existing research has not yet provided insight into the nature of relational problems that lead couples not to comply. The second case study exemplifies some relational issues that impact on compliance.

Step 1: The need for information is converted into an answerable question

The fertility counselor needs to consider the multifaceted case and select intervention targets consistent with the referral.

Amy and Petroc expressed a need for decisional support about fertility treatment uptake. The fertility counselor's role is therefore to help them negotiate and reach agreement about whether to undergo fertility treatment. Because concerns about the safety of the medical procedures were a central issue for Petroc, and therefore for decision-making for this couple, information about risk of malformations in children conceived with ART would need to be provided. The MHP would also have to support the couple in their deliberation process. One approach could be for the fertility counselor to recommend an effective decision-support tool designed to help individuals and/or couples make decisions about whether or not to comply with treatment recommendations from their doctor. Such a tool could be used as a basis to guide discussion in the consultation, ensuring that all relevant topics and information were covered. Therefore, the relevant questions for this case would be:

In couples referred for IVF...

a. ... are children conceived with IVF more likely to present malformations than children conceived spontaneously?
b. ... which decision-support tools are associated with high-quality decision-making about undergoing IVF?

Step 2: The best evidence with which to answer that question is identified

The MHP would need to use electronic databases to search for the best evidence for each question.

The fertility counselor would develop search procedures using search terms to be used for the case of Amy and Petroc (e.g., decision-making, decisional aid, IVF, children, malformations, birth defects) combined with terms indicating better-quality research designs. The MHP would find no relevant papers regarding decision-support tools for compliance in IVF, or more generally with fertility treatment, and would conclude that none had yet been developed. Two systematic reviews would be found concerning malformations in children conceived with IVF [42,43].

Step 3: The evidence is critically appraised for its validity, impact and applicability

Critical appraisal is the process by which one judges the trustworthiness of the research being examined.

a. ...are children conceived with IVF more likely to present malformations than children conceived spontaneously?

One meta-analysis was identified that estimated the risk of congenital malformations in IVF and ICSI infants. It included 19 studies with samples >100 children published after 1990, including 48 570 children conceived with IFV/ICSI and 3 202 346 conceived spontaneously. Congenital malformations were defined as a condition present at the time of birth that causes functional impairment or requires surgical correction (akabirth defects). Malformation rates across studies varied between 0 and 9.5% for IVF and between 1.1 and 9.7% for ICSI. The control group malformation rates varied between 0 and 6.9%. The meta-analysis indicated an increased risk of malformations in children conceived with ART compared to spontaneously conceived children (OR = 1.29, 95% CI 1.01–1.67).[2]

Another recent meta-analysis was found that included British and Chinese published studies reporting on birth defects of children conceived with IVF/ICSI [43]. A total of 46 studies, published from 1989 to 2011, compared data on 124 468 children conceived with IVF and/or ICSI with data on spontaneously conceived children. These studies also indicated an increased risk for malformations in ICSI/ICF conceived children (OR = 1.37, 95% CI 1.26–1.48). Sixteen studies comparing children conceived with IVF to spontaneously conceived children showed that the risk for the IVF group was higher. The authors could also compare data on birth defects in children conceived by IVF with children conceived with ICSI and no risk difference was found (OR = 1.05, 95% CI 0.91, 1.20). These results did not change according to analyses controlling for methodological characteristics (e.g., sample size, type of population) or confounding factors (e.g., maternal age, parity, sex, year of birth, social class and/or smoking). Averaged malformation rates for IVF, ICSI, IVF/ICSI or spontaneous conception were not reported in either study, therefore we do not know the estimated likelihood of an IVF/ICSI conceived children presenting a malformation.

Both meta-analyses provide confidence for the authors' conclusion that there is a significant increased

[2] An odds ratio (OR) is the probability of an event (e.g., pregnancy) occurring in one group over another. For example, suppose in XX group 30/100 women become pregnant whereas in YY group 15/100 become pregnant, then the OR would be 2.43 ((30/70)/(15/85)), representing 2.43 higher odds of pregnancy in group XX then group YY. An OR which falls below one is interpreted in percentage terms. Suppose in WW group 20/100 women became pregnant whereas in ZZ group 50/100 became pregnant then the OR would be ((20/80)/(50/50)) = .25, which would mean that the WW group had a 75% lower chance of pregnancy than the ZZ group. ORs are usually reported with a confidence interval (CI); if the interval includes the value of 1, then the increased risk is **not** significantly different from chance.

risk of malformation in infants conceived with ART. It should be noted, however, that the meta-analyses did not disentangle the risk associated with IVF/ICSI from the risk associated with the underlying infertility. To do this one would need a control group of infertile patients conceiving spontaneously or with other forms of treatment that require minimal intervention (e.g., insemination without ovulation induction).

b. ...which decision-support tools are associated with high-quality decision-making about doing IVF?

The lack of decision support tools that can be applied to Amy and Petroc's specific situation means that the fertility counselor will have to consider other ways of supporting the couple in their decision-making about the risks identified. Given the lack of research on decision-support tools for infertility (as described previously), decision-making theories and studies investigating predictors of high quality decisions in other contexts should be considered. What is a "high-quality decision" is debated within the general compliance and decision-making literature [5,44]. However, there is general agreement that it is a decision which is well informed (i.e., the individual has knowledge about the pros and cons of treatment and all alternatives available), consistent with individual values and preferences, and made with minimal decisional conflict and anxiety [44]. Therefore, the fertility counselor consulted a systematic review of decisional theories used to inform the design of decisional-support tools, and/or the selection of deliberation techniques, to be used in a counseling context [45]. This review provided multiple approaches to deliberation. For example, according to the Expected Utility Theory [46], a deliberation tool could be developed using a tree metaphor, where different branches correspond to different decisional options (e.g., doing more treatment, adoption, wait and see). The patient chooses by comparing the different tree branches (i.e., options) according to the likelihood of their expected benefits vs. costs happening (e.g., if I choose to do more treatment what is the likelihood of achieving parenthood vs. experiencing disabling treatment burden?). An example of such a decisional-aid tool is the Amniodex (http://www.amniodex.com), resulting from a collaboration between doctors and psychologists and designed to help pregnant couples/individuals deciding about whether to do amniocentesis [47].

Step 4: The critical appraisal is integrated with the clinician's clinical expertise and with their patients' unique psyche, values and circumstances

Facilitating effective couple communication to help in decision-making regarding the risks associated with IVF will be the central focus of psychological intervention.

The fertility counselor would have to consider first Petroc's concerns about the risks of ART because these were a main reason for him not to want to do treatment. Overall the meta-analyses seem to suggest that Petroc's concerns are justified. Therefore, the MHP would have to communicate the increased risk of malformation in IVF in a way that is clear, understandable and quantifiable to the couple. In addition, the fertility counselor would also explain that there is as yet no conclusion about whether the risk results from the treatment or from the medical condition. The couple would then have to decide on whether the risk level was an acceptable risk given their values (e.g., need for parenthood, attitudes to disability). In order to facilitate decision-making the fertility counselor could use the Expected Utility Theory tree metaphor. The branches would have to address both the treatment and its alternatives. The MHP would have to ensure that Amy and Petroc would have the necessary evidence about the probability of different positive and negative (i.e., benefits vs. costs) outcomes (at least achieving pregnancy with IVF and occurrence of malformations, as clearly important to them, but also discontinuing treatment, experiencing disabling treatment burden, etc.). Progress in deliberation could be monitored based on the level of decisional conflict experienced by the couple.

Step 5: Practitioners evaluate their effectiveness and efficiency in executing the EBM process and try to find ways to improve them

All aspects of the evidence-based process should be considered from formulation of questions to integration in the problem formulation.

The initial problem to note in this EBM process is the already mentioned use of a satisficing decision-making approach. The fertility counselor further identified that decision-making counseling and risk communication are specialist areas in their own right, which require a good understanding of odds ratios and how to interpret population-level data. The MHP also noted a deficit in knowledge regarding the different types of congenital malformations with the realization that if queried by the patient s/he would not be able to describe the more common disorders. Consequently, understanding of odds ratios and risk communication in counseling were targeted as areas of professional development. The fertility counselor also determined to learn the main malformations arising from the use of ART. During the process the MHP also noted that provision of information about malformations could be considered to be within the domain of the medical team. Consequently, the MHP resolved to discuss the issue of risk information with the medical team to determine how the team could best approach discussion of malformations with patients.

Reflections and conclusions

Compliance is a pressing problem in fertility care that needs to be addressed so patients can be enabled to achieve their parenthood goals with treatment [5]. However, evidence about the determinants of compliance and effectiveness of interventions to enable it are scarce. Despite these constraints, fertility counselors are still expected to provide psychological care with demonstrated effectiveness in complex decision-making scenarios [15]. This implies applying EBM principles in order to ensure that the best available evidence is used to inform practice decision-making.

In this chapter, we presented two case studies to illustrate the EBM process and its usefulness in supporting work with patients referred for treatment in fertility clinics. We acknowledge that applying EBM principles presents several challenges for MHPs working in both public and private practice. First, practitioners need to familiarize themselves with the EBM process and identify associated areas for professional development. Second, they need to be up-to-date on the research in the field. The EBM process requires a certain degree of tension between defining questions that are useful and finding answers from available sources and evidence. Managing this tension is facilitated when practitioners know the general research base. Third, fertility counselors need to diversify their interventions and their clients because, when the EBM process is followed, different strategies and targets are identified that go beyond those typically used in one-to-one counseling formats. As noted, patient and staff needs can sometimes identify areas for development (e.g., decision-support tools for treatment uptake). Fourth, the ability of practitioners to pursue these endeavors is dependent on their own motivation and effort, but also constrained by a multitude of factors, such as time and the organizational policy of the clinics that integrate them. For instance, practicing EBM may not be viable in a clinic without a research based culture or access to the Internet [48].

However challenging research and clinical work can be for fertility counselors, we strongly believe that in the long term the use of EBM principles can really contribute to improve psychological services in clinics and encourage clinics to make better use of MHP skills. For instance, EBM helps to clarify what can be done for each patient group or individual, while at the same time highlighting the genuine limits to the support that can be provided. For instance, the second case illustrated that sometimes validated interventions addressing the specific patient situation are not available. Fertility counselors have to make decisions about how to proceed in these cases to ensure that patients will still be supported. Therefore, the EBM process validates the support provided to each individual patient. It informs which interventions to use and how, and highlights when new solutions need to be developed, evaluated and implemented. This can also be very useful for troubleshooting. For instance, if a previously validated intervention does not produce the expected benefits, it is more likely that this is due to implementation problems than to the inefficiency of the therapeutic principles on which it is based.

EBM principles also provide a common reference frame for multidisciplinary communication and discussion about the therapeutic goals to be pursued. This may not always be easy because different health professionals will value different outcomes differently and these may be considered implicitly. The EBM process prompts explicit discussion about what can be considered best patient care. In the example discussed, the fertility team had to discuss who/when and how to address the provision of information about risk for malformations in children conceived with IVF/ICSI. Finally, it is a useful tool to identify areas for professional development (e.g., risk communication) that arise from patients needs and therefore will certainly be useful within the healthcare context.

We could point out many other benefits of EBM, including that it can be an enjoyable and rewarding process, despite the possibly challenging initial learning curve. The more one practices EBM, the more one increases his/her expertise in the field. In addition, EBM helps to justify the clinical decisions made for supporting patients. This can help build case support for the deliverance of specific interventions and/or services within the clinic. It can also help in coping with failure, which is bound to happen at some point in anyone's professional career. More importantly, it will help to identify and change those factors that contributed to failure and prevent it from happening again.

In summary, EBM is a feasible, efficient and useful tool designed to facilitate the task of supporting patients through their treatment experiences. For some it is a professional lifestyle: once you learn to see the world through its lenses, you cannot let go of it. Most of all, it can be extremely rewarding and fulfilling, as it allows professionals to go back to their patients, people like Faatima, Balaji, Amy and Petroc, and confidently assure them that they are receiving the best-quality support currently available.

References

1. Fauser BC, Tarlatzis BC, Rebar RW, Legro RS, Balen AH, Lobo R, et al. Consensus on women's health aspects of polycystic ovary syndrome (PCOS): the Amsterdam ESHRE/ASRM-Sponsored 3rd PCOS Consensus Workshop Group. *Fertil Steril.* 2012; 97(1): 28–38.
2. WHO. *Adherence to Long-term Therapies: Evidence for Action.* Geneva, Switzerland: World Health Organization; 2003.
3. Stern JE, Brown MB, Luke B, Wantman E, Lederman A, Missmer SA, et al. Calculating cumulative live-birth rates from linked cycles of assisted reproductive technology (ART): data from the Massachusetts SART CORS. *Fertil Steril.* 2010; 94: 1334–40.
4. Boivin J, Domar AD, Shapiro DB, Wischmann T, Fauser BC, Verhaak CM. Tackling burden in ART: An integrated approach for medical staff. *Hum Reprod.* 2012; 27(4): 941–50.
5. Gameiro S, Verhaak CM, Kremer JAM, Boivin J. Why we should talk about compliance with assisted reproductive technologies (ART): a systematic review and meta-analysis of ART compliance rates. *Hum Reprod Update.* 2013; 19(2): 124–35.
6. Gameiro S, Boivin J, Peronace LA, Verhaak CM. Why do patients discontinue fertility treatment? A systematic review of reasons and predictors of discontinuation in fertility treatment. *Hum Reprod Update.* 2012; 18(6): 652–69.
7. Brandes M, van der Steen JOM, Bokdam SB, Hamilton CJCM, de Bruin JP, Nelen WLDM, et al. When and why do subfertile couples discontinue their fertility care? A longitudinal cohort study in a secondary care subfertility population. *Hum Reprod.* 2009; 24(12): 3127–34.
8. Corrigan JM, Donaldson MS, Kohn LT, Maguire SK, Pike KC. *Crossing the Quality Chasm. A New Health System for the 21st Century.* Washington, DC: Institute of Medicine, National Academy of Sciences, National Academy of Press; 2001.
9. Pedro J, Canavarro MC, Boivin J, Gameiro S. Postive experiences of patient-centred care are associated with intentions to comply with fertility treatment: Findings from the validation of the Portuguese version of the PCQ-Infertility. *Hum Reprod.* 2013; 28(9): 2462–72.
10. van Empel IWH, Dancet EAF, Koolman XHE, Nelen WLDM, Stolk EA, Sermeus W, et al. Physicians underestimate the importance of patient-centredness to patients: A discrete choice experiment in fertility care. *Hum Reprod.* 2011; 26(3): 584–93.
11. Peddie VL, van Teijlingen E, Bhattacharya S. A qualitative study of women's decision-making at the end of IVF treatment. *Hum Reprod.* 2005; 20(7): 1944–51.
12. Rauprich O, Berns E, Vollmann J. Information provision and decision-making in assisted reproduction treatment: results from a survey in Germany. *Hum Reprod.* 2011; 26: 2382–91.
13. Boden J. When IVF treatment fails. *Hum Fertil.* 2007; 10: 93–8.
14. Peddie VL, van Teijlingen E, Bhattacharya S. Ending in-vitro fertilization: Women's perception's of decision making. *Hum Fertil.* 2004; 7(1): 31–7.
15. Boivin J. Evidence-based approaches to infertility counselling. In: Covington SN, Hammer Burns L, editors. *Infertility Counselling: A Comprehensive Handbook for Clinicians.* New York: Cambridge University Press; 2006.
16. Sackett D, Strauss SE, Richardson WS, Rosenberg W, Haynes RB. *Evidence-based Medicine: How to Practice and Teach EBM.* Edinburgh: Churchill Livingstone; 2000.
17. The Ethics Committee of the American Society for Reproductive Medicine. Fertility treatment when the prognosis is very poor or futile: a committee option. *Fertil Steril.* 2012; 98(1): e6–e9.

18. Malcolm CE, Cumming DC. Follow-up of infertile couples who dropped out of a specialist fertiliy clinic. *Fertil Steril.* 2004; 81(2): 269–70.

19. Gameiro S, Boivin J, Domar AD. Optimal IVF for 2020 should reduce treatment burden and enhance care delivery for patients and staff. *Fertil Steril.* 2013; 100: 302–9.

20. Shariff SZ, Math B, Bejaimal SAD, Sontrop JM, Iansavichus AV, Haynes RB, et al. Retrieving clinical evidence: A comparison of PubMed and Google Scholar for quick clinical searches. *J Med Internet Res.* 2013; 15(8): e164.

21. Bramer WM, Giustini D, Kramer BMR, Anderson FP. The comparative recall of Google Scholar versus PubMed in identical searchers for biomedical systematic reviews: a review of searches used in systematic reviews. *Systematic Reviews.* 2013; 2: 115.

22. Barry JA, Kuckmierczyk AR, Hardiman PJ. Anxiety and depression in polycystic ovary syndrome: a systematic review and meta-analysis. *Hum Reprod.* 2011; 26: 2442–51.

23. Dokras A, Clifton S, Futterweit W, Wild RA. Increased prevalence of anxiety symptoms in women with polycystic ovary syndrom: systematic review and meta-analysis. *Fertil Steril.* 2012; 97(1): 225–30.

24. Dokras A, Clifton S, Futterweit W, Wild RA. Increased risk for abnormal depression scores in women with polycystic ovary syndrome: a systematic review and meta-analysis. *Obstet Gynecol.* 2011; 117(1): 145–52.

25. Veltman-Verhulst S, Boivin J, Eikjemans E, Fauser BC. Emotional distress in women with Polycystic Ovary Syndrome: A systematic review and meta-analysis. *Hum Reprod Update.* 2012; 18(6): 638–51.

26. Boivin J, Griffiths E, Venetis CA. Emotional distress in infertile women and failure of assisted reproductive technologies: meta-analysis of prospective psychosocial studies. *BMJ.* 2011; 342(d223).

27. Matthiesen SM, Frederiksen Y, Ingerlev HJ, Zachariae R. Stress, distress and outcome of assisted reproductive technology (ART): a meta-analysis. *Hum Reprod.* 2011; 26: 2763–76.

28. Moran LJ, Hutchison SK, Norman RJ, Teede HJ. *Lifestyle Changes in Women with Polycystic Ovary Syndrome.* 06 July 2011 edn. Cochrane Library 2011.

29. Hartmann-Boyce J, Johns DJ, Jebb SA, Aveyard P, Behavioural Weight Management Review Group. Effect of behavioural techniques and delivery mode on effectiveness of weight management: a systematic review, meta-analysis and meta-regression. *Obes Rev.* 2014; 15: 598–609.

30. Phelps C, Bennett P, Hood K, Brain K, Murray A. A self-help coping intervention can reduce anxiety and avoidant health behaviours whilst waiting for cancer genetic risk information: results of a phase III randomised trial. *Psychooncology.* 2012; 22: 836–44.

31. Bennett P, Phelps C, Brain K, Hood K, Gray J. A randomized controlled trial of a brief self-help coping intervention designed to reduce distress when awaiting genetic risk information. *J Psychosom Res.* 2007; 63(1): 59–64.

32. Lancastle D, Boivin J. A feasibility study of a brief coping intervention (PRCI) for the waiting period before a pregnancy test during fertility treatment. *Hum Reprod.* 2008; 23: 2299–307.

33. Ockhuijsen H, van den Hoogen A, Eijkemans M, Macklon N, Boivin J. The impact of a self-administered coping intervention on emotional well-being in women awaiting the outcome of IVF treatment: a randomized controlled trial. *Hum Reprod.* 2014; 29: 1459–70.

34. Skiadas CC, Terry K, De Pari M, Geoghegan A, Lubetsky L, Levy S, et al. Does emotional support during the luteal phase decrease the stress of in vitro fertilization? *Fertil Steril.* 2011; 96: 1467–72.

35. Higgins J, Green S. Cochrane handbook for systematic reviews of interventions Version 5.1.0 [updated March 2011]. *The Cochrane Collaboration* 2011.

36. Lazarus RS, Folkman S. *Stress, Appraisal and Coping.* New York: Springer; 1984.

37. Lancastle D. *Reasons to be Cheerful: Part I, II, III. Dispositional Optimism, Positive Reappraisal Coping and Positive (Re)appraisals of the Situation: Effects on Emotional Well-being and Physical Outcomes.* ProQuest, UMI Dissertations Publishing: Cardiff University; 2006.

38. Pinborg A, Gaarslev C, Hougaard CO, Nyboe Anderson A, Kragh Anderson P, Boivin J, et al. The influence of female body weight on assisted reproductive technology (ART) procedures and live birth rates: A longitudinal multi-centre cohort study of 487 infertile couples. *Reprod BioMed Online.* 2011; 23(4): 490–9.

39. Rose SA, Poynter PS, Anderson JW, Noar SM, Conigliaro J. Physician weight loss advice and patient weight loss behavior change: a literature review and meta-analysis of survey data. *Int J Obes.* 2013; 37(1): 118–28.

40. Boivin J, Takefman J, Braverman A. Giving bad news: It's time to stop. In: Macklon N, editor. *Assisted Reproduction in the Complicated Patients.* London: Taylor & Francis; 2005. pp. 233–40.

41. Aarts JWM, van den Haak P, Nelen WL, Tuil WS, Faber MJ, Kremer JAM. Patient-focused intervent interventions in reproductive medicine: a scoping review. *Hum Reprod Update.* 2012; 18(2): 211–27.

42. Rimm AA, Katayama AC, Diaz M, Katayama KP. A meta-analysis of controlled studies comparing major malformation rates in IVF and ICSI infants with naturally conceived children. *J Assist Reprod Gen.* 2004; 21(12): 437–43.

43. Wen J, Jiang J, Chenyue D, Juncheng D, Liu Y, Xia Y, et al. Birth defects in children conceived by in vitro fertilization and intracytoplasmic sperm injection: a meta-analysis. *Fertil Steril.* 2012; 97(6): 1331–7.

44. Elwyn G, Miron-Shatz T. Deliberation before determination: The definition and evaluation of good decision making. *Health Expect.* 2009; 13: 139–47.

45. Elwyn G, Stiel M, Durand M-A, Boivin J. The design on patient decision support interventions: addressing the theory-practice gap. *J Eval Clin Pract.* 2011; 17: 565–74.

46. von Neumann J, Morgenstern O. *Theory of Games and Economic Behaviour.* Princeton, NJ: Princeton University Press; 1944.

47. Durand M-A, Boivin J, Elwyn G. Stakeholder field-testing of amnioDex, a person-centered decision support intervention for amniocentesis. *Int J Pers Cent Med.* 2012; 2(3): 568–76.

48. Jones ML, Cifu DX, Backus D, Sisto SA. Instilling a research culture in an applied clinical setting. *Arch Phys Med Rehabil.* 2013; 94(1): S49–54.

49. Centre for Evidence Based Medicine. Glossary 2014 [April 4th 2014]. Available from: http://www.cebm.net/?o=1116.

Chapter 20

Ethical aspects of fertility counseling

Joann Paley Galst and Judith E. Horowitz

Dr. Goodheart is a licensed psychologist who specializes in family therapy. Although Dr. Goodheart is not a member of the Mental Health Professional Group (MHPG) of the American Society for Reproductive Medicine (ASRM), she has promoted herself as an expert in infertility as she had personal experience with IVF, that is, she attempted IVF with her and her husband's gametes when she was in her early 40s, had a mid-trimester pregnancy loss, no subsequent pregnancies, and has since adopted two children.

Amanda, 37 years old, and her husband, Chuck, age 40, are currently in the first trimester of their first pregnancy, conceived through IVF. She and Chuck have seven frozen embryos remaining from this cycle. They wish to retain five and donate two of their embryos to their friends, Rebecca and Rick. Amanda and Rebeca work together and all live in the same city.

Rebecca, age 42, and Rick, age 50, have been married for five years with no children. They have attempted two cycles of intrauterine inseminations and two IVF cycles. Previously, Rebecca and Rick have used her oocytes and his sperm, but to no avail having both female and male factor diagnoses. They are both eager to receive two of the excess embryos and wish to use them for their next cycle, scheduled in one month. Amanda's reproductive endocrinologist (RE) has also been treating Rebecca, thus far unsuccessfully. Their RE, a solo practitioner, located in a mid-size cosmopolitan city not far from where the four patients reside, has requested Rebecca and Rick consult with a mental health professional (MHP) for their required recipient psychoeducational interviews. No request was made that Amanda and Chuck be seen for a psychoeducational session.

Dr. Goodheart, with whom Rebecca and Rick are scheduled to meet, called upon us in advance of their visit for consultation and described this very complicated case. Dr. Goodheart is a member of the two couples' church community and the only MHP available with any experience in the area of fertility counseling in the small city (population 100 000) in which they all reside. Dr. Goodheart does not personally know the RE. Rebecca and Rick selected her in consultation with Amanda and Chuck because they have all previously served together on several church committees.

The above vignette illustrates one of many possible ethical minefields encountered by fertility counselors. Revolutionary breakthroughs in scientific research have indisputably impacted and transformed reproductive technology over the past four decades. Although strides in biomedical technology have introduced significant treatment alternatives, they also have sparked controversy, public debate, political extremism and extensive ethical challenges. We begin by presenting information necessary for the resolution of a vast array of complex and ethically challenging situations, and will return to Amanda and Rebecca later. This chapter will discuss: principles and standards for ethical clinical practices; benefits and limitations of formal ethics committees; and a practical format that fertility counselors can implement to assist in ethical decision-making.

Ethical principles

It seems upon first blush that ethics are hardwired in humans, as most people know the difference between right and wrong. Moreover, we learn some variation of the *Golden Rule* before age 5. Across many cultures, children approaching their neighborhood sandbox are admonished to play nicely (beneficence), not

Fertility Counseling: Clinical Guide and Case Studies, ed. Sharon N. Covington. Published by Cambridge University Press.

to hit other children (nonmaleficence), share their toys (access and justice) and to take turns on the swings (fairness). However, as there are many perspectives to consider, consensus on the resolution of ethical dilemmas is elusive.

Ethical practice in fertility counseling requires MHPs to commit to the ethical code and standard of care of their individual professional societies, adhere to pertinent laws, policies and legislation in their jurisdictions, and utilize ethical principles most relevant to bioethics. Ethical principles help fertility counselors identify and analyze decisions regarding novel or complex dilemmas in reproductive medicine. Yet, despite referring to counseling in the ethics and practice guidelines of reproductive medical organizations worldwide, none delineate ethical principles specifically regarding fertility counseling, clearly leaving a void for MHPs bridging these fields.

However, there does appear to be a core of ethical standards approaching universal acceptance across various MHP affiliations worldwide. These include respect for individuals and cultures, competence to practice, informed consent, privacy, confidentiality, avoidance of conflict of interest and dual relationships and a focus on client well-being, all of which are consistent with ethical principles of beneficence and nonmaleficence [1–5].

The following five bioethical principles can aid fertility counselors to achieve balance in their resolution of ethical dilemmas [6–7]:

- ***Autonomy***: treating people with respect for their dignity, rights and capacity for self-determination as guided by their stated wishes, preferences and values. Client choices must be voluntary, free of coercion or controlling constraints by others, and informed, having been given full disclosure of all information available regarding treatment options. Within the area of assisted reproduction, multiple parties can be involved with the result that the autonomous needs or choices of the various participants can conflict. Autonomy, however, is neither absolute nor as highly valued universally as it is in Western cultures [8].
- ***Beneficence***: the obligation to contribute to the welfare of an individual. MHPs have a responsibility to do good, be proactive and prevent or minimize harm when possible, including harms to the potential children being created through the assisted reproductive technology (ARTs).
- ***Nonmaleficence***: MHPs are obligated not to intentionally or negligently cause harm. If nothing can be done to benefit a patient, at least do nothing that will harm him or her.
- ***Justice***: reflects fairness, such that all patients will be treated in a fair and impartial manner and goods and services will be distributed or accessed equitably.
- ***Fidelity***: involves integrity, loyalty, truthfulness and honoring one's commitments to the client enabling trust of the MHP and faith in their relationship. MHPs are expected to maintain confidentiality, advocate for and not abandon or threaten clients, nor leave obligations unfulfilled.

It is unreasonable to expect ethical principles to provide explicit guidance for resolving conflicts and balancing competing claims in every instance in which professional duties clash and create ethical dilemmas. Formats for ethical decision-making and consultation with an ethics committee and/or one's peers can be invaluable in providing assistance and a rationale for one's decisions.

Ethics committees

Healthcare ethics committees have evolved to become the primary formal mechanism for addressing ethical issues in clinical settings in pluralistic societies. Because of the multitude of complex, value-laden ethical issues raised within contemporary reproductive medicine, it has been suggested that fertility practices could benefit from having an in-clinic mechanism for ethical decision-making [9]. The advantages of in-house ethics committees are: they provide transparency throughout the decision-making process; committee members have the requisite expertise specific to reproductive medicine enabling them to consider the moral ramifications of the various ART treatments and are conveniently available for consultation when disagreement arises among staff members regarding the acceptance or rejection of patients who present for treatment; and members can educate their clinics' colleagues and staff members, as well as being able to provide detailed information which ultimately can generate clinical and practice policies and guidelines. These committees are able to prevent treatment that may be harmful to stakeholders, for example, potential offspring.

However, there are several notable limitations to in-house ethics committees: the assistance of in-clinic ethics committees may be too infrequently called upon to justify their cost; the scope and breadth of in-clinic committees may be too narrow in comparison to that of hospitals' general ethics committees [9]; and committee members may be defensive of their clinic's policies because of the members' dependence on the clinic for their employment.

Regardless of whether a fertility practice or fertility counselor has access to an in-clinic or hospital-based ethics committee or individual ethics consultants, it is useful to involve a variety of people who do not necessarily share the same values, yet incorporate multiple perspectives and insight, into the ethical discussion. The views of the patients (and their families, if appropriate) must also be included to prevent a return to a culture of paternalism.

Standards for the ethical practice of fertility counseling

MHPs have an important role in society as trusted experts with a duty to maintain the highest standards. Most national associations of MHPs (e.g., psychologists, social workers, marriage and family counselors, etc.) have explicit ethical standards to which their members abide. Yet, MHPs are not expected to blindly adhere to standards, but rather actively process and reason.

Furthermore, fertility counseling has become global in focus with MHPs working cross-nationally and clients crossing geographic borders to receive treatment. Ethics call upon fertility counselors to respect diversity and thus be aware of cultural, religious and ethnic differences in the meaning of family, kinship bonds, childlessness and the acceptability of fertility treatment in multicultural settings.

Ethical *standards*, unlike ethical *principles*, are enforceable. The following standards are found in the ethical guidelines of MHPs and reproductive medicine organizations throughout the English-speaking world. Their incorporation is essential for the ethical practice of fertility counseling.

Competence

The need for MHPs to offer counseling to fertility patients, rather than fertility nurses and physicians, has been recognized since the mid 1980s. Specialized knowledge of the psychosocial implications of infertility, complex medical treatments, alternative family building options, pregnancy and parenting issues, as well as legal and ethical issues that arise is necessary for those who counsel the infertile. Few MHPs have been adequately prepared by their graduate training to work with reproductive medical patients, particularly those considering undergoing third party reproduction. It is apparent that one needs more than personal experience with infertility and a graduate degree in a relevant mental health field to competently and ethically offer fertility counseling. However, at present, no uniform set of qualifications exists regarding education and/or experience that is either required or recommended.

The USA, Canada and Europe recommend, in addition to a graduate degree and license, certification, or registration to practice in a mental health field, that counselors should obtain training and/or supervision in the medical and psychological aspects of infertility [10–12]. The USA and Canada recommend continuing education in the medical and psychological issues in reproductive healthcare [10,12], and Canada recommends membership in a relevant professional body with a code of ethics [10]. However, these guidelines have no legal mandate to enforce them.

Confidentiality

There is worldwide agreement in the ethical codes of MHPs that confidentiality is a right of all those to whom services are provided and is essential to create trust in the relationship. It should be shared with clients that confidentiality is not absolute, due to legal and regulatory requirements placed upon the MHP, and written consent should be obtained for disclosures. Furthermore, confidentiality must also be upheld when MHPs seek consultation from colleagues or use clinical information for teaching purposes, as well as in the storage and disposal of clinical records.

Informed consent

Informed consent has three essential components. The patient should be fully informed, give his or her consent voluntarily, and have the requisite knowledge and capacity to make decisions. The concept of informed consent within the field of reproductive medicine involves very private, personal and often pivotal decisions about childbearing and is afforded great prominence. Fertility counselors must contribute to ensuring their clients receiving reproductive services are accurately informed.

One of the primary purposes of informed consent is to protect patient autonomy by encouraging ongoing and open communication of relevant, accurate and unbiased information, enabling patients to exercise personal choice. Fertility counselors may wear many different hats (e.g., therapist, counselor, evaluator, psychoeducational consultant) with varied stakeholders. It is important to inform clients prior to initiating an interaction of the specific role of the fertility counselor, the purpose of the interaction, to whom information will be disclosed and who will receive a copy of any notes or reports generated so as to allow the patient to make a clear decision to participate or decline participation.

Gamete donors, gestational carriers (GCs) and intended parents (IPs) must be given adequate information so they can give informed consent to treatment. Since gamete donors and GCs are assuming health risks for the benefit of others, a high level of informed consent regarding medical procedures and future psychosocial implications is required. Oocyte donors need to receive information that would include the medical risks of undergoing ovarian stimulation and oocyte retrieval, as well as the long-term risks of these procedures. Additionally, along with being informed of their right to withdraw at any time up to the moment of treatment, gamete donors should be given sufficient time to consider their decisions before treatment commences. All donors of oocytes, sperm and embryos, and GCs, should be informed of the psychosocial implications of undergoing their specific ART protocol and their lack of dispositional authority. Moreover, fertility counselors should discuss with anonymous donors that offspring conceived with their gametes may be able to contact their donor in the future using DNA testing, internet search capabilities and new technological developments.

Dual roles and/or conflicting relationships

The MHP has the obligation to follow ethical principles and consider the best interest of the patient receiving services and the client, if these differ, regardless of their role, for example conducting an evaluation, counseling, or psychoeducational consultation. Fertility counselors are often asked to perform multiple roles with multiple clients in the treatment(s) intended to create a child, thus the potential for dual roles exists. If asked to provide psychological services at the request of a third party (e.g., IP, referring RE, agency), prior to offering services fertility counselors should explain to all parties concerned: the nature of the relationship with each; the fertility counselor's role; the probable uses of information obtained; the limits of confidentiality; and when relevant, the financial arrangements regarding the provision of service.

Although international guidelines counsel against dual roles, in reality, particularly in less densely populated regions with fewer MHPs versed in fertility counseling, this may occur more often than is desired. Furthermore, clients may not be able to view a fertility counselor embedded within a reproductive medical practice as anything other than an evaluator. It is also questionable whether a MHP, who initially functioned as a counselor with fertility patients, later could be an objective evaluator.

Dual relationships can exploit the power differential inherent in the counseling relationship and harm the client. The more typical conflicts of interest in the practice of fertility counseling may occur between the MHP and the clinic or agency for whom they work or from whom they receive referrals. If a treatment team to whom the fertility counselor has reported ignores or disregards his or her recommendation, the fertility counselor may be confronted with the decisions of how vigorously to protest, whether to continue to work with this treatment team, as well as determining any additional responsibilities the fertility counselor may have to the client. Dual relationships may be unavoidable and, while not prohibited, fertility counselors are responsible for diligently keeping such multiple relationships harm-free.

Duty to care and not abandon patients

There are multiple situations in which a fertility counselor refuses to continue treatment with a client. However, to fulfill their professional duties, the MHP has responsibilities to the client to avoid abandonment or wrongful termination. If an assessment reveals an issue for which a donor or GC should seek further treatment, the fertility counselor has an ethical obligation to provide feedback and referrals so patients can secure care. Infertility patients have the right to access a copy of their test results, unless the fertility counselor believes releasing summaries of their test may cause substantial harm to the client or may be misused or misinterpreted.

Record keeping

Good records are the MHP's primary proof of having offered quality care and, with consent, can be useful to subsequent treating professionals. One must follow the laws and regulations of one's jurisdiction as well as professional guidelines regarding content and retention of the mental health record.

Generally, it is legally mandated that records be maintained a set number of years after the last date of service. However, in some circumstances, for example when donor gametes have been used to create a conception, it may be wise to retain records of both donors and recipients longer than is legislated, weighing the risks associated with obsolete or outdated information with the potential benefit associated with preserving the record.

Format for ethical decision-making

Ethical decision-making in fertility counseling, which often touches on an individual's deepest beliefs about the meaning of creating and sustaining life, requires thorough familiarity with the ethics codes and standards of one's profession, ethical guidelines published by organizations responsible for those who practice in the field of reproductive medicine, and the laws, policies and regulations of one's jurisdiction. Inevitably situations will arise where ethical principles are ambiguous or conflict with one another, relevant laws or regulations, clinic or agency policies, or ethical standards in allied professions. The judgment and discretion of the MHP must always fill the gap between abstract ethical principles, enforceable ethical standards and the reality of clinical practice [13].

The adoption of a structured strategy for ethical decision-making is imperative in providing a method for resolving ethical dilemmas. If the MHP follows such a strategy, considers the best interest of the client as well as other stakeholders in the situation, and documents the process, he or she can provide a professionally sound explanation for the chosen course of action should those decisions and actions be challenged [14]. Discussion with colleagues, that is professional peer advisory groups and supervision, about the difficult ethical choices we confront can add the insight and perspective of others.

We now return to the vignette about Amanda and Rebecca posed at the beginning of the chapter, and will use the following adaptation of Horowitz, Galst and Elster's structured framework for problem-solving (see Table 20.1) to guide our decision-making process for resolving the ethical dilemmas [15]. We will examine the different steps and discuss important issues for Dr. Goodheart's consideration. We will comment as consultants to this psychologist, who will be acting as the fertility counselor responsible for interviewing both couples prior to the commencement of Rebecca and Rick's potential embryo transfer. Additionally, where appropriate, we will proffer our personal opinions.

Table 20.1 Suggested format for ethical decision-making in fertility counseling [15].

1. Identify the ethical dilemma(s).
2. Review current literature.
3. Determine the relevant ethical principles and practice standards involved.
4. Review existing laws, policies and procedures.
5. Address practical considerations.
6. Balance multiple perspectives of all stakeholders.
7. Generate alternative courses of action.
8. Consider the anticipated consequences of each alternative.
9. Select and implement a course of action.
10. Evaluate the outcome. Implement changes, as needed.

Step 1: Identify the ethical dilemma(s)

What are the issues?

Maleficence

We would inform Dr. Goodheart of potential problems that may arise which could harm the participants. Amanda, the potential donor still in an early stage of pregnancy, has not completed building her family. Should Amanda miscarry or give birth to a child with physical or mental limitations, she may regret donating any of her remaining embryos, wishing to have them all for future IVF cycles. Conversely, Amanda may worry the embryos donated to Rebecca would develop into a child with disabilities. It is unknown whether the patients currently could address these issues other than on a hypothetical level. Dr. Goodheart should inform Rebecca about increased risk for fetal chromosomal abnormalities associated with Amanda's age, which is older than most accepted oocyte donors.

Hopefully, our consultation with Dr. Goodheart would alert her to any blind spots she may have as a result of her own infertility and subsequent failed treatments. Fertility counselors' personal reproductive histories and fertility experiences may influence their reactions to clients. If she were so inclined, prior to self-disclosure, we would advise Dr. Goodheart to consider her reasons for the disclosure and whether it would be beneficial to the clients. Whether a self-disclosure is ethical depends on many factors, including the therapist's rationale for the disclosure, the personality traits and psychological issues of the client to whom the disclosure is made, and the specific circumstances surrounding the disclosure. We would emphasize the importance of the MHP's careful documentation of her disclosure in her therapeutic records.

Conflict of interest

Neither of us prefers those situations where both the donor(s) and recipient(s) are being treated by the same RE. Larger practices employing two or more physicians are best able to accommodate designated sperm, oocyte and embryo donors and their recipients. However, for patients residing in less densely populated areas, it is not uncommon for both to use the same RE. One might also question if a conflict of interest exists when both donors and recipients meet with the same MHP. However, it is deemed preferable the two couples meet with the same MHP rather than not have an opportunity to obtain psychoeducational input from any MHP at all.

We would inform Dr. Goodheart that, where possible, it is preferable for each couple to be seen by different physicians so each doctor can advocate for his or her own patients. Considering Amanda and Chuck's best interest, their RE, following the ASRM practice guidelines [16], might be inclined to recommend they wait until they have completed building their family prior to embryo donation. Acting in Rebecca and Rick's best interest, their RE might recommend not using Amanda and Chuck's embryos, preferring they choose embryos from younger donors. Additionally, Rick and Rebecca's physician might want them to quickly proceed, because pregnancy complications often arise when the intended mother is of an advanced age.

Competence to practice

Although Dr. Goodheart has had fertility treatment, it is apparent she does not have the requisite expertise to practice as a fertility counselor. We believe Dr. Goodheart, with whom Rebecca and Rick have scheduled an appointment, lacks the necessary information and training to work with couples and/or individuals who are contemplating the use of designated donor embryos. On the most elementary level, she is ignorant of the fact that apart from her appointment with Rebecca and Rick, she needed to schedule an additional session to separately consult with Amanda and Chuck. Dr. Goodheart also needed to schedule a joint session, during which both couples would have the opportunity to discuss their expectations of this procedure.

The final conjoint session will usually include an in-depth discussion of potential problem areas for the donors and recipients. The fertility counselor will note red flags that might cause Amanda and Chuck, as well as Rebecca and Rick, to be uncomfortable moving forward with treatment. We both have experienced the dissolution of designated arrangements because the unspoken problems finally had been openly addressed with an objective party: the fertility counselor. During the final session the participants would also discuss their wishes regarding disclosure to the child created from Amanda and Chuck's embryo, the child Amanda is currently carrying, as well as to others, such as family members, friends and so on, and the impact this means of family building may have on their ongoing relationship during the potential pregnancy and long after. We routinely present our patients with a template for disclosure we personally have developed, which we would provide to Dr. Goodheart.

We don't believe many MHPs would be aware of the issue of compensation to known donors and GCs. Very frequently known donors or GCs state they do not wish to receive compensation and ASRM guidelines state that embryo donors should receive no compensation for the embryos [16]. As consultants, we could inform Dr. Goodheart that presents to known embryo donors are usually appreciated and ethically acceptable, especially when in the form of a gift to the donor's child.

Confidentiality and dual roles

All participants in this type of third party reproduction, as well as the MHP, live in the same community and are members of the same church. Can Dr. Goodheart be objective in assessing whether to continue treating these clients? What are the potential biases that can be ethically navigated? Both the limited competence to practice and the multiple roles of the clients and the MHP involved in this scenario need to be balanced against the potential for harm of not seeing these clients in advance of continuing this third party reproductive arrangement should they have no access to other fertility counselors.

Who are the stakeholders involved?

- Amanda, Rebecca, their respective spouses, the RE, and the potential offspring of each couple are all stakeholders.

Who will make the ultimate decision?

- In all likelihood, with the input of Dr. Goodheart, the RE will make the decision as to whether and when to proceed with the designated donation. This may create a conflict of interest as the RE is treating both Amanda and Rebecca.

What are the parameters of the situation, including contextual? What facts are known? What facts are not known?

- We would advise Dr. Goodheart to give the patients the opportunity to explore their feelings and think through the ramifications, both short and long term, of embryo donation. However, it is doubtful we could adequately educate Dr. Goodheart in such a brief period of time. We would ask Dr. Goodheart to inquire whether Chuck and Amanda intend to have additional children, and thoroughly discuss the timing of Rick and Rebecca's fertility treatment.
- There appears to be limited choice of MHPs with competence in fertility counseling in the geographic area in which the donors and recipients live.
- Without adequate consultation, Dr. Goodheart may have failed to offer the embryo donors and recipients available resources to help them decide whether this is an acceptable option to them. Dr. Goodheart, Amanda, Chuck, Rebecca and Rick are part of the same church community which may create dual roles and/or multiple relationships, as well as potential problems with maintaining appropriate boundaries and the confidentiality of all parties involved, including that of the MHP.

Step 2: Review current relevant scientific, medical and psychosocial literature

The medical literature suggests embryo freezing is safe, for both the embryo and the potential child/ren created, and is relatively successful [17–19].

- Amanda has not had to undergo any additional medical procedures in order to make this donation.

The available psychosocial literature has found individuals report high levels of ambivalence concerning the donation of surplus embryos.

- Disposition decisions are highly emotionally challenging and most couples, once they have completed their families, choose to dispose of their excess embryos, freeze them indefinitely, or abandon them [20]. Moreover, the majority of couples changed their disposition choices between the time their embryos were created and follow-up three to nine years later [21,22].

There is virtually no psychosocial research on embryo donor offspring or the offspring of the individuals or couples who have donated their excess embryos.

- It is uncertain whether research on offspring of gamete donation can be generalized to this population because of the psychological complexity of family creation by embryo donation. Designated donation involving two couples who reside near each other, work together and fraternize with one another adds to the potential for complications.

Step 3: Determine the relevant ethical principles and practice standards involved

Review relevant formal ethical codes and standards. If applicable, look to other professions and other countries for guidance. As consultants, we would provide Dr. Goodheart with the following information.

- **American Psychological Association Ethical Principles of Psychologists and Code of Conduct (2010)** [23]. Importance of autonomy, beneficence, competence to practice, obtaining voluntary informed consent and avoidance of dual roles/conflict of interest.

- **ESHRE Task Force on Ethics and Law III: Gamete and embryo donation (2002)** [24]. Careful counseling of both donor and recipients is indispensable for known donation; explanation by a MHP that parenthood increases the awareness of the meaning and implications of embryo donation and is strongly recommended for the donor who must also obtain consent of her partner; and focusing on welfare of future child(ren).
- **Practice Committee of the American Society for Reproductive Medicine and the Practice Committee of the Society for Assisted Reproductive Technology, (2013)** [16]. ASRM strongly recommends psychological consultation with a qualified MHP for all couples considering a designated donation. The committee opinion specifically states that it should occur after the donor couple has concluded their own attempts at reproduction, with the potential impact of the relationship between the donor and recipient explored; and a three-month waiting period with appropriate follow-up assessment between the time a couple signs the consent form to donate embryos and the actual donation to a recipient couple. This waiting period, however, is referencing excess frozen embryos that are donated after the individual(s) have completed building their family.

Try to define the problem in terms of the ethical principles and values that may conflict.

- Informed consent must be ensured, which is questionable because the MHP currently is not qualified to practice in the area of assisted reproduction and cannot adequately educate the couples about the multiple aspects of embryo donation. There is a conflict between autonomy vs. beneficence and nonmaleficence. We believe fertility counselors must consider patient autonomy; however, we must not harm those participating in this collaborative reproductive alternative, and must prevent harm to the potential children born to each couple. There are multiple relationships between the MHP, embryo recipients and donors (i.e., all reside in the same small town and are congregants of the same church), and potentially competing interests exist as the RE is providing services to both donor and recipient couple.

Rank the ethical principles and standards of practice to determine priorities when two or more are in conflict.

1. Competence and dual relationship.
2. Informed consent.
3. Autonomy versus nonmaleficence.
4. Conflict of interest.

Step 4: Review existing laws, policies and procedures

Review current standards and laws regarding professional qualifications for fertility counseling.

- Currently, there are no formal graduate programs in the specialized area of fertility counseling. It is doubtful this MHP could competently practice without continuing education about the many issues which ART raises, and particularly third party reproduction. However, until more clinicians worldwide are able to access and receive specialized training in fertility counseling, consultation with colleagues when facing clinical challenges and ethical dilemmas is advised.

Consult with legal colleagues practicing in the field of reproductive medicine, when necessary.

- Embryo donation for family building is regulated by government agencies in the United States [25] and other countries (e.g., the Human Fertilisation and Embryology Authority Code of Practice in the UK). In the USA, state laws on embryo disposition are tracked by the National Conference of State Legislatures [26]. This document indicates what is legally permissible in each state. We would provide Dr. Goodheart with either hard copies of such references or internet links so she could read the relevant information. Law review articles are particularly helpful.

Step 5: Practical considerations

Do discrepancies exist among applicable laws, government policies, employers and ethical principles that can jeopardize the welfare of clients?

- As consultants to Dr. Goodheart, we can attempt to ensure all parties to this embryo donation have explored the potential implications for their relationship and that of the prospective children involved. We expect the various aspects to be openly discussed so as not to jeopardize their friendship and the welfare of the children involved, who will have the same biogenetic progenitors. Knowing Rebecca and Amanda from church, Dr. Goodheart may be unable to be impartial to the donor and recipient who, as good friends, may wish to experience pregnancy together and raise children of approximately the same age. We would need to explore Dr. Goodheart's own feelings to reduce potential countertransferencial issues.

- It is unclear if the RE is pressing to proceed with embryo donation at this time. This would conflict with ethical guidelines. We would strongly recommend Dr. Goodheart obtain the informed consent of both couples so she may discuss with and evaluate the wishes of the RE, to assess whether conflicts exist.

Will doing what seems ethically right cost you time, money, referrals, prestige, a promotion, or your job?

- Fertility counselors may feel torn between the conflicting demands of those who pay for their services, their referral source, third party payers, employers, employees and colleagues. If the referring RE wants to expedite this donation for financial benefit or to please both the donor and the recipient, both of whom are her or his patients, this might create a conflict for Dr. Goodheart. If she follows the guidelines for embryo donation and recommends Amanda and Chuck conclude their own reproductive attempts first, and then wait an additional minimum of three months to reconsider their decision before agreeing to donate embryos to Rebecca, Dr. Goodheart may fear the loss of a potential referral source to her professional practice. We would encourage Dr. Goodheart to discuss the guidelines with the RE. Minimally, this would enable the RE to recognize Dr. Goodheart's earnest desire to become familiar with ASRM guidelines, as well as demonstrate a willingness to take into consideration the RE's reasoning. We would hope this would elevate the RE's opinion of Dr. Goodheart and would demonstrate her concerns for the welfare of the RE's current and future patients.

Step 6: Balance multiple perspectives and evaluate the rights, responsibilities, vulnerabilities and welfare of all parties

- All parties are vulnerable. Should Amanda lose her current pregnancy or have a child with some form of anomaly, disability, or serious illness, she may regret her decision to donate embryos to Rebecca. Also, as research suggests, Amanda and her husband may change their minds about embryo donation after they have given birth to a child. They may become uncomfortable with another genetically related offspring being raised by parents other than themselves, having no control over how their genetic progeny is being raised, as well as knowing that their own child has a donor-linked individual growing up in another family. With the passage of time and after experiencing parenthood, embryo donation may come to feel more like child relinquishment than gamete donation [27,28].
- Rebecca and Rick may be upset if the possibility of embryo donation is suddenly withdrawn, after previously experiencing two failed cycles of IVF. The child(ren) resulting from the donated embryos will have no genetic connection to the recipient parents, but may have a totally related genetic sibling living in another family. This relationship causes greater ethical complexity than either oocyte or sperm donation. The children of both the donor and recipient couple will likely know each other. If their parents have shared the information regarding genetic relatedness with their children, they are likely to have some complicated feelings.
- We are frustrated with the dearth of data generated from prospective studies regarding the donation of excess embryos. In our opinion, although embryo donation has become a more widely available family building option, little is known about the effects on the recipients' children or those to whom they are totally biogenetically related. Consequently, we are unable to provide reliable advice to Dr. Goodheart, as we believe more information is necessary to guide best practices for fertility counselors.
- The recipients are vulnerable to a change in relationship with Amanda and her husband should there be a treatment failure, a problem in

either of their pregnancies, or any conflict between them regarding their parenting style. Because of Amanda's advanced age, they also have greater risk of difficulty conceiving and/or having a healthy child. Rebecca and Rick being of advanced age also raises the issue of the welfare of the child should the demise of either or both of them occur before the child reaches adulthood. However, their ages fall within the limits acceptable to most IVF clinics for recipients of donor eggs.

Step 7: Generate alternative courses of action

Brainstorm.

- In this case, we would explain to Dr. Goodheart the necessity of meeting with all parties involved. We would strongly suggest she determine the reason for the urgency of this embryo donation, and confirm the absence of coercion, for example, should she learn Rebecca is Amanda's supervisor and/or boss at work. Both couples should be interviewed separately and then together as a group to ensure there is no coercion, and to discuss the implications of embryo donation and disclosure issues. Donor and recipient couples should be referred to different attorneys.
- Because Dr. Goodheart is unfamiliar with ASRM's recommended practices and the couples need to be seen immediately, we would recommend referral to a more qualified fertility counselor even if less geographically convenient. At the very least, we would urge her to have several consultations with qualified fertility counselors who could advise her about salient topics, guidelines and pertinent ethical issues. Additionally, acting as her consultants, we will provide Dr. Goodheart with a comprehensive reading list. According to the American Psychological Association [23] Standard 2.01, if a psychologist's boundaries of competence are exceeded and there is no other referral source with greater competence available who is geographically accessible to the client, the psychologist should make a reasonable effort to achieve competence by using relevant research, training and/or consultation with expert colleagues. Although this competency standard pertains to psychologists, similar rules are applicable to other mental health professions.
- It also may be preferable, if possible, to have a MHP whose roles vis-à-vis the participants in this vignette do not overlap (i.e., is not a member of their church), although boundaries are being increasingly blurred as a result of the Internet and social networking. Not all multiple relationships are considered unethical. Questions the MHP should address when a dual relationship exists include: (a) Does it have the potential to cause harm to the clients or disrupt the relationship between the MHP and the client? (b) Can the MHP objectively evaluate the matter at hand? The dual relationship should be openly discussed and proactively managed by Dr. Goodheart as part of the informed consent process, for example discussing how to handle inadvertent public encounters. If the multiple relationships might be reasonably expected to impair Dr. Goodheart's objectivity, or carry the potential for a risk of significant harm or exploitation of the client(s), the multiple relationships should be avoided and referral to another MHP is necessary.
- Discussion with the RE about his or her potential conflict of interest in working with both donors and participants is also recommended. However, discussions about ethical issues can be delicate and occasionally, we believe, unwelcome. Fertility counselors wishing to either remain employed by or consultant to REs may be hesitant to approach topics that could be considered a direct challenge to the physicians' integrity.

Assuming all parties appear to be adequately informed, and no exclusion criteria are present for either donors or recipients, the following alternative courses of action are possible:

- Recommend that Amanda complete her pregnancy and take a reasonable amount of time after the birth of her child (no less than three months) before she and Chuck re-visit their decision to donate embryos to Rebecca and Rick. An agreement stipulating Rebecca's payment of part of the embryo storage fee, if she does receive embryos at a later time, could be negotiated by their attorney.
- Recommend that Amanda and Chuck complete their family before deciding on disposition of any of the remaining embryos.
- Proceed at this time to thaw two of Amanda's embryos and transfer them to Rebecca.

Tap into the collective wisdom of associates by considering consultation with ethically sensitive, experienced and informed colleagues, as well as state or national professional associations.

- In all likelihood, colleagues would recommend Dr. Goodheart refer these patients to a qualified fertility counselor while she becomes proficient in the field. They would advise her to avoid practicing outside of her area(s) of competency, and may encourage her to join ASRM, avail herself of the MHPG's mentoring program, and receive supervision from a fertility counselor practicing within the field of reproductive health and medicine. We believe Dr. Goodheart should consider the measures she would need to take to ensure adequate training.

Step 8: Consider the anticipated consequences of each course of action

We would alert Dr. Goodheart to the various ramifications, and she, in turn, can help her patients weigh the risks against the benefits for each option.

- We could inform Dr. Goodheart about research that indicates how the passage of time and becoming parents can profoundly affect patients' beliefs about the proper use of their surplus embryos and the importance of genetic lines. She could explain one risk of moving ahead immediately with embryo donation is Amanda and Chuck may feel differently about their donation after they become parents. Thus, they cannot, at present, give their fully informed consent. The strong desire to have a child on Rebecca's part may overshadow the implications of using her friend's donor embryos. If the relationship between the two families suffers as a result, this would have an impact on both the adults and the children involved.
- Dr. Goodheart could explain by slowing down the process these possibilities could be avoided, giving the donation process a greater likelihood of a successful emotional resolution. However, there is a risk in reducing Amanda's decision-making autonomy. Moreover, abating the process of embryo donation may result in both couples believing their wishes were being thwarted by the RE, Dr. Goodheart, and medical personnel.

Step 9: Select and implement a course of action that is consistent with the ethical priorities that have been determined as central to the dilemma

Select a course of action.

- The MHP recommends that Amanda and Chuck complete their current pregnancy, consider completing their family, if possible, and then reconsider the decision to donate any surplus embryos to Rebecca and Rick.

  Implement the decision.

- Dr. Goodheart would clearly express her recommendations in this situation and document her reasons in her report to the IVF clinic. If the RE, who has the ultimate responsibility for the treatment plan, agrees with Dr. Goodheart's recommendations, she could meet with the donors and recipients and discuss the decision with all affected parties.

Document your decision and whether or not it was implemented as part of a good standard of care.

- We would advise Dr. Goodheart to keep a thorough record of her consultations with all involved, including professional consultants and the decision-making process, as well as the reactions of donors and recipients. Documentation of the content of communication with the RE should also be recorded.

What would be the implications of this decision if it was applied as a general rule?

- Couples wishing to donate their surplus embryos to others whom they know would need to complete their family first and re-visit their decision to donate at a later time (a minimum of three months and preferably longer between consent and actual donation). This would reduce patient autonomy. Agreement to a reasonable reimbursement of cryopreservation fees by the recipient to the donor would be allowed.

If you told your chosen option to a respected colleague or a newspaper or television audience, what would they say?

- We would not anticipate much, if any, disagreement with this decision based on the present research and professional ethical guidelines.

Identify the strongest counter-argument(s) to the option you are leaning towards. Can you rebut this argument?

- Probably the strongest counter-argument is the emphasis on patient autonomy in medical decision-making. In rebuttal we would note: although patient autonomy is reduced, before successfully completing the current pregnancy, Amanda and Chuck are unable to provide informed consent to donate excess embryos as they cannot know how they will feel about this decision until after they have given birth to their child. Having them wait until they have completed their family building efforts is consistent with following the guidelines promulgated by ASRM [16, p. 61].

Guard against becoming such a strident advocate of any position which causes you to fail to evaluate the needs of a particular individual and/or family regarding their values, culture, religious beliefs and social context.

- Of any of the possible reasons we hypothesized for the expedited embryo donation, including the desire, as friends, to share a pregnancy experience and parent children of similar age, none would appear to supersede the need for beneficence, that is, allowing the passage of time to minimize the possibility of regret. However, many of our patients try to become parents for a very long time. Any delay is seen as a huge obstacle thwarting their efforts. Amanda (at age 42) and Rick (age 50) would probably be loath to wait and therefore might wish to choose another option, for example, receiving other available embryos, availing themselves of oocyte and sperm donation, or attempting to adopt.

Consult with other resources (e.g., a hospital ethics committee or the ethics committee of your professional organization) and document this phase of decision-making should others challenge your rationale for your final decision and corresponding actions.

- Full documentation would be maintained for the number of years recommended by the state or jurisdiction within which the MHP is working or longer as recommended by ESHRE and ASRM when donor gametes are involved. We would inform Dr. Goodheart about the relevant guidelines during our consultation.

Step 10: Evaluate the outcome of the decision and implement changes, as needed

Assume personal responsibility for the consequences of your action. To what extent did your action bring about the intended consequence(s)? To what extent were there unforeseen consequences? Would you act again in the same way or choose a different response to the situation?

- We would hope Amanda, Rebecca and their respective spouses would be appreciative of Dr. Goodheart's discussion of the possible ramifications of proceeding with embryo donation during Amanda's pregnancy, as well as the psychoeducational discussion regarding suggested methods and timing of disclosure, both to the children involved and to family and friends. We have found it extremely difficult to gauge the outcome of our patients' actions, as fertility counselors are rarely informed about long-term consequences to the donors, recipients and the resulting children. We find this lack of feedback to be frustrating because the absence of relevant information diminishes our ability to facilitate better decision-making for patients in the future.

If your action brought about new ethical challenges, determine what steps you would need to take to address the consequences. Make every effort to correct any negative outcomes. Modify your course of action as required or re-engage in the decision-making process, if necessary. Consider the implications for future planning and prevention, for example, create new or modify existing clinic or practice policies.

- We recommend professional guidelines for embryo donation be amended to incorporate psychosocial research indicating time is needed between the initial decision to create embryos and the determination to donate excess embryos, even in the case of known recipients (i.e., designated embryo donation) to reduce the possibility of coercion, allow donors to reappraise their current situation and decision regarding supernumerary embryos, and provide current, voluntary informed consent.

Conclusions

MHPs act ethically when we operate within the boundaries of our professional competence. Fertility counselors, in accordance with ethical standards, allow their clients autonomy and self-determination, and treat patients with beneficence and nonmaleficence. If no ethical standards and ethical principles currently exist within fertility counseling, MHPs are governed to follow those of their specific profession (e.g., social work, marriage and family, psychology, etc.). Additionally, fertility counselors, mindful of following ethical standards and principles, provide patients with the information necessary to obtain their clients' informed consent.

Furthermore, ethical behavior requires fertility counselors to avoid dual roles and conflicting relationships, and when not possible, we are instructed to make sure our objectivity is not impaired. Ethics mandate fertility counselors to recognize their commensurate responsibility to all parties involved in third party collaborative reproductive arrangements. Additionally, adequate maintenance of patient records is required by ethical standards, as is the respect for patient diversity.

The authors, who have been practicing within the area of reproductive health and medicine for a combined total of more than 50 years, came to understand early on that our experiences influence our professional work. We acutely recognize the potential biases and/or ethical boundary transgressions that may be created by our personal childbearing and fertility experiences, and recommend to others they be cognizant of these factors in order to avoid unethical practices. We both employ structured decision-making strategies when confronting ethical dilemmas and take comfort from adherence to a formal procedure, as compliance guides ethical behavior.

A formal decision-making procedure is intended to reduce the incidence of impulsive, poorly considered decisions by encouraging consideration of all relevant factors. The best possible outcome when confronting ethical conflicts is more likely to be achieved if sufficient time has been allotted to collect all pertinent information; the individual or entity to whom one owes primary allegiance has been properly identified; all relevant stakeholders have been involved; ongoing evaluation of data and decisions is maintained to allow for mid-course corrections, if necessary; and the ethical decision-making process is properly documented [14]. Even though we may be frustrated that consideration of ethical dilemmas requires significant tolerance for uncertainty and yields no one correct answer, through our carefully reasoned attempts to resolve the various conundrums faced, MHPs can practice ethically in the field of fertility counseling, improve patient care and patient satisfaction, and contribute to the value of assisted reproductive technology to all parties involved.

Reflections

The field of reproductive health and medicine has greatly changed over the years. Evolving guidelines are regularly amended by those serving on practice and ethics committees of ASRM, ESHRE, and so on, which guide fertility counselors' best practices. Fertility counselors serve on many of these committees, and are able to inform committee members practicing within other specializations about psychological factors.

Some of the changes we have experienced include intergenerational oocyte donation from daughters to mothers, which has been generally abandoned as coercion can never be totally ruled out. Traditional surrogacy has almost vanished, and with it many of the protracted legal battles regarding parentage. The routine suggestion from physicians to sperm or oocyte recipients not to disclose their use of donated gametes still does occur, albeit less frequently. However, influenced by the wisdom of fertility counselors, we have been able to educate professionals and patients alike regarding the negative ramifications of family secrets and the benefits of offspring knowing their genetic histories. We are pleased to report professionals in the field more frequently treat gay and lesbian individuals and couples attempting to build their families through ART, and believe these advances have come about in no small part due to the influence of fertility counselors.

Moreover, we are very concerned about the practice of referrals to MHPs who do not specialize in fertility counseling. Generalists continue to conduct evaluations of potential gamete donors and GCs, as well as meet with recipients for their psychoeducational sessions. These patients, in our opinion, are not receiving adequate information and, consequently, cannot provide their legitimate, informed consent for treatment. Fertility counselors, unless they have received the necessary education, training and subsequent supervision, are equally unable to conduct neuropsychological evaluations for head trauma wounds or child custody evaluations for the judicial system. Similarly, a podiatrist could not perform testicular sperm extraction or embryo transfer. Licensure in social work, mental health counseling, or psychology does not prepare us to conduct all types of psychotherapy, and changes in our ethical guidelines to reflect the necessity for referral specifically to qualified fertility counselors, in our opinion, are long overdue.

References

1. International Union of Psychological Science. Universal Declaration of Ethical Principles for Psychologists. 2008. www.sagepub.com/cac6study/pdf/UniversalDeclaration.pdf. http://www.sagepub.coms (Accessed May 11, 2014.)
2. Hendricks BE, Bradley LJ, Southern S, Oliver M, Birdsall B. Ethical code for the International Association of Marriage and Family Counselors. *The Family Journal* 2011; 19: 217–24. http://www.iamfconline.org/public/department3.cfm (Accessed October 21, 2014.)
3. International Federation of Social Workers. Second Draft Document: Ethics in Social Work Statement of Principles. 2012. http://ifsw.org/policies/statement-of-ethical-principles/. (Accessed May 11, 2014.)
4. Leach MM, Glosoff HL, Overmier JB. International Ethics Codes-A Follow-up Study of Previously Unmatched Standards and Principles. IUPsyS Global Resource. 2009. http://e-book.lib.sjtu.edu.cn/iupsys/ethics/ethics2_info.htm. (Accessed May 11, 2014.)
5. Leach MM, Harbin JJ. Psychological ethics codes: A comparison of twenty-four countries. *Int J of Psychol* 1997; 32: 181–92. http://e-book.lib.sjtu.edu.cn/iupsys/ethics/ethics_info.htm. (Accessed May 11, 2014.)
6. Beauchamp TL, Childress JF. *Principles of Biomedical Ethics*, 6th edn. New York, Oxford University Press, 2009.
7. Kitchener KS. Intuition, critical evaluation and ethical principles: The foundation for ethical decisions in counseling psychology. *Couns Psychol* 1984; 12: 43–55.
8. Pettifor JL. Professional ethics across national boundaries. *Eur Psychol* 2004; 9: 264–72.
9. Frith L. The use of clinical ethics committees in infertility clinics. *Hum Fertil* 2009; 12: 89–94.
10. Canadian Fertility and Andrology Society. Counseling Special Interest Group of the Canadian Special Interest Group of the Canadian Fertility and Andrology Society. Assisted Human Reproduction Counseling Guidelines. 2009. https://www.cfas.ca/index.php?option = com_content&view = article&id = 936%3Aassisted-human-reproduction-counselling-practice-guidelines&catid = 999%3Aguidelines-counsellors-sig-&Itemid = 521 (Accessed May 11, 2014.)
11. ESHRE Psychology and Counselling Special Interest Group. Guidelines for Counselling in Infertility. 2001. http://www.eshre.eu. (Accessed on May 11, 2014.)
12. Mental Health Professional Group of the American Society for Reproductive Medicine. Qualification guidelines for mental health professionals in reproductive medicine. In: Covington SN and Burns LH, eds. *Infertility Counseling: A Comprehensive Handbook for Clinicians*, 2nd edn. New York, Cambridge University Press. 2006; 559–60.
13. Pope KS, Vasquez MJJ. *Ethics in Psychotherapy and Counseling: A Practice Guide*, 2nd edn. San Francisco, Jossey-Bass/Wiley, 2011.
14. Koocher GP, Keith-Spiegel P. "What Should I Do?" Ethical Risks, Making Decisions, and Taking Action. 2012. http://www.continuingedcourses.net/active/courses/course050.php. (Accessed May 11, 2014.)
15. Horowitz JE, Galst JP, Elster N. *Ethical Dilemmas in Fertility Counseling*. Washington, DC, American Psychological Association, 2010.
16. Practice Committee of the American Society for Reproductive Medicine and the Practice Committee of the Society for Assisted Reproductive Technology. Recommendations for gamete and embryo donation: A committee opinion. *Fertil Steril* 2013; 99: 47–62.
17. Bankowski BJ, Lyerly AD, Faden RR, et al. The social implications of embryo cryopreservation. *Fertil Steril* 2005; 84: 823–832.
18. Takahashi K, Mukaida T, Goto T, et al. Perinatal outcome of blastocyst transfer with vitrification using cryoloop: A 4-year follow-up study. *Fertil Steril* 2005; 84: 88–92.
19. Wennerholm UB, Soderstrom-Anttila V, Bergh C, et al. Children born after cryopreservation of embryos or oocytes: A systematic review of outcome data. *Hum Reprod* 2009; 24: 2158–72.
20. Bangsboll S, Pinborg A, Yding AC, et al. Patients' attitudes towards donation of surplus cryopreserved embryos for treatment or research. *Hum Reprod* 2004; 19: 2415–19.
21. Klock SC, Sheinin S, Kazer RR. The disposition of unused frozen embryos. *N Engl J Med* 2001; 345: 69–70.
22. Newton CR, Fisher J, Feyles V, et al. Changes in patient preferences in the disposal of cryopreserved embryos. *Hum Reprod* 2007; 22: 3124–8.
23. American Psychological Association. Ethical principles of psychologists and code of conduct,

including 2010 amendments. 2010. http://www.apa.org/ethics/code/index.aspx. (Accessed May 11, 2014.)

24. ESHRE Task Force on Ethics and the Law III. Gamete and embryo donation. *Hum Reprod* 2002; 17: 1407–8.

25. United States Food and Drug Administration. 21 CFR parts 210, 211, 820, 1271, Eligibility determination for donors of human cells, tissues, and cellular and tissue-based products; final rule and notice.

26. National Conference of State Legislatures. http://www.ncsl.org/issues-research/health/embryo-and-gamete-disposition-laws.aspx. (Accessed May 11, 2014.)

27. Brakman S-V. Embryo adoption. *The Lahey Clin Med Ethics J* 2005; 12: 1–2.

28. de Lacey S. Parent identity and 'virtual' children: Why patients discard rather than donate unused embryos. *Hum Reprod* 2005; 20: 1661–9.

Chapter 21

Legal issues for fertility counselors

Margaret Swain and William Petok

Blind woman sues fertility clinic [1]

DENVER – A woman who has accused a clinic of denying her fertility treatments because she is blind testified yesterday that she felt humiliated when doctors refused to help her become pregnant.

Kijuana Chambers, 33, testified at the start of her trial in federal court that doctors at the Rocky Mountain Women's Health Care Center performed four rounds of artificial insemination in 1999 but stopped when she refused to hire an occupational therapist to evaluate the safety of her home.

Her lawsuit seeks unspecified damages, claiming that the clinic violated the Americans with Disabilities Act.

Miss Chambers said she always wanted a child, but it had seemed impossible because she is a lesbian. She found another clinic to do the procedure and gave birth to a daughter, Laurina, on Jan. 1, 2001.

Introduction

Family building is seldom a straight-line march to the finish, even for those fortunate individuals who avoid a detour into the ethical and legal minefield of assisted reproductive technology (ART). The landscape has become ever more rugged, notably complicated by, among other issues, third party reproductive collaboration, accessibility to care, protections against exploitation of women, and concerns for the safety and well-being of children and potential children. The client is influenced by cultural mores and religious beliefs, as well as by general societal pressure, but also by more practical concerns such as affordability and accessibility of medical care, feasible aspects of participating in these arrangements and the like. Further, the client selects courses of action based not only on personal choice, but also upon the integrated influences of the surrounding local community, and in some sense, through the input of the larger global society. Most importantly, intended parents and their third party helpers often lack fundamental information about the parties' status to any child created – who is a parent, what rights the respective parties possess, and how those rights are protected. Unless appropriately addressed, these issues may contribute to misunderstandings, misperceptions and confusion, all of which may be laid at the feet of the fertility counselor.

Few other areas of clinical counseling are so intimately aligned with the law. The two disciplines grew in parallel tracks as the needs within ART developed. Sometimes, the intertwining provides for affirmative action and clear resolutions. Other times, the lack of qualified assistance from one or both fields is glaring, or simply, the "perfect storm" of circumstances arises and the need becomes excruciatingly apparent. This chapter will guide the fertility counselor in recognizing risky situations, analyzing them with a critical eye, practicing within the parameters of competence, ethics and legal sound stricture, and applying best practice principles.

Case discussion: "Blind women sues fertility clinic"

While no professional wants to practice looking over the shoulder in anticipation of legal action, certain cases do scream, "Look out!" We offer the opening

The addenda referred to in this chapter are available for download at www.cambridge.org/9781107643116. Password: AX164BKR7.

Fertility Counseling: Clinical Guide and Case Studies, ed. Sharon N. Covington. Published by Cambridge University Press.

case as one example of many that require a thoughtful approach and a strong adherence to legal, ethical and good clinical principles. The analysis, while tailored to the particular case, is applicable to other situations with complicated fact patterns and troublesome, sometimes unclear, issues.

This was a case where a legally blind woman sued several physicians and their practices for discriminating against her by refusing to provide infertility services because of her blindness. Further, she claimed discrimination because she was required to provide proof she was fit to be a mother after the defendant had provided those services previously without these assurances. Ultimately, evidence established that the plaintiff's blindness was not a motivating factor in the decision to defer treatment until medically appropriate concerns about her ability to care for the child were resolved. The patient also had a history of clinical depression, was emotionally abused as a child and subsequently demonstrated problems interacting with others. The defendants were able to show that Ms. Chambers consistently perceived that people were always trying to prevent her from following her plans and making her own choices. She admitted to jumping to conclusions about other's desires to interfere with her wishes and that she had a hard time understanding people's true intentions. She also dealt inappropriately with authority figures. A psychiatrist who examined her testified that she had traits of borderline personality disorder as well as major depressive disorder and narcissistic personality disorder [2].

The case is illustrative of a few of the myriad legal issues that a mental health professional (MHP) might consider in working with a patient who is seeking treatment for infertility. It highlights the impact of the law on the delivery of mental health services attached to reproductive medicine clinics. While most cases the MHP will face are not nearly as complex, it points out the multilevel nature of our work and the need for collaboration between knowledgeable professionals on both sides of the law–mental health axis. For example, this case requires a working knowledge of the Americans with Disability Act (the "ADA") [3]. Under the ADA, a disability means a physical or mental impairment that substantially limits one or more of the major life activities of an individual; this includes a disability that is reflected in a person's record, or that individual being regarded/perceived as having such an impairment. Employers may not discriminate against such persons based on their disability. An employer is defined, generally speaking, as an entity engaged in business affecting commerce and having 15 or more employees. Much of the act applies to discrimination in the workplace, but the law also applies to discrimination in housing, education and access to public services, including healthcare.

When a healthcare discrimination claim is filed by a qualified individual with a disability – that is, failing to offer health services in an accessible manner – courts are likely to view the dispute as one that falls within the ADA's remedial scope. Assuming that a plaintiff can show conduct considered discriminatory under the ADA, and a defendant entity cannot prove an affirmative defense – that is, cannot bring its conduct within a legally permissible exception to the rule of nondiscriminatory conduct – the ADA provides a remedy. In situations involving accessible care, the major social challenge is how to create remedies that foster accessibility without placing an undue burden on the program. An undue burden would be a remedy that forces the provider to make a fundamental change in its services.

And, all of these factors must be considered before evaluation of the issues around the patient's infertility!

W. D. Schlaff, MD, one of the physicians involved in this case routinely instructed his staff "don't do anything different for any case." [Oral communication, February 2014, Professor, Department of Obstetrics and Gynecology, Thomas Jefferson University, Philadelphia, PA.] In other words, if we require a psychological evaluation for heterosexual couples who wish to use donor sperm to conceive, then we apply the same standard to anyone wishing to use donor sperm. From an ethical point of view this guidance addresses the American Psychological Associations principles of beneficence, nonmaleficence, justice and respect for people's rights and dignity. (For an in-depth discussion of this topic, see Chapter 22.) It also gives the fertility counselor a clear path to follow when other factors such as personal feelings might come into play.

Ms. Chambers' combined history of abuse and diagnosis of several significant mental disorders gave clear substantiation for the treatment team to tread cautiously in this case. On the face of it, her blindness seems the least of the issues to be considered in determining whether or not fertility treatment was appropriate. However, because she was blind, an entirely new level of scrutiny was required, including the consideration of the aforementioned laws governing individuals with disabilities.

Lynn S. Blyth, PhD, the psychologist, who was part of the treatment team at one of the institutions, was involved in not only evaluating the patient but also working with the staff around the unusual challenges presented by her. She noted that during the initial donor sperm consult the patient had a "chip on her shoulder." [Oral communication, February 2014, Psychologist, Advanced Reproductive Medicine, University of Colorado, Denver, CO.] She had recently moved to Denver for a program that trained blind individuals in self-sufficiency skills and was living in a supported living arrangement. The team approved her to go forward because she originally had good ideas about child management and seemed to understand the medical issues involved in getting pregnant. However, as time went on, she never became self-supporting and her social support network dwindled. It became clear that she had difficulty reading the ovulation predictor kit and requested the nursing staff to do this task for her. The nursing staff, normally helpful and generous, felt burdened and mistreated due to the patient's demeanor towards them. They began to wonder how the woman would be able to care for a baby if she was unable to take care of these relatively less complicated tasks. The psychologist recalls acting as a support person for the nursing staff during this time.

The psychologist ultimately became a case manager of sorts, to the point of contacting various agencies for the blind in hopes of creating a resource team for the patient, but found nothing that would be useful. In fact, she was told that there was "no way" resources of the extent necessary would be available. It was at this juncture that the treatment team eventually decided to terminate treatment. When the lawsuit was brought against the clinic, the psychologist was deposed and noted that she felt confident that her documentation would corroborate her input into what appeared to be a reasonable decision to terminate care. The defendants were ultimately cleared of any wrongdoing [4].

A multidisciplinary approach to crisis management: the fertility counselor's role

Inherent in the highlighted case, but also typical for many situations in fertility counseling, are medical, psychological, nursing and legal issues, all of which influence the final outcome. Collaboration among the various professionals is the best plan to address the interests of the medical practice, the concerns of the professionals involved, and the safety, well-being and equitable treatment of the patient. Assigning possible resolutions and treatments according to the scrutiny suggested below should provide some protection to all the stakeholders. In the development of a team approach, the following guideposts should be in the forefront:

Professional standards of practice for counselors

Professional competency provides the basic theoretical approach of fertility counseling in the context of the law. Competency involves a collection of skills, abilities, habits, character traits and knowledge a person must have in order to perform a specific job well. An individual performs effectively within the professional construct when he/she possesses the skills, abilities and knowledge that constitute competence. Competency is based upon knowledge, training and standards that a profession has identified are necessary to perform a job effectively. These standards, with some variations, provide the bedrock for licensing, credentialing and discipline-specific regulations, both in the USA and abroad. Each fertility counselor is responsible for compliance with the requirements in the jurisdiction of practice.

Credentialing and licensure

In the United States, psychiatrist, psychologists, social workers, psychiatric nurses, counselors and marriage and family therapists are credentialed separately, typically under distinct legislative titles. State statutes provide for a licensing entity that specifies licensing and certification requirements, and enumerates prohibited actions, as well as penalties, for violations of the code. Standards of practice and ethical guidelines are typically promulgated by professional associations, and in some countries, are the basis for licensure. Once adopted by the organization, they may be viewed as the legal standards against which practitioners in each category may be judged. Of interest in the United States are the American Psychological Association's (APA) *Ethical Principles of Psychologists and Code of Conduct* [5], the National Association of Social Workers (NASW) *Code of Ethics* [6], and the National Board for Certified Counselors (NBCC) *Code of Ethics*

[7]. Also pertinent may be: the American Association for Marriage and Family Therapy (AAMFT), *Code of Ethics*; the American Psychiatric Association (the APA), Ethics Primer of the APA, *Opinions of the Ethics Committee on the Principles of Medical Ethics with Annotations Especially Applicable to Psychiatry* [8]; and the American Psychiatric Nurses' Association (APNA), *Scope and Standards of Psychiatric and Mental Health Nursing* [9].

In countries other than the United States, psychiatrists and psychologists are regulated separately from other MHPs, and systems for regulating social workers and other types of counselors are not uniform. For instance, statutory registration systems are used in some Canadian provinces, and in Japan, Hong Kong, Israel, Germany, France, South Africa and the Netherlands. England, Wales and Scotland regulate the training of social workers. In contrast, Australia allows social workers to self-regulate, based on an agreement between the profession, educators and employers. The majority of registration systems operate in tandem with a competency evaluation and a disciplinary procedure, and registration is defined by statute. In the United Kingdom, credentialing of fertility counselors is available through the British Infertility Counselling Association (BICA) and the British Fertility Society (BFS), but is not required [11]. The Infertility Counselling Award is a recently developed joint project of BICA and the BFS. Counselors in the reproductive and assisted conception field may earn this professional designation by completing workshops and other training seminars and by demonstrating the expected competency in professional conduct.

HFEA, in 1991, recommended that the minimum qualifications required for a counselor be a certificate of qualification of Social Work; an equivalent qualification recognized by the Central Council of Education and Training in Social Work; or an accreditation by the British Association of Counselling or Chartered Psychologist status. However, controversial new guidelines in 2009 excluded social workers from the list of "acceptable counseling professionals" [11].

Australia requires that working psychologists comply with registration requirements of the State and Territory Psychologists Registration Boards. Generally, all states or territories require completion of a four-year course of undergraduate study in psychology, and two full-time, additional years of postgraduate work or supervised fieldwork as a probationary/conditional registered psychologist. Social workers are expected to comply with the ethical requirements of state regulatory bodies, such as the South Australian Council on Reproductive Technology, established as a function of the Reproductive Act of 1998 [12].

Professional guidelines for the area of practice

The American Society for Reproductive Medicine (ASRM) Practice Guidelines, while mostly applicable to medical providers, are at least arguably applicable to fertility counselors and attorneys, as practitioners in both professions are accepted as members of the organization and both maintain separate professional groups within ASRM. In the absence of other established guidelines, these recommendations may be legitimately viewed as standards of care against which professional behavior is evaluated and judged. For fertility counselors, the specific standards of practice for each discipline, as well as the bylaws and guidelines of pertinent professional groups within parent organizations for reproductive medicine are critical (e.g., the Mental Heath Professional Group [MHPG] of ASRM). Since the MHPs have a separate professional group within ASRM, the guidelines established through this body do speak specifically to fertility counselors, as do those within ESHRE and its Psychology and Counseling Special Interest Group. Another similar organization is the International Infertility Counseling Organization (IICO). One of the goals of IICO is "...to establish professional standards and guidelines for the psychosocial care and treatment of infertile patients" [13]. The guidelines established by these professional groups fall short of enforceable rules, but nevertheless provide the framework for professional standards, competency, and possibly credentialing for fertility counselors.

Other professional pronouncements

Both ASRM and ESHRE Ethics Committee Opinions are available to members and are printed in the respective society's journals. For example, and of particular interest when considering the Chambers case discussed above, is the ASRM Ethics Committee Opinion regarding Child Rearing Ability and Provision of Fertility Services [14] which recognizes the potential moral responsibility of providers to consider the interest of a future child. The Committee concluded that it may be permissible to turn a fertility patient away if the provider reasonably concludes that patient is likely incapable of safely raising a child. Accordingly, it is possible to withhold services on the basis of *well-substantiated* judgments that patient cannot provide care for a child and does not have an adequate support system to assist him/her. (The Opinion was published after the Chambers case and was not considered in the resolution of the matter.) These types of considered and thoughtfully written opinions provide justification for professional decisions and, should a dispute arise, may provide a basis for defense of those actions.

Laws affecting outcomes for reproductive technology patients

While the fertility counselor is not expected to know and provide information about state and federal law, it is important to recognize that clients may be contemplating arrangements that are restricted or prohibited in their state or country. Acting in contravention to those laws can lead to unintended and highly problematic situations. Advising clients that such laws may exist and apply to their situations, and a consultation with an experienced reproductive law attorney is indicated, is both helpful and appropriate.

General principles of sound business practice

These drive institutional policy and procedure and should be part of the decision-making matrix. It is best practice to develop uniform and consistently applied formal policies for all parts of the fertility counseling practice: financial, process and practical. While counselors who are employed by institutions will be expected to adhere to institutional policies, independent practitioners should employ the same practices as may pertain to their individual businesses. For example, providers in the USA who are in solo practice must still adhere to the guidelines promulgated by the Health Insurance Portability and Accountability Act (HIPAA) [15] and provide policy statements to clients. In addition, anyone who uses a credit card processing machine to collect fees is required to complete a Payment Card Industry (PCI) compliance evaluation every year, adhere to the guidelines developed by the Security Standards Council and document such adherence [16]. As a general statement, informal policies invite misunderstanding and are typically indefensible in a lawsuit. (The recommendations of the Ethics Committee in its child-rearing statement acknowledge this principle.) To protect itself and, if part of a larger group, then to make certain that all members of the team are reliably following clear standards in a predictable manner, the practice should ensure that:

- Written and clear policy and procedures are maintained.
- Such policies are applied uniformly, and exceptions are not entertained without substantial and compelling reason and further review, preferably by an outside entity.
- Any evaluation is customary and usual and part of a standard protocol.
- Patients are informed at the outset that interviews may be conducted with an eye toward evaluating the intended parent's ability to safely participate.

Collaboration with other disciplines

Including members of all the related professions in an orchestrated manner provides for safeguards and protections, not just for the client, but for members of the treatment team, including the private practitioner. Typically, the group might include physicians, nurses, geneticists, embryologists, office managers and practice coordinators, matching program directors and coordinators, fertility counselors and attorneys. When the team members all practice within the same group, the various members should all meet periodically to review cases and patient information, update policy and assess the overall success of the team. Input of other professionals not part of the practice, such as independent fertility counselors and lawyers, should be solicited as needed. For problematic and more complex arrangements, it is wise to have access to an Ethics Review Board. If this is not part of a usual protocol within a facility, such a board could be convened on an ad hoc basis. If practicing as an independent provider, it is useful for the fertility counselor to have a "team" of trusted professionals from other disciplines who can be consulted when difficult issues arise. At a minimum, this team should include an experienced reproductive law attorney and another fertility counselor with comparable or greater experience. Additional consults with knowledgeable physicians and nursing professionals can be useful as well.

A primer for practice

The following are offered as minimal guidelines and suggestions for establishing oneself as a competent provider of fertility counseling services and carrying out those services.

Evidence of competency as a fertility counselor

Proper licensure to practice in the field as a psychologist, social worker, marriage and family therapist or other state sanctioned mental health provider. This would include proof of a degree in the field, the necessary supervised experience to become licensed and evidence of licensure from the state in which one practices. Membership in other professional certifying organizations, such as the National Register of Health Service Psychologists or status as a Certified Social Worker in Health Care (C-SWHC), provide further evidence of competency. Adherence to the minimum standards for training, such as those provided by the MHPG of ASRM or the Psychology and Counseling Special Interest Group of ESHRE, also offer skill-building and aptitude in this specialized field.

Membership in professional organizations devoted to the provision of mental health services to fertility patients. This would include the above mentioned as well as the British Infertility Counseling Association (BICA) and the Australian and New Zealand Infertility Counselors Association (ANZICA). These organizations offer continuing education opportunities not often found in other continuing education programs. In addition, access to current thought and practice in the medical aspects of infertility is available via membership in these organizations. Mentoring programs and the opportunity to consult with thought leaders in the field is available through membership in many of these organizations. Finally, ethical and practice guidelines for the profession are found within their publications.

Building blocks of sound business practice

Forms play an important role in documenting the professional relationship that exists between fertility counselor and clients, whether they are carriers, intended parents, attorneys or medical practices performing ART. Carefully worded, intentional documentation is the key to avoiding misunderstanding and legal mishaps. This would include but not be limited to written statements about policies on confidentiality, privacy (HIPAA) and fees. In the case of evaluations, forms should clearly delineate who is the client; the clinic, the agency, the individual being considered as a gestational carrier or the intended parents. Retainers establish the fertility counselor's role and limitations. The nature of the services to be provided and the compensation for those services are also contained here. These documents are useful in the general practice of providing therapy services and in the more specialized practice of evaluations and psychosocial educational consultations.

Documentation of therapy sessions is essential. There is an old rule in the law that states if it wasn't written down, it didn't happen. While it is impossible to write down everything that takes place in a session, it is possible to document many aspects of one. At a minimum the following information should be contained in a note following a session:

- date, time and length of session
- who was present
- diagnosis code (if appropriate)
- procedure code (ICD – 9, DSM-V or whatever standard is dictated by law and practice guidelines)
- mental status
- session behavior
- level of functioning and stressor levels
- medications
- treatment goals
- homework or recommendations
- narrative note
- signature of therapist.

Documentation becomes quite important should a problem develop. In the great majority of cases no problems do develop and the work goes smoothly. However, in the rare circumstance when something does go awry, having a well-documented record is invaluable to the counselor's professional and mental health! It will also provide valuable assistance for legal counsel, should you need it, and will substantiate your adherence to standards and policies.

An *informed consent* in psychotherapy grew out of a case of the late 1980s, Osheroff v. Chestnut Lodge, in which a client alleged that he was not given access to all available treatments and would have improved dramatically had he been prescribed medication sooner [17]. ASRM practice guidelines address informed consent when conducting psychological screening for ART, as well as when counseling clients about the ART process [18]. A good informed consent will outline the fertility counselor's role with the client during the process, what process and procedures might take place with the context of the interactions, and what the client can expect from the counselor. It will also describe the limits of confidentiality that the counselor must adhere to by law and ethics.

Conflict of interest waivers can ameliorate the difficulty of one fertility counselor representing two parties in an ART arrangement. These documents make it clear that conflicts may exist and a fertility counselor may give advice that is contrary to the wishes of one of the parties. Clients should be given the option of accepting this arrangement, or opting out of treatment or evaluation by the same fertility counselor as is involved with the other party. Professional liability, however, cannot be waived within such documents.

Retainers are often employed by attorneys for similar purposes and will be well understood by the legal professionals with whom you work. A good retainer will outline what action will take place in the event of a dispute [18], as well as describe the services to be performed.

Reports and evaluations are a necessary part of an integrated team approach that includes evaluating and counseling participants in third party arrangements. They are equally present when the counselor is part of a team or an independent practitioner. In either case, the fertility counselor should be certain to document the client's understanding of the nature of the consultation, what information will be contained in any report and that he or she may be disqualified from participation in fertility treatments by the evaluation.

The question of how and by whom those reports may be used, and to whom they may be released, is an irksome one and, among other things, turns on the intent and language in the fertility counselor's consents and releases. Generally speaking, the records belong to the person whose private health information they contain. The client is entitled to those records. If an appropriate, HIPAA-compliant release has been presented and voluntarily and knowingly signed by the client, then the records (or whatever portion of them is designated) may be shared with whomever the client designates. Absent very specific, written restrictions, if someone other than the client has paid for the evaluation, the consent of that payor is not required. If, however, the fertility counselor has an agreement with a referral source that limits release of the report to the fertility center and/or matching program, this must be carefully reviewed with the participant and stated in plain language in the document. Such an agreement may limit release of the records to the client, and will limit release as to any outside parties. In regard to psychological testing, raw test data from the report is not released to clients, clinics or other practitioners in the same way test materials themselves are not to be released according to the APA's ethics guidelines.

Evaluations, as well as other written or electronically generated reports or notes, should be stored in compliance with HIPAA, state law and professional guidelines. In many cases that means these records are to be maintained, securely, for seven years after the end of therapy or, in the case of a minor, three years after the minor reaches the age of majority [19]. Many counselors maintain records in perpetuity as a matter of course. However, it is easy to see how a busy practice could generate significant paper and have a need for off-site storage that is HIPAA compliant. One suspects that as time and technology go forward many of these records will be converted to electronic or digital format, thereby reducing the amount of space they require for maintenance. The question of storage "on the cloud" will become an increasingly important consideration as this happens and one can be sure that the law and professional standards will evolve rapidly.

Disclaimers: wise or waste of time?

A disclaimer is a statement limiting or providing specifics about a scope of responsibility in a legally recognized relationship. Examples of those relationships might be landlord–tenant, host–guest, common carrier–passenger, or parties to a contract. Typically, disclaimers are introduced when there is a risk inherent in the relationship.

Disclaimers may or may not be enforceable. Their enforceability turns on the nature of the disclaimer, the laws of the particular jurisdiction, and whether the aggrieved party consented to the risk or uncertainty addressed in the disclaimer. For instance, if the language of the disclaimer is not clear and unambiguous or if it is not visible or apparent to the concerned party, a court may decide that the party suffering harm never consented to that risk. Additionally, a party seeking the protection of a disclaimer should be certain that the statement includes the specifics of the matter, as opposed to a blanket statement of no liability. Further, if the party is seeking protection from misrepresentation of omission within a contract and it is demonstrated that the party knew that certain facts were misrepresented or omitted, the disclaimer is likely to be set aside.

Fee agreements and similar documents

That said, a careful, unambiguous and specific disclaimer may provide a measure of protection in a contract or other document, but, in the event of a dispute, it does not guarantee recognition and enforceability of its terms. Overly general, boilerplate statements, tacked onto an agreement or other document may potentially be viewed as a mechanism to escape any responsibility whatsoever by the author. These are not useful and may place the writer in a more vulnerable position of scrutiny by a court.

A disclaimer is not likely to protect a professional from a claim of professional malpractice. For example, in many states, a clause in an attorney's fee agreement that attempts to limit his liability or exculpate him for his own negligence, thereby avoiding a claim for legal malpractice, is prohibited. However, laws do vary from state to state. The fertility counselor should be aware of the laws governing the mental health profession and particular licensure regulations or rules.

Reports of evaluations and testing

The fertility counselor should include a particular disclaimer in anticipation of the following situation: an evaluation is conducted and a report issued for a gestational carrier and a set of, or an individual, intended parents. For some reason, the arrangement does not move forward, or is indefinitely postponed. The agency or participant requests that (or simply uses without asking) the report, specifically issued and pertaining only to the gestational carrier and a particular set of intended parents, be recycled for use in a new match, or even for a subsequent arrangement with the same parties. This is concerning because, of course, the relationship between gestational carrier and the intended parents, at that specific point in time, is a critical component. To address this concern, and to protect the fertility counselor, the report should include, in bold writing, the following or similar language:

> *The evaluation documented in this report was conducted for the specific purpose and intent of (name of gestational carrier) acting as a gestational carrier for (name of intended parent/s), in an arrangement to proceed within a reasonable time period from the date of this report. The writer makes no recommendation as to any other circumstance or arrangement that may arise in the future, including the parties entering into a similar situation with another gestational carrier or intended parent. Further, circumstances may change among the parties, which may make this recommendation inappropriate and void as to any future arrangement, even between the same parties.* ***The following comments, opinions and recommendation are limited to the parties evaluated at this time and are only applicable for a reasonable time period within which to complete the presently-contemplated arrangement."***

In summary, it may be wise, and is some circumstances very important, to include disclaimers in certain client documents, such as fee agreements, retainers and reports. If doing so:

- Ensure the language is bold and conspicuous.
- Explain the risks that the disclosure addresses.
- Ask the clients to initial the disclaimer section.
- Use specific and unambiguous language when writing a disclaimer.

Legal consultation

Attorneys and counselors are necessarily involved in third party ART arrangements and working collaboratively serves the best interests of the clients. It is helpful to the legal professionals to understand the evaluation process, the time involved and the timeline for the evaluation to be completed, the cost and the nature of the reports that the fertility counselor provides. The attorney should also understand that the fertility counselor will need an authorization from the client to share the report or other communications.

Fertility counselors may be surprised to learn that many ART agreements, especially gestational surrogacy contracts, require the parties to meet with a counselor if a dispute arises during the term of the agreement, or may require that a party seek counseling if the other party requests it. Should such a consultation be requested, it benefits everyone for the fertility counselor and the attorneys involved to discuss the situation, if for no reason other than the fertility counselor being forewarned that the client(s) will likely be unsettled and perhaps angry. The fertility counselor should ask the client which attorneys are representing the parties in the contract drafting, review and finalization, and request the relevant language for dispute resolution.

In the course of preparing consent forms for the fertility counseling practice, it makes good sense to consult with a qualified and experienced legal

Table 21.1 How to avoid a lawsuit.

Do	Don't
Practice within the scope of your competence	Make exceptions
Follow professional code of ethics	Skip steps
Obtain adequate consents	Fail to document phone calls and other communications
Consult when you have a question	Be afraid to turn down a questionable referral
Be aware of the law and legal implications	Answer legal questions or give legal advice
Establish policies and follow them	Fail to clarify your role to all parties
Follow ASRM/ESHRE practice guidelines	
Refer client for legal consultation with a qualified attorney in third party cases	

professional. Reference examples of consent forms are contained in the addendums, but state-specific requirements should be reviewed with your practice attorney.

Examples of the following documents are contained in the Addendums:

21.1 Release of records
21.2 Informed consent for donors and surrogates
21.3 Informed consent IP
21.4 Authorization to contact attorney
21.5 Attorney letter
21.6 Consent and waiver regarding conflict of interest.

Table 21.1 provides helpful guidance on what fertility counselors need to consider regarding how to avoid legal conflicts.

Dilemmas in policy implementation

An example of how many of the above points can place the fertility counselor in a sticky situation is the following: Many fertility counselors have faced a call from a clinic coordinator, or an attorney representing a gestational carrier or intended parent, requesting an evaluation "quickly." Often these calls indicate that a cycle is about to happen and the psychological evaluation is the only thing holding up the process. The individuals involved are likely under a great deal of stress to complete the process and their urgency is obvious. What do you do under these circumstances? Do you feel compelled to assist the process to move rapidly or do you take a more reasoned approach? Working in this field requires not only an understanding of the medical issues (e.g., "we've got day 3 embryos and need to transfer within 2 days!") as well as the psychological problems inherent in the overall process. Rush situations have unnecessary stress attached to them and undermine the goals associated with the evaluation (i.e., making sure all parties understand the long-range implications of assisted reproduction, are making an informed decision and are at the best place possible to move forward treatment). Are you going to point this out to the parties when you decline the evaluation? Will it have a negative impact on your practice if you do decline or will the parties gain respect for your concern for a best-case outcome and want to work with you in the future? If you accept the case, will you include a disclaimer indicating there is no guarantee that your work will be concluded within the posited time frame? Attorneys also face this pressure, with the same consequences and issues. Your consideration of these types of requests should include a visit to the previously stated business practice guidelines, particularly those addressing exceptions. While circumstances vary from case to case, it is almost always better to adhere to your own internal policies and procedures when addressing these requests.

While this kind of situation provides an opportunity for a "teaching moment," the coordinator, the legal professional or other parties involved may not be open to learn! You may decide that on a one-time basis you'll take the evaluation, turn it around quickly and have a subsequent conversation with the professionals explaining why you can't do it again under future, similar circumstances. Fertility counselors early in their careers who are eager for work may be willing to take the evaluation regardless and worry that to not take the case would not only impact their future reputation, but might well constitute an improper refusal to provide services. Does your state law require that you provide service to anyone who requests it or do you have the ability to refuse a case? In all likelihood you have the right to be selective. It would be unreasonable to expect that every professional has a schedule that permits taking every case opportunity. Furthermore, borrowing from the medical code of "do no harm," you may be colluding to increase stress and reduce positive outcomes. Would it be better for the recipients to have their treatment team plan thoroughly for these situations so no one is subjected to undue pressure and encouraged by the timeline to do shoddy work? Most of us would answer in the affirmative!

Other, more specific issues can give rise to procedural and ethical dilemmas for the fertility counselor. A call came from a couple asking to conduct a psychological evaluation for a gestational carrier (GC). The couple was referred by their reproductive endocrinologist (RE), who was known to the fertility counselor. The wife noted in her call that she had been working with the RE for nine years and that it was clear that they needed a GC. She mentioned that the fertility counselor might want to know that there are "extenuating circumstances." It turned out that those circumstances included the fact that the GC was a single woman who had never given birth. The couple had identified her via an internet advertisement and the physician thought she might make a good candidate because she had a cranial abnormality and would likely never marry or have children.

The fertility counselor not only saw a "red flag" but also heard sirens wailing! This couple was most likely very frustrated by their long treatment without a successful birth. Furthermore, the physician sounded like he was equally frustrated and desperately wanted to help the couple in any way possible. The physician clearly felt that the proposed GC's physical problem was more cosmetic and that created a mitigating circumstance for not observing the ASRM practice guideline that all GCs have given birth before becoming a GC.

On questioning, the fertility counselor ascertained that the couple had not yet retained an attorney but were "looking into it." The fertility counselor explained that an evaluation would be impossible because it violated the practice guidelines of ASRM. The absence of a pregnancy carried to term was a "rule out" for GCs and the counselor adhered to those guidelines. The guideline existed to ensure that the GC could give informed consent and the lack of a prior birth precluded her ability to give it. The explanation went further to include the rationale that, particularly in this case where the GC was unlikely to marry or have a child of her own, she was even more vulnerable to develop an attachment to the fetus and have a difficult time following through with her intention to place the baby with the intended parents. The potential long-term psychological consequences for her were too significant. In fact, what appeared to be a reason to the couple and the physician to use her was a glaring reason to exclude her from consideration. Finally, the fertility counselor advised that the couple seek legal advice sooner rather than later as they pursued a suitable GC. The wife said she understood the fertility counselor's position and thanked the counselor for being frank with her.

Knowing and adhering to the practice guidelines and the possibility of legal complications averted a potential disaster for at least three and possibly four individuals: the GC, the couple and the potential child.

Conclusion

As practices in this area have developed, and science continues to push the limits of the possible, the problematic issues have become even more multifaceted and complex. Our responses must be reasoned, measured and frequently crafted *after* the science has leapt forward. It seems that the interface of law and mental health with regard to reproductive medicine is always playing catch up!

Fertility counselors who pay attention to the issues outlined in this chapter will have tools to reduce their own stress and potential liability, and presumably provide a better service to not only their clients but also to the professionals in other disciplines who refer to them.

Reflections on a combined half-century of practice

WP: Providing mental health services in the field of reproductive medicine has provided a unique opportunity for collaborative work with some of the brightest and most creative professionals with whom I've been able to work. The ability to create families when hope has been severely damaged is truly remarkable. Not only the medical aspects but the complicated legal arrangements necessary can be mind-boggling, as evidenced by the cases we've discussed above. And, since the practice of helping individuals create families is an expensive, time-consuming and stressful proposition, I've had to develop nonjudgmental responses to a degree never discussed in graduate school! Clients are frequently engaged in a process they never anticipated in their worst nightmare. The task of helping them navigate the emotional roller coaster of their infertility is compounded by the frustration they can experience when the complexity of the process prevents speedy resolution. Clients are often upset that their physician or attorney isn't understanding or empathic enough to respond to their emotional needs. Explaining that these highly trained and competent individuals are handling a different aspect of their treatment has become a regular part of the care I provide. This is in no way a knock on either the professionals or the clients involved. Rather, it highlights just how stressful the process is and how much clients expect of all their care providers. Normally rational, thoughtful and competent individuals can become so focused on their goal of having a child that they forget that we specialize rather than generalize in various aspects of reproductive care. And I believe the "confusion" they experience in this area is compounded because we do have to know an extraordinary amount about multiple disciplines, most of which are beyond the scope of our licensure or practice. And if we don't have a good working knowledge of the legal and medical aspects we aren't providing the highest level of care possible. Who in their right mind would sign up for this set of conditions for practice?!

As MHPs, I believe we have another set of conditions to deal with that impacts our practice, generated by media portrayals of reproductive medicine and law in general. Clients read popular press, watch television and movies and receive messages indicating that all physicians, especially "fertility doctors" make enormous sums of money. Furthermore, attorneys are often portrayed as wealthy from their work as well. Certainly, some practices in law and medicine generate significant wealth for their owners. But experience says that a comfortable living is more likely for many and some are doing less well, especially in reproductive law where there is a limit to what one can bill and no third party ever picks up the tab. No one has ever claimed that MHPs get wealthy from this work! And so when I quote a price for an evaluation, which is based on my time and expertise, there is often a push back. Clients have already incurred tens of thousands of dollars in medical and legal fees. My fee is paltry in contrast but it is hard for many clients to appreciate the value when no medical procedure or contract arises out of it. It just seems like an unnecessary add-on to them. It's not concrete and they literally can't get their hands on it. I doubt that there is an easy solution to this but I sure wish there was one! Helping clients understand the highly collaborative nature of our work is a challenge unique to this discipline.

MS: ART lawyers deal with many facets of ART on a daily basis, including policy and professional issues that are not directly client based. Because we spend much time considering the more global aspects of this field, it may be easy to neglect the very real emotional burden that clients bring to us. We are, of necessity, focused on crafting solutions, and not officially assisting with emotional adjustment. However, our clients come to us as a product of their experiences and not in a vacuum. No one begins planning their family by asking for referrals to a reproductive attorney and no one wants to need our services. Recognizing and acknowledging the grief, the emotional exhaustion and financial cost of infertility, and the loss of control regarding their family building journey has, I think, allowed me to better serve my clients. After all, stripping our work down to the bare bones, we are taking what is normally a human act of intimacy and reducing it to a business transaction. This can't feel right to the client sitting across from us, and remembering this can drive a more empathetic approach to the legal aspects of the fertility treatment.

One more lesson dovetails with my co-author's reflections. Throughout the years, many of us have occasionally been asked to assist with or provide legal advice for situations that were unusual and pushing the limits of not just our own comfort levels but sometimes also of widely held ethical tenets. Although none of these various suggested actions may have technically been illegal, they could be best described as questionable. In the earlier years of practice, I would torture myself thinking about them, turning them over and over, trying to find a way to help the client without disregarding my own moral compass, or frankly, jeopardizing my practice. In the end, I would just report that I didn't have the time to devote to the case and, yes, that would be a total avoidance of the core issues. Now, I am much more likely to spend time explaining that I believe something is unacceptable, and why I think it is wrong and simply say I won't accept the referral for those reasons. I might not make new friends or clients that way, but maybe I've helped someone from taking a disastrous step in the wrong direction (and, that "someone" may well have included me!).

References

1. Blind woman sues fertility clinic. *Washington Times* (Internet) 2003 Nov 12 [cited 2003 Nov 12]. Available from: http://www.washingtontimes.com/news/2003/nov/12/20031112-115222-2089r/?page=all
2. Colorado Cross-Disability Coalition, "Rocky Mountain Women's Health Care," Accessed

February 27, 2014,. Available from http://www.ccdconline.org/case/196.

3. Harkin T. *Americans with Disabilities Act of 1990, Title 4, Chapter 126*. Washington (DC). The United States Senate; 1990, July 26.
4. Morian K (ed.) Kijuana Chambers v. Rocky Mountain Women's Health Care Center [Internet]. 2003. Accessed April 3, 2014. http://www.morelaw.com/verdicts/case.asp?n=00-CV-1794&s=CO&d=26278.
5. American Psychological Association. *Ethical Principles of Psychologists and Code of Conduct*. Washington: The American Psychological Association; 2010.
6. National Association of Social Workers. *Code of Ethics [pamphlet]*. Washington: National Association of Social Workers; 1996.
7. National Board for Certified Counselors. *National Board for Certified Counselors (NBCC) Code of Ethics [pamphlet]*. Washington: 2013.
8. Klemmer H. et al. *Principles of Medical Ethics with Annotations Especially Applicable to Psychiatry 2013 Edition*. Arlington, VA: American Psychiatric Association; 2013.
9. 2012 Workgroup. *Scope and Standards of Practice, Draft*. Silver Spring, MD: American Nurses Association; 2012.
10. *British Infertility Counseling Association Accreditation Scheme [Internet]*. Sheffield, UK: British Infertility Counseling Association; 2009 [cited 2014 May 31]. Available from: http://www.bica.net/accreditation-scheme.
11. Human Fertilisation Embryology Authority. *Code of Practice, 8th Edition [Internet]*. London: Human Fertilisation Embryology Authority; 2009 [Cited 2014 May 18]. Available from: http://www.hfea.gov.uk/code.html.
12. Norman RJ. Enquiry into scientific, ethical and regulatory aspects of human cloning. *House of Representatives Standing Committee on Legal and Constitutional Affairs (Australia)*. 2000, Feb. 4 p.
13. Mission statement for IICO [Internet]. [Cited 2014 May 22]. Available from: http://www.iico-infertilitycounseling.org/kinderbuecher/
14. Ethics Committee of the American Society for Reproductive Medicine. Child-rearing ability and the provision of fertility services. *Fertil Steril*. 2009; 92: 864–67.
15. Health Insurance Portability and Accountability Act of 1996, *Public Law 104–191*. Washington (DC). The United States Senate; 1996, August 2.
16. PCI SSC Data Security Standards Overview [Internet]. [Cited 2014 May 29]. Available from: https://www.pcisecuritystandards.org/security_standards/index.php.
17. Hanafin H. Surrogacy and gestational carrier participants. In: Covington SN and Burns LH, Eds. *Infertility Counseling: A Comprehensive Handbook for Clinicians (2nd Edn.)* Cambridge: 2006; 374.
18. Swain ME. Legal issues in infertility counseling. In: Covington SN and Burns LH, Eds. *Infertility Counseling: A Comprehensive Handbook for Clinicians (2nd Edn.)* Cambridge: 2006; 530.
19. The American Psychological Association. Record keeping guidelines. *Am Psychol*. 2007; 62: 993–1004.

Chapter 22

Cross-border reproductive services and fertility counseling

Petra Thorn and Eric Blyth

Simon (42) and Sally (40) have had several failed treatment cycles with donor sperm. They had always assumed that Simon's diagnosis of a low sperm count was the only factor limiting their fertility. As a result of treatment taking several years, Sally has also been diagnosed with infertility due to poor ovarian response. She was advised that it has become very unlikely that she will conceive using her own oocytes. The couple is now considering oocyte donation in combination with ICSI. As oocyte donation is prohibited in their home country, they have to travel abroad. In addition, they only find very limited information and are uncertain which country and which clinic to travel to. They feel confused by the infinite amount of information they find online and have the impression that much of this information is unreliable. At the same time, they feel time is pressing, and they want to continue treatment as soon as possible and hopefully finally conceive.

Traveling to another country for medical and for fertility treatment is not a new phenomenon. For centuries, couples have traveled to places considered conducive to infertility, such as spas, fertility shrines and specific landmarks in the hope that these will have a positive impact on their fertility. The development of in vitro fertilization (IVF) has brought hope to many experiencing infertility and, together with quick and affordable international travel, has provided the momentum for cross-border reproductive services (CBRS). Those experiencing fertility problems who faced limited access to, or availability of, appropriate services in their own countries started to consider travel abroad to access services that they hoped would realize their family building aspirations. Although IVF and related procedures have become available quickly in many developed and developing countries, various factors have contributed to individuals and couples traveling for treatment. Key amongst these are:

- law evasion in jurisdictions with restrictive legislation (e.g., prohibition of oocyte donation in Italy and Germany; prohibition of sperm donation in jurisdictions subject to Sharia law; prohibition of either commercial or altruistic surrogacy in many jurisdictions);
- lengthy waiting lists for, or unavailability of, specific services (e.g., oocyte donation in the United Kingdom, sperm donation for couples in a same-sex relationship or single women in several jurisdictions);
- the wish to undergo fertility treatment without the knowledge of family or friends;
- the wish to undergo treatment in the individual's or couple's country of origin; and
- beliefs that treatment in another country may be more successful and/or less costly.

As a consequence, although accurate and robust data are not available, the number of individuals and couples engaging in CBRS is believed to have risen significantly over the last 20 years [1–3]. According to a pilot study carried out by ESHRE (European Society of Human Reproduction and Embryology), 24 000 to 30 000 treatment cycles alone were provided annually to foreign patients in the following six destination countries: Belgium, the Czech Republic, Denmark, Slovenia, Spain and Switzerland [4]. Patients had travelled from 49 different "home" countries, with approximately two-thirds of patients coming from Italy (31.8%), Germany (14.4%), the

Fertility Counseling: Clinical Guide and Case Studies, ed. Sharon N. Covington. Published by Cambridge University Press.

Netherlands (12.1%) and France (8.7%). It is not surprising that country-specific associations were observed. The majority of Italians traveled to Switzerland and Spain, most Germans to the Czech Republic, most Dutch and French patients traveled to Belgium and – to a lesser extent – Spain. The nature of these flows can be explained largely by the relatively easy access provided by shared national borders. French, Norwegian and Swedish patients were the most likely to travel for sperm donation, while Denmark, Belgium and Switzerland were the most popular destinations for sperm donation. Patients from Germany and the UK were the most likely to travel for oocyte donation, and Spain and the Czech Republic were the most popular destination countries for both oocyte and embryo donation. Extrapolating the data relevant for Germany, we can assume that approximately 2000 German couples travel annually mainly for egg donation. (See Table 22.1 for a listing of patient's home countries and the destination country for treatment.) Survey data from the United States indicate that 4% of all fertility treatments (around 6000 cycles p.a.) is provided for non-US domiciliaries [12,13]. The largest groups of incoming patients are from Latin America (39%) – as with the European findings, geographical proximity contributing to a significant extent – and Europe (25%). By contrast, the incidence of patients from the US traveling abroad for care is estimated to be far lower than the rate of incoming patients [6,12].

On an international level, Blyth et al. [14] have shown that:

- patients travel from more or less anywhere to everywhere, although not all destination countries have a reputation for high-quality service provision;
- a number of countries are both home and destination countries; and
- although, in general, patients report a relatively high level of satisfaction with the services they have received, clinical experience also suggests that some clinics leave questions unanswered. For example, there can be little transparency regarding recruitment strategies and financial compensation for donors and surrogates, and counseling is seldom available. In addition, treatment contracts may be minimal and only cover issues relevant for the clinic.

While not all CBRS arrangements give major cause for concern, those that are potentially most problematic remain under-researched. There is emerging evidence of potentially serious risks to patients, donors, surrogates and children, such as high numbers of multiples, unknown quality of medical services for donors and surrogates, and offsprings' lack of access to their gamete or embryo donor or surrogate (see, for example, [3,15]). Furthermore, there has been criticism regarding the dearth of available information. Despite the growth of the CBRS industry, there is only minimal international monitoring and little is known of the services provided by, and remuneration of, intermediary

Table 22.1 CBRS: Home and destination countries (compiled by the authors based on data from recent studies [3–11]).

Home Country	Destination Country	Service
Australia	Thailand	Sex selection
Canada	USA	Donor oocytes
Denmark	Baltic States, Czech Republic, Greece, Russia, Span	Donor oocytes
Egypt	Spain, other European countries	Donor oocytes
France	Belgium	Donor sperm
Germany	Spain, Czech Republic	Donor oocytes
Hungary	USA	Surrogacy
India	Europe, USA, United Arab Emirates	Standard IVF
India	Thailand, USA	Sex selection
Israel	Romania	Donor oocytes
Italy	Austria, Belgium, Czech Republic, Greece, Slovenia, Spain, Switzerland, UK	Donor oocytes, donor sperm, embryo cryopreservation, PGD
Japan	USA	All services
Macedonia	Belgium	ICSI-TESE
Macedonia	Czech Republic	Donor oocytes
Middle East	Jordan	Sex selection
Netherlands	Belgium	Donor sperm
Norway	Denmark	Donor sperm
Portugal	Russia, Spain	Donor oocytes
Sweden	Denmark	Donor sperm
Sweden	Baltic States, Finland, Russia	Donor oocytes
Switzerland	Austria	Standard IVF
Switzerland	Eastern Europe, Spain	Donor oocytes
UK	Czech Republic, Spain	Donor oocytes
USA	India	Surrogacy

agencies. These organizations symbolize the interface of medicine and business in this field and the Internet has become a "virtual site" of CBRS activities. Utilizing CBRS to evade domestic restrictions and/or to restrict other people's knowledge of recourse to assistance with family building in turn promotes secrecy. This ensures that many of the practices relating to CBRS remain "hidden," with significant potential psychosocial, ethical and legal consequences [16]. However, the secrecy has also impacted on the uptake of counseling. CBRS is only beginning to emerge as a theme for infertility counseling and little has been published by experts in this field, with the German Society for Fertility Counselling being the only organization that has developed CBRS guidelines for counselors [17].

Lack of a framework for CBRS

Due to different and sometimes contradictory cultural and ethical values, the harmonization of legislation between different jurisdictions is unlikely to occur. It has also been argued that harmonization may not be desirable as it denies ethical, cultural and religious pluralism. Thus, "harmonization" may actually result in "uniformization" and CBRS could be considered a "safety valve" that helps to avoid conflicts [18]. On the other hand, the current situation lends itself to the exploitation of vulnerable parties, above all, the donors, surrogates and children born from these services. Their voices so far have not been heard to any significant degree. Furthermore, with the exception of a small British study relating to the impact of overseas multiple-embryo transfer during single IVF cycles [15] no research has been conducted on or with children born as a result of CBRS, especially on the psychosocial impact of their mixed cultural/ethnic background. Last but not least, worries have been expressed that CBRS could create demands and burdens on both the home and the destination countries [15].

These concerns have led to the development of practice guidelines by two professional bodies, ESHRE and ASRM, respectively. ESHRE's "Good practice guide for cross border reproductive care for centers and practitioners" [19] and the ASRM Ethics Committee's "opinion" [20] are both welcomed for making a start in acknowledging the challenges as well as the opportunities presented by CBRS. However, the scope of both documents as regards infertility counseling practice is modest. The ESHRE guidelines identify the need of foreign patients to receive the same level of medical care, information, counseling and psychosocial support as are provided for domestic patients; the need to minimize health risks for donors and surrogates; and the possibility of professional collaboration in those countries where this does not pose a legal problem. However, it fails to acknowledge the problematic areas: the interests of donors or surrogates, or the possibility for children born as a result of treatment to be able to access information about themselves.

The committee opinion of the Ethics Committee of the American Society for Reproductive Medicine [20] summarises what is currently known about the incidence of, and the key reasons for, utilizing CBRS. It describes the potential benefits of travel to access fertility services and acknowledges the potential harms of CBRS. It focuses only on the responsibilities of physicians; there is no mention of the roles of counselors. Physicians in departure countries are not considered to have any duty to be informed about or disclose risks and benefits of treatment elsewhere and physicians in destination countries are seen to have a duty to deliver the same quality of care required for all domestic patients. The ASRM does not consider that the physician is obliged "to discuss the patient's circumvention tourism."

In order to expand on these existing practice guides, minimum standards of care have been proposed [21] that could be implemented on a voluntary basis by clinics, professionals and research institutions, and thus provide a degree of transparency to other professionals as well as to potential patients, donors and surrogates. Most importantly, they could contribute to national and pan-national discussion of the challenges in CBRS. These minimum standards cover the following issues:

1. Voluntary commitment to the standards to be followed as well as voluntary oversight by a national or supra-national body. This is especially pertinent for those countries that have not yet established legislation.
2. A commitment to altruistic donation and surrogacy and a ban on commercial procedures. It is difficult to say the least to determine a just price for services such as donation or surrogacy. There should be national and pan-national discussions regarding financial compensation in order to agree on a "just" price.
3. Gamete donors and surrogates should receive the same level of care as recipients. They should be provided with full healthcare coverage to enable

them to access free medical treatment required after potential complications and they should be insured for any (long-term) health impairment resulting from the donation or surrogate service.

4. Since donors and surrogates undergo health risks for the benefit of others, a high level of informed consent should be ensured. They should receive comprehensive and accurate information regarding the medical procedure and the psychosocial implications in an unbiased manner. This should also include legal information such as the status of the donor/surrogate, her husband (in the case of a married surrogate or female donor) and the recipients/intended parents. An independent ombudsman or a donor/surrogate advocate can be established to represent the interests of these parties.
5. All parties involved should have access to psychosocial counseling prior to, during and post treatment. Psychological assessment may be necessary in some cases, but this should neither be confused with, nor substituted for, counseling.
6. In complex cases, prior to new and/or innovative treatment, multi-disciplinary ethics committees installed in the clinic providing treatment should be involved.
7. In order to avoid conflicts of interest, the recruitment of donors and surrogates should be carried out independently from those institutions that are responsible for the informed consent procedure, the psychosocial counseling and the legal advice.
8. There has been a lot of controversy regarding the anonymity and ability to identify donors and surrogates. From a moral perspective, offspring should be granted as much autonomy as possible, including the possibility of accessing full information about their biological and genetic origins, if they wish to do so. Therefore, clinics should document records for a minimum of 80 years and offspring should be entitled to access this information. As a complementary requirement, donors should be able to learn about the outcome of their donation and the number of offspring conceived with their gametes, if they wish. Registers should also enable contact between half-siblings, if mutually agreed upon.
9. All countries should strive towards self-sufficiency as regards ART services so as to reduce the need for patients to travel. Donors and surrogates do not need to provide their service to recipients from abroad (usually with a higher living standard) in order to generate income. In accordance with national cultural and ethical principles, ARTs should be regulated so that this aim is achieved.
10. There are a number of international regulations and conventions on human rights such as the Convention of Human Rights and Biomedicine of the Council of Europe [22], the Convention for the Protection of Human Rights and Fundamental Freedoms [23], the Ethical Issues in Obstetrics and Gynecology [24] or the International Alliance of Patients' Organisations (IAPO) – Declaration on Patient-Centered Healthcare [25] that can serve as a framework for CBRS.

While adherence to such minimum standards can contribute towards more ethical and respectful treatment, considerable challenges lie in the way of their acceptance. However, they can form the basis of discussion and collaboration between different professional groups, and between professionals in different countries, to ensure that patients, donors, surrogates and the children born as a result of CBRS are not exposed to unnecessary risks.

Counseling in cross-border reproductive services

The provision of appropriate counseling as an integral part of fertility services has been well documented (for an overview see [26–28]) and qualification guidelines have been issued by several organizations [29]. There is agreement that professionals offering fertility counseling should:

1. hold a graduate-level qualification in a psychosocial profession;
2. hold a relevant professional license to practice;
3. demonstrate relevant training in the medical and psychosocial aspects of infertility;
4. demonstrate a minimum level of relevant clinical experience; and,
5. demonstrate engagement in continuing professional education.

When counseling in CBRS, additional requirements arise for professionals. These include: knowledge and information regarding the legislation of typical destination countries; awareness of societal attitudes and their impact on patients; attentiveness for ethical issues, such as commodification, and the potential of exploitation of donors and surrogates, and its effect on patients; as well as being able to raise these issues with patients.

Given that counseling is non-directive, supports the decision-making process of patients, and explores the implications of family building options rather than recommends specific treatments, counseling does not direct patients towards treatments that may not be allowed in their home country. Whether counseling in this area may entail punitive consequences, however, is dependent upon national legislation and/or case law. Fertility counselors, therefore, need to be informed about the implications of relevant legislation and proceed with care, even though supra-national bodies such as ESHRE [30] endorse evasion of domestic law by a medical professional as in the interest of patient autonomy by providing information on treatment options abroad.

Fertility counselors also need to explore their personal and professional attitude regarding CBRS, especially regarding treatment options that are controversial in their country and that raise moral dilemmas. There is a risk of exploiting donors and surrogates, especially when CBRS takes place between countries with very different living standards and customs (e.g., North America and Europe on the one hand, and Eastern Europe and South East Asia on the other). Counselors need to explore their professional attitude towards such challenging issues, beware of transference issues and make use of professional supervision to clarify these. Patients deserve understanding and respect for their family building plans. This does not imply that counselors should refrain from raising controversial issues. In fact, it is often a relief for patients to be able to explore these in a supportive and empathetic environment, and counseling often affords the only possibility to provide time and space for this. The counseling process, however, should not be influenced by the attitude of the fertility counselor.

The case of Simon and Sally presented at the beginning illustrates many common matters presented in CBRS counseling: patients pursuing treatment that is not available in their home country, dealing with limited information, resources and a sense of time. The following section will further examine these clinical issues and provide case vignettes when working with (a) patients, (b) donors and surrogates and (c) the resulting children [17]. Given that CBRS is a relatively new phenomenon, there is little research on which these issues can be based. Therefore, counseling interventions are based on existing knowledge in the area of fertility counseling, especially third party reproduction, although the focus will be on issues that are relevant where treatment takes place outside the patients' country of residence. For specific counseling in third party reproduction, reference should be made to the relevant chapters in this book.

Preparing for CBRS

Fertility counselors should respect the reproductive autonomy of all parties involved, including the interest of offspring created, resulting in a well-considered and measured use of reproductive medicine. Counseling should be accessible prior to, during and after fertility treatment in a language that patients can use to explore emotional issues; counseling in the country of residence is most likely to fulfill these conditions. Providing counseling *prior* to treatment may mitigate the risk of accepting treatment that could entail physical or psychological risks for patients or the future child. However, clinical experience indicates that many patients take up counseling after failed treatment cycles, and, in the area of CBRS, after having decided on a clinic and thus the country of treatment.

> Susan and Richard sought counseling after they had signed a contract with a clinic and had already made payments towards their first treatment cycle. During the counseling sessions, they raised their frustration regarding the lack of communication by the clinic. Their emails remained unanswered, the responsible staff could not be reached by telephone and they were unable to clarify several issues in the treatment protocol they did not understand. This could not be rectified by counseling. We focused one session on this frustrating situation and this helped the couple develop a greater understanding of the gullibility their emotional situation had resulted in when signing the contract. They developed more confidence and were able to proceed with much more assertiveness during medical treatment.

From a counseling perspective, this is frustrating from several perspectives. This situation is indicative of the importance of pre-treatment counseling. Although fertility counselors are not in a position to recommend specific clinics, even though there may be no adverse legal consequences for doing so where the treatment planned is possible in the "home" country, we firmly believe that patients who have considered their needs prior to medical treatment and have developed their personal "check-list" for the clinics they consult, are more likely to choose a clinic that fulfills their needs. In the case of CBRS, this "check-list" includes issues such as reliable communication via email or telephone and the possibility of contacting staff in emergency situations. This is one of the tasks of counseling before treatment: preparing patients for what lies ahead of them and supporting them to make informed choices.

Exploring infertility always includes a critical appraisal of limits in life, limits of medical treatment and limits of emotional suffering. It therefore may also result in patients deciding against pursuing treatment abroad, in which case counseling focuses on developing strategies for a life without children.

As many patients who intend to undertake treatment abroad have already experienced treatment failure in their home country, fertility counselors should explore whether they have sufficient psychological, emotional and financial resources to continue treatment, and whether this is feasible given their physical, psychological and emotional health. Furthermore, treatment abroad can be associated with moral qualms, especially if the treatment intended is prohibited in the patients' home country. Careful exploration is necessary in order to assess whether the patients are sufficiently confident to proceed. Moral doubts can also result in keeping the treatment a secret from family members and friends, and thus vital emotional and practical support may be absent during treatment. In some cases, time off treatment may be indicated to work through and resolve some of these issues; in others, patients may decide not to proceed with treatment altogether. For those who proceed, fertility counseling should include the exploration of general issues, issues related to the use of their own gametes and issues related to third party reproduction.

Treatment issues

Patients need to ensure that they fully understand the information regarding the treatment planned and counselors should advise patients of the importance of being as fully informed as possible before they embark on overseas treatment. Patients who are not sufficiently proficient in the language of destination countries, or where competence in a common language with service providers is limited, may often struggle to understand details. If a translation and/or interpretation service is required, patients should ensure – as well as they can – that the translation is correct. They should resist any pressure to sign consent forms they do not fully understand. Patients can request clinics to provide treatment plans, consent forms and contract drafts prior to their first visit. This gives them the opportunity to read them through and make arrangements for independent translation, if necessary. They should also ensure that there are no medical counter-indications against the treatment planned and that there are adequate success rates.

In order to facilitate the flow of necessary information, clinics in both home and destination countries should be provided with relevant medical records, which patients may have to facilitate on their own. In some countries there are restrictions, such as oocyte donation can only be carried out for medical reasons, and clinics need to have documentation confirming this. Medical documents may also be important in case of complications or malpractice. Patients, however, should be aware that it may be difficult to take effective legal action in the case of medical malpractice in a destination country, especially where no protective regulation or legislation is in place.

Under certain conditions, patient health insurance may reimburse costs for treatment abroad. This is dependent upon the legal status of the treatment and upon the state or the individual insurance policy. Patients should be encouraged to clarify any available reimbursement prior to treatment. Clinics should provide a transparent and legally binding treatment plan, which also details the cost (including the compensation or payment for donors and surrogates, if applicable). Couples should be aware that several treatment cycles may be necessary to achieve pregnancy and that carrying out treatment abroad also entails traveling, accommodation and incidental costs (such as visas, for example). For costs during pregnancy and for birth, the country of conception is irrelevant; reimbursement is dependent upon the parent's/parents' health insurance scheme.

Patients may be more willing to risk multiples after having experienced recurrent treatment failure in their home country. Although the high number of multiples following CBRS has been criticized [15,31], and recent European data indicate that the general rate of multiple pregnancy is decreasing within Europe, there are significant national differences, with four and more embryos regularly transferred in several countries (e.g., Bulgaria, Lithuania, Moldova, Romania and Serbia) [32]. Similar practices may be prevalent in other countries, especially in the absence of formal policies or guidelines restricting the number of embryos that may be transferred in a single IVF cycle [31]. For example, one American study found that at least half of the clinicians surveyed would deviate from ASRM embryo transfer number guidelines in certain situations [33].

Couples should be made aware of this risk whenever more than one embryo is transferred or hormonal induction is used to stimulate the growth of oocytes, and be informed that current guidelines seek to minimize the risk of multiples by only transferring one or two embryos [31,34,35].

> After five failed IVF cycles, Steven and Joyce, both in their mid-30s, were very frustrated as the clinic would only transfer two embryos per treatment cycle in order to minimize the risk of multiples. They had contacted a clinic abroad that offered to transfer a higher number of embryos with the promise of a higher pregnancy rate. As their financial resources were such that they could afford only one more cycle, they contemplated having four embryos transferred, hoping to increase their chances of conceiving.

It is easy for the fertility counselor to develop empathy for couples who have had to experience so many "mini losses," as couples often described failed treatment. The couples' desire to "put all their eggs into one basket" (pun intended) is also understandable. At the same time, the counselor's emotional distance allows a greater degree of reflection and enables him/her to understand the risks of transferring three or more embryos to such a relatively young woman. The issues here are two-fold: to use professional knowledge in a way that helps clients to make informed decisions and to appreciate that the information of transferring a certain number of embryos was given by medical doctors who tend to be afforded a higher professional status than mental health professionals.

One way of avoiding a professional power struggle (for oneself as well as for patients who would find themselves in between two professional views) is to focus on the psychosocial issues. Fertility counselors can and should inform couples like Steven and Joyce of the medical and physical consequences of multiple pregnancies. Focus should be on questions regarding the scope of social support typically required after multiples are born, the realistic options of both partners to share child care, and equally important, the financial burden multiples can result in.

Counseling prior to treatment using the patients' own gametes

Many patients travel in the hope that less restrictive legislation will enable medical practitioners to offer different or innovative treatment that may result in higher pregnancy rates. Such treatment can include PGD or blastocyst transfer with selected embryo transfer. Others travel in the hope that treatment is less costly outside their country of residence. Patients considering traveling abroad should be informed that it is vital that treatment adheres to international standards and they should satisfy themselves regarding the standards of care available; caution is advised if independent confirmation of standards is not readily available. Should innovative treatment be offered, patients should be adequately informed about the implications, including the financial cost, as well as any risks this treatment may entail for themselves or the resulting child. This requires fertility counselors to continuously stay up-to-date with medical and scientific developments.

Counseling prior to third party reproduction

Patients need to be knowledgeable of the legal regulations, guidelines or common practice regarding anonymity or identifiability of the donor. In many countries, legislation mandates anonymity [31] and patients are given little or no non-identifiable information about their donor(s). Clinical experience indicates that at the time of treatment, for several reasons, many patients pay little attention to legal regulations. They are unaware of legislation, they naively follow recommendations of their previous clinic, or their desire is focused on the short-term need to conceive and have a child rather than on long-term issues relevant for the child.

Once the child is born and parents consider disclosure, however, having undergone treatment in a country where donors or surrogates remain anonymous may result in a dilemma: parents can disclose the use of a donor or surrogate, but the child will not be able to access any information about his/her biological background. Furthermore, in many countries, it may be legally possible for clinics to provide non-identifiable information, although they are reluctant to do so. It is important for fertility counselors to explore with patients their intentions regarding disclosure and draw attention to the need for selecting a country and a clinic that provides the future child with the possibility to access information about the donor or surrogate, should he/she wish so.

Counseling should also explore the values and attitudes of patients regarding the circumstances of the donor(s) and/or surrogate(s). Whether the donation was altruistic and/or an autonomous decision or the result of a financial need, the fact that gamete donors and surrogates are typically young and healthy men and women, who take medical risks for the benefit of others, usually are considerations that impact on the patients' moral assessment. Although these issues cannot be resolved, in many cases, counseling is the only opportunity that provides time and space to raise them:

> After cancer of the uterus and a hysterectomy, Julie and Ben were confident that surrogacy was a positive choice for them to have children. They had explored clinics in several countries and were unable to decide which clinic and country to choose. They struggled most with what they called "belly-buying," the concept that, as a couple from a developed country in a comfortable financial situation, they were able to "buy" the "belly" of a woman who would use this payment for life necessities. The agencies they had contacted described their payment as "a wonderful gift to the surrogate and her family" and failed to acknowledge the couple's different perspective. Although the issue of payment could not be resolved in counseling, it was a relief for Julie and Ben to have time and space to explore their feelings and their moral concerns.

Surrogacy arrangements may be most challenging for counselors' ethical values. In these situations, typically young women make available their body and risk the potential side effects of ART treatment, pregnancy and birth. Whereas historically these were women often known to the patients and had altruistic motives, nowadays commercial agencies around the globe are involved, collaborating with clinics and legal advisors. In many, if not most, cases we can assume that the costs paid to the professionals involved are higher than the compensation or payment the surrogate receives. In some countries there is contact between the surrogate and the intended parents, which allows intended parents to show their gratitude and appreciation beyond the financial transaction that takes place. In others such contact is banned. Our experience shows that intended parents can struggle with the concept of payment to donors and surrogates. They find it difficult, if not impossible, to "fix a price" for oocytes, semen or pregnancy. If this exchange is anonymous, they also struggle with the concept that they cannot show any appreciation for this "gift of life." Some have written a letter to donors and surrogates in which they describe their experiences and gratitude and hoped that the clinics passed them on.

In some cases, these issues only become relevant to patients once pregnancy has been established and having a child becomes a reality. In other cases, they become acute after the child is born or starts to ask questions about her/his conception. It is therefore important for counseling to be available at every stage of treatment and after the child is born, to be available in the parents' home country, and for parents to be informed about further resources, such as support organizations.

Although fertility counselors are not in a position to provide binding legal advice, they should raise the legal implications of gamete and embryo donation and surrogacy. The legal implications of international surrogacy are very complex, and intended parents should ensure that they have all the relevant information relating to the country of treatment. In most jurisdictions, the woman giving birth is the legal mother and her husband or partner the legal father. Consequently, the intended parents, even if their gametes were used, are not the legal parents. Intended parents, who are single or in a same-sex relationship, should be informed about the legal status of the donor in relation to the child. In cases where there is no male partner to automatically assume legal paternity, in some jurisdictions the donor may both run the risk of assuming parental obligations and be able to claim visitations rights. Fertility counselors should encourage legal consultation in these situations.

Regardless of their genetic relationship to the child, intending parents may need to apply to adopt him/her or take other available legal measures to ensure a transfer of parentage from the surrogate to themselves [36]. In some jurisdictions, transfer of legal parentage is stipulated in legally enforceable contracts prior to treatment (see Chapter 9), although in most jurisdictions such contracts are not legally enforceable.

In some international surrogacy arrangements there have been disputes about the nationality of the child [14], especially in those cases where surrogacy is prohibited in the intended parents' country of residence, and embassies have been reluctant to issue birth certificates, passports, or other legal documents which are required for the intending parents' to return home with the child [37]. It is therefore vital for intended parents to be knowledgeable about the documents they need in the country of treatment, the documents they need in order to travel home with the baby and those required for the legal proceedings in their home country to transfer parentage.

It is also advisable for intended parents not to rely on the legal information provided by the clinic or the agency, but to seek independent advice from a legal expert experienced in this area. The legal information should also entail details about the documents regarding donors and surrogates, such as what information is recorded, how long and where these records are kept. Countries belonging to the European Union, for example, must keep documents for a minimum of 30 years [38]. However, there is currently no evidence that this document retention period is adhered to in all EU member countries. The right of offspring to access these documents is subject to national legislation. Intended parents should also be informed that these records may be relevant beyond the 30-year period and that it may be necessary in the case of medical complications to have access to the identity of the donor or the surrogate.

Counseling donors and surrogates

In many destination countries, there is no evidence that counseling is available for donors and surrogates. Therefore, in addition to the general counseling interventions for donors and surrogates described in Chapters 8 and 9, fertility counselors need to raise issues specific to CBRS. These include issues such as the question whether donors are aware of, and have consented to, the use of their oocytes or their semen for recipients from other countries; in this case, their future children will have half-siblings living in other countries. There is little international agreement regarding the number of offspring per semen donor [39], and there is no international agreement regarding the number of offspring per oocyte donor, let alone the maximum number of treatment cycles to which she should be subjected. In those jurisdictions where there are no legal limits, donors should be informed about national guidelines applicable to them and be encouraged to determine the number of offspring they wish to contribute to. Similarly, surrogates should be informed about relevant national guidelines regarding the maximum number of embryos to be transferred (in order to minimize the risk of multiples for surrogates and any consequent multifetal reduction) and of pregnancies or, if there are no guidelines, be encouraged to determine themselves the number of pregnancies they are willing to carry out for others.

The meaning of financial compensation or payment should be carefully explored in order to assess financial coercion. Although this is especially pertinent in developing and emerging countries, such as India and Thailand, it is also relevant in countries such as Spain, the Czech Republic or the USA where donors and surrogates typically are young women with (considerably) less financial resources than patients [40]. Last but not least, more research is required on the short- and long-term implications for donors and surrogates. There is a dearth of information on how these groups fare with their decision in later life and what their needs are regarding information about and contact to offspring they have helped to conceive.

Counseling offspring

The psychosocial needs of offspring conceived via donated gametes, embryos and via surrogacy in a foreign country is another issue the fertility counselor should address with intended parents, ideally prior to treatment [41]; this is covered in detail in Chapter 18. For offspring conceived abroad, there may be additional issues, such as exploring the meanings of having a dual cultural/ethnic background. In inter-country adoption, racial, ethnic and cultural awareness have been found to be essential ingredients for successful identity formation [42]. Currently, there is little evidence either from formal research or from clinical practice that this issue is considered at all by those providing services for individuals and couples traveling for treatment. It is highly likely, however, that similar issues will apply to offspring following CBRS whose parents may be of different races or cultures. More research is also required for this group, especially if conceived via CBRS, in order to understand both the short- and long-term needs of these children.

Counseling resources

Information on legislation and international guidelines

As the policy situation in many countries is dynamic and many countries do not have legislation pertaining to ART or to specific aspects of ART, such as the establishment of legal parenthood following [43] surrogacy or the number of offspring a donor can help to conceive or the right of offspring to access biological information, it will be difficult for counselors to stay abreast of these developments. An overview has been put together by ESHRE (http://www.eshre.eu/Guidelines-and-Legal/Legal-documentation.aspx and http://www.eshre.eu/Guidelines-and-Legal/Legislation-for-MAR-treatments.aspx), the website "Biopolicywiki" (www.biopolicywiki.org) and the German Max-Planck Institute for International Penal Law (http://www.mpicc.de/meddb/show_all.php, only available in German).

Patient organizations

It can be helpful to refer to patient organizations in the country of treatment where they exist. These are generally knowledgeable not only in the legal area but can also provide information regarding the medical practice in their country. In addition, they can help to establish contact with other patients in their country to provide support. The international umbrella organization iCSi (International Consumer Support for Infertility; www.icsicommunity.org) and the European organization "Fertility Europe" (www.fertilityeurope.eu) have compiled a list of national patient organizations.

Fertility counseling organizations

In several countries, specialist fertility counseling organizations have been founded. These can provide information for counselors regarding national legislation, guidelines and practices and also provide a list of counselors that can be contacted by patients. The international umbrella organization IICO (International Infertility Counseling Organization – http://www.iico-infertilitycounseling.org/about-us/iico-members) provides links to national organizations.

Guidelines for counseling in the area of CBRS

The German Fertility Counselling Organisation has published guidelines for counseling in the area of CBRS. These guidelines have also been published in English [17]. In addition, Table 22.2 provides questions for fertility counselors to consider regarding counseling issues occurring in the context of CBRS.

Table 22.2 Questions for fertility counselors to consider on counseling issues arising in the context of CBRS.

- What do I know about the implications of legislation relevant to me when providing counseling to patients who travel for treatment, especially those who intend treatment prohibited in my country of practice?
- What type of legal and medical information can I provide as a psychosocial professional? Are there any restriction/limitations by professional bodies or by legislation? (Typically, counselors can provide basic medical and legal information but are not in a situation to provide binding information.)
- What is my attitude towards treatment prohibited or not offered in my country? Do I think patients have a right to exert their reproductive autonomy even if they engage in an activity that is illegal if carried out at home? Does my attitude vary according to the type of treatment; if yes, can I describe why?
- How do I feel about women who undergo invasive procedures for the sake of others (oocyte donors, surrogates)?
- How do I feel about these groups receiving financial compensation/payment for these procedures? Should there be a lower and/or upper limit for such payment? What or who should determine the amount of this payment?
- How do I feel about the need or right of offspring conceived by third party reproduction to access information about the donor and/or surrogate?
- How do I feel if this is possible in my country, but not the treatment country of patients (or vice versa)?

Reflections

PT: I think all infertility counselors worldwide have seen tremendous changes in our field in recent years. Working in Germany, it is fascinating to see how many couples travel in order to obtain treatment, mainly oocyte donation, which is prohibited in Germany. Whereas six or seven years ago, I hardly did any counseling in this area, I now usually have several clients every week. These counseling sessions can pose challenges, for both the clients and myself. Many German couples are considering treatment in Spain, which is considered to be the hub for oocyte donation in Europe. This is also the country suggested by many medical professionals. From a psychosocial perspective, however, treatment in Spain cannot be recommended. Legislation is such that all donors remain anonymous and children born as a result from third party treatment in Spain will not be able to access their biological origins. In a sense, this is a déjà vu situation: Many years ago, there were controversial discussions regarding sperm donor anonymity in Germany.

This is now – to a large degree – resolved and offspring are able to access the identity of the donor. Now, we are having very similar discussions with patients considering treatment in Spain (and any other country that grants anonymity to donors and/or surrogates). Often, couples know very little about the legal implications and are not aware of the rights and possibilities of their future children. Often, too, the needs of their children are so far in the future that they are not taken into consideration before or during treatment. The couples' focus is on getting pregnant and it can be a challenge to raise long-term implications that do not affect them, but their future child. Given the legal situation in Germany, counselors are also concerned about potential legal issues if they counsel in an area that is prohibited; they fear criminal penalties. At the same time, there is little discussion about counseling issues in this area and thus little awareness. This is the reason why, as chair of the German Society for Fertility Counselling, I have been involved in issuing guidelines for counseling in third party reproduction as well as for counseling individuals and couples traveling for treatment. Both guidelines provide psychosocial professionals with background of the international scientific discussion in this area and describe issues relevant for counseling in these areas.

As fertility counselors, we work in a dynamic area, both technically and ethically. We have seen and will continue to see many changes, both in the way infertility is treated and regarding the groups that access medical treatment. I am certain that the future will hold new challenges for us – and I hope that we will continue professional development and exchange so that our role in the provision of treatment will continue to grow.

EDB: It is now almost a decade since I first commented on what was then generally referred to as "reproductive tourism" [44]. This paper has now become a routinely cited work in this field (89 citations according to Google Scholar as of March 31, 2014). Over that time I have also undertaken further research, commentary and professional practice [3,12,14,45–48]. What has become apparent over this period is both increased professional and academic interest in the field and increased media interest in the more exotic/problematic examples of cross-border reproductive travel. The effect of this appears to be increasing awareness of both the opportunities and the hazards associated with cross-border reproductive travel and realization of the need to ensure the effective protection of the interests of patients, donors, surrogates, the children to be born as a result of the procedures undertaken, as well as any existing children that the patients, donors or surrogates may already have. It is gratifying to have been able to contribute to policy developments in this area [20], a report that incidentally credits me with drawing attention to unscrupulous "bait and switch" practices. I did, indeed, refer to the plight of some parents and their children once the children started to grow up and it was evident from the children's physical characteristics that a different donor had been used to the one stated by the clinics. I wish I had also been sufficiently inventive to come up wth the "bait and catch" phrase. Unfortunately I didn't!

References

1. Thorn P. Reproduktives Reisen – eine Expertise für den Pro Familia Bundesverband. *Pro Familia Bundesverband.* 2008 http://www.profamilia.de/fileadmin/publikationen/Fachpublikationen/expertise_reproduktives_reisen.pdf. (Accessed 14 April, 2014.)
2. Inhorn MC, Patrizio P. Rethinking reproductive "tourism" as reproductive "exile." *Fertil Steril* 2009; 92: 904–6.
3. Blyth E. Fertility patients' experiences of cross-border reproductive care. *Fertil Steril* 2010; 94: e11–15.
4. Shenfield F, de Mouzon J, Pennings G, et al. Cross border reproductive care in six European countries. *Hum Reprod* 2010; 25: 1361–68.
5. Bergmann S. Reproductive borders, agency, and imagination: the experience of Germans seeking egg donation abroad. *Reprod Biomed Online* 2011; 23: 600–8.
6. Hughes E, DeJean D. Cross-border fertility services in North America: a survey of Canadian and American providers. *Fertil Steril.* 2010; 94: e16–e19.
7. Infertility Network. *The Infertility Network UK Fertility Tourism Survey Results.* Unpublished survey results. 2008.
8. Inhorn MC, Shrivastav P. Globalization and reproductive tourism in the United Arab Emirates. *Asia-Pacific J Pub Health/Asia-Pacific Academic Consortium for Public Health* 2010; 22(3 Suppl): 68S–74S.
9. Kilani Z, Shaban M, Haj Hassan L. Gender selection. In: Hédon B, Mettler L, Tinnneberg HR. eds. *Proceedings of the IFFS 2th World Congress on Fertility*

and Sterility. München, Lukn Verlagsgesellschaft. 2010; 110–14.

10. Smerdon UR. Crossing bodies, crossing borders: international surrogacy between the United States and India. *Cumberland Law Rev* 2008; 39: 15–85.
11. Whittaker AM. Reproduction opportunists in the new global sex trade: PGD and non-medical sex selection. *Reprod Biomed Online* 2011; 23: 609–17.
12. Hudson N, Culley L, Blyth E, et al. Cross-border reproductive care: a review of the literature. *Reprod BioMed Online* 2011; 22: 673–85.
13. Centers for Disease Control & Prevention. U.S. Department of Health and Human Services, 2008 assisted reproductive technology success rates: national summary and fertility clinic reports 13. 2010. http://www.cdc.gov/art/artreports.htm. (Accessed April 14, 2014.)
14. Blyth E, Thorn P, Wischmannn T. CBRC and psychosocial counselling: assessing needs and developing an ethical framework for practice. *Reprod Biomed Online* 2011; 23: 642–51.
15. McKelvey A, David A, Shenfield F, et al. The impact of cross-border reproductive care or "fertility tourism" on NHS maternity services. *BJOG* 2009; 116: 1520–3.
16. Inhorn MC, Patrizio P. The global landscape of cross-border reproductive care: twenty key findings for the new millennium. *Curr Opin Obstet Gynecol* 2012; 24: 158–63.
17. Thorn P, Wischmann T. German guidelines for psychosocial counselling in the area of "cross border reproductive services." *Arch Gynecol Obstet* 2012; 287: 599–606.
18. Pennings G. Legal harmonization and reproductive tourism in Europe. *Hum Reprod* 2004; 19: 2689–94.
19. Shenfield F, Pennings G, De Mouzon J, et al. ESHRE's good practice guide for cross-border reproductive care for centers and practitioners. *Hum Reprod* 2011; 26: 1625–7.
20. Ethics Committee of the American Society for Reproductive Medicine. Cross-border reproductive care: a committee opinion. *Fertil Steril* 2013; 100: 645–50.
21. Thorn P, Wischmann T, Blyth E. Cross Border Reproductive Services – suggestions for an ethically based minimum standard of care in Europe. *J Psychosom Obstet Gynecol* 2012; 33: 1–6.
22. Council of Europe. *Convention for the Protection of Human Rights and Dignity of the Human Being with Regard to the Application of Biology and Medicine: Convention on Human Rights and Biomedicine*. CETS No: 164. 1997. http://conventions.coe.int/Treaty/en/Treaties/Html/164.htm (Accessed April 14, 2014.)
23. Council of Europe. *Convention for the Protection of Human Rights and Fundamental Freedoms*. CETS No: 005. 1950. http://conventions.coe.int/treaty/en/treaties/html/005.htm. (Accessed April 14, 2014.)
24. International Federation of Gynecology and Obstetrics. *Ethical Issues in Obstetrics and Gynecology by the FIGO Committee for the Study of Ethical Aspects of Human Reproduction and Women's Health*. 2012. http://www.glowm.com/pdf/English%20Ethical%20Issues%20in%20Obstetrics%20a (Accessed October, 2014.)
25. International Alliance of Patients' Organisations. *What is Patient Centred Health Care? A Review of Definitions and Principles*. 2007. http://www.patientsorganizations.org/pchreview. (Accessed April 14, 2014.)
26. Blyth E, Hunt J. A history of infertility counselling in the United Kingdom. In: Jennings S. ed. *Infertility Counselling*. Oxford, Basil Blackwell. 1994; 175–90.
27. Blyth E. 1988–2008: twenty years of BICA [British Infertility Counselling Association. *J Fertil Counsel* 2008; 15(1): 15–28.
28. Kleinschmidt D, Thorn P, Wischmann T. *Kinderwunsch und professionelle Beratung. Das Handbuch des Beratungsnetzwerkes Kinderwunsch Deutschland (BKiD)*. Stuttgart, Kohlhammer. 2008.
29. Blyth E. Guidelines for infertility counselling in different countries: is there an emerging trend? *Hum Reprod* 2012; 27: 2046–57.
30. Pennings G, de Wert G, Shenfield F, et al. ESHRE task force on ethics and law 15: cross-border reproductive care. *Hum Reprod* 2008; 23: 2182–84.
31. International Federation of Infertility Societies. IFFS Surveillance 2013. http://www.iffs-reproduction.org/?page = SurveillanceHidden. (Accessed April 14, 2014.)
32. Ferraretti, A.P., Goossens, V., Kupka, M., et al. Assisted reproductive technology in Europe, 2009: results generated from European registers by ESHRE. *Hum Reprod* 2013; 28: 2318–31.
33. Jungheim, E, Ryan, GL, Levens, ED, et al. Embryo transfer practices in the United States: a survey of clinics registered with the Society for Assisted Reproductive Technology. *Fertil Steril* 2010; 94: 1432–36.
34. American Society for Reproductive Medicine. Guidelines on number of embryos transferred. *Fertil Steril* 2006; 86(5 Suppl): S51–52.
35. The ESHRE Task Force on Ethics and Law. 6. Ethical issues related to multiple pregnancies in medically assisted procreation. *Hum Reprod* 2003; 18: 1976–9.
36. Trimmings K, Beaumont P. *International Surrogacy Arrangements*. Oxford, Hart Publishing. 2013.

37. Spiewak M *Verbotene Kinder. Die Zeit.* 2010, April 22;17. http://www.zeit.de/2010/17/Leihmutterschaft?page = all. 07.05.2010. (Accessed April 14, 2014.)
38. European Parliament and the Council of the European Union. Directive 2004/23/EC of the European Parliament and of the Council of 31 March 2004. http://eur-lex.europa.eu/LexUriServ/LexUriServ.do?uri = OJ:L:2004:102:0048:0058:en:PDF. (Accessed April 14, 2014.)
39. Janssens PM, Nap AW, Bancsi LF. Reconsidering the number of offspring per gamete donor in the Dutch open-identity system. *Hum Fertil* 2011; 14: 106–14.
40. Pfeffer N. Eggs-ploiting women: a critical feminist analysis of the different principles in transplant and fertility tourism. *Reprod Biomed Online* 2011; 23: 634–41.
41. Thorn P, Wischmann T. German guidelines for psychosocial counselling in the area of gamete donation. *Hum Fertil* 2009; 12: 73–80.
42. Triseliotis J. Identity-formation and the adopted person revisited. In: Treacher A, Katz I. eds. *The Dynamics of Adoption. Social and Personal Experiences.* London, Jessica Kingsley Publishers. 2000; 81–98.
43. Dickens B. Cross-border reproductive services: FIGO Committee for the Ethical Aspects of Human Reproduction and Women's Health. *IJ Gynecol Obstet* 2010; 111: 190–1.
44. Blyth E, Farrand A. Reproductive tourism – a price worth paying for reproductive autonomy? *Crit Soc Pol* 2005; 25: 91–114.
45. Blyth E, Auffrey M. *International Policy on Cross Border Reproductive Services.* Geneva, International Federation of Social Workers. 2008. http://ifsw.org/policies/cross-border-reproductive-services/ (Accessed April 14, 2014).
46. Culley L, Hudson N, Rapport F, et al. Crossing borders for fertility treatment: motivations, destinations and outcomes of UK fertility travellers. *Hum Reprod* 2012; 26: 2373–81.
47. Culley L, Hudson N, Rapport F, et al, 'What are you going to do, confiscate their passports?' Professional perspectives on cross-border reproductive travel. *J Reprod Infant Psychol.* 2013; 31(1): 46–57.
48. Palattiyil G, Blyth E, Sidhva D, et al. Globalisation and cross-border reproductive services: ethical implications of surrogacy in India for social work. *I Soc Work* 2010; 53: 686–700.

Glossary

Assisted hatching: an *in vitro* procedure in which the zona pellucida of an embryo is either thinned or perforated by chemical, mechanical or laser methods to assist separation of the blastocyst.

Assisted reproductive technology (ART): all treatments or procedures that include the *in vitro* handling of both human oocytes and sperm, or embryos, for the purpose of establishing a pregnancy. This includes, but is not limited to, *in vitro* fertilization and embryo transfer, gamete intrafallopian transfer, zygote intrafallopian transfer, tubal embryo transfer, gamete and embryo cryopreservation, oocyte and embryo donation, and gestational surrogacy. ART does not include assisted insemination (artificial insemination) using sperm from either a woman's partner or a sperm donor.

Biochemical pregnancy (preclinical spontaneous abortion/miscarriage): a pregnancy diagnosed only by the detection of HCG in serum or urine and that does not develop into a clinical pregnancy.

Blastocyst: an embryo, five or six days after fertilization, with an inner cell mass, outer layer of trophectoderm and a fluid-filled blastocoele cavity.

Cancelled cycle: an ART cycle in which ovarian stimulation or monitoring has been carried out with the intention to treat, but did not proceed to follicular aspiration or, in the case of a thawed embryo, to embryo transfer.

Clinical pregnancy: a pregnancy diagnosed by ultrasonographic visualization of one or more gestational sacs or definitive clinical signs of pregnancy. It includes ectopic pregnancy. *Note: Multiple gestational sacs are counted as one clinical pregnancy.*

Clinical pregnancy rate: the number of clinical pregnancies expressed per 100 initiated cycles, aspiration cycles or embryo transfer cycles. *Note: When clinical pregnancy rates are given, the denominator (initiated, aspirated or embryo transfer cycles) must be specified.*

Clinical pregnancy with fetal heart beat: pregnancy diagnosed by ultrasonographic or clinical documentation of at least one fetus with heart beat. It includes ectopic pregnancy.

Congenital anomalies: all structural, functional, and genetic anomalies diagnosed in aborted fetuses, at birth or in the neonatal period.

Controlled ovarian stimulation (COS) for ART: pharmacological treatment in which women are stimulated to induce the development of multiple ovarian follicles to obtain multiple oocytes at follicular aspiration.

Controlled ovarian stimulation (COS) for non-ART cycles: pharmacological treatment for women in which the ovaries are stimulated to ovulate more than one oocyte.

Cryopreservation: the freezing or vitrification and storage of gametes, zygotes, embryos or gonadal tissue.

Cumulative delivery rate with at least one live born baby: the estimated number of deliveries with at least one live born baby resulting from one initiated or aspirated ART cycle including the cycle when fresh embryos are transferred, and subsequent frozen/thawed ART cycles. This rate is used when less than the total number of embryos fresh and/or frozen/thawed have been utilized from one ART cycles. *Note: The delivery of a singleton, twin or other multiple pregnancy is registered as one delivery.*

Delivery: the expulsion or extraction of one or more fetuses from the mother after 20 completed weeks of gestational age.

Delivery rate after ART treatment per patient: the number of deliveries with at least one live born baby per patient following a specified number of ART treatments.

Delivery rate: the number of deliveries expressed per 100 initiated cycles, aspiration cycles or embryo transfer cycles. When delivery rates are given, the denominator (initiated, aspirated or embryo transfer cycles) must be specified. It includes deliveries that resulted in the birth of one or more live babies and/or stillborn babies. *Note: The delivery of a singleton, twin or other multiple pregnancy is registered as one delivery.*

Early neonatal death: death of a live born baby within 7 days of birth.

Ectopic pregnancy: a pregnancy in which implantation takes place outside the uterine cavity.

Elective embryo transfer: the transfer of one or more embryos, selected from a larger cohort of available embryos.

Embryo: the product of the division of the zygote to the end of the embryonic stage, eight weeks after

Glossary reproduced with permission from International Committee for Monitoring Assisted Reproductive Technology (ICMART) and the World Health Organization (WHO) revised glossary of ART terminology, 2009* Zegers-Hochschild, F. et al. Fertil Steril 2009; 92(5):1520–24 and Hum Repr 2009; 24(11): 2683–87.

fertilization. (This definition does not include either parthenotes – generated through parthenogenesis – nor products of somatic cell nuclear transfer.)

Embryo donation: the transfer of an embryo resulting from gametes (spermatozoa and oocytes) that did not originate from the recipient and her partner.

Embryo recipient cycle: an ART cycle in which a woman receives zygote(s) or embryo(s) from donor(s).

Embryo/fetus reduction: a procedure to reduce the number of viable embryos or fetuses in a multiple pregnancy.

Embryo transfer (ET): the procedure in which one or more embryos are placed in the uterus or Fallopian tube.

Embryo transfer cycle: an ART cycle in which one or more embryos are transferred into the uterus or Fallopian tube.

Extremely low birth weight: birth weight less than 1,000 grams.

Extremely preterm birth: a live birth or stillbirth that takes place after at least 20 but less than 28 completed weeks of gestational age.

Fertilization: the penetration of the ovum by the spermatozoon and combination of their genetic material resulting in the formation of a zygote.

Fetal death (stillbirth): death prior to the complete expulsion or extraction from its mother of a product of fertilization, at or after 20 completed weeks of gestational age. The death is indicated by the fact that, after such separation, the fetus does not breathe or show any other evidence of life such as heart beat, umbilical cord pulsation, or definite movement of voluntary muscles.

Fetus: the product of fertilization from completion of embryonic development, at eight completed weeks after fertilization, until abortion or birth.

Frozen/thawed embryo transfer cycle (FET): an ART procedure in which cycle monitoring is carried out with the intention of transferring a frozen/thawed embryo or frozen/thawed embryos. *Note: A FET cycle is initiated when specific medication is provided or cycle monitoring is started with the intention to treat.*

Frozen/thawed oocyte cycle: an ART procedure in which cycle monitoring is carried out with the intention of fertilizing thawed oocytes and performing embryo transfer.

Full-term birth: a live birth or stillbirth that takes place between 37 completed and 42 completed weeks of gestational age.

Gamete intrafallopian transfer (GIFT): an ART procedure in which both gametes (oocytes and spermatozoa) are transferred to the Fallopian tubes.

Gestational age: age of an embryo or fetus calculated by adding 2 weeks (14 days) to the number of completed weeks since fertilization. *Note: For frozen/thawed embryo transfers, an estimated date of fertilization is computed by subtracting the embryo age at freezing from the transfer date of the FET cycle.*

Gestational carrier (surrogate): a woman who carries a pregnancy with an agreement that she will give the offspring to the intended parent(s). Gametes can originate from the intended parent(s) and/or a third party (or parties).

Gestational sac: a fluid-filled structure associated with early pregnancy, which may be located inside or outside the uterus (in case of an ectopic pregnancy).

Hatching: the process by which an embryo at the blastocyst stage separates from the zona pellucida.

High-order multiple: a pregnancy or delivery with three or more fetuses or neonates.

Implantation: the attachment and subsequent penetration by the zona-free blastocyst (usually in the endometrium) that starts five to seven days after fertilization.

Implantation rate: the number of gestational sacs observed, divided by the number of embryos transferred.

***In vitro* fertilization (IVF):** an ART procedure that involves extracorporeal fertilization.

Induced abortion: the termination of a clinical pregnancy, by deliberate interference that takes place before 20 completed weeks of gestational age (18 weeks post fertilization) or, if gestational age is unknown, of an embryo/fetus of less than 400 grams.

Infertility (clinical definition): a disease of the reproductive system defined by the failure to achieve a clinical pregnancy after 12 months or more of regular unprotected sexual intercourse.

Initiated cycle: an ART cycle in which the woman receives specific medication for ovarian stimulation, or monitoring in the case of natural cycles, with the intention to treat, irrespective of whether or not follicular aspiration is attempted.

IntraCytoplasmic Sperm Injection (ICSI): a procedure in which a single spermatozoon is injected into the oocyte cytoplasm.

Live birth: the complete expulsion or extraction from its mother of a product of fertilization, irrespective of the duration of the pregnancy, which, after such separation, breathes or shows any other evidence of life such as heart beat, umbilical cord pulsation, or definite movement of voluntary muscles, irrespective of whether the umbilical cord has been cut or the placenta is attached.

Live birth delivery rate: the number of deliveries that resulted in at least one live born baby expressed per 100 initiated cycles, aspiration cycles or embryo transfer cycles. When delivery rates are given, the denominator (initiated, aspirated, or embryo transfer cycles) must be speciied.

Low birth weight: Birth weight less than 2,500 grams.

Medically Assisted Reproduction (MAR): reproduction brought about through ovulation induction, controlled ovarian stimulation, ovulation triggering, ART procedures, and intrauterine, intracervical, and intravaginal insemination with semen of husband/partner or donor.

MESA: Microsurgical Epididymal Sperm Aspiration.

MESE: Microsurgical Epididymal Sperm Extraction.

Micromanipulation: a technology that allows micro-operative procedures to be performed on the spermatozoon, oocyte, zygote or embryo.

MicroTESE: Microsurgical Testicular Sperm Extraction.

Mild ovarian stimulation for IVF: a procedure in which the ovaries are stimulated with either gonadotropins and/or other compounds, with the intent to limit the number of oocytes obtained for IVF to fewer than seven.

Missed abortion: a clinical abortion where the embryo(s) or fetus(es) is/are non-viable and is/are not expelled spontaneously from the uterus.

Modified natural cycle: an IVF procedure in which one or more oocytes are collected from the ovaries during a spontaneous menstrual cycle. Drugs are administered with the sole purpose of blocking the spontaneous LH surge and/or inducing final oocyte maturation.

Multiple gestation/birth: a pregnancy/delivery with more than one fetus/neonate.

Natural cycle IVF: an IVF procedure in which one or more oocytes are collected from the ovaries during a spontaneous menstrual cycle without any drug use.

Neonatal death: death of a live born baby within 28 days of birth.

Neonatal period: the time interval that commences at birth and ends 28 completed days after birth.

Oocyte donation cycle: a cycle in which oocytes are collected from a donor for clinical application or research.

Oocyte recipient cycle: an ART cycle in which a woman receives oocytes from a donor.

Ovarian Hyper Stimulation Syndrome (OHSS): an exaggerated systemic response to ovarian stimulation characterized by a wide spectrum of clinical and laboratory manifestations. It is classified as mild, moderate or severe according to the degree of abdominal distention, ovarian enlargement and respiratory, haemodynamic and metabolic complications.

Ovarian torsion: the partial or complete rotation of the ovarian vascular pedicle that causes obstruction to ovarian blood flow, potentially leading to necrosis of ovarian tissue.

Ovulation Induction (OI): pharmacological treatment of women with anovulation or oligo-ovulation with the intention of inducing normal ovulatory cycles.

Perinatal mortality: fetal or neonatal death occurring during late pregnancy (at 20 completed weeks of gestational age and later), during childbirth and up to 7 completed days after birth.

PESA: Percutaneous Epididymal Sperm Aspiration.

Post-term birth: a live birth or stillbirth that takes place after 42 completed weeks of gestational age.

Preimplantation Genetic Diagnosis (PGD): analysis of polar bodies, blastomeres or trophectoderm from oocytes, zygotes or embryos for the detection of *specific* genetic, structural and/or chromosomal alterations.

Preimplantation Genetic Screening (PGS): analysis of polar bodies, blastomeres or trophectoderm from oocytes, zygotes or embryos for the detection of aneuploidy, mutation and/or DNA rearrangement.

Preterm birth: a live birth or stillbirth that takes place after at least 20 but before 37 completed weeks of gestational age.

Recurrent spontaneous abortion/miscarriage: the spontaneous loss of two or more clinical pregnancies.

Reproductive surgery: surgical procedures performed to diagnose, conserve, correct and/or improve reproductive function.

Severe Ovarian Hyper Stimulation Syndrome: severe OHSS is defined to occur when hospitalization is indicated. (see definition of Ovarian Hyper Stimulation Syndrome)

Small for gestational age: birth weight less than 2 standard deviations below the mean or less than the 10th centile according to local intrauterine growth charts.

Sperm recipient cycle: an ART cycle in which a woman receives spermatozoa from a donor who is someone other than her partner.

Spontaneous abortion/miscarriage: the spontaneous loss of a clinical pregnancy that occurs before 20 completed weeks of gestational age (18 weeks post fertilization) or, if gestational age is unknown, the loss of an embryo/fetus of less than 400 grams.

TESA: Testicular Sperm Aspiration.

TESE: Testicular Sperm Extraction.

Total delivery rate with at least one live birth: the estimated total number of deliveries with at least one live born baby resulting from one initiated or aspirated ART cycle including all fresh cycles and all frozen/thawed ART cycles. This rate is used when all of the embryos fresh and/or frozen/thawed have been utilized from one ART cycles. *Note: The delivery of a singleton, twin or other multiple pregnancy is registered as one delivery.*

Vanishing sac(s) or embryo(s): spontaneous disappearance of one or more gestational sacs or embryos in an ongoing pregnancy, documented by ultrasound.

Very low birth weight: Birth weight less than 1,500 grams.

Very preterm birth: a live birth or stillbirth that takes place after at least 20 but less than 32 completed weeks of gestational age.

Vitrification: an ultra-rapid cryopreservation method that prevents ice formation within the suspension which is converted to a glasslike solid.

Zygote: a diploid cell resulting from the fertilization of an oocyte by a spermatozoon, which subsequently divides to form an embryo.

Zygote Intra-Fallopian Transfer (ZIFT): a procedure in which zygote(s) is/are transferred into the Fallopian tube.

Index

36326292R00193

Printed in Great Britain
by Amazon